Contents

Contributors

James Barnett BSc BVSc MRCVS
Vetlab Services, Unit 11, Station Road, Southwater, Horsham, West Sussex RH13 7HQ
and British Divers Marine Life Rescue, 13 Ford Road, Arundel, West Sussex BN18 9DX

Dick Best BVSc MRCVS
Vale Vets, Portishead Veterinary Centre, 32 West Hill, Portishead, North Somerset BS20 6LN

Steve Bexton BVMS MRCVS
RSPCA Norfolk Wildlife Hospital, Station Road, East Winch, Norfolk PE32 1NR

Matthew G.I. Brash BVetMed MRCVS
Battle Flatts Veterinary Clinic, 38 Main Street, Stamford Bridge, York YO41 1AB

John R. Chitty BVetMed CertZooMed MRCVS
Strathmore Veterinary Clinic, 6 London Road, Andover, Hants SP10 2PH

Stephen W. Cooke BVSc MRCVS
Veterinary Advisers, Braywood Orchard, Ascot Road, Maidenhead, Berks SL6 3SY

John E. Cooper DTVM FRCPath FIBiol FRCVS
School of Veterinary Medicine, Faculty of Medical Sciences, The University of the West Indies,
St. Augustine, Trinidad and Tobago

Margaret E. Cooper LLB FLS
School of Veterinary Medicine, Faculty of Medical Sciences, The University of the West Indies,
St. Augustine, Trinidad and Tobago

Neil A. Forbes BVetMed CBiol MIBiol Diplomat ECAMS FRCVS
Avian and Exotic Animal Department, Clockhouse Veterinary Hospital, Wallbridge, Stroud,
Glos GL5 3JD

Frances M. Harcourt-Brown BVSc FRCVS
30 Crab Lane, Bilton, Harrogate, North Yorks HG1 3BE

Peter Green BVSc CertEO MRCVS
Fellowes Farm Equine Clinic, Abbots Ripton, Huntingdon, Cambs PE28 2LL

Emma J. Keeble BVSc CertZooMed MRCVS
Royal (Dick) School of Veterinary Studies, Small Animal Hospital, Easter Bush Veterinary Centre,
Roslin, Midlothian EH25 9RG

Michael A. King BVM&S CertZooMed MRCVS
53 Henver Road, Newquay, Cornwall TR7 3DQ

James K. Kirkwood BVSc PhD FIBiol MRCVS
Chief Executive and Scientific Director, Universities Federation for Animal Welfare,
The Old School, Brewhouse Hill, Wheathampstead, Herts AL4 8AN

Becki Lawson BA VetMB MSc MRCVS
Veterinary Editor, Wildlife Information Network, Royal Veterinary College, Royal College Street,
London NW1 0UT

Paul Llewellyn MPhil CBiol MIBiol
104 Manselfield Road, Murton, Swansea

Elizabeth Mullineaux BVM&S CertSHP MRCVS
Quantock Veterinary Hospital, Quantock Terrace, The Drove, Bridgwater, Somerset TA6 4BA

Ian Robinson BVSc CertSHP CertZooMed MRCVS
RSPCA Norfolk Wildlife Hospital, Station Road, East Winch, Norfolk PE32 1NR

Andrew Routh BVSc CertZooMed MRCVS

Anthony W. Sainsbury BVetMed CertLAS CertZooMed MRCVS
Zoological Society of London, Regent's Park, London NW1 4RY

Richard Saunders BVSc CertZooMed MRCVS
32 Lee Warner Road, Swaffham, Norfolk PE37 7GD

Victor Simpson BVSc CBiol FIBiol DTVM MRCVS
The Wildlife Veterinary Investigation Centre, Jollys Bottom Farm, Chacewater, Truro, Cornwall TR4 8PB

Katherine E. Whitwell BVSc DipECVP FRCVS
Equine Pathology Consultancy, 19 Brookside, Moulton, Newmarket, Suffolk CB8 8SG

Foreword

Although veterinary surgeons in the UK have had a long-standing policy of treating wildlife casualties *gratis*, this area of welfare work has also been characterized by the efforts of those members of the public who have developed a special interest in treating casualties in one or more of our wildlife species, often running sanctuaries for them. Information on the treatment of such a diverse range of species has gradually been accumulating, through the work of these individuals and via specialist veterinary societies. Latterly, the Internet has also been a source of much valuable information. Notwithstanding, there has been a place on the practice bookshelf for a textbook dealing with this issue.

BSAVA is proud and pleased to present this latest manual, on the treatment of wildlife casualties. The initial chapters outline basic treatment of wildlife casualties, rehabilitation and release, clinical pathology and post-mortem examination and the law relating to British wildlife casualties. Species-specific chapters follow dealing, I think, with every British mammal and all classes of birds, a staggering achievement.

We are grateful for the time and efforts of all those who have contributed to this manual, and to the efforts of Publications Committee and our Publishing Manager, who have brought it to fruition.

I am sure it will be a great success.

Richard G Harvey BVSc PhD DVD MRCVS
BSAVA President 2002–2003

Preface

The British countryside has a wide variety of wild birds, mammals, reptiles, amphibians and fish. Unfortunately, many of these species are presented to veterinary surgeries by the general public as a result of injury, disease or being found apparently abandoned. The Royal College of Veterinary Surgeons suggests that all veterinary surgeons provide emergency service for wildlife casualties and that such care enhances the public perception of the profession.

Wildlife casualties provide the veterinarian with a wide range of problems. Success depends not only upon the clinical skills of the practitioner, but also encompasses nursing staff and those involved in the rehabilitation and release of the casualty. Knowledge of the natural history of the species directs the choice of suitable handling facilities and accommodation that are essential to the successful outcome. This manual will be of special interest to veterinarians, veterinary nurses and those people dedicated to the care and rehabilitation of wildlife.

The manual has drawn together scientists, specialist wildlife veterinarians, general practitioners and rehabilitators to produce a source of information, not only on treating individual casualties but also covering the ethical and practical aspects of their care. The book addresses those circumstances where casualties should be euthanased for welfare reasons. It also provides a vital source of information on infectious diseases that are of importance not only in the health of wild populations but also of farmed livestock and humans.

Chapters on ethical considerations, basic treatment and feeding principles, rehabilitation, clinical biochemistry, pathology, and legal considerations are followed by chapters dedicated to individual species or groups. These chapters outline the species' natural history, providing critical information to assess whether the casualty is likely to be able to return to a normal life back in the wild, and whether treatment should be considered. Practical guidelines detail the capture and handling of casualties and the diagnosis and treatment of common disabilities with, at all stages, an emphasis being given to their assessment for return to the wild. The editors hope that this manual will stimulate debate on wildlife issues and they welcome contributions for the updated version, which will undoubtedly follow.

In addition to thanking the authors and the staff at BSAVA for all their assistance in the production of the manual, and the many colleagues who have assisted the authors with their chapters, the editors wish to acknowledge the help and advice given by Nigel Harcourt-Brown BVSc FRCVS, Tim Thomas MBE and Paul Holmes BVSc MSc MRCVS.

Elizabeth Mullineaux
Dick Best
John Cooper
February 2003

Introduction: wildlife casualties and the veterinary surgeon

James K. Kirkwood

Veterinary technology has developed to the stage at which it can be applied very effectively to curing a wide range of infections and injuries in wild animals. This is relatively new: the claim could not have been made convincingly until the latter years of the 20th century. The technology is increasingly being applied for three distinct reasons (and by communities that have often tended to work in isolation from one another): for species conservation; for the welfare of casualties; and to control, in wildlife, reservoirs of infections that threaten domestic animal or human health.

To list a very few examples from each category:

1. Free-living mountain gorillas (*Gorilla berengei*) have been treated for sarcoptic mange and vaccinated against measles because these were judged to pose added threats to the viability of the species (Kalema *et al.*, 1998; Sholley, 1989).
2. Motivated by a concern for their welfare, rehabilitators and others now treat large numbers of common species for diseases and injury, of anthropogenic or natural causes, in Britain and in other countries (e.g. Peeters, 1991; Kirkwood and Sainsbury, 1996; Tribe and Brown, 2000).
3. As part of a public health programme, the number of rabies cases in wild foxes (*Vulpes vulpes*) has been greatly reduced in continental Europe by oral immunization administered via baits (Rupprecht *et al.*, 2001). If bovine tuberculosis could be prevented effectively in badgers (*Meles meles*) by their vaccination, it seems very likely that this would be explored as a method of controlling the disease in cattle in the UK.

This Manual is largely concerned with just one of these three reasons for intervention for wildlife health: the treatment of wildlife casualties for their welfare.

On an evolutionary time scale, compared with diseases and injuries (which are as old as life itself – 4 billion years – and have played a very major part in shaping it), the possibility of intervention by one species to cure the ills of another is a very new factor in the struggle for existence. Like many technological advances, the development of wildlife medicine brings with it new dilemmas. We can now cure many types of disease and injury in wild animals, but under what circumstances is it right to intervene?

And which types of problems should be tackled and when? Although this is a technical book, some consideration of these questions is appropriate here, since they impinge upon decisions about the way in which cases should be handled in practice at every stage of the process.

Charles Darwin saw very clearly the redness of nature's teeth and claws but in *On the Origin of Species by Means of Natural Selection, or the Preservation of Favoured Races in the Struggle for Life* (Darwin, 1859) he strove to take an optimistic point of view:

"All that we can do, is to keep steadily in mind that each organic being is striving to increase at a geometrical ratio; that each at some period of its life, during some season of the year, during each generation or at intervals, has to struggle for life and to suffer great destruction. When we reflect on this struggle, we may console ourselves with the full belief, that the war of nature is not incessant, that no fear is felt, that death is generally prompt, and that the vigorous, the healthy, and the happy survive and multiply."

Perhaps, in the last sentence, he was trying to protect his readers a little from the full, jarring force of the implications of his theory: that life can be explained by the action of a blind, uncaring and aimless process, rather than as part of a divine and benevolent purpose (as had largely been believed hitherto, at least in Judaeo-Christian societies). Darwin was a meticulous observer and must have been acutely aware, in spite of his words above, that death was often not very 'prompt'. Furthermore, his comment that 'no fear is felt' seems at odds with his view, expressed later (Darwin, 1871), that:

"The lower animals, like man, manifestly feel pleasure and pain, happiness and misery ... Terror acts in the same manner on them as on us."

Although it seems unlikely that animals other than humans fear impending death *per se*, they may well experience fear on being chased or caught by a predator.

In the final paragraph of *On the Origin of Species*, he wrote:

"Thus from the war of nature, from famine and death, the most exalted object which we are capable of conceiving, namely, the production of the higher animals, directly follows."

This 'war of nature' leads to casualties on a vast scale. The resulting suffering may appal us and seem to demand that where possible we should intervene; but, on the other hand, should we not be duly cautious about tampering with the machinery that produces 'the most exalted object which we are capable of conceiving'?

The present state of knowledge about animals includes much that supports the widely held belief that the capacity for conscious awareness of pleasant and unpleasant feelings (e.g. pain and fear) may be quite widespread in the animal kingdom, at least in its vertebrate branch – though, as reviewed by Kirkwood and Hubrecht (2001), not all subscribe to this view. Based on consideration of the clinical and pathological effects of many of the harms that can befall free-living wild animals, there is good reason to believe that their diseases and injuries often cause suffering and that this can be both prolonged and severe (Sainsbury *et al.*, 1995). Sarcoptic mange, for example, causes severe, chronic disease in many species of wild mammals around the world (Bornstein *et al.*, 2001) and the lesions and behaviour of affected animals are often such that it seems reasonable to conclude that the disease causes a very severe welfare insult through discomfort, pain and overstress. The same can be said of many other diseases and injuries.

In short, science has provided good evidence that suffering due to disease and injury is common in wild animals and it has provided the technology to alleviate or prevent some of this. However, it has also given us the knowledge that it is the very 'war' of nature that has driven the evolution of animals. The consequences of any interference with the process may be hard to predict, for, as Darwin (1859) noted, regarding the pressures that limit population sizes: 'Lighten any check, mitigate the destruction ever so little, and the number of the species will increase to any amount.'

There are reasons, then, to think hard before applying veterinary medicine to prevent or treat disease in wild animals living in their natural state. There are finite resources of food energy, space and other requirements on earth and it is inevitable that there must be winners and losers in the struggle to obtain them. We can certainly, if we wish, influence which particular individuals or which particular species survive but it is not clear that it would be possible, through wildlife medicine, to raise the net life quality of wildlife, since a gain to one individual may inevitably lead to loss by another of the same or a different species.

We should, therefore, be careful about intervening to treat injuries and diseases where these are part of natural ecological processes. It is a different matter when the diseases or injuries have been caused through human agency. In these cases, providing treatment and restoration to the wild does not further harm the casualty's welfare; it seems an entirely justifiable effort to right a wrong.

These are complex issues and ones that may not be the first to spring to mind when an injured wild animal is presented for treatment by a well-meaning member of the public who expects that the full force of modern veterinary therapy will promptly be brought to bear. However – and the debate simplifies to this – unless the animal is of a species so endangered that its treatment and rehabilitation can be justified on the grounds of species preservation (which is very rarely the case), its welfare is the prime, if not only, consideration. We should strive to make this, and whatever decisions it leads to, clear to all concerned.

The history of wildlife treatment and rehabilitation

It is part of human biology that animals, or at least some species of them, have a strong appeal to us. For thousands of years, no doubt, interested individuals have been moved by the plight of sick and injured wild animals and have tried to care for them. However, wildlife treatment and rehabilitation only really began to emerge as a distinct branch of veterinary medicine in the 1970s (e.g. Cooper and Eley, 1979; McKeever, 1979). At this time, there was growing public concern about threats to wildlife conservation and welfare; and developments in veterinary technology, notably in the fields of chemical restraint and antibiotic therapy, had reached a stage that opened the way to effective wildlife medicine. Interest in the subject grew and during the 1980s there were moves to set standards and to establish guidelines by organizations in several countries, such as, in the UK, the British Wildlife Rehabilitation Council (BWRC, 1989), the Wildlife Hospital Trust, the National Federation of Badger Groups, the Bat Conservation Trust and Raptor Rescue, and in North America, the International Wildlife Rehabilitation Council and the National Wildlife Rehabilitators Association (IWRC and NWRA, 1989). Since then, an increasing volume of publications has emerged on technical aspects (e.g. Stocker, 2000), on standards (e.g. Miller, 2000) and on research into various aspects of wildlife rehabilitation, including survival of released animals (e.g. Morris and Warwick, 1994; Robertson and Harris, 1995; Wernham *et al.*, 1997). Wildlife rescue is now an established interest in many countries, involving many thousands of people (Tribe and Brown, 2000).

Wildlife casualties in the UK: numbers, species and causes

In the UK, as in other countries (Tribe and Brown, 2000), wildlife rescue is not undertaken on a nationally coordinated basis but, mostly, by a network of individuals and locally based organizations acting autonomously. Obtaining information on the scale of the 'industry' is difficult but, since 1993, the British Wildlife Rehabilitation Council (BWRC) has collected data on the numbers and types of casualties treated by BWRC supporters each quarter of the year (Best, 1993). These statistics show that the total number of animals submitted each year to the centres and individuals who report their findings to the BWRC is well in excess of 15,000 (Figure 1.1). Since only a relatively small number of units (around 35) (Kirkwood and Best, 1998) regularly submit returns to the BWRC, the national total is almost certainly very much greater than this.

Class	Total recorded	Immature	Survived 48 hours	Released
Birds	10,979	5,453	6,874	5,143
Mammals	5,330	2,872	3,066	1,668
Amphibians and reptiles	68	8	38	33
Totals	16,377	8,333	9,978	6,844

1.1 British Wildlife Casualty Recording Scheme: summary of statistics on taxa of casualties during the year 2000.

The BWRC statistics in Figure 1.1 suggest that about 67% of casualties rescued are birds and about 33% are mammals. Most are of common species, with hedgehog (*Erinaceus europaeus*), feral and racing pigeons (*Columba livia*), woodpigeon (*Columba palumbus*), blackbird (*Turdus merula*) and collared dove (*Streptopelia decaocto*) comprising over 40% of the total (Kirkwood and Best, 1998). Some 50% of the 16,377 casualties recorded during 2000 were immature, 60% survived 48 hours and about 42% were released (Figure 1.1). This release rate is within the ranges reported for Australian wildlife in an extensive survey by Tribe and Brown (2000).

The BWRC has also attempted to gain information on the causes of wildlife casualties – the reasons why they arrived at rehabilitation centres. Again, it is difficult to obtain highly accurate information because determination of causes of sickness or injury often depends on very detailed clinical and post-mortem examinations, which cannot in most cases be afforded. However, there is no reason to suppose that the results in Figure 1.2 give a misleading summary. These suggest that some 30% of casualties during 2000 were due to parental abandonment. A large proportion of these were young birds – not all of which, in reality, may have been truly abandoned. Of the remaining 11,855 casualties recorded during the year, only 1103 (9%) were considered to have been due to natural causes; 14% were injured by cats and a further 44% were injured by other unnatural (i.e. anthropogenic) causes, including 3% that were poisoned.

There is, therefore, good evidence that a large proportion of the animals recorded at wildlife rehabilitation units have been injured through human agency (74% if injuries caused by cats are included). This is consistent with the findings of similar surveys in Australia and in the USA (Tribe and Brown, 2000). Conversely, these results suggest that interventions to treat casualties that are due to natural causes (i.e. those judged not to be linked to human agency) are in a minority – about 10%, if the 'abandoned' group is rather arbitrarily excluded from consideration.

Diversity of rehabilitation centres and the role of the veterinary surgeon

Wildlife treatment and rehabilitation centres in the UK range from large, modern, custom-built, lavishly equipped veterinary hospitals with highly qualified and experienced staff, to small garden-shed type operations run by enthusiasts with limited resources. In contrast to the keeping of wild animals in zoos or for research, there is no specific legislation that sets standards and regulates the running of wildlife treatment and rehabilitation centres in the UK (though the possibility of such legislation has recently been discussed in Parliament). In order to promote good practice and good welfare standards, the BWRC produced a booklet providing guidelines on aspects of husbandry, treatment, release, records and the law (BWRC, undated). In a number of countries wildlife rehabilitation can only be undertaken under licence.

Although a small number of organizations and centres have full-time veterinary surgeons, most rely on a local practice for veterinary expertise. The BWRC encourages lay rehabilitators to develop close working relationships with interested veterinary surgeons and also to produce a statement of facilities, outlining the maximum capacity and working practices. The latter is important, because there are often times when more casualties arrive than can be cared for to high standards, in which circumstances recognition that there is a limit to capacity helps to maintain a realistic perspective focused on quality.

At present, wildlife medicine in Britain comprises almost exclusively the treatment of wildlife casualties on an individual case-by-case basis. Whilst there are various programmes to investigate wildlife diseases (Sainsbury *et al.*, 2001) and to prevent some of these (e.g. the prevention of lead poisoning in wildfowl by a voluntary ban on use of lead shot), there

	Injury[a]	Poisoning	Abandoned	Natural causes	Cat injury	Other	Total
Birds	3,058	254	3,310	409	1,373	1,857	10,261
Mammals	1,201	73	1,305	690	264	1,300	4,833
Amphibians and reptiles	24	—	—	4	17	26	71
Totals	4,283	327	4,615	1,103	1,654	3,183	15,165

1.2 British Wildlife Casualty Recording Scheme: summary of statistics on types of casualty during the year 2000.
[a] Injuries caused by unnatural (anthropogenic) agency.

are no corresponding nationally coordinated programmes for treating particular wildlife diseases or for dealing with casualties. It seems possible that the approach to some diseases (e.g. mange in foxes) could become more strategic in the future, with attempts to control disease on a population-wide basis. The greater the scale of intervention, the more carefully should the larger issues, about altering the balance of factors that naturally regulate populations, be considered.

Ethical considerations: the potential welfare costs and benefits of wildlife rehabilitation

There is a strong moral and, in most countries, legal obligation to provide prompt treatment for diseases or injuries that befall the animals for which we are responsible. Truly free-living wild animals are not owned and it is generally believed that we do not have a corresponding responsibility for them (e.g. Norton *et al.*, 1995). Opinions differ (see reviews by Cooper, 1989; BWRC, 1989; Sikarskie, 1992; Tribe and Brown, 2000) but, as briefly outlined above, there are practical and philosophical reasons for not intervening to deal with naturally occurring casualties other than to destroy them humanely to prevent unnecessary suffering (Kirkwood, 1992, 2000; Kirkwood and Sainsbury, 1996). However, as the results of the surveys by Sainsbury *et al.* (1995) and the BWRC (described above) have revealed, many insults to the welfare of wild animals are caused by human agency, and endeavours to treat these cases in order to redress the harm caused seem entirely justifiable. In these circumstances, the motive for intervening – except in very rare cases in which rehabilitation may benefit species conservation – is to restore or to improve the welfare of the animal (and its dependents, if it has any). Therefore, assuming the necessary resources are available for treatment and rehabilitation, the decision whether or not to employ these resources should be based solely on cool and realistic assessment of the welfare costs and benefits. As suggested by Kirkwood and Best (1998):

"For an animal with little realistic chance of being returned to the wild in a fit state to survive and facing a prolonged period in captivity and possibly stressful handling and treatment, euthanasia at an early stage may be the most humane course of action."

Some potential costs and benefits to welfare are listed in Figure 1.3. They have been discussed at some length elsewhere (e.g. Cooper, 1989; Sikarskie, 1992; Kirkwood and Sainsbury, 1996; Morris, 1997; Kirkwood, 2000; Tribe and Brown, 2000) and there is no room to expand upon them here. Although the list relates largely to welfare aspects (which are the focus of this chapter), a wider perspective has also to be taken in planning wildlife treatment and rehabilitation work. It should encompass human health risks from injuries or zoonotic diseases, economics, the legal framework and other relevant issues.

Potential costs

- Welfare costs associated with captivity
- Welfare costs associated with treatment
- Welfare costs associated with release and failure to re-establish
- Welfare risks to conspecifics on release through:
  - introduction of infection
  - competition for resources
- Welfare risks to other species on release (as above)
- May prevent or delay selection for natural defences (e.g. immunity)
- May favour selection of the less fit (with welfare consequences to offspring)

Potential benefits

- Restoration of good health and welfare of the individual
- Opportunities for detecting/monitoring threats to wildlife populations
- Stimulation of public interest and support for wildlife protection
- Contributions to development of technology that may have wider application
- Education in wildlife veterinary care
- Pleasure to humans from close encounters and caring for wildlife

 Potential welfare costs and benefits of wildlife treatment and rehabilitation.

Assessment of the balance between welfare costs and benefits is often difficult. In addition to the problem of the unpredictability of responses of individual cases to treatment, there are few robust yardsticks for use in judging, for example, whether any stress or pain that may be associated with captivity and treatment does or does not outweigh potential welfare benefits to the animal. The task is not made easier by the paucity of information on outcomes of wildlife rehabilitation cases. Although increasing numbers of studies are being undertaken, data on survival of released animals remain rather scant (but see, for example, Morris and Warwick, 1994; Robertson and Harris, 1995; Wernham *et al.*, 1997; Sweeney *et al.*, 1997; Fajardo *et al.*, 2000; Bennett and Routh, 2000). In time, sufficient data may be collected on clinical and post-release histories to provide a basis for detailed analyses of welfare costs and benefits in some species.

To conclude, judgements about when to intervene (i.e. whether or not to bring a casualty into captivity for treatment), and then whether to initiate therapy or to euthanase, are less straightforward than many assume. In addition to applying their clinical knowledge and expertise, veterinary surgeons have an important role in these ethical assessments and in helping to determine priorities and focus in interventions for wildlife welfare. Finally, close veterinary involvement is crucial to making full use of the opportunity presented, through dealing with casualties, for playing a major front-line role in detecting new anthropogenic threats to the health, welfare and population status of wild animals. To capitalize on this requires detailed diagnostic work, good record-keeping and publication of findings.

References

Bennett JA and Routh AD (2000) Post-release survival of hand-reared tawny owls (*Strix aluco*). *Animal Welfare* **9**, 317–321

Best JR (1993) Wildlife casualty recording scheme. *Rehabilitator* **1**, 5

Bornstein S, Mörner T and Samuel WM (2001) *Sarcoptes scabiei* and sarcoptic mange. In: *Parasitic Diseases of Wild Mammals*, 2nd edn, ed. WM Samuel *et al.*, pp. 107–119. Iowa State University Press, Ames, Iowa

BWRC (1989) *Ethics and Legal Aspects of Treatment and Rehabilitation of Wild Animal Casualties*. British Wildlife Rehabilitation Council, c/o RSPCA Wildlife Department, Horsham

BWRC (undated) *Guidelines for Wildlife Rehabilitation Units*. British Wildlife Rehabilitation Council, c/o RSPCA Wildlife Department, Horsham

Cooper JE (1989) Care, cure or conservation: developments and dilemmas in wildlife conservation. In: *Proceedings of the Inaugural Symposium of the British Wildlife Rehabilitation Council, 19th November 1988, London*, ed. S Harris and T Thomas, pp. 14–23. British Wildlife Rehabilitation Council, c/o RSPCA, Horsham

Cooper JE and Eley J (1979) *First Aid and Care of Wild Birds*. David and Charles, Newton Abbott

Darwin C (1859) *On the Origin of Species by Means of Natural Selection, or the Preservation of Favoured Races in the Struggle for Life*. John Murray, London

Darwin C (1871) *The Descent of Man, and Selection in Relation to Sex*. John Murray, London

Fajardo I, Babiloni G and Miranda Y (2000) Rehabilitated wild barn owls (*Tyto alba*): dispersal, life expectancy and mortality in Spain. *Biological Conservation* **94**, 287–295

IWRC and NWRA (1989) *Wildlife Rehabilitation Minimum Standards and Accreditation Program*. International Wildlife Rehabiltation Council, Suisun, California

Kalema G, Kock RA and Macfie E (1998) An outbreak of sarcoptic mange in free-ranging Mountain gorillas (*Gorilla gorilla berengei*) in Bwindi Impenetrable National Park, South Western Uganda. *Proceedings of the American Association of Zoo Veterinarians/ American Association of Wildlife Veterinarians Joint Conference, Omaha, Nebraska, 17–22 October, 1998*, p. 438

Kirkwood JK (1992) Wild animal welfare. In: *Animal Welfare and the Environment*, ed. RR Ryder, pp. 139–145. G Duckworth & Co., London

Kirkwood JK (2000) Interventions for the conservation or welfare of wild animals. In: *Veterinary Ethics: an Introduction*, ed. G Legood, pp. 121–128. Continuum, London

Kirkwood JK and Best JR (1998) Treatment and rehabilitation of wildlife casualties: legal and ethical aspects. *In Practice* **20**, 214–216

Kirkwood JK and Hubrecht R (2001) Consciousness, cognition and animal welfare. *Animal Welfare* **10s**, 5–17

Kirkwood JK and Sainsbury AW (1996) Ethics of intervention for the welfare of free-living wild animals. *Animal Welfare* **5**, 235–243

McKeever K (1979) *Care and Rehabilitation of Injured Owls*. WF Rannie, Lincoln, Ontario

Miller EA (ed.) (2000) *Minimum Standards for Wildlife Rehabilitation, 3rd edn*. National Wildlife Rehabilitators Association, St Cloud, Minnesota

Morris PA (1997) Animal medicine or human therapy? *Biologist* **44**, 288

Morris PA and Warwick H (1994) A study of rehabilitated juvenile hedgehogs after release into the wild. *Animal Welfare* **3**, 163–177

Norton BG, Hutchins M, Stevens EF and Maple T (1995) *Ethics on the Ark: Zoos, Animal Welfare and Wildlife Conservation*. Smithsonian Institution Press, Washington DC

Peeters H (1991) Birds and oil pollution. In: *Wild Bird Mortality in the Netherlands 1975–1989*, pp. 23–30. Netherlands Society for the Protection of Birds/Central Veterinary Institute, Zeist and Lelystad, The Netherlands

Robertson CPJ and Harris S (1995) The condition and survival after release of captive-reared fox cubs. *Animal Welfare* **4**, 295–306

Rupprecht CE, Stöhr K and Meredith C (2001) Rabies. In: *Infectious Diseases of Wild Mammals, 3rd edn*, eds ES Williams and IK Barker, pp. 3–36. Iowa State University Press, Ames, Iowa

Sainsbury AW, Bennett PM and Kirkwood JK (1995) Welfare of free-living wild animals in Europe: harm caused by human activities. *Animal Welfare* **4**, 183–206

Sainsbury AW, Kirkwood JK, Bennett PM and Cunningham AA (2001) Status of wildlife health monitoring in the United Kingdom. *Veterinary Record* **148**, 558–563

Sholley CR (1989) Mountain gorilla update. *Oryx* **23**, 57–58

Sikarskie JG (1992) The role of veterinary medicine in wildlife rehabilitation. *Journal of Zoo and Wildlife Medicine* **23**, 397–400

Stocker L (2000) *Practical Wildlife Care*. Blackwell Science, Oxford

Sweeney SJ, Redig PT and Tordoff HB (1997) Morbidity, survival and productivity of rehabilitated peregrine falcons in the upper midwestern US. *Journal of Raptor Research* **31**, 347–352

Tribe A and Brown PR (2000) The role of wildlife rescue groups in the care and rehabilitation of Australian fauna. *Human Dimensions of Wildlife* **5**, 69–85

Wernham CV, Peach WJ and Browne SJ (1997) *Survival Rates of Rehabilitated Guillemots*. BTO Research Report No 186. British Trust for Ornithology, Thetford

2

Basic principles of treating wildlife casualties

Dick Best and Elizabeth Mullineaux

Introduction

Wildlife casualties present the veterinary practitioner with a fascinating and challenging range of clinical problems, from those of handling, housing and nursing, to those of diagnosis and treatment. Although the range of problems may be extensive, the actual veterinary techniques required should be well within the scope of most veterinary practices. However, success in treating casualties often depends not only on the clinical skill of the practitioner but also on the experience and patience of the nursing staff and the availability of suitable accommodation and handling facilities.

The process of dealing with a wildlife casualty can be divided into a series of stages from initial location, through treatment, to release. The term 'rehabilitation' is often used to describe the whole process of treating and returning a casualty to the wild. At each stage the casualty needs to be monitored and its condition and progress assessed. The accuracy of this assessment has an important effect on the welfare of the animal and, ideally, should be made with professional veterinary expertise. On welfare grounds, euthanasia must be considered if at any stage in this process it is considered that the treatment is causing excessive distress, or if it is apparent that the casualty is unlikely to be returned safely to the wild. The health of people handling a casualty must also be considered and the animal euthanased if the risk of contracting a serious zoonotic infection (e.g. tuberculosis from badgers) is high.

Stages in dealing with casualties

The stages of dealing with a casualty are:

1. Initial location, capture and transportation
2. Examination and assessment for rehabilitation
3. First aid and stabilization
4. Treatment (including diagnostic investigations, anaesthesia, and medical and surgical treatment)
5. Recuperation and rehabilitation
6. Release.

The aim of this book is to provide the practising veterinary surgeon with the information required to treat a wildlife casualty and with the background information needed to be aware of the requirements of the patient during its convalescence and its preparation leading up to release. This chapter covers the basic principles of handling a casualty from capture through to the completion of treatment (i.e. stages 1–4). Although many of these basic principles are common to all wildlife casualties, this chapter deals with mammals and birds; the specific management of reptile, amphibian and fish casualties is described in Chapter 26. The basics of the final two stages, rehabilitation and release, are covered in Chapter 3.

Initial location, capture and transportation

Wildlife casualties are usually found by members of the public. Their welfare at this stage will depend on general public awareness (principally gained through the media) of the correct action to be taken when faced with a casualty and where to seek further information and assistance.

Although the animal welfare societies receive many wildlife casualties, local veterinary practices are likely to be the first source of assistance to which the public will turn. Practice staff should be prepared to give general advice on the best way to deal with a wildlife emergency, including advice on capture and safe handling and, if available, the sources of local assistance (some rehabilitation units offer a recovery service for casualties). As a precaution, a written note should be made of any advice given to the public and retained as evidence for any possible litigation that could follow an accident in handling a wildlife casualty (see Chapter 5).

Figures 2.1 and 2.2 give an indication of the advice that might be given by reception staff of a veterinary practice to a member of the public seeking information on the handling of a casualty.

When a casualty is first found, the priority is to establish whether the animal is in need of assistance and, if so, to capture it, or to prevent it from escaping (or from sustaining further injury, especially with road traffic accidents), until assistance arrives. The action to be taken will vary with each case and with the materials available at the time, but the main objective must be restraint of the casualty without causing excessive distress or risking injury to the patient, the handlers or onlookers. If the casualty is to be taken into captivity, the exact location should be recorded and kept with the case notes, allowing the animal to be released later where it was found.

Group	Dangers	Capture techniques	Transportation
Small birds	Few physical risks Zoonotic infections	Cover with cloth Catching net	Small dark box with air holes and non-slip floor Pillowcase
Medium-sized birds (pigeon, crow)	Bites and scratches Zoonotic infections	Cover with cloth, coat or blanket Catching net	Short journeys: hand-hold in covering cloth. Dark box or cardboard pet carrier with air holes and non-slip floor covering Pillowcase or hessian sack
Seabirds (gulls, gannet)	Painful bites Gannets stab at face Zoonotic infections	Prevent re-entry to water Cover with blanket or coat Angler's landing net Immobilize head	Short journeys: hand-hold in covering material Dark box or cardboard pet carrier with air holes and non-slip floor covering Hessian sack
Large water birds (swans, geese, herons)	Painful bites Swans strike with wings Herons stab at face Zoonotic infections	Prevent re-entry to water; if on water seek expert assistance Immobilize head	Restrain body in blanket or sack 'Swan bag'
Raptors (falcons, hawks, owls)	Painful bites Serious injury from talons of larger species Zoonotic infections	Cover with cloth, coat or blanket Angler's landing net Allow to grip material with talons Restrain legs	Short journeys: hand-hold in covering material Dark box or cardboard pet carrier with air holes and non-slip floor covering.

2.1 Advice for the general public on the capture and transportation of avian wildlife casualties.

Group	Dangers	Capture techniques	Transportation
Small rodents	Bites Zoonotic infections	Leather gloves or cover with cloth	Escape-proof box with air holes
Bats	Bites Zoonotic infections	Leather gloves or cover with cloth	Escape-proof box with air holes Pillowcase or cash bag
Rabbits, hares, hedgehogs	Bites, scratches Zoonotic infections	Cover with cloth or towel Thick gloves Angler's landing net	Dark box or cardboard pet carrier, with non-slip floor or soft bedding
Mustelids, squirrels	Bites, scratches Zoonotic infections	Thick leather gloves Angler's landing net	Plastic box or dustbin with fitting lid Plastic or fine-meshed wire carrier cage (covered)
Foxes, badgers	Serious injury from bites Zoonotic infections	Approach with caution Shocked animals appear tame Prevent escape (with loop around animal's neck) Seek expert assistance	Once restrained lift with care into plastic dustbin with fitting lid or stout hessian sack Wire crush cage
Deer	Serious injury from antlers and feet	Approach with caution Shocked animals appear tame Cover animal's head, legs and feet Seek expert assistance	Do not attempt to move without expert advice or assistance
Marine mammals	Serious bites from seals Zoonotic infections	Seek advice from marine mammal specialists, animal welfare society, police wildlife liaison officer	Do not attempt to move without expert assistance

2.2 Advice for the general public on the capture and transportation of mammalian casualties.

Bird casualties

Capture

Due to weakness, entrapment or injury, most avian casualties will be unable to fly and, if still mobile, can usually be pursued for a short distance until they can be restrained or encouraged into a corner or an enclosed space. Waterfowl and seabirds on land must be prevented from returning to the water, as capture on open water requires expert assistance.

For most species, capture is best performed by covering and completely enclosing the bird with a suitable fabric object, such as a cloth, towel, coat or blanket. Once a bird is enclosed in this way, with its wings and legs held closely to the body and its head covered, it will usually stop struggling. This is particularly important for birds with limb injuries, as immobilization of any fractures by such restraint will prevent further damage from flapping and struggling.

Larger birds, especially swans and geese, are best caught initially by the neck – using hands or, if available, a 'swan hook' – and then the body is restrained within a large blanket, sack or 'swan bag'. Handling raptors requires special care, as the talons of the larger species can cause serious injuries. Advice must be given to inexperienced handlers to ensure that the bird's legs are restrained at all times, either by completely enclosing the bird in a thick towel or blanket or, for short journeys, holding the legs firmly. Diurnal species are easier to catch in darkness and this could be used in certain circumstances, such as a bird trapped in a building, or an injured raptor roosting in a tree.

Lengths of mist-netting (fine nylon mesh nets used to trap wild birds for ringing) can be used to catch birds trapped within large enclosed buildings, or long lengths of coarser netting may be used across open ground or even on the water to catch larger flightless birds. Larger birds, especially birds of prey when chasing quarry, frequently become trapped inside large buildings. The majority of such birds will eventually escape through an open door if left undisturbed and attempts to catch them should be mounted only if non-intervention is impracticable. The capture of free-living animals is controlled by law (see Chapter 5).

Transportation

Once restrained, the casualty can be examined and, if necessary, moved to safety or taken for further examination. Over short distances, birds can be moved quite safely wrapped in fabric – the main concern being overheating, which can occur if the casualty is wrapped tightly and with its head totally covered.

* Small birds can be safely moved in dark cloth bags or pillowcases, in which they will lie quietly
* Boxes can be used for transportation of small to medium-sized birds, seabirds and raptors; they should be of a secure design and darkened, with suitably sized air holes, and have a non-slip floor covering to prevent the casualty from sliding (pieces of short-pile carpeting are ideal)
* Medium-sized to large birds with wing or leg injuries should not be transported loose in boxes without immobilization of any affected limb
* Larger species of waterfowl may be safely transported with their bodies restrained within a blanket or sack and the head and neck free, or in a 'swan bag' as used by animal welfare societies.

Transportation methods may be influenced by legal constraints (see Chapter 5).

Mammal casualties

Capture

Small rodents (mice, voles) and insectivores (shrews) can be lifted by the base of the tail or by covering them with a cloth and lifting by the scruff of the neck. Medium-sized rodents (rats, squirrels) and smaller mustelids

(stoats, weasels) need to be handled with great care, preferably using thick leather gloves, in view of the danger from bites. Hedgehogs, with their sharp spines and the risk of contracting ringworm infection, are more safely lifted wearing gloves or by using a thick cloth.

Larger mammals (foxes and badgers) should be approached with caution; apparently comatose or very tame animals may suddenly attack and bite. The casualty should be prevented from escaping by restraint with a loop of rope, a dog-catcher or a similar device around the neck; then, by carefully taking a grip on the scruff (if sufficiently loose) and supporting the weight of the body with a hand under the hindquarters, the handler can lift the animal into a secure container or a sack, possibly leaving the neck restraint in place to make it easier when removing the animal from its container. If available, a suitably sized crush cage is the ideal secure container in which to hold and transport a badger or fox.

Lengths of coarse-mesh netting held between a row of helpers or fixed to poles may be used to trap disabled larger mammals. Baited traps can be used for casualties known to visit a site regularly.

Transportation

* Transportation of smaller mammals requires secure darkened boxes with air holes and a non-slip floor covering or plenty of bedding (straw, shredded paper)
* Larger mammals can be carried in containers such as plastic dustbins with fitted lids or in hessian sacks. Open cages need to be covered to give the casualty darkness and seclusion
* Handling and transportation of seals and deer require expert assistance, especially from trained staff of the animal welfare societies. Injured deer can be very dangerous when flailing their legs or antlers, but may be quietened and restrained if their heads and limbs are covered.

Under livestock disease legislation, movement of animals may be controlled and would then need authorization. Further details on the capture and transportation of mammals are given in the group or species-specific chapters.

Examination and assessment for rehabilitation

Assessment

The overriding aim in any attempt at rehabilitation of a wildlife casualty must be its successful return to the wild. To be successful, the casualty must be released with a chance of survival equivalent to that of other free-living members of its species. This does not mean that the casualty must be in perfect physical condition, but in a condition that will not prejudice its survival. Each case must be assessed on its own merits, in the light of the animal's natural history and, where available, on the basis of experience gained from the monitoring of casualties after release. The alternatives to rehabilitation and release are either permanent captivity or euthanasia.

Decisions about the future of the casualty (Figure 2.3) can only be made after a careful assessment of the individual casualty, its disabilities and its natural requirements. In assessing the suitability of a casualty for rehabilitation the main consideration must be, at all times, the welfare of the animal. The role of the veterinary surgeon is important in making a decision but there is also heavy reliance on competent wildlife rehabilitators, with their experience of handling casualties, and on naturalists with knowledge of local wildlife and the local environment.

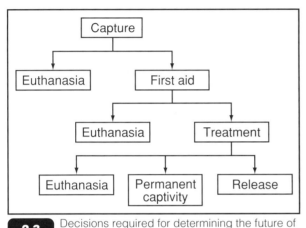

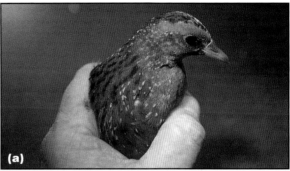

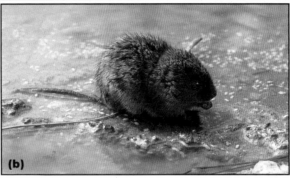

2.4 Two rare species: (a) spotted crake; (b) water vole. ((b) Courtesy of Andy Purcell/Conservation Education Consultants © CEC.)

2.3 Decisions required for determining the future of a casualty.

Each casualty should be assessed individually. The circumstances surrounding each case will vary and it is not possible to give criteria that will apply to every case, but the following points should be considered:

1. Natural history of the species and the age and sex of the individual
2. Body condition
3. Health status, nature of the disability and the prognosis
4. Psychological status
5. Facilities for treatment and aftercare
6. Availability of suitable release sites.

Natural history, age and sex

A prerequisite to the assessment of a casualty must be accurate identification of its species, its age and, whenever possible, its sex. Without this information, and knowledge of the natural history of the species, it is difficult to house and feed the patient adequately and impossible to make the correct decisions regarding its rehabilitation and release. Rare and unexpected species are occasionally presented as wildlife casualties, e.g. spotted crake (Figure 2.4a). Such findings might well be an indication of the presence of an otherwise unrecognized species in an area (i.e. a useful source of information on the biodiversity of that area).

The ability to identify small mammals is important. For example, the water vole (Figure 2.4b), an endangered species, may be confused with the brown rat (see Figure 8.6a), which is considered to be vermin.

A casualty that requires only a brief period in captivity for stabilization and can then be returned to the site where it was found (if the site is still suitable)

presents few practical and ethical problems. However, for species with specialized feeding behaviour (e.g. insectivorous birds that are aerial feeders; cetaceans) or that are highly active (e.g. raptors that hunt on the wing; deep-diving seabirds), it may be very difficult to keep the casualty alive or to retain its state of physical fitness if it is kept in captivity for extended periods. Some very nervous mammals, especially fox and deer, may become very stressed and show behavioural problems leading to self-trauma. Migratory birds present problems if kept beyond their normal periods of residency.

Persistent abnormalities: The significance of a persistent abnormality in a casualty following the treatment of an injury (especially a skeletal injury) varies with the lifestyle of the species. With birds, raptors that hunt on the wing by speed and agility (e.g. peregrine, hobby, sparrowhawk) or by hovering (e.g. kestrel) require near-perfect wing function to survive, whereas more sedentary and resident species that fly only short distances to find new feeding locations or territories (e.g. mute swan, resident mallard) or use cryptic camouflage or a skulking behaviour to evade predators (e.g. moorhen, resident passerines) may survive with restricted wing function.

Similarly in mammals, less active species (e.g. hedgehog) may survive with one partially functional limb, whereas bats and larger more mobile species (e.g. badger, fox) require fully functional limbs to survive. An attempt to repair a fractured long bone in a highly mobile species when the possibility for return to full function of the limb is poor compromises the welfare of the animal, unless there are adequate provisions for keeping the casualty in permanent captivity.

Pelvic fractures in female mammals may lead to deformity of the pelvic canal and predispose a pregnant animal to dystocia. Although it is possible to perform a hysterectomy or ovariohysterectomy, this might have consequences on the social structure of a group (e.g. in badgers, Chapter 11).

Juveniles: The recognition of a dependent juvenile casualty is essential for the correct assessment of its feeding and nursing requirements. Many 'orphaned' juveniles of both avian and mammalian species are brought into captivity unnecessarily. They are found without any apparent evidence of protective parents and, therefore, assumed to be abandoned. However, it is normal for fawns to be left in thick cover, fox cubs to leave the earth whilst the vixen is away or seal pups to appear on beaches; they are usually still being attended by their parents.

Many altricial (nest-reared) birds on the point of fledging leave the nest before they can fly and remain for several days in the safety of the tree canopy or surrounding vegetation, where they can be displaced by strong winds or predators. In this way many fledgling passerines are found in urban gardens or juvenile tawny owls in woodland. If uninjured, it is better to replace juvenile passerines in the cover of vegetation, preferably within a small, darkened box to which the adults can gain access, than to keep them in captivity to be reared by hand and given a very uncertain future. Juvenile birds of many species can be fostered into nests holding young of the same age and species, and this requires the cooperation and expertise of local naturalists. Grounded juvenile tawny owls are able to climb trees and regain safety, but will benefit from being assisted by being placed as high and as close as possible to the site where found.

Hand-reared animals may have difficulty in adapting to feeding in the wild and avoiding predators. A lot of care and skill is needed to prepare them for returning to the wild, which might be beyond the scope of most veterinary practices – and even many rehabilitation units. It is important to appreciate these problems when assessing an appropriate course of action with apparently abandoned young wildlife casualties.

Body condition
Casualties in poor body condition should be critically assessed and the possible cause of the weight loss determined. If the likely cause is a genuine failure of a food resource (e.g. abandoned juvenile, storm-driven seabird, hedgehog in a drought) or as a sequel to an injury that may respond favourably to treatment (e.g. territorial fight wound in a young animal, wing with a closed ulnar fracture), temporary captivity and supportive feeding may be justified. However, if no cause of the weight loss is apparent, it is likely to be due to either physical problems (e.g. unidentified infectious or non-infectious disease) or behavioural problems (e.g. inability to establish a feeding territory) that would prevent the casualty from surviving in the wild. Such animals are possibly the failures of the process of natural selection. Attempts

at rehabilitating and releasing such casualties may compromise their welfare, as they are unlikely to survive if given a 'second chance' (see 'Emaciated casualties', below).

Health status and nature of disability
Attention should be paid to the possibility of a casualty introducing to a naïve wild population a novel pathogen, either acquired whilst in captivity or because the casualty is released at a location and into a wild population distant from its capture site. Identification of such infections requires special investigations (see Chapter 4).

The extent of any injuries or disease processes and their significance regarding the possibility of releasing a casualty will be apparent only after a thorough clinical examination and, if indicated, further ancillary investigations (see Chapter 4).

Psychological status
To survive in the wild, a rehabilitated casualty must be fit both physically and behaviourally (see Chapter 3). It must be able to react to its environment and to locate and deal with its natural food source. It must also be able to relate and react normally to individuals of its own species and to potential predators.

Facilities for treatment and after-care
The welfare of casualties of species that have specialized feeding requirements (e.g. suckling mammals, avian insectivores) or require specialized accommodation (e.g. larger mammals, marine mammals, waterfowl) can be safeguarded only if they are cared for in rehabilitation units that are suitably equipped and staffed with experienced personnel. Similarly, funds must be available to ensure that the treatment and husbandry of the casualty is adequate. If the required financing or facilities are not available, euthanasia is the most humane course of action.

Availability of suitable release sites
For most short-term casualties, the ideal release site is the place where it was found; it is then returned to a familiar area, preferably its own territory. This is sometimes not possible, usually because the original site cannot be located, or the site may be unsuitable for release (e.g. storm-driven seabirds found inland; badger cubs from a disturbed sett). The lack of a suitable release site with adequate food resources and free of conflict with conspecifics, or the length of time a casualty might have to be kept in captivity before a suitable site is found, might affect the assessment of the best course of action for the animal.

The selection of a suitable release site for medium-term or long-term casualties is a critical factor in their rehabilitation. Territorial animals will have lost their territory in the meantime and a suitable release site with adequate food resources yet free from territorial conflicts would need to be found. As with short-term casualties, these factors (discussed in Chapter 3) influence an assessment of the welfare of the casualty and a decision on its treatment.

Examination

Handling for clinical examination

Bird casualties: The nature of a wild bird casualty and its method of presentation often prevent an inspection from a distance, and reliance has to be put on an examination in the hand. A method of handling has to be adopted that will allow an examination of the animal without causing it excessive distress or additional injury, whilst at the same time preventing injury to the handlers. The examination should be made in a quiet and possibly darkened room.

- Small passerines are most easily held with bare hands using the 'ringer's grip', with the bird's neck between the first and second finger and its body gently enclosed within the hand (Figure 2.5a)
- Medium-sized passerines and pigeons are more easily handled using the 'pigeon-fancier's grip', with the bird's body supported in the palm of the hand and its legs secured between the first and second fingers (Figure 2.5b)
- Large passerines, seabirds, waterfowl and raptors are capable of inflicting painful injuries and are more safely handled with the help of an assistant. Once the bird's body and wings have been enclosed in a towel or blanket (Figure 2.5c), the assistant should restrain its head and (especially in the case of raptors) its feet.

Sedation may be of value in attempts to catch a wild bird trapped in an enclosed building, using baited food (under a permit from English Nature or its counterparts in Scotland and Wales), but it is rarely necessary to sedate a wild bird in order to perform a clinical examination. However, some birds may be extremely distressed on being handled and sedation might be essential to allow a thorough examination.

General anaesthesia is indicated for most radiographic examinations and also for ophthalmic examination in larger birds that have received trauma to the head (see Chapter 22).

Mammalian casualties: In many cases the clinical examination of small mammal casualties – especially those that bite – is greatly facilitated by sedation or anaesthesia, which will reduce the stress of handling to the animal and also reduce the risk of injury to the handlers.

Further details of clinical examination for specific groups of mammals are given in the species chapters.

Categorization by length of stay in captivity

It is possible, in clinical terms, to categorize wildlife casualties on the basis of their disabilities, the resulting length of time that they will need to be kept in captivity, and the facilities that they will require to ensure their welfare and to aid their recovery (Figure 2.6). An early diagnosis of the cause of a disability and an assessment of general condition will allow, in many cases, a prediction of the outcome of treatment and the time required in captivity and, therefore, the potential for the humane handling of the casualty. Juvenile casualties (see 'Examination and assessment for rehabilitation: Juveniles', above) require careful consideration.

Permanently disabled casualties

In assessing the significance of a physical disability or an abnormal behaviour pattern, the possibility must be considered that, although the condition might not be immediately life-threatening, it would by its nature permanently prevent the animal from surviving in the wild. In such cases the alternative to euthanasia would be permanent captivity, which can be envisaged only if the animal can be guaranteed for the foreseeable future a reasonable quality of life in captivity and if there is a sound justification for this action.

Justifications for retaining permanently disabled casualties in captivity include the following.

Captive breeding programmes: Permanently disabled adults might be used in breeding programmes either to produce offspring for use in regulated release schemes of endangered species or to supply birds for legitimate uses such as falconry or aviculture. The use of permanently disabled wild animals reduces the demand for individuals taken from the wild population and will add new genetic material to existing captive breeding stock. However, candidates for captive breeding schemes must be chosen carefully to ensure that the risk of introducing significant pathogens or genetic problems is greatly reduced.

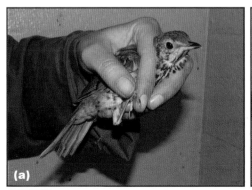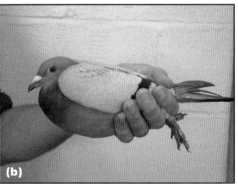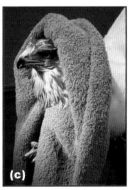

2.5 Handling birds: (a) ringer's grip; (b) pigeon fancier's grip; (c) holding a large bird.

Category	Length of stay and requirements	Examples
Short-term casualties	Can be released within days, or sometimes hours, of capture; require only stabilization and minimal treatment	Stunned but uninjured casualty following collision Exhausted bird or mammal caught in netting Storm-driven seabird Displaced juvenile being translocated Reptile or amphibian trapped in drain
Medium-term casualties	Requiring treatment and hospitalization lasting no more than several weeks and able to be released without any special preparation	Soft tissue injuries following trauma Poisoning Oil pollution Emaciation following starvation, due to displacement Simple fractures
Long-term casualties	Requiring prolonged treatment and captivity, usually lasting months, and needing additional management in preparation for release	Skeletal damage Abandoned juveniles, especially raptors and larger mammals Migratory species of bird
Permanently disabled	Unable to be released for physical or behavioural reasons yet able to maintain health and quality of life in captivity	Loss of limb function through severely misaligned fractures of long bones Partial wing amputees Loss of sensory perception Social imprints

2.6 Categorization of casualties by length of stay in captivity.

Education: Trained animals, especially birds, are widely used in displays and talks given to the general public on aspects of conservation. Permanently disabled casualties are frequently employed for such purposes and can be used successfully, provided that their disabilities do not cause significant welfare problems.

Imprint models: Permanently disabled adults can be used successfully as imprint models for young animals of the same species when reared in captivity with the minimum of human contact (see Chapter 3).

Zoonotic risks

Although the list of possible zoonotic infections from British wildlife might appear long, the actual risk to those handling wildlife casualties seems to be low. In a small anecdotal survey, veterinary surgeons working with British wildlife were asked for their experiences with zoonoses acquired from wildlife. The majority had little or no experience of confirmed zoonotic infections. The commonest infection encountered was ringworm, presumed to have been caught from hedgehogs; a few others had experienced occasional cases of chlamydophilosis, yersiniosis and sarcoptic mange, and 'seal finger' occurred in those working with marine mammals (J.R. Best, unpublished). Significant zoonotic diseases are set out in Figure 2.7 and are discussed in more detail in the species chapters.

It is important that those who handle wildlife casualties are made aware of the potential hazards and that health and safety risk assessments are made within veterinary practices and rehabilitation units (see Chapter 5). Possible modes of infection determine risk assessments for procedures involving a particular species, as follows:

Zoonotic infection	Carrier species
Tuberculosis	Badgers, deer, foxes
Seal pox	Seals
'Seal finger' (infection by *Mycoplasma* spp.)	Seals
Ringworm	Foxes, hedgehogs
Rabies	Bats, foxes
Sarcoptic mange	Foxes
Lyme disease	Deer, foxes
Toxoplasmosis	Rabbits
Salmonellosis	Most species
Campylobacteriosis	Most species
Coliform infections	Most species
Chlamydophilosis (ornithosis)	Pigeons and other birds

2.7 Significant zoonotic infections of British wild animals.

- Dermal irritation from fleas and lice (most species)
- Dermal contact (e.g. ringworm from hedgehogs)
- Contact with blood, faeces or urine (e.g. *Borrelia* infection from deer, *Campylobacter* spp. from birds, mycobacteriosis from badgers, parasitic infections)
- Respiratory aerosol spread (e.g. psittacosis or ornithosis from birds)
- Trauma and non-specific infection from bites and scratches (most species)
- Specific infections from bites and scratches (e.g. *Mycoplasma* infection from seals).

Suitable precautions to avoid zoonotic risks include:

- Risk assessments for common procedures involving veterinary and nursing staff
- Training in correct handling techniques for all staff and members of the public involved in handling wildlife casualties (basic handling techniques have been given above; suitable techniques for different species are given in the relevant chapters)
- Use of gloves (e.g. latex), protective clothing and masks as necessary when handling wildlife
- Use of protective clothing and suitable hygiene precautions when carrying out post-mortem examinations
- Vaccination as appropriate (e.g. rabies vaccines for those involved in frequent handling of bats; Heaf testing and BCG vaccination for those involved frequently with badgers)
- Rapid appropriate medical attention as necessary.

Techniques for euthanasia
Euthanasia, within the terms of this manual, can be defined as the killing of an animal with the minimum of physical and mental suffering. It may be the most humane course of action for a wildlife casualty with little chance of a speedy and successful return to the wild. Methods are summarized in Figure 2.8.

Physical methods: Any physical method of euthanasia must ensure immediate loss of consciousness, which can be ensured only if performed by a trained, confident and competent operator.

- Dislocation of cervical vertebrae:
  - in small fledgling birds: by sudden firm pressure between thumb and first finger across the neck;
    - in birds up to 500 g: with the bird held upside down by its legs, by sharp downward pull on the head with the cranial vertebrae fully extended (bent backwards)
- Skull crush: with a suitably heavy and blunt instrument, a blow over the back of the skull, with sufficient force to fracture the skull severely and cause extensive brain damage
- Use of firearms: only trained personnel should use firearms for euthanasia of larger mammals to ensure a shot to the head, using either a free bullet or captive bolt that will give instant loss of consciousness (see Chapter 16).

Chemical: Lethal injections, using barbiturates (normally pentobarbital), can be given by a variety of routes. In many cases the preliminary use of an injectable or oral sedative will minimize any problems in giving the lethal injection.

Volatile anaesthetic agents may be used to euthanase smaller casualties by administering a fatal overdose in an anaesthetic chamber or to induce anaesthesia, which is then followed by a lethal injection or death by a suitable physical method.

Most injection sites are described later (see 'First aid and stabilization'). Details of intrahepatic injection in birds are given in Chapter 25; details of intracranial injection are given in Chapter 20.

Emergency euthanasia by non-veterinary personnel
Whenever possible, euthanasia of wildlife casualties should be performed by veterinary surgeons, veterinary nurses or trained staff of animal welfare societies. However, there will be occasions when emergency humane destruction of a casualty needs to be performed by workers at rehabilitation units. Veterinary surgeons attending rehabilitation units should be prepared to give

Group	Physical methods	Chemical methods
Small birds (up to crow size, approx. 500 g)	*Dislocation of cervical vertebrae *Skull crush	Inhalation anaesthesia followed by suitable physical method or lethal injection Lethal injection: intrahepatic, intravenous, intraosseous
Large birds	*Skull crush	Lethal injection: intravenous, intracardiac, intrahepatic, intracranial, intraosseous
Small mammals (up to juvenile rabbit)	*Skull crush	Inhalation anaesthesia followed by suitable physical method or lethal injection Lethal injection: intravenous, intracardiac, intrahepatic, intrarenal, intraperitoneal, intraosseous
Medium-sized mammals (adult rabbit)	*Skull crush	Lethal injection, possibly pre-sedate: intravenous, intracardiac, intrahepatic, intrarenal, intraperitoneal, intraosseous
Large mammals (fox, badger, deer)	Firearms, head shot	Lethal injection, possibly pre-sedate: intravenous, intracardiac, intraperitoneal
Reptiles and amphibians	*Skull crush Do not use decapitation alone Special care must be taken to ensure animal is indeed dead	Lethal injection (usually without pre-sedation): intraperitoneal, occasionally intravenous
Fish	*Skull crush Do not use decapitation alone Special care must be taken to ensure animal is indeed dead	Lethal injection: intraperitoneal or overdose of MS222 or benzocaine

2.8 Methods of euthanasia for wildlife casualties. ★ These techniques are also suitable for demonstration to non-veterinary workers for use in an emergency.

instruction in appropriate techniques to be used in an emergency, i.e. on occasions when it is impossible to get immediate professional assistance and where delay would prolong the pain and suffering of a severely injured animal whose chances of return to the wild are clearly non-existent. Figure 2.8 indicates some physical methods of euthanasia that would be suitable for demonstration to non-veterinary personnel.

First aid and stabilization

Many casualties have been disabled for a while before they are found and brought into captivity. During this time they may have been unable to take food and water and may have become dehydrated and cachectic. The first step must be to give emergency treatment to any injuries or urgent medical problems; the second is to stabilize the animal with administration of fluids, energy and heat.

Emergency trauma management

Soft tissue injuries
Standard first aid procedures for cleansing of the wound, and haemostasis if required, can be followed but problems may occur with the application and maintenance of dressings for protecting wounds from further infection and damage (see 'Wound management', below).

Orthopaedic injuries
Fractures of long bones require immediate immobilization of the fragments to minimize further soft tissue damage.

Wing fractures in birds: Immobilization of the fractured wing is imperative, especially in cases involving the humerus. As this bone is pneumatized (the medulla contains an extension of an air sac) with a thin cortex, a fracture invariably results in the formation of long, sharp fragments of bone that may puncture the skin and cause other soft tissue damage as the bird flaps its injured wing. The wing must be immobilized as soon as possible. Depending on the site and nature of the fracture, various emergency bandaging methods can be employed:

- Fractures of the manus or fractures of either the radius or ulna alone may need only simple support of the wing by using masking tape to tape together the primaries of the closed wing (Figure 2.9a,b)
- Fractures of the radius and the ulna can be supported with a 'figure-of-eight' dressing, using a conforming bandage, which will hold the ulna and radius against the humerus for support (Figure 2.9c)
- Fractures of the humerus must be held against the body to give temporary immobilization and this can be achieved with a 'figure-of-eight' dressing, again using a conforming bandage, that includes the body but leaves the opposite wing free (Figure 2.9d,e).

It should be noted that these techniques are for emergency immobilization of the wing and such dressings should not be left in place for more than 2–3 days initially, as the joints of the avian wing stiffen when held in flexion.

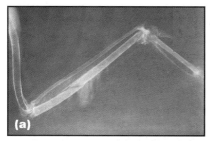
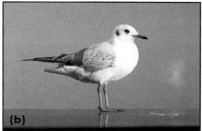
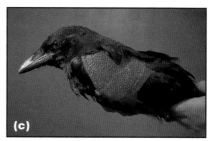
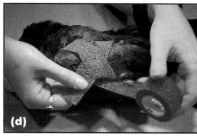
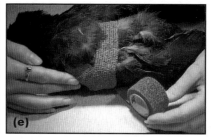

2.9 Bandaging a fracture. (a) Radiograph of black-headed gull with well aligned closed fracture of the ulna. (b) Masking tape is securing the primaries to the tertial wing feathers; it will be left in place initially for no more than 2–3 days. (c) Carrion crow with figure-of-eight bandage supporting a closed fracture of the ulna (the bandage holds only the carpal and elbow joints flexed; it does not include the body). (d) Conforming bandage used to form a figure-of-eight support for a fractured humerus. The bandage is holding the carpal and elbow joints flexed. (e) The humerus is then immobilized by passing the bandage completely around the body, passing beneath the opposite wing.

Leg fractures in birds: Fractures of the leg in birds must be immobilized temporarily to prevent further damage, especially in active larger birds that are free to jump and struggle inside an inappropriate container.

- Fractures of the tarsometatarsus in larger birds can be splinted using suitable rigid materials held with tape. In passerines the use of an Altman splint formed from masking tape, to include the intertarsal joint, is tolerated extremely well (see Chapter 25)
- Fractures of the tibiotarsus in larger species can be supported with Robert Jones dressings, whereas femoral fractures are usually well supported by the surrounding muscle mass and supporting bandages are of little help
- Fractures of the toes in larger species can be immobilized using a 'ball' bandage made by placing a firm ball of cotton wool within the grasp of the foot and taping the toes to the ball with a conforming tape.

Limb fractures in mammals: In small mammals, fractures may need no immediate support. In the larger species, standard methods of emergency immobilization are appropriate, possibly with the need of sedation in some cases. The risks of further damage at the fracture site and self-trauma need to be considered; if appropriate, a rapid move to surgery may be indicated.

Fluids and energy replacement

Assessment of dehydration

The standard approach to rehydration is similar to that used in small animal practice, though the methods of administration may need some modification. Assessment of the degree of hydration of a mammalian casualty can be achieved with standard clinical criteria, i.e. skin pliability, moistness of mucous membranes, capillary refill time, and position of the eyeballs within the orbit. Similar criteria do not apply to all avian casualties; for example, some birds have coloured mucous membranes. An assessment of the state of hydration of a bird can be made by measuring the refill time of the basilic vein; if it is longer than 1–2 seconds it might indicate a dehydration level of 7% from normal (Rupley, 1998). Laboratory examination of blood to determine the packed cell volume will give an indication of the state of hydration but it is safe to assume that any casualty received in poor body condition has been starving and will benefit from the administration of fluids and energy.

Fluid and energy requirements

For clinical purposes, the daily maintenance requirement of fluid in the majority of birds and mammals is regarded as being approximately 50 ml/kg bodyweight (5% of bodyweight). This figure varies with the body mass of the animal: it is lower for larger animals and higher for smaller ones (Kirkwood, 1983b), increasing considerably in very small animals. For example, birds weighing above 100 g need 5% of their body mass in fluids per day, whereas this rises to 50% of the body mass for small birds weighing 10–20 g (Sturkie, 2000).

Similarly, daily energy requirements vary with the bodyweight of the animal. Larger birds can survive without food for many days; for example, common buzzards (1100 g) might lose 15% of their bodyweight after 7 days of starvation, while the smaller common kestrels (250 g) might lose 12% of their bodyweight in only 3 days of starvation (Kirkwood, 1981). Small passerines such as blue tits may not survive for more than 48–72 hours without food (Perrins, 1979).

It is safe to assume that a casualty in a debilitated state will have lost at least 10–15% of total body fluids. Ideally, this deficit should be replaced within the first 48–72 hours of hospitalization and given in addition to the animal's calculated daily fluid maintenance requirement.

Hypovolaemic shock: Following severe trauma, many casualties will be suffering from hypovolaemic shock and will require an immediate increase in their circulating volume by intravenous infusion of a suitable solution at doses extrapolated from the standard techniques applying to small animal practice (see King and Hammond, 1999).

Choice of suitable fluid

The choice of an appropriate fluid for a particular case is often complicated by the lack of an accurate clinical history on matters such as starvation or the presence of vomiting and diarrhoea affecting the acid/base balance, or an increased respiratory rate accelerating dehydration. To be suitable, the fluid must replace the fluid deficit, maintain the composition of the intercellular fluid and, possibly, provide an immediate source of energy.

In general terms, fluids suitable for different routes of administration are as follows:

- Injection: a sterile, isotonic, balanced crystalloid mixture, such as a lactated Ringer's (Hartmann's) solution or an isotonic 4% glucose and 0.18% saline solution. Hypertonic solutions and colloids may be used to treat clinical shock in the larger mammals
- Oral administration: either of the above isotonic fluids, proprietary hypotonic oral rehydration electrolyte and glucose mixtures (e.g. Lectade or Lectade Plus, Pfizer; Ion-aid, Merial: when prepared, these solutions contain 2%, 3% and 2.5% glucose, respectively) or, in an emergency, a freshly prepared 5% glucose solution. Proprietary preparations of hydrolysed starch are available and promoted as sources of energy by companies supplying the aviculture trade (e.g. Polyaid, Birdcare Company; Rapidaid, Vetrepharm).

Routes of fluid administration

The choice of a suitable route for administration of the fluid is dictated by the nature of the animal and its disabilities: the species, the degree of debilitation, the nature of the casualty's injuries and the facilities available (Figure 2.10). Severely debilitated

Method of administration	Birds	Mammals
Oral	Unassisted drinking Syringing directly into mouth Gavage to crop or thoracic oesophagus	Unassisted drinking Syringing directly into mouth Gavage to stomach Nasogastric tube Pharyngostomy
Rectal/colonic	Possible route in emergency	Useful route in emergency
Subcutaneous injection	Medial aspect of the thigh	Loose skin of scruff or lateral thorax
Intraperitoneal injection	Danger of injecting fluid into air sacs	Suitable for small mammals
Intravenous injection	Tarsal vein Ulnar or basilic vein Jugular vein	Cephalic vein Jugular vein Saphenous vein
Intraosseous injection	Proximal or distal ulna, proximal tibiotarsus	Femur, tibia or humerus

2.10 Administration of fluids to avian and mammalian casualties.

and dehydrated animals may have a poor blood supply to peripheral tissues and the gastrointestinal tract, making oral and subcutaneous administration of fluids less effective than intravenous or intraosseous administration. In all cases the fluid should be warmed to the approximate body temperature of the casualty before it is administered.

Birds:

Crop or stomach tubing: All native British birds have a buccal cavity with a simple anatomy (Figure 2.11), which facilitates the passage of a gavage tube through the pharynx and down the oesophagus to the crop, or to the proximal portion of the cervical oesophagus in those species that do not have a well developed crop (e.g. owls, gulls). Rigid gavage tubes are available commercially in several sizes and are suitable for most small passerines; alternatively, semi-rigid tubes can be made from cut-down urinary catheters, care being taken to round off the cut edges over a flame to prevent damage to the oesophageal mucosa.

This technique is suitable for demonstration to lay workers as a standard first aid procedure:

* With the bird suitably restrained by an assistant, its mouth is opened and the tube is introduced along the roof of the mouth, into the oesophagus and then into the crop
* In larger birds the beak is most easily, and safely, kept open with a finger inserted in the commissure of the mandibles; it is often easier in such birds to introduce the tube on the left side of the pharynx
* The progress of the tube can be checked by palpation of the neck
* The correct position is identified when the tip of the tube is at the thoracic inlet.

Approximate volumes of fluid that can safely be deposited at one time into the crop or proximal cervical oesophagus of some fully grown common birds are given in Figure 2.12.

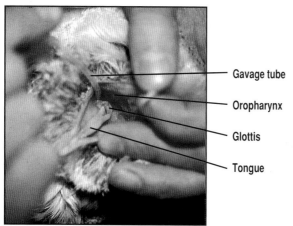

— Gavage tube
— Oropharynx
— Glottis
— Tongue

2.11 Buccal cavity of a barn owl, showing the anatomical features and a gavage tube being passed into the oesophagus.

Species	Approximate volume of fluid to be given by single gavage administration (ml)
Robin (*Erithacus rubercula*)	1
Blackbird (*Turdus merula*)	2
Feral pigeon (*Columba livia*)	5
Carrion crow (*Corvus corone*)	10
Common buzzard (*Buteo buteo*)	30
Grey heron (*Ardea cinerea*)	100
Mute swan (*Cygnus olor*)	500

2.12 Approximate volume of fluid to be given by single gavage administration to common species of British birds

Rectal fluids: The mucosa of the coprodeum (the cranial compartment of the cloaca) and of the rectum has the additional function of resorbing water and electrolytes from the urine and the faeces. In an emergency, when other routes are unavailable, it is possible to administer fluids to a bird by the rectal route. Hypotonic fluids can be administered by repeated infusion into the coprodeum and rectum by use of a syringe and a short length of tubing (Lumeij and Ephrati, 1997).

Subcutaneous injections: The site of choice is the loose skin on the medial aspect of the thigh in the groin, which appears to cause little discomfort to the patient. Lay workers may be taught this technique for use in emergency situations.

The bird is restrained in lateral recumbency, with the leg extended; the site is disinfected (and at the same time made more visible) by wetting the feathers with a swab carrying surgical spirit. Injections can be made bilaterally and the use of a small needle (25 or 27 gauge) will reduce the amount of fluid leaking through the needle puncture in the thin, inelastic skin.

The maximum volume of warmed fluid to be injected at each site varies with the size of the bird (e.g. 0.5 ml in a small passerine, 10 ml in a common buzzard, 20 ml in a pheasant). If the patient is warmed (see 'Maintenance of optimal temperature'; below), the fluid is absorbed quickly from the site and may have disappeared within 30–60 minutes.

Intravenous injections: This is the preferred route in a severely debilitated and dehydrated patient requiring rapid correction of circulating fluid volume and acid/base balance. The most accessible sites for intravenous injection (and collection of blood samples maximum safe volume in birds is 1% of bodyweight) are as follows (Figure 2.13):

- Medial tarsal vein: accessible in most birds weighing over 100 g (preferably using a 27 gauge needle). The vein runs medially along the length of the tarsometatarsus and over the craniomedial aspect of the intertarsal joint. With the bird restrained in a cloth and held in lateral recumbency, its leg can be extended caudally and the vein raised by pinching the muscles on the caudal aspect of the tibiotarsus. The vein will be seen more clearly if the overlying skin is wetted with a swab carrying surgical spirit. In species with a scaled tarsus, the vein is well supported by the surrounding connective tissue and will allow repeated venepuncture

- Ulnar/basilic vein: located on the ventral aspect of the wing, crosses the radius and ulna just distal to the elbow and then extends along the humerus. The vein is most easily found with the bird restrained in a cloth and held in lateral recumbency (with the head covered and the feet securely held in larger species) and the wing extended. It is a very fragile vein and usually forms a haematoma following venepuncture, which limits its repeated use

- Right jugular vein: in most species, lies under a featherless tract of skin on the lateral aspect of the neck directly in line with the external auditory meatus. The bird is restrained in a cloth in dorsal recumbency, with its tail facing away from the operator, who can hold its head to expose the right side of the neck. The vein can be raised with gentle pressure applied to the neck slightly distal to the thoracic inlet. Occasionally a full crop or a subcutaneous air sac needs to be pushed caudally to reveal the length of the vein. Some species (pigeons, gamebirds) have very dense feathering on the neck, making this site difficult to locate.

Fluids can be administered either as an intravenous bolus or by continuous infusion. The bolus, which should be approximately 1% of the bird's bodyweight, can be injected slowly into any available vein and repeated as necessary. Continuous infusion is given through an indwelling intravenous catheter and can only be performed satisfactorily in a very debilitated and sedentary bird or a sedated patient. Gravity-fed drip-sets are difficult to use in any other than the larger species, as the very slow delivery rate required is difficult to achieve without the risk of overhydrating the patient. Mechanical syringe drivers, especially those in which the delivery rate can be set as low as 1.0 ml/h, are the preferred method of intravenous infusion of fluid.

Intraosseous injection: This is possibly the most useful route in severely debilitated birds with poor peripheral circulation, especially in the larger species. A non-pneumatized long bone must be used and the most commonly selected are the ulna (proximal or distal) and tibiotarsus (proximal). Intraosseous needles with stylettes are available but in most birds an 18 or 20 gauge hypodermic needle attached to a syringe can be driven into the medulla. Once the patency of the needle and its correct location have been confirmed, it can then be connected to a delivery system and infusion performed in a similar manner to that used with intravenous catheters (see above).

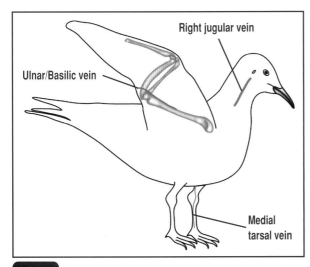

2.13 Sites for venepuncture in a bird.

Mammals:

Oral fluids: Successful passage of a stomach tube in conscious mammals is generally difficult. Although this might be a technique attempted by lay carers, there is a risk of the tube being chewed or fluids being inadvertently administered into the trachea. Nasogastric tubes may be placed in some species under light sedation and local anaesthesia but these are rarely tolerated for long in unsupervised mammals.

Oral fluids for mammals are usually restricted to commercial electrolyte solutions or liquid diets (e.g. Reanimyl, Virbac; Hill's a/d diet, Hill's Pet Nutrition). Few casualties will drink readily when first admitted.

Subcutaneous injection: These may be used where the animal is mildly hypovolaemic and oral or intravenous administration of fluid is not possible. Lay carers can easily be taught the technique. Fluids should be sterile, isotonic and warmed to body temperature. Only small volumes of fluid should be given at one site (up to 10 ml). Suitable sites in most species are the scruff of the neck or over the shoulders. The casualty should be warmed slowly, to encourage peripheral vasodilation. Repeat administration of fluids should be avoided as this can lead to local tissue necrosis.

Intraperitoneal injection: Intraperitoneal injections have an increased absorption rate over subcutaneous injections for fluid therapy, but are still only suitable for mildly hypovolaemic patients where oral fluids cannot be administered. Volumes of around 10 ml/kg at a time are suitable. The patient should be kept warm, to encourage vasodilation and fluid uptake. The technique may be taught to lay people for emergency situations but care should be taken to make them aware of the risks of infection and organ damage. The standard technique of angling a needle cranially just behind the umbilicus in a patient supported vertically is appropriate in most cases.

Intravenous injection: This is the preferred route of administration of fluids in moderate to severely hypovolaemic mammalian casualties. In many of the larger mammals (foxes, badgers) the cephalic or saphenous veins are usually accessible and easily catheterized. Jugular veins may be used in other species such as deer and some small mammals, or the ear vein in rabbits and hares. Over-the-needle catheters are the most appropriate for most species. Catheters are usually well tolerated in animals requiring fluid therapy. Baskerville-type muzzles can be placed on the larger mammals to prevent chewing of drip-lines. Fluid types and rates can be adapted from domestic mammal fluid therapy.

Intraosseous injection: This is the preferred method of fluid administration in moderate to severely hypovolaemic mammals where intravenous access is not possible. The humerus, tibia and femur are all possible sites for administration; the most practical is usually the trochanteric fossa of the femur. The site of penetration should be clipped as necessary and surgically prepared. Small volumes of local anaesthetic may be used as necessary. The density of mammalian bone means that spinal or intraosseous needles are the most suitable for these procedures, but hypodermic needles of an appropriate size (usually 18–20 gauge) can be used in the smaller species.

Maintenance of optimal temperature

Many casualties (especially those that are debilitated) will be hypothermic. All mammalian and avian casualties will benefit from being kept at an environmental temperature that lies within their thermoneutral range (the range of environmental temperatures within which an animal needs to expend no energy, in addition to its maintenance requirements, to maintain a stable body temperature). For most mammals this is 15–24°C. For birds the optimal temperature varies with their body mass (Figure 2.14).

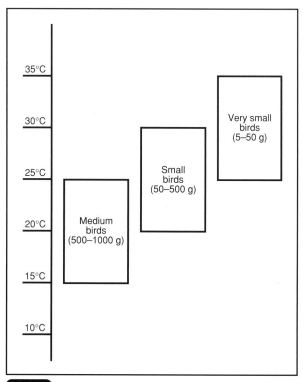

2.14 Avian thermoneutral ranges.

Heat loss from a debilitated or shocked casualty can be limited by wrapping the animal in an insulating blanket but correction of a heat deficit will need an external source of heat to raise the body temperature.

- Hot-water bottles and heated plastic or grain bags may be useful as a temporary source of heat in an emergency but their use needs to be closely monitored: they cool rapidly and can then draw warmth from the patient
- Electric heat pads are helpful for immobile mammals but, with some types, need to be covered to prevent the risk of overheating (or even burning) of the animal through direct contact with the pad; the pads may also need protection to prevent damage from being bitten

- Heat lamps and electric heaters can be suspended within walk-in pens, or over cages, or attached to the outside of smaller cages. They are ideal for mobile patients, as they create a heat gradient that allows the animal to select a position giving itself an optimal temperature. Care must be taken when positioning a heat lamp to ensure that the patient is not overheated. Some heat lamps can be controlled with a thermostat
- Hospital cages and brooders, with built-in thermostatically controlled heating, are commercially available and are suitable for small mammals and small to medium-sized birds, as are ex-hospital paediatric incubators.

With all forms of heated accommodation, the provision of a thermometer (preferably a maximum/minimum one) to measure the temperature within the immediate environment of the patient is valuable.

Analgesia

The provision of pain relief is part of first aid for an injured casualty. The administration of analgesics will increase the comfort of the casualty and reduce the amount of 'stress' suffered by the animal. Analgesics are discussed in more detail later (see 'Analgesia, sedation and anaesthesia'). Details of the doses of suitable analgesics are to be found in each of the mammal chapters and in the avian formulary in Appendix 1.

Hospitalization

Special requirements for hospitalized casualties

It is worth repeating that the aim of treating wildlife casualties is to enable them to return to the wild physically fit and able to relate normally to their own and other species. This means that their 'wild' state must be respected and retained whilst in captivity, which requires a system of husbandry that differs considerably from that used for companion animals and domesticated exotic species. The requirements are as follows:

- As much seclusion as is practicable, especially from the sight and sound of humans and other potential predators, particularly dogs and cats
- Secure, escape-free accommodation, designed to minimize the risk of injury to the casualty
- Means of capture and handling that minimize stress and risk of injury to the patient and to the handler
- A diet that resembles, as closely as possible, the natural diet
- Strict attention to hygiene to prevent any cross-infection from other wildlife casualties or domesticated animals held within the hospital
- For long-term patients, means of maintaining their physical fitness prior to release.

In most general veterinary practices it may be impossible to fulfil these requirements, especially for the larger species of mammals and birds. In these circumstances, after initial primary care, a close working relationship with a wildlife rehabilitation unit that has the required facilities will greatly benefit the welfare of the patient and the outcome of the treatment.

Housing for hospitalization and short-term care

The design of suitable accommodation for hospitalization and short-term care for casualties is covered in detail in the group and species-specific chapters. The basic requirements of suitable accommodation are as follows.

Size

The accommodation should give the animal enough space to be able to move freely within the limits of its disability, but with some species (especially deer) an ability to reduce the space available will facilitate handling. Mammals must have a sleeping area that is separate from the feeding and lavatory areas. All birds should have sufficient room to extend their wings in all directions and to be able to turn without damaging their plumage. In addition, perching birds should be provided with blocks or perches suitable for their size and habits, placed in such a way that the bird can reach and use them and that damage to the plumage is avoided.

Seclusion

Most casualties will benefit from seclusion from any contact (be it sight, sound or smell) with potential predators, including dogs and cats. There should also be minimal human contact and disturbances, such as banging doors, voices and telephones.

Generally it is unwise to house individuals of different species in the same accommodation. Some gregarious animals will benefit from contact with members of their own or related species, as will developing juveniles. Great care must be taken in mixing animals from different populations, due to the risk of cross-infection with potential pathogens.

Design

Where possible, the design of the accommodation should allow for the food and water containers to be reached from outside and also for the floor covering of cages for perching birds to be changed from the outside. The design and layout should allow for the swift and safe capture of the animal for examination and for the administration of medication, when this cannot be performed by remote methods. For example, bird cages should have a minimal number of perches that obstruct capture and should be in rooms where the lighting can be reduced. Most perching birds will select a high perch and placing perches and cages as high as possible (at least above human eye level) might give the bird a greater sense of security.

Security

Accommodation must be of secure design to prevent escape, especially during routine cleaning, feeding and handling of the patients. Rooms holding caged casualties must also be escape-proof. Many mammalian species are highly destructive and are capable of chewing their way out of wooden, plastic or cardboard boxes; foxes and badgers are capable of destroying poor-quality metal cages or wooden doors and at the same time causing themselves dental and pedal damage.

Warmth

Initially, debilitated casualties will benefit from being kept at a temperature within their thermoneutral range (see 'Maintenance of optimal temperature', above). Once stabilized and feeding well, native species will only require a stable ambient environmental temperature. Excessive heat for prolonged times requires a period of acclimatization to ambient temperatures before release.

Hygiene

Accommodation must be designed to allow cleaning of floors or bedding and food and water containers with minimal disturbance to the patient. It must also be capable of being physically cleaned and effectively disinfected between patients, to prevent cross-infection.

Observation

Methods of discreet observation of the patient should be incorporated, so that the behaviour of the animal can be monitored without disturbance. Security spy-holes in doors and closed-circuit television, if practicable and available, are ideal (see Chapter 3).

Feeding

The feeding of wildlife casualties whilst in care presents the problem of designing a diet that is both acceptable to the animal and nutritionally sound. The ideal diet is as close to its natural diet as possible, balanced in its constituents and free from potential pathogens. Initially, an 'unnatural' diet may be acceptable – or even essential – in order to start improving the animal's nutritional status (e.g. liquidized food given by gavage tube). Total intravenous nutrition can be of value in casualties unable to feed independently. Details of diets for specific groups of casualties are dealt with in the group and species-specific chapters. Much of the skill shown by experienced rehabilitators is in their patience in assisting a casualty to feed and then encouraging it to eat on its own.

Diets for medium-term to long-term casualties require supplementation with vitamins and minerals. Seed-eating birds need a source of insoluble grit.

With a stabilized yet anorectic casualty, nutritional support can be given using commercial feeding preparations (e.g. Reanimyl, Virbac; Hill's a/d diet, Hill's Pet Nutrition; Critical Care Formula, Vetark Animal Health) or the intended diet in a liquidized form administered by gavage tube. This is routine practice in avian patients but more difficult with larger, adult mammals.

Provision of water

Fresh drinking water should be available at all times and failure to provide access to water contravenes welfare laws (see Chapter 5). Some birds (notably raptors) and small mammals drink very little, as they obtain their fluid from food and metabolic water; however, water should be available as a casualty may not be obtaining sufficient to fulfil its fluid requirements. For larger mammals, water should be provided in heavy bowls that cannot be knocked over. Waterfowl feed more easily if their food is given in large containers of water. Although not all bird casualties will be able to bathe, water should be made available (if appropriate) in suitable shallow containers.

Weighing

Obtaining an accurate weight of the casualty gives an indication of its condition and enables calculation of the dosage of medication. Bodyweight must be considered together with body condition (i.e. the prominence of the keel of the sternum in a bird and the bones of the spine in a mammal) and with body size.

Monitoring bodyweight gives a useful indication of the animal's progress during treatment. Comparisons can be made only if the animal is weighed at the same time of day and at the same time in relation to feeding.

Small birds and mammals can be restrained in closed boxes or wrapped in cloths and weighed on electronic scales (animals weighing less than 30 g are more accurately weighed on scales registering in intervals of 1 g or less). 'Pesola' spring balances, designed for use by field biologists, are suitable, especially for passerines and also for small mammals. Larger birds and mammals can be suspended in hessian sacks for weighing on spring balances, or placed on 'step-up' weighing scales after being either sedated or restrained in a suitable container that has been pre-weighed.

Analgesia, sedation and anaesthesia

The nature of wildlife casualties, and the circumstances under which they are brought into veterinary care, provide the veterinary anaesthetist with numerous problems. There is a lack of pre-anaesthetic history, limited knowledge of concurrent disease and often a need to anaesthetize before proper clinical examination is possible. This, together with the small size of many patients and limited intravenous access for anaesthetic drugs, can make anaesthetizing wildlife difficult. If basic principles are adhered to, however, risks can be limited.

Pre-anaesthesia

Where possible, casualties should be weighed. Age, size and body condition should also be taken into consideration in the choice and dose of anaesthetic agents. A pre-anaesthetic assessment of cardio-respiratory function, hydration status and ability to thermoregulate should be made, even if only by careful observation from a distance. In some casualties, closer examination and the collection of blood for pre-anaesthetic screening may be possible. More specific details of such testing are given in the species chapters that follow.

Monitoring

In addition to a knowledgeable designated veterinary nurse, standard monitoring methods used in general practice (oesophageal stethoscopes, pulse oximeters, blood pressure, respiratory and cardiac monitors) can easily be adapted for use in many species.

Provision of heat during and after anaesthesia is an important factor in survival of casualties, especially those that are very small or have a lack of ability to thermoregulate. Temperatures should be monitored throughout the anaesthesia and recovery periods.

Oxygen

Provision of oxygen during and after anaesthesia will increase survival rates. Many of the sedative and anaesthetic drugs used in mammals (see below) will have negative effects on cardiorespiratory function and this, together with pre-existing problems, can lead to hypoxia and hypotension in all species. Anaesthetizing casualties by masking with inhalation agent/oxygen will suffice, but where possible endotracheal tubes should be placed to maintain a patent airway and allow positive pressure ventilation, if necessary.

Avian casualties

Analgesia

Non-steroidal anti-inflammatory drugs (NSAIDs), especially carprofen, ketoprofen and butorphanol, can be safely administered to avian casualties (see Appendix 1).

Local anaesthesia

Birds are sensitive to some local anaesthetic agents, and these should be used with caution, especially in smaller species.

Sedation

Restraint during a clinical examination or simple procedure such as redressing a wound, collecting blood samples or radiography, can be achieved using injectable sedative agents or light inhalation anaesthesia. Injectable sedatives have the advantage of requiring minimal equipment or trained assistance for their administration (they are, therefore, ideal for use in the field) but do not have the advantage of the versatility and, especially when using isoflurane, the greater safety of inhalation anaesthesia. Details of injectable sedative/anaesthetic agents and combinations are given in the avian formulary in Appendix 1.

General anaesthesia

General anaesthesia can be obtained using injectable agents, as discussed above and detailed in Appendix 1, but inhalation anaesthesia is more commonly used in current avian practice. Although halothane and methoxyflurane were widely used in the past, the agent of choice at present is isoflurane. It gives a rapid induction and recovery, good analgesia and muscle relaxation, and has a very wide therapeutic index. Food should be withheld for several hours before anaesthesia, especially in those species possessing crops. Anaesthesia is induced with a flow rate of oxygen of 1.5–2.0 l/min and an isoflurane concentration of 4–5%, and is then maintained at 2–3%. In larger species that may be difficult to restrain, anaesthesia can be induced by gradually increasing the concentration of isoflurane.

Most species of bird can be induced by 'masking down', using a circuit with sufficient reserve in a reservoir bag or wide-bore tubing to accommodate the patient's tidal volume. Avian anaesthetic masks are available commercially but a variety of sizes is needed for the range of avian species and effective masks can be adapted from Hall's rubber masks or from plastic cases for disposable syringes. To be effective, a mask must be large enough to accommodate the head of the bird comfortably but also needs an airtight seal around the neck to prevent leakage of anaesthetic gases or inspiration of fresh air.

Tracheal intubation is an advantage in most cases, other than short periods of anaesthesia, as it will reduce the leakage of anaesthetic gases, allow access to the head and, if required, allow assisted ventilation. Tracheal intubation is a simple procedure in most species. Uncuffed tubes are preferred in smaller species, as over-inflation of a cuff could damage the tracheal rings, which in birds are complete and, in larger species, ossified.

The depth of anaesthesia can be assessed by the relaxation of the limbs, the loss of digital and (later) corneal reflexes and the rate and depth of respiration. Respiration is most effectively monitored by a trained nurse, possibly assisted by a respiration monitor. The heart rate is most simply monitored with an oesophageal stethoscope; however, the use of cardiac monitors and pulse oximeters is becoming more readily available in general practice.

As the body temperature of an anaesthetized bird will drop during prolonged procedures, the use of insulating material on the operating table and the provision of additional heat during recovery are important. In dorsal recumbency the viscera will compress the air sacs and so reduce the available tidal volume. Similarly, the venous return to the heart may be compromised by compression from the viscera with the bird held on its back. Care must be exercised with a bird in this position for any length of time. Administration of intravenous fluids is advocated, wherever practicable, for avian patients undergoing prolonged anaesthesia.

Air sac cannulation: Anaesthetic gases can also be administered to a bird through cannulation of an air sac and this is of great value in a bird requiring prolonged surgery to the head or upper airways. Air sac cannulae are available commercially or can be made from endotracheal tubes of a suitable size. They are generally placed into the caudal thoracic air sac through the last intercostal space, sutured *in situ* and connected to an anaesthetic machine.

Post-anaesthesia: A bird recovering from an anaesthetic must be protected from hypothermia and injury during any post-anaesthetic excitement. It should be loosely wrapped or covered with a towel or blanket and allowed to recover in a quiet, heated pen, devoid of any perches or obstructions.

Mammalian casualties

Analgesia

Most analgesics suitable for use in domestic mammals can be used safely in wild mammalian casualties. The most common of these are the NSAIDs. It is generally assumed that the cyclo-oxygenase-2 (COX-2) selective agents, such as meloxicam and carprofen, have reduced renal and intestinal side effects in all species. Opioid analgesics have been used in some species (see specific chapters) and are the best agents for producing good quality long-lasting analgesia, especially in surgery. Care should be taken with species variation and respiratory suppression when using pure opioids. Where possible, NSAIDs and opioids should be given before surgery to gain maximum analgesic benefit.

Other injectable agents such as xylazine, medetomidine and ketamine (see below) provide some analgesia which, in the case of alpha-2 agonists, will be lost on reversal. The use of inhalation agents such as nitrous oxide can provide additional analgesia during surgical procedures but should not be used in cases with evidence of respiratory disease. Nitrous oxide should be switched off 5 minutes before the end of surgery to prevent diffusion hypoxia, making the duration of its analgesic effects limited to approximately the end of surgery.

Local anaesthetic agents such as lidocaine, bupivacaine and mepivacaine can be useful in wild mammals but total doses should be calculated carefully based on bodyweight.

Injectable sedatives and anaesthetics

Propofol: Intravenous agents such as propofol and thiopental can be used in most mammalian casualties, provided that intravenous access is possible. The rapid metabolism and elimination of propofol make it the agent of choice in most cases. Propofol can also be used for continuous intravenous anaesthesia. Alfaxalone/alfadolone (Saffan, Schering-Plough Animal Health) has been used in some wild mammals but histamine release can be a problem in some species (see species chapters).

Ketamine: The most commonly used injectable agent in wild mammals is probably ketamine. This drug has minimal negative cardiorespiratory effects, giving it high safety margins in most cases, and it can be used as the sole anaesthetic agent. However, hallucinogenic effects and other side effects (e.g. salivation, seizures and sneezing) are seen in some species at the doses of ketamine required for anaesthesia; muscle relaxation is poor for surgical procedures and sudden noises can rouse patients to a dangerous level of consciousness. For these reasons, ketamine is usually combined with a benzodiazepine (diazepam or midazolam) or an alpha-2 agonist such as medetomidine or xylazine. In most cases the drugs are given in the same syringe without problems. Most combinations should be given by the intramuscular route and this can be achieved by careful restraint, or through the bars of a crush cage or, rarely, via dart or syringe-firing methods. In all cases, a period of peaceful induction time, ideally in a darkened room or a box covered with a blanket, is necessary. The loss of blink reflexes can result in corneal damage and so a suitable ocular preparation should be used as soon as the animal is anaesthetized. The negative effects on cardiorespiratory function of the alpha-2 agonist drugs means that care should be taken in their use, and oxygen and warmth should be provided where possible. Xylazine and medetomidine can be reversed with yohimbine

and atipamezole, respectively; the timing of such reversal should be made so as to minimize ketamine-related effects. Specific details and doses of anaesthetic drugs are given in the species chapters.

Tiletamine: Tiletamine, an alternative dissociative anaesthetic to ketamine, is available in combination with zolazepam, a benzodiazepine, as the commercial products Zoletil 20 (Parke Davis) and Telazol (Eskins-Sinn, USA). These provide a useful, easily reconstituted drug for wildlife work with most of the advantages of ketamine/benzodiazepine combinations. Unfortunately Zoletil and Telazol are currently not commercially available in the UK.

Immobilon: A commercially available mixture of etorphine and acepromazine (Large Animal Immobilon, Vericore) is recommended for the euthanasia of stranded cetaceans (see 'Methods of euthanasia' in Chapter 17) and may be used occasionally by suitably qualified and licensed operators for the remote capture (darting) of large land mammals.

Gaseous agents

Gaseous agents can be used as the sole anaesthetic in small mammalian species or those that can be handled easily. An anaesthetic chamber connected to a vaporizer is most suitable for species up to the size of rabbits. Chambers should be constructed such that gas is ducted into the chamber at the bottom and removed from the top. Masks, ideally scavenged, can be used with care to induce larger mammals. The dangerously high levels of anaesthetic released from pads soaked in volatile agents and dropped into boxes makes this method suitable only for field situations and euthanasia. Health and safety aspects should be considered when using volatile agents in open systems.

The gaseous agent of choice for most species at present, because of its high safety margins, is probably isoflurane. Halothane and methoxyflurane can be used safely in most cases. All may be superseded in the future by newer agents such as sevoflurane.

Gaseous agents can also be used to prolong or deepen anaesthesia induced by injectable drugs as described above. Endotracheal tubes (generally cuffed) can easily be passed in most of the larger mammalian species. Smaller species can be maintained on a mask, as described in the avian anaesthesia section.

Treatment stage

Once the casualty has been stabilized, attempts may be made (where indicated) to reach a clearer diagnosis with a thorough clinical examination, possibly under sedation or general anaesthesia, and by using ancillary techniques, especially radiography and laboratory examinations. Armed with such information a tentative prognosis can be reached. If this is favourable, a programme of treatment can be instituted.

The techniques of veterinary medicine and surgery that apply to the treatment of wildlife casualties are, in general, well within the scope of any competent small animal practice.

Assessment of the significance of any disease condition at this stage must ensure that the disability is likely to resolve, that the treatment will not expose the animal to excessive pain and distress and that, once the disability has been resolved, the animal will be able to be released to the wild.

Pharmacology

It should be noted that no pharmaceutical products available in the UK are licensed for use in indigenous wild birds and mammals and that the choice of a drug should follow the recommendations made in various professional codes of practice and guidelines on the use of medicines (see Chapter 5).

Allometric scaling

It is recognized that the calculation of dose rates for smaller animals cannot be simply scaled down from the doses for larger domesticated mammals. The smaller a warm-blooded animal is, the higher is its metabolic rate; therefore, to obtain effective levels of a medication, either a higher dose rate or more frequent administration is required. Accurate dosages can be calculated using a formula described by Kirkwood (1983 a,b) but, as described by Cooper (1991), a general rule for warm-blooded animals weighing less than 500 g would be to double the recommended dose for a dog or cat. Such recommendations do not take into account the variations (species or individual) in the pharmacokinetics of different medications.

Parasite control

Although a normal, healthy wild animal is likely to be 'in balance' with its parasites, a captive casualty is likely to be showing stress-induced immunosuppression, which could cause its parasite infestation to increase to the point of causing disease. The routine treatment of wildlife casualties for parasites is a contentious point and a pragmatic approach would be to monitor the presence of ectoparasites with routine clinical examinations and intestinal parasites with routine faecal examinations and then to treat as and when indicated.

As blood-sucking ectoparasites such as ticks and mites, fleas and louse flies (Hippoboscidae) may be vectors of pathogens, routine treatment of hospitalized casualties on admittance and regular treatment of the animal accommodation with suitable insecticides would be indicated (see species chapters and Appendix 1).

Trauma

The majority of injuries sustained by wildlife in Britain are caused either by human activity (e.g. road traffic accidents, collisions with power lines and windows, entrapment in netting, firearm and trapping injuries) or from attack by predators or conspecifics in territorial disputes.

Wound management

Many simple soft tissue injuries, such as abrasions from entangled netting, may require only first aid treatment. For more severe wounds, standard procedures of management (i.e. debridement, drainage and closure) are appropriate but ideally subsequent nursing should involve a minimum of handling. A minimal amount of hair should be clipped or feathers plucked. If wounds are closed, absorbable sutures or subcutaneous sutures patterns could be used. In many cases dressings will be tolerated when held in place with bandages, but care must be taken with adhesive tape – especially in birds, where the adhesive could damage the feathers. In birds, dressings are best held in place using cohesive bandages or masking tape, the adhesive of which will not damage the plumage. Many birds may well tolerate dressings being sutured to feathers or skin, especially on the wings.

Self-trauma to wounds or interference with dressings may be controlled with collars or muzzles. Some birds will tolerate either Elizabethan collars, made to measure from plastic sheeting/radiographic film or available commercially, or neck braces, made from lengths of plastic-foam water-pipe cladding. Most mammals tolerate Elizabethan collars poorly, but collars or Baskerville-type muzzles can be used for short periods in some situations.

Thoracic and abdominal injuries in mammals: Following road traffic accidents, mammalian casualties may present with a range of injuries similar to those seen in domestic species. Common thoracic injuries include rupture of the diaphragm, lung contusions, pneumothorax and haemothorax. These can be confirmed from a combination of radiography, ultrasonography and chest drainage. Drainage of air or fluid from the chest cavity can easily be carried out under appropriate sedation or local anaesthesia using a needle, syringe and three-way tap or appropriate-sized chest drain. Most species will not tolerate chest drains left *in situ* and any cases requiring repeated drainage are best euthanased. Diaphragm ruptures may be repaired in the standard way in mammals that are large enough to be ventilated during surgery (especially foxes and badgers). The chest should be drained as above at the end of surgery. As with any other surgical procedure, careful assessment of the casualty for other injuries and general suitability for release must be made before surgery is carried out. Additionally good surgical skills, time and some costs will be required; if these are not available, euthanasia is the preferred option.

Common abdominal injuries are abdominal wall rupture (with or without prolapse of abdominal contents) and haemoperitoneum. Animals with prolapsed abdominal contents require immediate first aid (protection of the prolapsed material, analgesics and fluids), followed by general anaesthesia and surgery. The abdominal wound should be opened to allow examination of all the structures involved. If there is any chance of loss of tissue vitality or contamination with gut contents, the patient should be euthanased. Bleeding into the abdomen can be diagnosed from radiographs, ultrasonography and peritoneal tap. Whilst bleeding may be controlled by body wrapping in some species, this does not allow for assessment of abdominal contents for future release. Where bleeding is significant, therefore, patients should be stabilized and exploratory surgery performed. Bleeding from minor organs can be surgically controlled. Euthanasia is preferred where there is damage to vital organs. Splenectomy in wild mammals is easily performed but may predispose the animal to problems with recovery from infection in the future and should be considered carefully.

Gunshot wounds: See Chapter 18.

Management of skeletal injuries

Fractures of long bones, especially wing bones in birds, are very common disabilities and present many problems with their management and treatment. Assessment of the significance of a fracture requires an accurate diagnosis of the site and nature of the fracture, of the extent of soft tissue damage and of the risk of infection. In deciding the suitability for treatment of an individual case, consideration should be given to the following.

Species and natural habits: Animals, especially predatory species that rely on speed and agility to hunt, need to be fit and have a fully functional musculosketetal system. Any persisting skeletal abnormality, especially of the axial skeleton and limbs, might prejudice the ability of the animal to hunt successfully. On the other hand a small mammal, such as a hedgehog, or a small species of waterfowl, may survive adequately in the wild with a semi-functional leg.

Age: Young animals and smaller animals heal quickly and, with support, a well aligned closed fracture could heal and be functional before the animal is old enough to be independent. An adult animal may need a prolonged period of hospitalization to repair a fracture requiring surgical intervention. In this time the breeding and feeding territory of the animal might have been lost and its ability to regain a territory or find an alternative site could be compromised by its loss of fitness resulting from the hospitalization.

Site of the fracture: Uncomplicated fractures of some bones may heal spontaneously, requiring only restricted activity (e.g. fractured digits and ribs, coracoid fractures in birds). Other fractures may require only minimal support (e.g. fractures of the avian ulna with an intact radius, fractures of distal limb bones in passerine fledglings or small immature rodents).

Fractures of limb bones require the greatest care with assessment and repair, as in most cases the resulting union must ensure restoration to perfect, or near perfect, function of that limb. If this cannot be achieved, the animal may never be fit for release. As with all species, the prognosis is better with a mid-shaft fracture than one adjacent to a joint, and better in a long bone with a straight shaft than one with a curved shape, notably the 'S'-shaped avian humerus.

Nature of fracture: Simple, closed fractures present no additional complications to treatment but in wildlife casualties the fractures are frequently old, comminuted, open and infected (Simpson, 1996) (Figure 2.15). In fractures of the limb bones in birds, especially the pneumatized bones (the humerus and, in some species, the femur), the thin cortex shatters to produce

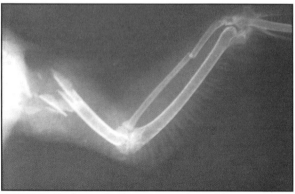

2.15 Radiograph of open comminuted fractured humerus in a barn owl RTA casualty, showing severely splintered humerus. The extent of skeletal and soft tissue damage in this bird precluded any chance of a successful return to the wild.

a severely comminuted fracture with sharp fragments that can cause extensive soft tissue damage. Many such fractures are beyond satisfactory repair.

Practicalities of fracture repair: Careful consideration must be given to the welfare implications of exposing a casualty to a prolonged period of hospitalization with extensive surgical interventions and restrictive, uncomfortable aftercare, especially when the prognosis for release is poor. Techniques for fixation must be carefully selected, as some species (such as foxes) commonly interfere with dressings and external fixators, whereas most birds appear to tolerate them well. Ideally, the selected technique should allow for the removal of all metal implants before the release of the casualty.

Specific fractures

Some fractures that are commonly seen in wildlife casualties but may not be regularly encountered in general practice are as follows.

Wing fractures in birds: The avian wing is a vertebrate forelimb that is highly developed to give a sturdy, yet lightweight, highly mobile structure, the bones of which will fracture readily when, in flight, they are brought to an abrupt halt against a solid object.

In attempting to repair a fracture in a wild bird's wing it is essential to preserve not just the patient's ability to fly but also its agility, by retaining the original anatomy as closely as possible. The degree of agility in flight that is required is obviously greatest in species that hunt or feed on the wing but all free-living birds need a high degree of agility to avoid predators and other dangers. Many species, even apparently resident species, may make migratory movements, especially in adverse weather conditions. A very careful assessment must therefore be made, both before and after treatment, of an individual casualty's expectations for survival in the wild (see Chapter 3).

Intramedullary pins and external fixators can be used to immobilize fractures but the use of bone plates is rarely possible, as the cortices are too thin to accept screws. The wing does have the advantage that it is not weight-bearing and so is free from some of the post-operative complications that occur in legs; however, immobilization of wing joints with dressings for periods exceeding 10–14 days may lead to a permanent restriction of mobility. A detailed description of the management of fractures of the wing of birds of prey can be found in Chapter 22 and in Simpson (1996).

Pectoral girdle: The complex pectoral girdle is vulnerable to impact fractures caused by collisions in flight, a common injury being fracture of the coracoid bone. Birds with such an injury are unable to fly and are often presented with the wing tilted so that primaries of the affected wing are held higher. An absence of palpable lesions along the length of the wing would indicate a closer investigation of the pectoral girdle. Palpation on the lateral borders of the thoracic inlet may reveal crepitus but radiography is required to confirm the fracture and the degree of displacement of the fragments. If the fragments are in apposition, healing will occur with cage rest, and the bird is very likely to regain an adequate power of flight. Fractures with poor apposition of the fragments can be immobilized surgically with intramedullary pins but the technique does involve sectioning the overlying pectoral muscle (see Chapter 22).

Humerus: Fractures of the humerus are possibly the commonest wing fractures seen in wild birds and usually have a poor prognosis. Many are open, infected, several days old and seriously comminuted, making retention of the original anatomy difficult. In suitable cases intramedullary pinning is effective, the pins placed exiting the medulla at a site along the shaft that will allow the 'S' shape of the bone to be retained. Placing two intramedullary pins can prevent rotation of the major fragments, and cerclage wires are often required to stabilize viable bone fragments. The use of tie-in or hybrid fixator techniques may be preferable for the repair of some fractures of the humerus (see Chapter 22). The use of intramedullary plastic 'shuttle' pins (Cook, UK) allows alignment of the major fragments but needs additional support in the form of external fixators.

Radius and ulna: The fracture of either the radius or ulna can occur without damage to the other bone; as long as the fragments are in alignment, healing will go ahead with simple support of the wing for the first 7–10 days using a figure-of-eight bandage or simply taping the primaries together (see Figure 2.9). If both bones are fractured only the ulna usually needs to be stabilized, preferably with an intramedullary pin driven through the length of the medulla and entering on the convex, caudal aspect of the bone just distal to the elbow.

Carpometacarpus: A fractured carpometacarpus can be stabilized with external support, using dressings in smaller birds or external fixators in larger species. The fractures frequently offer a poor prognosis, as they are usually open, infected and associated with soft tissue damage.

Elbow: Luxation of the elbow, though easy to reduce, is often difficult to stabilize without reduced mobility of the joint.

Complications: Complications for repair of a wing fracture include:

- Infection in open fractures, requiring adequate local and systemic antibiotic treatment
- Damage to soft tissue structures, tendons, ligaments, muscles, nerves and blood vessels
- Avascular bone fragments forming sequestra
- Callus formation at the fracture site interfering with soft tissue structures, especially tendons, and (if in the proximity of a joint) causing ankylosis.

Pelvic limb fractures in birds: Details of management of leg fractures are given in the 'First aid' section earlier in this chapter. Surgical repair of fractures to the long bones can be performed using standard techniques of intramedullary pinning (stack pinning will prevent rotation of fractures to the tibiotarsus), external fixation (using tubing filled with quick-setting resin as lightweight connecting bars) or combinations of both.

Fractures of the beak: Any damage to the skeletal structure of the beak is likely to result eventually in a malformation that could affect the bird's ability to feed and preen. Although such patients may survive well in captivity, they are not suitable candidates for release.

Fractures in mammals:

Long bones and pelvis: Long bone and pelvic fractures are common in mammals, especially following road traffic accidents. Pelvic fractures are difficult to manage: they require long healing periods, there are pain management problems and, if surgically corrected, there are problems with the removal of metal-work before release. Additionally, complications of pelvic canal narrowing have to be considerable, especially in female animals. The repair of long bone fractures depends on species, fracture type and suitability of the individual for release. Young animals that are otherwise physically fit and heal well are usually the most suitable candidates for surgery. Additionally, younger animals also appear to tolerate fixators, plasters and dressings much better than adults.

Jaw: Jaw fractures are commonly seen in some species (especially the larger land mammals) following road traffic accidents and occasionally baiting or snaring injuries. Provided that adequate jaw conformation, strength and satisfactory dentition can be maintained, such fractures can be repaired successfully. The fixation methods used (wire or screws) need to allow the patient to eat soon after surgery and must be removable before its release.

Planning of fracture fixation techniques can be difficult, as the most suitable techniques for the fracture type may not be tolerated well by the patient (e.g. external fixators) or may require excessive post-operative surgery to remove implants (e.g. plates). Metalwork should, where at all possible, be removed prior to release. There are no grounds for second-rate treatment of orthopaedic problems in wildlife. If the skills, facilities and finances are not available for the best possible care, the patient should be euthanased.

Emaciated casualties

Emaciation will occur in wildlife casualties through the lack of an adequate supply of food, the inability to feed or as the result of a debilitating disease process. It is important to investigate the cause of the emaciation, as this will give an indication of the prognosis. A full and thorough clinical examination, including laboratory investigations, is essential to identify any significant lesions.

If starvation is likely to have been caused by temporary food shortage due to a short-term local climatic problem (e.g. prolonged cold weather or drought), the animal needs to spend time in captivity with nutritional support until conditions improve and then be released at a suitable location. Such animals will regain weight rapidly with supportive feeding, indicating the absence of any underlying debilitating disease processes. Anabolic steroids may be helpful in some cases (J. Lewis, personal communication).

An inability to find sufficient food might be associated with an injury or a behavioural problem. Such animals might regain weight with adequate supportive feeding in captivity but will succumb on release unless the underlying problem has been identified and corrected. Animals with a confirmed disease process that is leading to emaciation, or animals that have received adequate supportive feeding yet have failed to gain weight, are likely to be poor candidates for release and very careful consideration should be given to whether they are treated or euthanased.

Weight loss associated with heavy parasitic infestations (ectoparasites and endoparasites) should be approached with caution, as it is likely that the infestation is associated with an underlying physical or behavioural problem, which is reducing the animal's immune status, thus upsetting the natural host/ parasite balance.

Abandoned young

The hand-rearing of abandoned young animals is both an art and a science. It requires a detailed knowledge of the natural history of the species and a wealth of patience and ingenuity to feed and nurture the animals in such a way as to prevent their becoming imprinted on humans (see Chapter 3) and to enable them to develop sufficient independence and survival skills to be released successfully to the wild. Details of rearing abandoned young are dealt with in each group chapter.

Poisoning

Generally, wild animals have an innate ability to avoid most natural toxic substances, due to the evolution of selective feeding habits; however, they cannot avoid toxins introduced accidentally or intentionally into their environment by human activity.

Classification

Poisoning incidents can be classified as follows:

- **Natural**: toxins released by naturally occurring microorganisms, such as *Clostridium botulina* (botulism), blue-green algae, dinoflagellates ('red tides'), mycotoxins (fungi) and venom from higher vertebrates and invertebrates
- **Accidental**: spillage, mishandling or poor storage of pesticides, herbicides and rodenticides; industrial and marine accidents leading to pollution
- **Intentional**: legitimate use in controlled pest control schemes and illegitimate uses, mostly in attempts to destroy (protected) predators on shooting estates or destructive pest species.

In cases where the illegal use of poisons is suspected, a Wildlife Incident Investigation Scheme is run by DEFRA through the Central Science Laboratory.

Diagnosis

The problems of dealing with a potential poisoning incident are often compounded by the difficulty in rapidly establishing a diagnosis and, even if an accurate diagnosis is made, by the lack of an effective specific antidote for many poisons. Also, by the time a poisoned casualty is captured and presented for treatment, it may be that a large amount of the toxic agent has already been absorbed into the body. Assistance may then be limited to symptomatic and supportive treatment of the less severely affected cases and euthanasia of the hopeless ones.

An accurate diagnosis of poisoning requires the following:

- A suggestive history. For example, several dead raptors, crows or foxes found in the same vicinity might indicate the illegal use of pesticides
- Suggestive clinical signs or post-mortem lesions (e.g. dead or paralysed waterfowl on a shallow pond during hot weather might suggest botulism)
- Detection of the toxic agent (e.g. radiographic evidence of lead in the gizzard of a mute swan showing weakness and loss of weight).

Treatment

Acute poisoning is always an emergency, with no time to wait for laboratory investigations. Treatment can be considered under three stages:

1. Prevent further absorption of the poison.
2. Treat acute symptoms.
3. Give specific antidotes.

Prevention of further absorption: Most poisons that are likely to affect wildlife are taken by mouth. Prevention of further absorption requires removal from the alimentary canal, which in fairly early cases means removal from the stomach of mammals and the crop or stomach of birds. However, more often than not, by the time a casualty has been captured any ingested material will have already moved from the stomach into the intestines.

Emetics: In mammals that can vomit (i.e. carnivores and omnivores with a simple single stomach), the use of oral emetics (sodium chloride, mustard or crystals of sodium carbonate, i.e. washing soda) or parenteral emetics (apomorphine) may be helpful in the first few hours. Dangers of inhalation of vomited material will arise if the animal is made to vomit while it is convulsing. Irrigation of the stomach under sedation or general anaesthesia is an alternative to the use of emetics in severe cases.

Crop washing: In birds with a full crop it is possible, with care, to manipulate and expel the contents through the mouth in a conscious patient. The crop can be irrigated, preferably in an anaesthetized and intubated bird, using a wide-bore rubber or plastic tube (as wide a tube as possible) passed down the oesophagus. Warm water is repeatedly run into the crop through the tube, agitated and then removed by lowering the bird's head to allow it to run out by gravity.

Adsorbents and astringents: In casualties with chemical or oil pollution of the coat or plumage, it is important to remove as much as possible to prevent local damage to the skin and to minimize the amount swallowed when the animal licks or preens itself.

Once a poison has entered the intestine, it is possible to attempt to limit further absorption into the body by the use of adsorbents and astringents. Mixtures such as BCK granules (Fort Dodge Animal Health), containing activated charcoal (wood charcoal), kaolin (natural aluminium silicate as a very fine powder) and bismuth salts, are used as adsorbents. Astringents, such as tannic acid, may possibly precipitate alkaloids, or form insoluble salts of heavy metals, and so prevent their adsorption.

The following general adsorbent/astringent mixture (Greenwood, 1979) can be used in suspected cases of oral poisoning, with a dose of 2–50 ml (depending on size of patient): 10 g activated charcoal; 5 g kaolin; 5 g light magnesium oxide; 5 g tannic acid; 500 ml water.

If the toxic agent is known to be fat-soluble (e.g. fuel oil), liquid paraffin will mix with the agent and dilute its effects.

Treatment of acute symptoms, and supportive care: If the casualty is suffering from an acute poisoning, the cause of which is unknown, the relief of symptoms and supportive care may be the only course of treatment available whilst (it is hoped) the poison is being excreted.

The symptoms displayed by an acutely poisoned animal might include nervous signs, haemorrhage, vomiting and diarrhoea. If there are nervous signs, including tremors, convulsions and coma, it is an emergency, especially if the animal is convulsing continuously. The animal will become exhausted by the muscle activity and develop hyperthermia, requiring treatment to control the convulsions and reduce the body temperature.

Vomiting occurs in most single-stomached mammals but rarely in ruminants, whilst birds can regurgitate their crop and stomach contents. Vomiting is advantageous initially to remove toxins from the stomach but, if it persists, it becomes exhausting and will lead to dehydration and alkalosis. Birds and mammals showing persistent diarrhoea certainly need fluid replacement. If the casualty is continuously losing blood from internal haemorrhage, it is likely to be in hypovolaemic shock.

Specific antidotes: Specific antidotes are available for some poisons and these must be given, together with the supportive and symptomatic treatment, as early as possible in the treatment of the patient.

Further details on some specific poisonings can be found in the following chapters:

- Oil pollution: Chapter 18
- Lead poisoning: Chapter 20
- Botulism: Chapter 20
- Pesticides: Chapter 22.

Vaccination of wildlife casualties

Although the subject of vaccinating free-living wild animals might be contentious, there are situations when wildlife casualties held in captivity for treatment are exposed to infectious agents.

A vaccination policy should be considered only if the presence of a potential pathogen is confirmed and if a vaccine is available that has proven efficacy, with minimal side effects, in the species of casualty (or in members of the same taxonomic group) considered to be at risk. The major concern with the use of vaccines in wildlife casualties is the risk that an infectious agent to which wild populations have had no previous exposure will be introduced in the vaccine and carried by a vaccinated animal when it is released. The use of inactivated vaccines wherever possible should reduce these risks.

Examples of situations where vaccination of casualties have been advocated include:

- Distemper vaccine in the face of an outbreak of morbillivirus infection in common seal pups held in rehabilitation units
- Myxomatosis and viral haemorrhagic disease vaccine in hand-reared wild rabbit neonates held in rehabilitation units
- Duck viral enteritis vaccination of mute swans in contact with wild mallards in rehabilitation units.

References and further reading

Cooper JE (1991) Introduction. In: *BSAVA Manual of Exotic Pets*, eds PH Beynon and JE Cooper. BSAVA, Cheltenham
Greenwood AG (1979) In: *First Aid and Care of Wild Birds*, eds JE Cooper and JT Eley. David and Charles, Newton Abbot
Jordan WJ and Hughes J (1982) *Care of the Wild*. Macdonald, London
King L and Hammond R (1999) *BSAVA Manual of Canine and Feline Emergency and Critical Care*. BSAVA, Cheltenham
Kirkwood JK (1981) Maintenance energy requirements and rates of weight loss during starvation in birds of prey. In: *Recent Advances in the Study of Raptor Diseases*, eds JE Cooper and AG Greenwood. Chiron Publications, Keighley
Kirkwood JK (1983a) Dosing exotic species. *Veterinary Record* **112**, 486
Kirkwood JK (1983b) Influence of body size on health and disease. *Veterinary Record* **113**, 287

Knobel DL, du Toit JT and Bingham J (2002) Development of a bait and baiting system for delivery of an oral rabies vaccine to free-ranging African wild dogs (*Lycoan pictus*). *Journal of Wildlife Diseases* **38**, 352–362

Lumeij JS and Ephrati C (1997) Theory and practice of rectal fluid therapy in birds. *Proceedings of the 1997 European Conference on Avian Medicine and Surgery*, London

Paddleford RR (1999) *Manual of Small Animal Anaesthesia, 2nd edn.* WB Saunders, Philadelphia

Perrins C (1979) *British Tits.* Collins, London

Rupley AE (1998) Critical care of pet birds, procedures, therapeutics and patient support. *Veterinary Clinics of North America: Exotic Animals Practice.* **1,** 11–41

Simpson G (1996) Wing problems. In: *BSAVA Manual of Raptors, Pigeons and Waterfowl,* eds PH Beynon *et al.* BSAVA, Cheltenham

Stocker L (2000) *Practical Wildlife Care.* Blackwell Scientific, Oxford

Sturkie PD (ed) (2000) *Avian Physiology, 5th edn.* Academic Press, San Diego, California

Wildpro® (April 2002) *UK Wildlife First Aid and Care.* Wildlife Information Network, Royal Veterinary College, London, www.wildlifeinformation.org

Acknowledgements

Acknowledgements are due to James Barnett, Neil Forbes, Dan Holden, Tony Sainsbury and John Lewis for their contributions to early drafts of this chapter.

3

Rehabilitation and release

Paul Llewellyn

Introduction

With more people becoming involved in the rescue of injured wild animals, the veterinary profession is expected to deal with all manner of ailments. The purpose of this chapter is to establish best practice by setting out feasible criteria for assessment of physical and mental fitness of wild casualties prior to release – whatever the species, be they birds, mammals or reptiles.

There is a need to draw a line between the domestic animal casualty (which can be kept alive in relative comfort with the use of surgery, modern medication and the loving care of the owner) and the wild casualty, where the ultimate goal is rehabilitation and release back to the wild. The wild environment is harsh, with many factors influencing survival and population density – predominantly food availability, predation and disease.

In order to survive in the wild, animals have to be wholly fit so that they can:

- Locate food resources and catch and kill prey species
- Avoid predators
- Compete with their own and other species
- Defend and maintain feeding and breeding territories
- Withstand fluctuating climatic conditions or undertake migrations.

To meet these challenges they need to:

- Appreciate which species they are themselves, in order to socialize and procreate
- Be able to identify naturally occurring food items and prey species
- Be able to locate and identify suitable feeding and breeding habitats.

These factors are not always innate and early learning from the parents during development and maturation is essential, with genetic predisposition also playing a part (Hess, 1973; Ridley, 1986; Krebs and Davies, 1987; Llewellyn, 1987; Fox, 1995).

Rehabilitators have legal and ethical obligations to ensure that any casualty being prepared for release has its mental and physical fitness properly assessed and that the release site is suitable. Therefore, any advice given by the veterinary profession can have legal ramifications (Chapter 5).

Housing facilities for assessment and rehabilitation

After the initial veterinary treatment and confinement during recuperation, casualties must be placed in suitable rehabilitation housing in order to regain fitness and coordination and to be assessed and prepared for release procedures. Some suitable types of housing for casualties are suggested in Figures 3.1 to 3.4.

The rehabilitation enclosure must:

- Be of adequate size for the species concerned, allowing enough space for the casualty to exercise

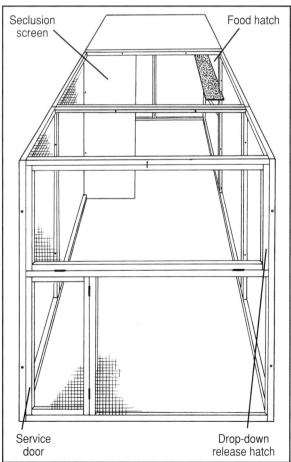

Seclusion screen

Food hatch

Service door

Drop-down release hatch

3.1 Sectional rehabilitation and release flight with solid back and sides. Dimensions, mesh size and furniture will depend on the species being housed.

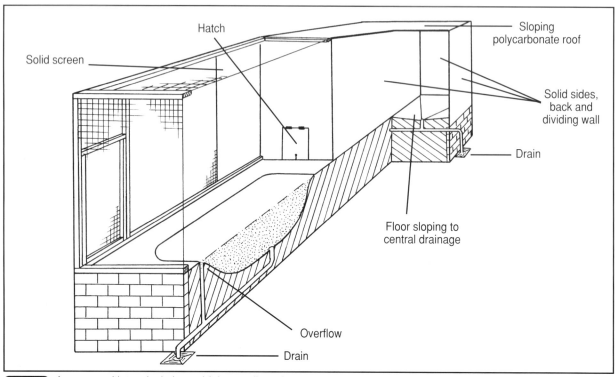

3.2 Aquapen with two isolation cubicles to allow cleaning without stressing the residents. The design also allows two groups or species to access the water independently.

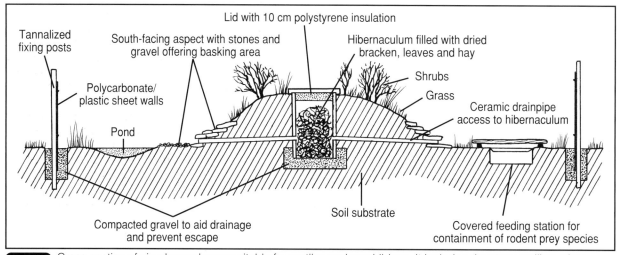

3.3 Cross-section of circular enclosure suitable for reptiles and amphibians. It includes dry-stone walling, plant cover, log piles and open areas to maximize foraging potential and temperature gradients for recovering casualties. (Designed after Kelleway, 1980, unpublished.)

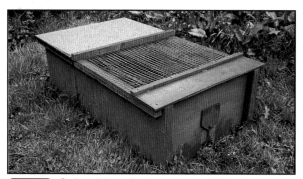

3.4 Collapsible soft-release pen suitable for a hedgehog, with the release hatch (front) opened. Designed by Gower Bird Hospital. (Courtesy of C. Gryniewicz.)

- Contain suitable substrate or perches to enable the casualty to improve movement and coordination, flying, walking, climbing or digging (e.g. swinging perches for birds are a form of physiotherapy) (Parry-Jones, 1988)
- Be constructed of suitable material to minimize physical damage to the housed casualty and to exclude pest species and facilitate easy cleaning and disinfecting
- Be escape-proof, with double doors for access into aviaries and sunken fences or solid substrate for digging mammals
- Include a refugium or retreat area so that the casualty can escape observation (to reduce stress)

- for reptiles and mammals, use boxes or pipes, or include a purpose-built hibernaculum
- for birds, place the highest perch (usually used for roosting) under cover in the refugium area
- Have observation facilities to aid unintrusive assessment of condition and progress prior to release, such as closed-circuit television (CCTV) (Llewellyn, 1987) or, where finance is limited, strategically placed peepholes (but the patient will usually be aware of the observer's presence)
- In skylight-and-seclusion aviaries (usually used in busy locations and comprising four solid sides and a mesh roof), have a suitable observation window with an adjacent perch for the casualty to see the surrounding area in order to reduce stress and fear response (Llewellyn, 1987)
- For aquatic species, give access to a suitable body of water to allow natural behaviour such as bathing and swimming to take place (essential for improving fitness and aiding waterproofing, particularly in avian species).

Overstocking of any aviary or housing pen can cause undue stress and adversely affect the survival potential of the casualty concerned, even with juvenile passerines, fox cubs and hedgehogs (Gower Bird Hospital, personal communication).

Assessment of condition

One of the main problems with all animals that have undergone treatment and confinement is the loss of condition and general fitness, with medium-term and long-term detainees suffering from disuse muscle atrophy. Although the overall bodyweight can be brought back to acceptable parameters (average weight for size, sex and age of species), the muscle-to-fat ratio might be incorrect (Fox, 1980, 1995). This would most certainly have an adverse effect on the survival potential of the individual in the wild, as stamina and manoeuvrability would be impeded.

Rehabilitators must have an understanding of what constitutes natural behaviour, in particular the movement, posture and feeding behaviour of the casualty being prepared for release. This can be a problem if the rehabilitator only sees injured and disabled wildlife in confined conditions. There must be rigorous assessment of the casualty's mental and behavioural fitness throughout its care, together with regular monitoring of the casualty's general health and screening for external and internal parasite infestation and for any other organisms likely to cause problems (for the casualty and for the receiving populations) after release. Assessment can be carried out by:

- Observing the animal's progress during recuperation and the preliminary process of rehabilitation in the aviary, hack flight (an aviary that doubles as a feeding station for birds being prepared for independence) or rehabilitation pen
- Using falconry techniques for raptors (Glazier, 1978; Parry-Jones, 1988; Fox, 1995), such as flying to the lure, flying to the fist or flying with the aid of a long leash (creance) (see Chapter 22).

For both nocturnal and diurnal species the observational process in the aviary or enclosure is greatly aided by using CCTV throughout confinement, as the casualty's behaviour is greatly affected when an observer is present – even at a discrete distance. A much more realistic assessment of general behaviour can be obtained by remote observation or by playing back a videotape recording (Llewellyn, 1987; Gower Bird Hospital, personal communication). CCTV is also an essential tool in assessing conflict or stress due to overcrowding (Gower Bird Hospital, personal communication; and P Llewellyn, personal observation) (Figure 3.5). Social stress can adversely affect birds, mammals and reptiles, limiting their growth and ultimately their survival potential.

Item	Function
Weatherproof bullet camera kit (black-and-white) with 20 m cable, power supply and universal connectors	Black-and-white cameras essential when using infrared light source at night The lower the lux rating, the better sensitivity for night application (typical values 0.1–0.5 lux) Higher resolution gives sharper image during daylight monitoring
Weatherproof camera (colour) with 20 m cable, SCART connectors and power supply	Will not work with infrared illuminators Useful for identifying individuals with colour markings but will need to be high resolution (cost is prohibitive)
Covert camera cable	Various types available designed with 75 ohm core for video and additional cores to carry power and audio
Infrared light source	Can be from LEDs built into camera housing but give limited range of illumination Tungsten halogen illuminators (12 v), available in weatherproof housings, give more useful light
Quad processor	Displays up to four cameras at a time on split screen and allows recording on to VCR Loss of resolution
Multiplexer	Can display up to 16 (or more) cameras on split screen and allows recording on to VCR When playing back tape, individual cameras may be selected for full frame observation without loss of resolution but may have 'silent film' effect as not all frames are recorded
TV monitor	Domestic colour TV with AV SCART facilities
VCR	Domestic VCR with one or more SCART inputs, LP (long play) mode and ability to select AV input in timer mode

3.5 Closed-circuit television (CCTV) systems.

Condition	Reason
Any animal with congenital defect	Likely to impede survival or be passed on through genes
Any animal sexually imprinted on humans or excessively socialized showing redirected sexual behaviour	Danger to humans and conspecifics Would fruitlessly occupy good breeding territories
Amputees (wings or limbs, partial or full)	Impeded mobility, affecting survival
Restricted mobility caused by callus or arthritic formation, secondary to fracture or dislocation	Unable to hunt successfully, avoid predation or migrate
Feather (and fur) condition not natural comparable to wild counterpart (taking seasonal moult into account)	Unable to hunt successfully, avoid predation, migrate or properly regulate body temperature
Any medical condition likely to need ongoing treatment	No veterinary support in wild
Loss of sight, hearing and smell	Unable to locate food and avoid predation
Female mammals with pelvic fractures	Possible problems with dystocia

3.6 Criteria for casualties unsuitable for release.

The findings of previous and current research on birds and mammals provide the criteria that must be met in order to avoid suffering and inappropriate releases and have resulted in the establishment of conditions under which casualties should not be released (Figure 3.6). Criteria regarding suitability for release have been outlined by Cooper *et al.* (1980), Llewellyn and Brain (1983), Llewellyn (1987) and Fox (1995); they are largely based on raptors but many of the factors are fundamental and are relevant to other classes of animal.

Problems associated with human contact

Animals that have extensive contact with people can develop behavioural problems. The degree of susceptibility can depend on species, age and type of contact. Juvenile mammals and fledglings are most vulnerable, particularly if their natural development is disrupted.

The period between birth and maturation is the time when sexual imprinting and early learning take place and survival skills develop (Slukin, 1972). Filial imprinting takes place in many species of birds and mammals, particularly those with extensive parental care (Ridley, 1986). The word 'imprinting' is used as an all-embracing term for these complex but related processes. In simplistic terms, the likely developmental stages and associated learning phases under natural conditions are as follows:

1. Imprinting sexually on parent image (species identity); this will be reinforced with first breeding.
2. Imprinting on siblings; this will be followed by a fear response to other species.
3. Identifying the nursery area, nest type and site.
4. Recognizing habitats.
5. Recognizing food species (developing a search image).

With precocial birds (e.g. ducks and waders), the process is rapid as the young are able to feed themselves as soon as they hatch. In altricial birds (e.g.

raptors and corvids), the process is protracted and young have to be fed by the parents after hatching and throughout early development.

In some species, the processes are innate. For example, cuckoos reared by unrelated species have an innate self-identity mechanism; and swifts, abandoned in the nest by their parents prior to fledging, are able to hunt for food instinctively.

When young casualties are taken into care, permanent psychological damage can be caused by imprinting on an inappropriate species – for example, sexual imprinting on the human image. Once the imprinting mechanism has taken place, it is irreversible. Subadult and adult animals can also develop problems if excessive socialization takes place with inappropriate species (including humans) and this can manifest itself in redirected sexual behaviour.

It is illegal knowingly to imprint a wild animal on humans, as this would prevent the possibility of its release into the wild. Every precaution must be taken to alleviate this possibility:

* Contact with humans should be minimized at all times, even during initial clinical care
* Fledglings or juvenile mammals should be returned to the wild parents whenever possible
* In other cases, juvenile mammals or fledglings should be fostered with suitable receptive captive animals of the same species. They should not be cross-fostered, even within the same genus, as the reared animal will imprint on the foster parent image (Bird, 1981).

Casualties needing prolonged clinical care or rearing by hand should be reared with members of their own species and should be fed by means of a puppet glove that represents the parent. If only one individual of a species is in care, every attempt should be made to place it with another of compatible age, possibly in a different wildlife unit. Once the individual is feeding itself, it must be placed in suitable rehabilitation accommodation and rearing by hand should be stopped.

It is necessary to assess a casualty's mental state, particularly if its case history is suspect or unknown or if the casualty shows signs of abnormal behaviour, such as being too tame for a wild animal or openly aggressive towards people. Abnormal behaviour can be the result of a pathological condition, conditioning or disruption of natural development. Observations should be made of reactions to the handler, to other humans and to its own species. The assessment of maladaptive (abnormal) behaviour in raptors, e.g. those sexually imprinted on humans, is outlined in Jones (1981).

In hand-reared individuals, varying degrees of abnormal behaviour can be observed. This depends on the age and species of the animal, in combination with the husbandry techniques involved. Abnormal behaviours might include:

- Prolonged infantile behaviour, such as food begging, constant vocalization (screaming) and mantling over food parcels
- Pair-bonding, such as preening and grooming the handler
- Males attempting to mate with humans or submissive posturing by females
- Aggressive behaviour by both sexes, such as attacking the handler and any other people in view (possibly a territorial reaction or sexual frustration)
- Attempting to feed the handler or another person.

Habitat assessment

Whatever the species or its clinical history, or the time scale involved, suitable areas for release must be found. The requirements for such areas include the following:

- A suitable habitat with foraging areas for the species concerned, with available prey species or other food resources
- No resident members of the individual's own species or genus, or of conflicting species (although this is not always the case with small mammals and passerines)
- A secure site for rehabilitation procedures to be carried out without public interference and influence
- Not situated where herbicides, insecticides or rodenticides are or have been extensively used
- For captive-reared juveniles and long-term patients, at least 2 km from the nearest motorway or major trunk road.

The rehabilitator must ensure that the release site is used only with the agreement of the landowner and after all relative permissions have been obtained (see Chapter 5).

For many species the habitat can differ between seasons, especially summer and winter, and also during migration. Reference to relevant literature on natural history should be made prior to release. Information on the status of potential release sites can be obtained from local naturalists, rehabilitators, conservation organizations such as the local county wildlife trust, or county bird, mammal, invertebrate and plant recorders. Information may also be obtained from biological scientists at the local university and from environmental consultants. Liaison with regional authorities is advised and the Countryside Council for Wales (CCW), English Nature and Scottish National Heritage must be consulted, where Phase I habitat survey information should be made accessible (this is a standardized method of habitat classification outlining basic habitat types, e.g. 'woodland, broad-leaved, semi-natural', 'calcareous grassland, semi-improved', 'wet dwarf scrub heath'). Rehabilitators wishing to conduct their own surveys of potential release sites should refer to the relevant literature suggested in the References section, covering habitat and species identification and survey techniques.

Release methods

The method chosen for release will depend on:

- The species concerned
- Type of injury or ailment
- Age of the animal being released (juvenile, subadult, adult)
- Length of time the animal has been in captivity
- Location chosen for release
- Time available
- Experience of the rehabilitator.

Time of release
The time of year for release will depend on the age and clinical problems of the casualty.

Short-term casualties
Short-term casualties suffering from minor trauma (e.g. mild concussion or caught in fishing line) that need only superficial first aid should be released as soon as they recover and as near as possible to where they were found, in order to maximize their survival potential because they are familiar with the geography and the habitat's feeding areas. The time of day for release must be taken into account with nocturnal or diurnal species. No formal rehabilitation process is required, provided that careful assessment of the casualty's condition has been carried out. This might not be possible if the details of capture were not recorded on arrival; therefore a suitable release site must be found.

Medium-term to long-term casualties
These casualties should ideally be released during the summer months, when juveniles are naturally dispersing. Territoriality is less intense and food abundance is at its highest. This gives the individuals the best chance of survival and to gain fitness, enabling them to survive the winter or migrate.

Migrating species
Migrating species should be released well before migration starts, as the period between fledging and migration is used to gain fitness and build up reserves for the long trip ahead.

Categories of rehabilitation

Rehabilitation can be divided into two categories: hard release and soft release.

Soft release

The casualty is gradually introduced into the wild and food is made available until the individual gains independence. This should be done during periods of natural dispersal, which usually means summer and early autumn.

Soft-release pens or hack flights can be collapsible so that they can be moved to suitable release areas each season (see Figures 3.1 and 3.4). The enclosure should be placed at the chosen site, together with the casualty, well before release is intended. With birds, this should be as soon as the casualty is capable of feeding itself.

Released animals have to be reprogrammed to recognize naturally occurring prey items (as opposed to the white mice, day-old chicks or commercial food pellets on which they were fed during captivity). For the correct search image to develop, therefore, natural food items must be used (Figure 3.7) and these can be obtained in a number of ways, depending on species (Figure 3.8). Food should be dropped into the

flight or enclosure without the handler being seen (e.g. via a food chute). If this is not possible, a seclusion screen should be in place to allow the casualty access to visual seclusion.

The timing of any release programme must allow the casualty to become familiar with the geography of the surrounding area and establish visual references for relocation of the food resource during reintroduction. For some species (passerines), the flight should have suitable internal plant cover; bushes in pots will suffice. To encourage food searching, an area of natural substrate should be provided – for example, turf and leaf litter or forest bark – where live invertebrate food (mealworms, crickets, gentles) should be scattered. Mixing adult and subadult passerines with fledglings of the same species improves the learning process and greatly improves food searching (Gower Bird Hospital, personal communication; personal observation) but mixing of species should be avoided at all costs because of the possibility of conflict and stress.

The release hatch on the enclosure or flight can be situated on the roof or the top half of the front for birds and at floor level for mammals. The timing of the opening has to be carefully assessed. With birds, it

Group	Food items	Means of collection
Carnivorous mammals	Bird and mammal prey	Road kills; cat kills; Longworth trap for small rodents
	Fish, shrimps, etc.	Dip nets; push nets; fish traps
Terrestrial insectivorous mammals (e.g. shrews)	Ground-dwelling invertebrates	Sweep net; pitfall trap; digging
Bats	Free-flying insects	Sweep net; moth trap
Carnivorous birds	Bird and mammal prey	Road kills; cat kills; Longworth trap for small rodents
	Fish, shrimps, etc.	Dip nets; push nets; fish traps
Hirundines (swallows, martins)	Free-flying insects	Sweep net; moth trap
Passerines (e.g. songbirds)	Ground-dwelling and arboreal insects and snails	Sweep net; beating tray; pitfall trap; log turning
Wading birds	Ground-dwelling and aquatic invertebrates	Sweep net; pitfall trap; digging; push net; dip net
Reptiles and amphibians	Free-flying and ground-dwelling invertebrates	Sweep net; pitfall trap; log turning; moth trap; beating tray

3.7 Natural food items to be fed to insectivorous and carnivorous species prior to release.

Technique	Method	Target species
Digging and log turning		Worms, fly larvae, slugs and beetles
Sweep net	Butterfly net or similar drawn rapidly across low vegetation	Flies, beetles, spiders etc.
Beating tray	White sheet or upturned umbrella, held underneath bushes that are beaten with a stick to dislodge arboreal insects	Spiders, caterpillars, beetles etc.
Pitfall trap	Jar or tin buried in soil, top level with ground, with raised cover – any invertebrate falling in cannot escape	Beetles, amphipods and any other mobile ground-dwelling species
Moth trap	Box trap with light above entrance funnel (usually ultraviolet)	Night-flying species of moths or other species attracted to light
Push net	Flat-bottomed net pushed along sea bed or open ponds	Fish, shrimps and other mobile aquatic species
Dip net	Circular, rectangular or pear-shaped net in ponds or rock pools	Fish, shrimps or other mobile species

3.8 Techniques for collection of natural food items.

usually takes place when they are fully feathered, flying and feeding independently. Mammals should be feeding themselves and of adequate size and weight for their age. The hatch should be removed quietly at night so as not to panic the occupant, which could be driven out of the area before becoming fit enough to catch its own wild food and disperse properly.

Chapter 22 gives information on falconry-based soft-release techniques. Relevant information may also be found in Glasier (1978), Llewellyn (1987), Parry-Jones (1988) and Fox (1995).

Hard release

This is usually practised with short-term casualties, where the animal is simply released into the wild after treatment.

With medium-term to long-term patients, even where their general condition is considered good, the chances of survival following hard release are much reduced because of lack of familiarity with the release site and its feeding areas and roosts, conflict with resident species and lack of physical fitness.

Release should be carried out as close as practicable to the capture site, because the animal is familiar with the habitat and foraging areas and because the territory that it previously occupied might still be vacant, thus reducing conflict.

The release of excessive numbers of rehabilitated animals in any one site must be avoided for the following reasons:

- It could cause predator/prey oscillations by over-exploiting food resources locally
- There could be serious conflict with members of the same species or genus and with conflicting species
- The survival of the released casualty could be seriously affected by stripping the available food resource
- There could be a deleterious effect on other biological communities.

Post-release monitoring

The purpose of rehabilitation is to ensure that the released casualty becomes an integral part of the wild breeding population. The aims of monitoring casualties during and after their release are as follows:

- To establish success rates and percentage survival of species that are handled
- To improve assessment techniques and rehabilitation procedures
- To prevent unnecessary suffering by releasing unsuitable or inappropriate casualties
- To monitor the behavioural interactions and conflict between the rehabilitated casualty and the wild resident population.

Monitoring methods

The following methods are those that are most frequently used, sometimes in combination, in order to gather both short-term and early post-release information and long-term data regarding survival.

Radio-tracking

Radio-tracking uses tail-mounted, harness-held or glued-on transmitters (Kenward, 1978; Johnson *et al.*, 1991; Reeve, 1994). The casualty is located in the field by a hand-held receiver and directional antenna (Figure 3.9). Where finance permits, satellite-tracking is a possibility. The length of surveillance depends on battery life or moult patterns and is usually just a few months.

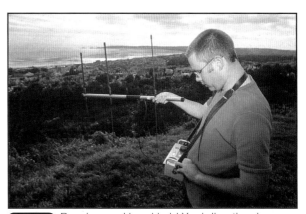

3.9 Receiver and hand-held Yagi directional antenna. (Gower Bird Hospital. Photograph courtesy of Chinch Gryniewicz.)

Microchips

Microchips are ideal for long-term monitoring; for example, for hedgehogs (Gower Bird Hospital, personal communication).

Leg rings

British Trust for Ornithology leg rings, combined with coloured plastic rings, give easy visual identification and are ideal for long-term monitoring.

Dyes

Colour dye, systematically placed on different parts of the casualty, allows easy visual identification. It is used only for short-term monitoring, as dyes fade or disappear during moult. Substances include, for example, rhodamine B or possibly a bleaching agent, depending on the colour of the feathers or fur.

Marking mammals

Additional methods for marking mammals include ear tagging, fur clipping and tattooing (Gurnell and Flowerdew, 1994).

Licences and standards

Although technically it may not be necessary to obtain a licence to monitor wildlife casualties if the method being used is not invasive, it is essential that all relevant authorities are contacted prior to embarking on any release monitoring programme in order to undergo appropriate training for the technique chosen and to establish whether other researchers are conducting similar research on the same species using the same techniques. This could result in incorrect data being collected, which might invalidate both research programmes.

References and further reading

Arnold EN and Burton JA (1978) *A Field Guide to the Reptiles and Amphibians of Britain and Europe*. Collins, London

Bibby CJ, Burgess ND and Hill DH (1993) *Bird Census Techniques*. Academic Press, London

Bird D (1981) Influence of cross-fostering on mate selection in captive kestrels. In: *Recent Advances in the Study of Raptor Diseases. Proceedings of the International Symposium on Diseases of Birds of Prey, 1st–3rd July 1980, London*, eds JE Cooper and AG Greenwood, pp. 41–59. Chiron Publications, Keighley

Chinnery M (1993) *Insects of Britain and Western Europe*. Collins Pocket Guide. Harper Collins, London

Cooper JE, Gibson L and Jones CE (1980) The assessment of health in casualty birds of prey intended for release. *Veterinary Record* **10**, 340–341

Corbet GB and Harris S (eds) (1996) *The Handbook of British Mammals, 3rd edn*. Blackwell Science, Oxford

Corbett K (1989) *The Conservation of European Reptiles and Amphibians*. Christopher Helm, London

Fitter R and Fitter A (1984) *Collins Guide to the Grasses, Sedges, Rushes and Ferns of Britain and Northern Europe*. Collins, London

Fitzner RE and Rogers LE (1977) Techniques useful for determining raptor prey species abundance. *Raptor Research* **11**(3), 67–71

Fox NC (1980) Condition in hawks. *The Falconer* **7**(4), 263–270

Fox N (1995) *Understanding the Bird of Prey*. Hancock House Publishers, Surrey, BC

Gibbons DW, Reid JB and Chapman RA (1993) *The New Atlas of Breeding Birds in Britain and Ireland: 1988–1991*. Poyser, London

Glasier P (1978) *Falconry and Hawking*. Batsford, London

Gurnell J and Flowerdew JR (1994) *Live Trapping Small Mammals. A Practical Guide, 3rd edn*. Occasional Publication No. 3. The Mammal Society, London

Hess EH (1973) *Imprinting*. Van Nostrand, Reinhold, New York

Johnson GD, Pebworth JL and Krueger HO (1991) Retention of transmitters attached to passerines using a glue-on technique. *Journal of Field Ornithology* **62**(4), 486–491

Jones CG (1981) Abnormal and maladaptive behaviour in captive raptors. In: *Recent Advances in the Study of Raptor Diseases. Proceedings of the International Symposium on Diseases of Birds of Prey, 1st–3rd July 1980, London*, eds JE Cooper and AG Greenwood, pp. 53–59. Chiron Publications, Keighley

Kenward RE (1978) Radio transmitters tail-mounted on hawks. *Ornis Scandinavia* **9**, 220–223

Krebs JR and Davies NB (1987) *An Introduction to Behavioural Ecology, 2nd edn*. Blackwell Scientific, Oxford

Lack D (1954) *The Natural Regulation of Animal Numbers*. Oxford University Press, Oxford

Lack P (1986) *The Atlas of Wintering Birds in Britain and Ireland*. Poyser, London

Langton T (1989) *Snakes and Lizards*. Whittet Books, London

Lawrence MJ and Brown RW (1974) *Mammals of Britain, their Tracks, Trails and Signs*. Blandford Press, London

Llewellyn P (1987) Assessing conditions prior to raptor release. In: *Breeding and Management in Birds of Prey. Proceedings of the Conference held at University of Bristol, January 24–26, 1987*, pp. 103–119

Llewellyn PJ and Brain PF (1983) Guidelines for the rehabilitation of injured raptors. In: *International Zoo Yearbook, Vol. 23*, ed. PJ Olney, pp. 121–125. Zoological Society of London

Mitchell A (1974) *A Field Guide to the Trees of Britain and Northern Europe*. Collins, London

Nature Conservancy Council (1990) *Handbook for Phase I Habitat Survey*. Nature Conservancy Council, Peterborough

Parry-Jones J (1988) *Falconry. Care, Captive Breeding and Conservation*. David and Charles, Newton Abbot

Reeve N (1994) *Hedgehogs*. Poyser, London

Ridley M (1986) *Animal Behaviour: a Concise Introduction*. Blackwell Scientific, Oxford

Rose F (1981) *The Wild Flower Key, British Isles – NW Europe*. Frederick Warne, London

Sherrod SK, Heinrich WR, Burnham WA, Barclay JH and Cade TJ (1981) *Hacking: a Method for Releasing Peregrine Falcons and Other Birds of Prey*. Peregrine Fund Inc., Cornell University, Ithaca, NY

Slukin W (1972) *Imprinting and Early Learning*. Methuen, London

Snow DW and Perrins CM (eds) (1998) *The Birds of the Western Palearctic. Vol. 1. Non-Passerines, Concise Edn*. Oxford University Press, Oxford

Snow DW and Perrins CM (eds) (1998) *The Birds of the Western Palearctic. Vol. 2. Passerines, Concise Edn*. Oxford University Press, Oxford

Stace C (1997) *New Flora of the British Isles, 2nd edn*. Cambridge University Press, Cambridge

Sutherland WJ (ed.) (1996) *Ecological Census Techniques*. Cambridge University Press, Cambridge

4

Principles of clinical pathology and post-mortem examinations

John E. Cooper

Introduction

Clinical ability and acumen play an important part in the treatment of wildlife casualties, because these patients are wild animals and therefore detailed examination is often hampered by difficulties of handling or the undesirability of using anaesthesia. Nevertheless, there are limitations on the amount of information that can be gained from clinical work alone. Aids to clinical examination, such as endoscopy and radiography, contribute substantially but there often remains a need to obtain more information in order to make a diagnosis.

Laboratory investigations, therefore, have an important role to play in the treatment of wildlife casualties. They may be restricted to investigation of samples from live animals, or involve post-mortem examination (sometimes alternatively referred to in this chapter as 'necropsy') of casualties that fail to survive or have to be euthanased.

Value of laboratory investigations

Laboratory tests on live animals can contribute substantially to the making of a diagnosis and thus effecting appropriate treatment. In addition, such tests provide valuable information about the health status of a casualty, which can be of great value prior to release.

Post-mortem examination of a wild animal may help to determine the cause of death, throw light on the cause of an injury, or reveal factors that could have contributed to its being presented as a casualty. Necropsy can also permit the detection of changes in organs and thus provide background information (see below) about the health of that individual, or of the group or population from which it came or its species (Cooper, 1989).

Many biologists bemoan the fact that so little scientific information about British wildlife emanates from rehabilitation centres or from the numerous veterinary practices where casualty animals are seen. It is perhaps not surprising that so many authors of chapters in this manual state that 'little is known about the diseases of the species'. If this situation is to be rectified, those who carry out wildlife rehabilitation (or, like veterinary surgeons, work with those who do) should endeavour to ensure that data are collected. In the context of this chapter, that means that a gross post-mortem examination at least is carried out on any animal that dies or has to be euthanased.

Laboratory investigations on live animals

General considerations

Although the examination of blood and other samples from casualty animals can provide a great deal of valuable information, this must be balanced against the stress that can be caused to a casualty through restraint and sampling. A careful cost/benefit analysis of each case is essential. Whenever possible, a non-invasive or minimally invasive technique should be used (Cooper, 1998).

Even when a relatively invasive method is deemed necessary, every effort should be made to reduce the adverse effect of this on the animal and to obtain optimal results. Ways of so doing include the following:

- Ensure that all the equipment that is likely to be needed for sampling is available *before* the animal is restrained
- Take the *correct* samples and then transport and process them proficiently
- In some cases, there should be prior discussion with the pathologist or laboratory staff regarding appropriate sample collection and presentation.

Sampling methods

A sample can be defined as a 'representative portion of the original' and this definition is a reminder that a sample should reflect, as closely as possible, the material or site from which it came. A sample has to be collected; it has to be transported to the laboratory; and there it has to be examined. Errors can occur at each of these stages and as a result the findings and conclusion may not accurately reflect the situation in the live or dead animal. Therefore, standard techniques should be used and equipment of high quality employed.

Samples from wildlife casualties can present additional problems. First of all, they are often taken under difficult circumstances – a wild animal, for example, that is struggling, stressed and not amenable to restraint. Some samples from wild animals are taken in the field, where conditions are unpredictable, facilities are limited and improvisation is often necessary.

The main sampling methods that are likely to be employed in wildlife casualties are:

- The collection of freshly voided faeces or of material from the rectum or cloaca
- Taking blood samples with a needle and syringe (or perhaps a vacutainer) from a vein or occasionally from an artery or a sinus
- Taking smaller samples of blood from a vessel by pricking with a needle, or (with care, depending upon the species) by pricking the skin elsewhere or short-cutting a claw
- Collecting urine, either voided naturally or removed with a catheter or syringe (cystocentesis)
- Skin scrapings
- Collecting hair, feather, scales or shed skin (sloughs)
- Biopsies, either external (e.g. skin) or internal (via endoscopy or laparotomy)
- Swabs for bacteriology, mycology, cytology, etc.
- Post-mortem sampling to include many of the above, plus (for example) specimens of tissues (for histology, electronmicroscopy, etc.) or stomach contents for toxicology.

Sample-taking is carried out in a similar way to that followed for domestic animals. Where differences exist, these are referred to and described in more detail in the relevant species' chapter in this book. It is often good practice to perfect a technique first on either a domesticated species or a *dead* wild animal before attempting to do so on a frightened and stressed living casualty.

Precautions must always be taken to minimize pain and distress to the animal and to reduce the risk of injury or spread of infection to human beings. There are also legal implications (see Chapter 5).

Processing of samples

Methods of processing samples from wildlife casualties are not significantly different from those used for comparable samples from domestic animals or 'exotic' species (Meredith and Redrobe, 2002). In most cases there are no reference values for 'healthy' wildlife, although some examples are given in different chapters of this manual. The collation of such data is most important but care has to be taken that the procedures used are in accordance with the law (see Chapter 5). Pre-anaesthetic (operative) screening of animals can provide useful samples but they may not be 'normal' (see Chapter 2). Therefore extrapolation from other species, preferably those that are closely related to the one under investigation, is often necessary.

Opinions differ as to which parameters are most important in assessing health and there are strong constraints (financial and practical) on carrying out too many tests. Nevertheless, the 'screening' of wildlife prior to release or translocation is now a well established procedure and there is strong pressure (sometimes legal, often moral) on those involved in rehabilitation to follow established guidelines (Woodford, 2001) in the interests of both the animal to be released and the population that it is to join. Important health monitoring tests are listed in Figure 4.1.

Microbiological examination

Microbiological examination is of great importance when dealing with wild animal casualties, especially when it is linked with antimicrobial sensitivity tests. Ideally, both aerobic and anaerobic culture should be performed; where this is not feasible, perhaps on the grounds of cost, aerobic culture can be coupled with cytological examination of the lesion – which may reveal anaerobes as well as providing information on cellular changes.

Sample	Investigations	Comments
Faeces	Presence/absence and numbers of endoparasites Aerobic (sometimes anaerobic) bacteriological examination Other microbiological investigations Contents: food remnants Contents: abnormalities, such as free blood or excessive undigested food (e.g. starch or fat)	Wet preparations in saline should be examined first, followed by flotation methods and smears
Blood	PCV and smears (for differential blood cell counts and parasitological examination) Other haematological investigations (where practicable) Biochemical estimations, including enzymes Serology	Choice of anticoagulant is important Bird blood is best taken in lithium heparin rather than in EDTA
Urine	Standard 'dip-stick' investigations Specific gravity (using refractometer) Centrifugation and cytological examination of deposit	Similar procedures are used for mammal samples as for dogs and cats. Bird and reptile samples usually comprise urates; interpretation of results is not always easy
Skin	Parasitological, microbiological, cytological and histopathological examination	Standard procedures are used for mammals Plucked feathers of birds, scales of reptiles and skin mucus of amphibians or fish often give good results
Swabs from various sites (including orifices)	Microbiological and cytological examinations	Standard procedures

4.1 Important health monitoring tests.

Biopsies

Biopsies can provide very useful information (Cooper, 1994) and should always be considered, despite the costs involved. A rapid diagnosis using biopsy is preferable to drawn-out investigations on (say) skin scrapings, as it can reduce the amount of stress and pain caused to a casualty wild animal and accelerate its return to the wild.

Other samples

A whole range of other specimens may be examined to advantage. Water analysis can assist in the diagnosis of disease or detection of environmental problems when dealing with fish, amphibians and aquatic birds and mammals. Examination of feathers (Cooper, 1987, 2002) can throw much light on causes of skin disease and help in the assessment of plumage prior to release. Feathers and hair can be analysed for heavy metals. Sloughed skins of reptiles can also provide useful information, as can preparations from the gills of fish or of larval amphibians.

Interpretation

Interpretation of results is not easy (Fudge, 2000). They should be analysed in discussion with colleagues, in the light of the particular animal and the plans for its future. For example, the presence of small numbers of intestinal nematodes may not be a reason for declining to release a patient if those same parasites are present in the free-living population. A slightly lowered PCV may be acceptable if the animal is to be given a 'soft release' (see Chapter 3) and thus will have an opportunity to improve in condition and to be fed prior to total independence.

It is important that the veterinary surgeon who is working with wildlife builds up a close relationship with a laboratory that has an interest in non-domesticated species. Consultation *before* taking and submitting samples is always wise.

Recording and dissemination

A vital part of laboratory testing is to ensure that results are recorded, stored and – whenever possible – published or otherwise disseminated to interested people. There is an acute shortage of reliable information on laboratory values of wild animals that might aid rehabilitators and others. The overall value of having such data and making information available cannot be overemphasized.

Post-mortem examinations

Post-mortem examination (necropsy) is a very useful and important way of building up information on wild animal casualties and obtaining data on the causes of morbidity, mortality and failure to thrive. However, such data are really only of long-term value if the examinations are carried out in a systematic way and the findings are properly recorded.

Ideally a post-mortem examination should be carried out on every wild animal casualty that dies or has to be euthanased. In addition, full supporting laboratory tests should be performed and material such as serum and tissues retained for reference.

In practice, because of the constraints of time and money, this approach is rarely feasible. It is usually necessary to restrict the examination to a gross necropsy with retention of some specimens in case they are needed at a later date.

Procedures

The post-mortem examination itself should follow standard procedures (Woodford, 2000), which often do not differ greatly from those used for domestic animals. Where unusual species are involved (e.g. marine mammals) it may be wise to seek specialist help. Some special features relevant to different groups of wildlife are listed in Figure 4.2.

Group	Special features
Mammals	Many variations in external and internal anatomy (e.g. presence or absence of tail, structure of gastrointestinal tract, wing of bats, specialized features of cetaceans) All mammals have mammary glands and some hair
Birds	Variations in external and internal anatomy (e.g. presence or absence of preen gland, crop, caeca) Certain specialized features (e.g. modified syrinx in male ducks) All birds have feathers All are oviparous
Reptiles	Much anatomical variation but lizards and snakes essentially very similar All reptiles have scaled skin Most are oviparous; some are viviparous All have a cloaca Melanin often abundant in internal organs
Amphibians	Marked distinction in most species between immature (larval/tadpole) stage with gills and other modifications to aquatic lifestyle, and mature (adult) with lungs and terrestrial lifestyle All amphibians have unscaled mucous skin Melanin often abundant
Fish	Often variation in external and internal anatomy associated with life cycle and habitat (including whether freshwater or marine) Most fish have (mesodermal) scales, fins, gills and swim bladder

4.2 Special features relevant to post-mortem examination of wildlife.

An important consideration is health and safety (see Chapters 2 and 5), as dead wild animals may be a source of infectious organisms. As a general rule, it should be assumed that a carcass is dangerous and, following a risk assessment, appropriate precautions should be taken. Useful data on zoonoses are to be found in Cooper (1990) and Palmer et al. (1998).

Whatever the type of animal to be examined, the following general rules apply:

- As full a history as possible should be obtained
- Whenever feasible, the environment from which the animal came and (where applicable) the management to which it was subjected should be evaluated
- If several animals are available for post-mortem examination, particularly if there may be a common aetiology for the deaths, a series of examinations comparing and contrasting the findings is necessary; a pattern may emerge. Such necropsies may need to be coupled with microbiological and chemical investigation of, say, water samples
- The circumstances of death, including the method of euthanasia, must be ascertained and taken into account
- Biological data must be obtained.

Even basic information such as measurements and bodyweight (mass) are of value to biologists and others who are studying the species. At the same time, those data can be of assistance in assessing the health of the animal. Recording only the bodyweight (mass) of the animal is not satisfactory: it gives no indication of condition, size or configuration. For example, a stoat weighing 200 g may be a very fat, small (young) animal or a very thin, large (adult) animal. Standard measurements are used by field biologists and these should be followed when examining wild animal casualties. The key ones are listed in Figure 4.3.

Group	Standard measurements
Mammals	Crown–rump length Specific measurements (e.g. wings and digits of bats)
Birds	Carpal length Tarsal length
Reptiles	Snout–vent (SV) (rostrum–cloaca) Vent–tail-tip (VT)
Amphibians: tailed (Urodela)	Snout–vent (SV) (rostrum–cloaca) Vent–tail-tip (VT)
Amphibians: tailless (Anura)	Snout to end of body
Fish	Total body length

4.3 Standard measurements.

Some wild animal casualties are small (e.g. rodents, nestling birds, lizards, frogs) and it can be difficult to carry out a meaningful necropsy. A useful approach here is to perform a 'mini necropsy' using a magnifying lens or loupe and microsurgical instruments and, if histological examination is to be carried out, to embed either the whole specimen or a block of tissues.

The most important samples that may be taken from post-mortem cases are listed in Figure 4.4.

Samples	Comments
Tissues in 10% formalin for histology	Have the advantage that they can be stored indefinitely and examined at a later stage General rule should be to take lung, liver and kidney (LLK), plus any organs that show abnormalities or are considered important because they may provide information about the animal's health or biology (e.g. bursa of Fabricius, of young birds, can yield data on immune status) Small carcasses can be fixed whole, following opening for processing
Cytological preparations	Easy to take, cheap to process (readily done in any veterinary practice or in the field) and produce rapid results Usually consist of touch preparations or impression smears, which can give valuable information about tissues within a few minutes Should be retained after examination in case they are needed later
Swabs, organ/tissue samples and other specimens for microbiological and other investigations	Usually comprise swabs (in transport medium if to be sent elsewhere), portions of tissue or exudates/transudates If culture proves impossible for financial or other reasons, impression smear stained with Gram or other stains often provides some useful information
Tissues for toxicological examination	Need to be taken routinely from casualties Usually frozen and can be analysed at later date As with formalin-fixed samples, should be taken and stored even if there is no immediate prospect of their being analysed

4.4 Samples from post-mortem cases.

Toxicology

Some casualties will have been exposed to toxic chemicals. These may be the cause of death or could have contributed to the animal's ill health, either directly or by increasing its susceptibility to infectious disease. It is important that samples from casualties are taken routinely for toxicological analysis; this not only assists with diagnosis but also contributes to scientific study and understanding of environmental pollution.

Other investigations

Collection of samples for other investigations may or may not be feasible. If there is a suspicion of a particular disease (e.g. a viral infection), appropriate specimens should be collected so that the relevant examination can be carried out. The selection and collection of samples require careful coordination between the rehabilitator, the veterinary surgeon and the laboratory.

Retention of material

An important rule (often overlooked) is to retain as much material as possible after the post-mortem examination. A whole carcass can be kept for up to 7 days at 4°C. After this time it is wiser to freeze it, even though this can result in tissue damage that will hamper histological investigations. If it is not realistic to retain the whole carcass frozen, selected tissues or all the viscera can be kept.

The reason for not discarding material immediately after necropsy is that the veterinary surgeon can return to the material later if necessary – for example, if further tests are needed or if samples are required for forensic (legal) purposes (see Chapter 5).

Disposal of carcasses

Quite apart from the point made above, those who examine dead wild animals should not discard carcasses and tissues too hastily. Such material is part of the database for that individual and for that species which, as emphasized many times earlier in this chapter and elsewhere in this manual, can contribute substantially to our knowledge of wildlife health and disease.

Sometimes, especially if the animal examined is of a rare species, a museum may ask to have the whole body, the skin or representative portions of the carcass. It is important to ascertain whether this is likely to be the case *before* the necropsy is carried out, because it may influence how the examination is performed – for example, how much damage is done to the skull. In some such cases it may be wise to have the examination carried out by a specialist pathologist.

It is always good practice to offer material from wildlife cases to museums (another part of building bridges with non-veterinary scientists). The establishment of reference collections, which can be used by the veterinary profession and others in retrospective and research studies, should also be considered, especially in the case of rare species (Cooper *et al.*, 1998). Retention of skins, bones and soft tissues from animals that are protected by law is unlikely to require a licence as such (see Chapter 5) but the veterinary surgeon who carries out the post-mortem examination and stores material is well advised to keep a written record of origin and to provide notice of this to anyone who receives any of it for whatever purpose.

References and further reading

Cooper JE (1987) Pathology. In: *Raptor Management Techniques Manual*, eds BA Giron Pendleton *et al.* National Wildlife Federation, Washington DC

Cooper JE (ed.) (1989) *Disease and Threatened Birds*. Technical Publication No. 10. International Council for Bird Preservation (now BirdLife International), Cambridge

Cooper JE (1990) Birds and zoonoses. *Ibis* **132**, 181–191

Cooper JE (1994) Biopsy techniques. *Seminars in Avian and Exotic Pet Medicine* **3**, 161–165

Cooper JE (1998) Minimally invasive health monitoring of wildlife. *Animal Welfare* **7**, 35–44

Cooper JE (2002) *Birds of Prey: Health & Disease.* Blackwell Science, Oxford

Cooper JE, Dutton CJ and Allchurch AF (1998) Reference collections in zoo management and conservation. *Dodo* **34**, 159–166

Fudge AM (ed.) (2000) *Laboratory Medicine. Avian and Exotic Pets.* WB Saunders, Philadelphia

Meredith A and Redrobe S (eds) (2002) *Manual of Exotic Pets, 4th edn.* BSAVA, Gloucester

Palmer SR, Soulsby, Lord, and Simpson DIH (eds) (1998) *Zoonoses.* Oxford University Press, Oxford

Woodford MH (ed.) (2000) *Post-mortem Procedures for Wildlife Veterinarians and Field Biologists.* Office International des Epizooties, Paris

Woodford MH (ed.) (2001) *Quarantine and Health Screening Protocols for Wildlife Prior to Translocation and Release into the Wild.* OIE, VSG/IUCN, Care for the Wild International and EAZWV, Paris

5

The law affecting British wildlife casualties

Margaret E. Cooper

Introduction

The legislation discussed in this chapter is that applying to England and, generally, Wales. In most cases this also applies in Scotland but this is not always so. For example, the deer laws are separate (and there may be increased divergence on account of devolution). It is therefore important to check separately the legislation in force in England, Wales and Scotland. Northern Ireland has its own, comparable, legal provisions.

It is important to keep up to date with developments in the law, since it can always be subject to change. Those using this chapter must also apprise themselves independently of the current state of the law. A number of organizations committed to wildlife conservation and animal welfare are very well informed and closely follow current developments regarding the law that relates to the species in which they are specifically interested. It is, therefore, worth referring to their staff or to their literature mentioned in this chapter. There are also books on animal law, such as Brooman and Legg (1997), Cooper (1987, 1991), Lorton (2000) and Palmer (2001). Publications on rehabilitation or related subjects may also cover the law relevant to wildlife rehabilitation, such as Corbet and Harris (1991), Porter (1989), Stocker (2000) and Thomas (1990). For information on wildlife law enforcement, see Department of the Environment, Transport and the Regions (DETR) (1996).

The process of rehabilitation falls into three stages: rescue, rehabilitation and release. Each of these stages is affected by legislation.

Rescue

Access to the casualty

The land
A casualty in the wild may be readily accessible in a place to which the public has access; however, if it is found on private land the landowner's permission to enter should be obtained, to avoid trespassing.

The animal (ownership)

- Normally, a free-living wild animal does not belong to anyone until it is 'reduced into possession', i.e. someone takes it into captivity. It

then belongs to the person who takes it. There are a few exceptions to this principle; for example, young animals that are not yet independent belong to the landowner, and the law on game species that is based on the issue of poaching (see below).
- Some methods of taking an animal (such as by nets or traps) are illegal, restricted or require a licence (see below).
- Once a free-living wild animal has been taken into captivity, it has the same status in law as other property. To steal it is an offence under the **Theft Act 1968**. Also, it becomes the property of the owner, whose consent must be obtained if the animal is to undergo treatment or to be disposed of in any way. The finder can keep the animal, provided that the acquisition was in conformity with the **Wildlife and Countryside Act 1981** (WCA) (see below). The scope of any treatment given must comply with the **Veterinary Surgeons Act 1966** (VSA) (see below). If the animal is taken to a rehabilitator for attention, the latter should obtain ownership from the finder so that the relevant provisions regarding treatment by non-veterinarians can apply and the rehabilitator, as the owner, can authorize a veterinary surgeon to treat the animal.
- A rehabilitator should obtain a history and written agreement to transfer the ownership, signed by the finder. This should form part of the rehabilitator's records that can be used to demonstrate conformity with the WCA and other legislation.

Taking the casualty: wildlife law

- ❖ **Wildlife and Countryside Act 1981** (as amended) **(WCA)**
- ❖ **Conservation (Natural Habitats, etc) Regulations 1994**

Taking casualties

- The WCA provides that it is permissible to take from the wild a sick or injured wild bird or other protected creature for the purpose of tending it until it is fit to be released.
- If it is injured or diseased beyond hope of recovery, it may be killed.

- Legislation regarding deer, badgers and seals (see below) has similar provisions.
- The right to keep a disabled protected species lasts only until it is no longer disabled. It should not be kept in a manner that would inhibit its capacity to return to the wild (e.g. by deliberate imprinting).

Species protection

The rehabilitator often needs to know the general principles of species protection. The WCA provides various degrees of protection for British wild birds and some other animals, as summarized below:

- All wild birds are protected. The WCA defines a 'wild bird' as 'any bird of any kind that is ordinarily resident in or is a visitor to Great Britain in a wild state'. It does not include poultry or gamebirds (i.e. 'any pheasant, partridge, grouse (or moor game), black (or heath) game or ptarmigan', but see below). The basic protection of the WCA (see below) does not apply to a bird that has been bred in captivity, i.e. both its parents were lawfully in captivity when the egg was laid.
- Mammals, reptiles, amphibians and invertebrates that are listed in Schedule 5 of the WCA are also protected. The Schedule is amended from time to time and a current list can be obtained from English Nature or the naturenet website (see Specialist Organizations). All reptiles and amphibians have some level of protection (e.g. the grass snake and common toad can be taken and kept but not sold) and the rare ones, such as natterjack toad and great crested newt, are fully protected. Badgers are covered by a specific Act (see below and Chapter 11).

The basic protection that is given to wild birds and Schedule 5 animals (together referred to as 'protected species') can be summarized as follows:

- The WCA provides that it is an offence to:
  - take, injure, kill or sell a protected species
  - disturb a protected species in its nest or place of shelter
  - possess a protected species
  - release a barn owl to the wild without the authorization of a licence from DEFRA
  - deliberately release or allow to escape into the wild any non-indigenous species or a species (already established in the wild) that is listed on Schedule 9 (such as the grey squirrel, edible frog, African clawed toad, Canada and Egyptian geese, chukar partridge and muntjac deer).
- There are various additional forms of protection. These include:
  - Close seasons for listed gamebirds (see Chapter 23)
  - Special penalties in respect of offences involving rare birds listed on Schedule 1 of the WCA
  - Provisions for ringing and registration with the Department for Environment, Food and Rural Affairs (DEFRA) in respect of the diurnal birds of prey and other rare species listed on Schedule 4

- Special provisions to protect bats and bat roosts from damage (Bat Conservation Trust (BCT), undated).
- Methods such as nets and traps for taking animals are either prohibited (in respect of birds and Schedule 6 animals) or restricted, as are certain hunting methods (such as specified firearms and pursuit with vehicles). The use of self-locking snares is also illegal; see Parkes and Thornley (1997) and Stocker (2000) for the distinction between these and free-running snares.
- Many activities that are *prima facie* prohibited can be authorized by the grant of a licence from the appropriate authority (DEFRA or English Nature, Scottish Natural Heritage or the Countryside Council for Wales) if they are for specified purposes, such as scientific studies, aviculture or crop protection.
- DEFRA issues Information Sheets providing guidance on the foregoing, lists of the birds affected and information on other aspects of the WCA (DETR, various dates). An RSPB booklet and leaflet cover the complexities of the wild bird legislation (RSPB, 2000 and undated).
- For Scottish wildlife law, see Scottish Natural Heritage (1998).
- A number of British species (such as bats, marine turtles, wildcat and natterjack toad) are also protected under the Conservation (Natural Habitats) Regulations 1994 as 'European protected species'.

Legislation protecting other species

❖ Protection of Badgers Act 1992

- Badgers are given protection comparable to that for Schedule 5 species (see above) together with additional provisions relating to cruelty and protection of their setts (see Chapter 11). A leaflet by the National Federation of Badger Groups (NFBG, 2000) provides a good summary of the badger legislation.
- The provisions of the WCA restricting methods of killing or taking wild animals (see above) also applies to badgers, as this species is included in Schedule 6 of the WCA.

❖ Deer Act 1991 and Deer (Scotland) Act 1996 (and related legislation)
❖ Conservation of Seals Act 1970
❖ Salmon and Freshwater Fisheries Act 1975
❖ Game Acts (various) (rabbits, hares, gamebirds) (also see WCA above)

Close season protection

- Animals such as gamebirds, deer (red, fallow, roe, sika; see also Chapter 16), seals (see also Chapter 17) and fish are protected during a specified close season and by the fact that certain methods of capture and killing are prohibited by the relevant legislation. There are provisions for deer and seals comparable to those in the WCA whereby casualties may be killed or taken for rehabilitation (Palmer, 2001; Parkes and Thornley, 1997).

- Gamebirds (pheasant, partridge, grouse, black game and ptarmigan) are not protected by the WCA apart from the provisions relating to methods of killing and taking (see above).

- In common law, free-living wild game (including gamebirds that have been reared and released) that is not enclosed or captive does not belong to anyone until a person takes or kills it. Taking and killing are regulated by the game laws and normally have to be authorized by a game licence, the legal right to take the game (usually given by the landowner or tenant) and legal access to the land where the game is situated. Killing or taking in other circumstances may constitute poaching when trespass or taking at night is involved (Lorton, 2000; Parkes and Thornley, 1997).

- The specific implications of the legislation relating to fish are discussed by Millichamp (1987), Parkes and Thornley (1997) and Scott (1992).

Unprotected species

- Many species of wild mammal are not protected by the WCA, such as hedgehog, fox, weasel and numerous invertebrates.

- The **Protection of Animals Act 1911** (which makes cruelty an offence; see below) does not apply to free-living wildlife. However, the **Wild Mammals (Protection) Act 1996** (see below) provides some protection against specified forms of inhumane treatment in respect of wild mammals.

- Various laws, including the **Pests Act 1954** and the **Spring Traps Approval Order 1995** (and similar legislation in Scotland), permit the use of specified kinds of traps to deal with pest animals. There are requirements about the placing and checking of traps and snares (Lorton, 2000; Palmer, 2001; Parkes and Thornley, 1997). The British Association for Shooting and Conservation codes of practice on trapping pest birds and mammals and the snaring of foxes are useful guides (BASC, 2001 and various).

- Various laws make the poisoning of animals an offence but permit certain kinds of poison to be used in specified ways to control pest animals (Parkes and Thornley, 1997; Lorton, 2000; Palmer, 2001).

- Certain sporting and other activities are not affected by these Acts, but:
  - There are limits on the type and use of firearms and other methods of taking and killing (see above)
  - Since February 2002, hunting with dogs is no longer allowed in Scotland (**Protection of Wild Mammals (Scotland) Act 2002**) and the issue is under debate in England and Wales.

Emergency care of the casualty

Veterinary law

Any person can give emergency first aid to an animal for the purpose of saving life and relieving suffering. The owner of an animal may give minor medical treatment (see below). Otherwise, veterinary surgery must be carried out by a registered veterinary surgeon or, in some respects, by a registered veterinary nurse.

Ownership

In principle, if it is obvious that an animal has an owner, that person's consent should be obtained before treatment is carried out by someone else. Hence, the rehabilitator who accepts a wild animal should ensure that ownership is transferred at the same time.

Rehabilitation

Right to keep the animal

This also includes the question of ownership, as discussed above under 'Rescue'.

Wildlife law aspects (WCA)

- The WCA provides that a casualty of a species protected by that Act may be kept only for the purpose of tending it and until it is no longer disabled. A casualty that is so severely disabled that there is no reasonable chance of recovery may be killed.

- Schedule 4 birds that have been taken for rehabilitation must be ringed and registered forthwith unless they are held (in accordance with general licences issued for England, Wales and Scotland) as follows:
  - RSPCA inspectors and experienced keepers of registered Schedule 4 disabled wild birds may keep disabled wild-bred Schedule 4 birds for up to 15 days for rehabilitation provided that they notify DEFRA within 4 days of receipt and keep specified records.
  - A veterinary surgeon may keep for up to 6 weeks without registration *any* Schedule 4 bird that is receiving professional veterinary treatment. The veterinary surgeon must keep records of each bird.

- Many activities that are *prima facie* prohibited, such as trapping, shooting or selling, can be authorized by the grant of a licence from the appropriate authority (DEFRA or English Nature) if they are for purposes such as scientific studies, aviculture or crop protection.

- The WCA does not apply to captive-bred animals (see above). In addition, a few species listed on Schedule 3 Part I, such as blackbird, barn owl, magpie and chaffinch, can be sold or exhibited if they have been captive-bred and ringed.

- Anyone in possession of an animal protected by the WCA must be able to prove that he/she is legally in possession of it – for example, that the animal is captive-bred, or has been imported, sold or taken in accordance with the Act (e.g. as a casualty) or under a licence. In this situation the burden of proof falls on the person (including any wildlife rehabilitator) who has such an animal in his/her possession. It is therefore essential to keep good records of any animals that are acquired and their provenance. This point also applies to parts and derivatives of a protected species, such as bones or feathers retained for reference, research or educational or sentimental purposes.

- If endangered species are kept for display or other purposes that include some commercial use, the CITES legislation (see below) may apply.
- Keeping (and releasing) certain pest species, such as mink, grey squirrel or rabbits (other than European rabbit), requires a licence under the **Destructive Imported Animals Act 1932**. There has been some debate in the veterinary press about the appropriateness of the continued application of these restrictions to the grey squirrel, since injured specimens are nevertheless rehabilitated.

CITES (Convention on International Trade in Endangered Species of Wild Fauna and Flora) conservation controls

- ❖ **Council Regulation EC No. 338/97**
- ❖ **Commission Regulation EC No. 1808/2001, 2087/2001** and associated legislation
- ❖ **Control of Trade in Endangered Species (Enforcement) Regulations 1997**

- The many species that are listed in Annexes A to D of Regulation 338/97 are subject to import and export controls.
- The CITES Regulation also requires the sale or commercial display of CITES Annex A species, including all European birds of prey and owls, to be authorized by an Article 10 (or Article 30) certificate. This provision also applies to parts and derivatives of Annex A species.
- Annex A species in commercial use must be permanently marked with a microchip or, for birds, with a closed ring. It is also good practice to mark all animals in permanent captivity so that they can be identified for the purpose of record keeping or if an animal is stolen.
- These and other provisions are described in Guidance Notes that are issued by DEFRA (various dates) or available through its website or enquiry point.

The regulation of keeping animals in captivity
Wildlife rescue facilities that admit the public to see their animals or occasionally admit dangerous species need to be licensed by the local authority (Cooper, 2002).

- ❖ **Dangerous Wild Animals Act 1976 (DWAA) (as amended by The Dangerous Wild Animals Act 1976 (Modification) Order 1984)**

The only UK species subject to the Act are the wildcat and the adder (viper).

- ❖ **Zoo Licensing Act 1981**
- ❖ **Zoo Licensing Act 1981 (Amendment) (England and Wales) Regulations 2002**
- ❖ **Council Directive EC No 22/1999**

- The Zoo Licensing Act applies to all zoos and other collections (including rehabilitation centres) of non-domesticated animals that are open (whether or not for a fee) to the public on 7 or more (formerly more than 7) days in any 12-month period.
- The Regulations extend zoos' responsibilities in conservation and public education, and for the behavioural needs of their animals, good animal husbandry, veterinary care and record keeping.

Medical

- ❖ **Veterinary Surgeons Act 1966 (VSA) (and supplementary legislation)**
- ❖ **The Veterinary Surgeons Act 1966 (Schedule 3 Amendment) Order 2002**

- Only veterinary surgeons and veterinary practitioners registered with the Royal College of Veterinary Surgeons have the right to practise veterinary surgery (i.e. diagnosis, treatment and surgery, and advice based thereon) in respect of mammals (including marine mammals), birds and reptiles.
- There are several exceptions to this general rule whereby other people may carry out certain levels of treatment.
- Anyone may treat fish, invertebrates and possibly amphibians, since they are not mentioned in the VSA. Any treatment given is nevertheless subject to the provisions of the Protection of Animals Acts (see 'Welfare').
- Anyone may give first aid in an emergency to save life or alleviate suffering. This term has not been legally defined but some people use it as a guide to the provision of care until a veterinary surgeon can attend to the animal.
- Owners of animals (and their employees and families) may give minor medical treatment.
- Veterinary students may provide diagnosis, treatment and surgery under specified levels of supervision.
- Veterinary nurses (VNs) may carry out medical treatment and minor surgery not involving entry into a body cavity. As from 10 June 2002 this provision is no longer restricted to pets and companion animals; both VNs and student VNs may give such

levels of care to any category of animal, provided that they act under the levels of supervision laid down in the amendment to Schedule 3.

Medicines legislation

❖ **Medicines Act 1968**
❖ **The Medicines (Restrictions on the Administration of Veterinary Medicinal Products) Regulations 1994 and 1997**
❖ **The Medicines (Veterinary Drugs) (Prescription Only) Order 2001** and associated legislation

Points of particular importance in respect of wildlife are as follows:

• Procedures for complying with the medicines legislation, such as the requirements that apply to prescribing, supplying and labelling prescription-only medicines (POMs), also apply to non-domesticated species, including reptiles, amphibians and fish.
• Veterinary surgeons may prescribe POMs only for 'animals under their care'. This phrase is amplified in the *Guide to Professional Conduct* (RCVS, 2000).
• Relatively few drugs are licensed for wildlife species, though where they have a domesticated counterpart (e.g. rabbits or pigeons) the species may appear on the data sheet. The 'cascade' should therefore be followed when prescribing outside the terms of the marketing authorization for a drug and the client's informed consent should be obtained (BVA, 2000; Veterinary Medicines Directorate (VMD), 1998).

Notifiable diseases

A person who finds an animal that is suspected of having a disease (such as tuberculosis, Newcastle Disease, foot-and-mouth disease, anthrax or rabies) that is notifiable under an Order made under the **Animal Health Act 1974** must isolate the animal and report the fact to the police. It should also be reported to DEFRA.

Drug-dart weapons

• Possession of any firearms or weapons, such as a dart-gun, crossbow or blowpipe, that can be used to discharge tranquillizing drugs must be authorized by a Firearms Certificate issued by the police.
• The use of a crossbow (with or without drugs) for wild animals requires a licence under the WCA.

Civil law responsibility for damage caused by non-domesticated animals

• The keeper (whether or not the owner) of non-domesticated animals is responsible for any damage that they cause (**Animals Act 1971**) (North, 1972; Parkes and Thornley, 1997).

• Liability for death, personal injury or damage to property can give rise to claims for compensation in civil law under the heads of negligence and other forms of civil liability such as nuisance (e.g. excessive noise or smell), trespass, or the escape of animals.

Health and safety

❖ **Health and Safety at Work etc. Act 1974**

• Rehabilitation and rescue centres should make risk assessments of their work and develop appropriate codes of practice. This may also include the provision of specialized guidance, training and working procedures. Attention should be given to matters such as the need to adapt existing items (e.g. nebulizers and facemasks), or to provide specialized equipment, facilities and protective clothing and to address the hazards involved in catching, handling and treatment of animals and the risk of zoonoses associated with wildlife (see also Chapter 6).
• Risk assessments and guidelines should be reviewed and revised regularly in order to provide for new or changed risks (such as that arising from the recent (2002) human fatality associated with lyssavirus infection acquired from a bat).
• There is a specific code of practice for zoos (Health and Safety Commission, 1985) that is currently under revision.

Welfare

❖ **Protection of Animals Act 1911**
❖ **Protection of Animals (Scotland) Act 1912 (PAAs)** (supplemented by various subsequent Acts)

• It is an offence to treat any domestic or captive species of animal cruelly or to cause it any unnecessary suffering. There is no definition in the Acts of the latter term but it could involve failure to provide necessary food, water, care and veterinary attention or any other act that amounts, in the opinion of a court, to unnecessary suffering.
• Killing an animal is not an offence under these Acts provided that it is carried out humanely.
• These provisions on cruelty do not apply to free-living wildlife but once any vertebrate is brought into captivity it becomes subject to the Acts. It has been held, however, that mere temporary restraint does not amount to captivity.

❖ **Wild Mammals (Protection) Act 1996**

• This Act provides that it is an offence to carry out specified acts that cause suffering, such as kicking, beating, burning or drowning a wild mammal, with the intent to inflict unnecessary suffering.

❖ **Protection of Wild Mammals (Scotland) Act 2002**

With certain exceptions, it is an offence deliberately to hunt a wild mammal with a dog.

❖ Protection of Animals (Anaesthetics) Acts 1954 and 1964

- Anaesthesia must be used in procedures that interfere with sensitive tissues or bones of an animal, with the exception of minor procedures such as injections.
- Although these Acts expressly do not apply to birds, fish or reptiles, anaesthesia should be used to fulfil the general requirements of the main PAAs which require an operation to be carried out with due care and humanity and without unnecessary suffering.

❖ Wildlife and Countryside Act 1981

- Section 8 of the WCA provides that it is an offence to keep *any* bird in a cage that is not large enough to allow the bird to stretch its wings freely.
- A smaller cage is permitted for use only while transporting or exhibiting a bird or while it is undergoing examination or treatment by a veterinary surgeon. Consequently, a rehabilitator who wishes to use a hospital cage that does not comply with Section 8 should put the casualty under the care of a veterinary surgeon.

❖ The Welfare of Animals (Transport) Order 1997

- Animals of any sort, including invertebrates, must not be transported in any way that causes or is likely to cause them injury or unnecessary suffering.
- In the case of commercial or non-private transportation of animals, additional requirements apply to the provision of suitable containers and vehicles, food, water, ventilation, temperature and attendance (see Chapter 2).

Additional provisions on transport and movement

- Public road and rail carriers may also have their own requirements or may decline to transport animals.
- Airlines apply the International Air Transport Association (IATA) Live Animals Regulations relating to methods of transport, especially standards for containers (IATA, annually).
- The CITES Secretariat has issued guidance for the transportation (by any means) of CITES species (CITES, 1980).
- The 1997 Order (above) makes it a legal requirement to comply with the IATA Regulations and CITES Guidelines where they are applicable.
- The Post Office forbids the transport by post of living animals, apart from a few species of invertebrate, such as bees. There are also precise requirements for the mailing of animal pathogens either within Britain or internationally, including special packaging and labelling.

❖ Animal Health Act 1981

Subsidiary legislation made under this Act provides powers for the control and prevention of spread of diseases such as foot-and-mouth disease and rabies and the monitoring of chlamydophilosis. When restrictions are in force, the movement of wildlife casualties may be controlled.

Codes of practice

In addition to the legal requirements to prevent cruelty, there are many voluntary guides and codes that promote good practice, animal welfare and the responsible care and management of animals in captivity and in the wild. These include: British Association for Shooting and Conservation (BASC, 2001, various); British Field Sports Society (BFSS, undated); British Wildlife Rehabilitation Council (BWRC, 1989); Cooper and Sinclair (1990); and the World Conservation Union (IUCN) guidelines on translocation, reintroduction and health monitoring (available on the WCU/IUCN website) (see also Woodford, 2001).

Release

Wildlife law

The rehabilitator is obliged by the WCA and by the deer, badgers and seals legislation to return a casualty to the wild as soon as it is no longer disabled.

Welfare law

❖ Abandonment of Animals Act 1960 (AAA)

- Animals should not deliberately and without good cause be abandoned in circumstances likely to cause them unnecessary suffering.
- Although this Act is aimed primarily at pets, it should be taken into consideration when assessing the suitability of wild creatures for release.

It is necessary to strike a balance between the obligations under the WCA and the AAA and any pre-release assessment should be made with both in mind. Sometimes a veterinary surgeon is asked to provide an assessment, particularly in the case of Schedule 4 birds, to support a decision to release or retain in captivity.

Although there is no legislation relating specifically to long-term permanent casualties, these animals should always be kept in compliance with the laws relating to welfare and wildlife discussed above.

Non-indigenous and pest species

- Non-indigenous species listed in Schedule 6 may not be deliberately released to the wild.
- The **Destructive Imported Animals Act 1932** provides that it is illegal to keep or release mink, grey squirrels, rabbits (other than the European rabbit) and coypu without a licence.

- Consideration should also be given to the effect of releasing species that are or will become a pest in the area. Owners and occupiers of land can be required under various laws to control a variety of wildlife (e.g. rabbits, deer, wild birds) if they become pests (Lorton, 2000; Palmer, 2001; Parkes and Thornley, 1997).

Conclusion

The aim of this chapter has been to provide veterinary surgeons with a summary of the British law that is particularly relevant to wildlife rehabilitation. It is hoped that it will enable them to extend their existing knowledge of the legislation that is generally applicable to the veterinary care of wildlife, thereby adding a further dimension to the service that they provide for their clients and those who are active in wildlife rehabilitation. At the same time, they are helping to protect themselves and rehabilitators from finding themselves in breach of the law.

Specialist organizations

CITES:
www.ukcites.gov.uk
www.cites.org

DEFRA:
wildlife.licensing@defra.gsi.gov.uk

English Nature:
www.english-nature.org.uk

Naturenet:
www.naturenet.net

WCU/IUCN:
www.iucn.org/themes/ssc/pubs/policy/index

References and further reading

BASC (2001) *Trapping Pest Birds: a Code of Practice.* British Association for Shooting and Conservation, Wrexham

BASC (various dates) *Lamping (Night Shooting): a Code of Practice. Ferreting: a Code of Practice. Fox Snaring: a Code of Practice.* (Also other subjects.) British Association for Shooting and Conservation, Wrexham

BCT (undated) *Bats and the Law. What to Do When the Law is Broken.* Bat Conservation Trust, London

BFSS (undated) *Code of Welfare and Husbandry of Birds of Prey and Owls.* British Field Sports Society, London

Brooman S and Legge D (1997) *Law Relating to Animals.* Cavendish Publishing, London

BVA (2000) *Code of Practice on Medicines.* British Veterinary Association, London

BWRC (1989) *Ethics and Legal Aspects of Treatment and Rehabilitation of Wild Animal Casualties.* British Wildlife Rehabilitation Council, London

CITES (Convention on International Trade in Endangered Species of Wild Fauna and Flora) (1980) *Guidelines for Transport and Preparation for Shipment of Live Wild Animals and Plants.* International Union for Conservation of Nature, Gland, Switzerland

Cooper ME (1987) *An Introduction to Animal Law.* Academic Press, London

Cooper ME (1991) British mammals and the law. In: *The Handbook of British Mammals*, eds GB Corbet and S Harris. Blackwell Scientific, Oxford

Cooper ME (2002) British legislation. In: *BSAVA Manual of Exotic Pets, 4th edn*, eds A Meredith and S Redrobe, pp. 288–292. BSAVA, Gloucester

Cooper ME and Sinclair DA (1990) Wildlife rehabilitation and the law: an introduction. In: *Proceedings of the Third Symposium of the British Wildlife Rehabilitation Council, Stoneleigh, 1990*, ed. T Thomas, pp. 63–65. British Wildlife Rehabilitation Council, London

Corbet GB and Harris S (1991) *The Handbook of British Mammals.* Blackwell Scientific, Oxford

DEFRA (various dates) Information Sheets (on aspects of the Wildlife and Countryside Act). Department for the Environment, Food and Rural Affairs, Bristol

DEFRA (various dates) Guidance Notes (on aspects of the CITES Regulations). Department for the Environment, Food and Rural Affairs, Bristol

DETR (1996) *Wildlife Crime: A Guide to Wildlife Law Enforcement in the UK.* The Stationery Office, London

Health and Safety Commission (1985) *Zoos – Safety, Health and Welfare Standards for Employers and Persons at Work. Approved Code of Practice and Guidance Notes.* HMSO, London

IATA (annual) *Live Animals Regulations.* International Air Transport Association, Montreal and Geneva

Lorton R (2000) *A–Z Countryside Law.* The Stationery Office, London

Macdonald AA and Charlton N (2000) *A Bibliography of References to Husbandry and Veterinary Guidelines for Animals in Zoological Collections.* Federation of Zoological Gardens of Great Britain and Ireland, London

Meredith A and Redrobe S (eds) (2002) *BSAVA Manual of Exotic Pets, 4th edn.* BSAVA Publications, Gloucester

Millichamp RI (1987) *Anglers' Law In England and Wales.* A&C Black, London

NFBG (2000) *Badgers and the Law.* National Federation of Badger Groups, London

North PM (1972) *The Modern Law of Animals.* Butterworth, London

Palmer, J (2001) *Animal Law: a Concise Guide to the Law Relating to Animals.* Shaw and Sons, Crayford

Parkes C and Thornley J (1997) *Fair Game, 3rd edn.* Pelham, London

Porter V (1989) *Animal Rescue.* Ashford, Southampton

RCVS (2000) *Guide to Professional Conduct 2000.* Royal College of Veterinary Surgeons, London

RSPB (2000) *Wild Birds and the Law.* Royal Society for the Protection of Birds, Sandy, Bedfordshire (booklet)

RSPB (undated) *Information about Birds and the Law.* Royal Society for the Protection of Birds, Sandy, Bedfordshire (leaflet)

RSPCA (1999) *Principal UK Animal Welfare Legislation; a Summary.* Royal Society for the Prevention of Cruelty to Animals, Horsham (booklet)

Scott PW (1992) Legal aspects. In: *BSAVA Manual of Ornamental Fish*, ed. RL Butcher. BSAVA, Cheltenham

Scottish Natural Heritage (1998) *Scotland's Wildlife: The Law and You.* Scottish Natural Heritage, Perth

Stocker L (2000) *Practical Wildlife Care.* Blackwell Science, Oxford

Thomas T (ed.) (1990) *Proceedings of the Third Symposium of the British Wildlife Rehabilitation Council, Stoneleigh, 1990.* British Wildlife Rehabilitation Council, London

VMD (1998) *Guidance to the Veterinary Profession. Animal Medicines European Licensing Information and Advice Guidance Notes 8 (AMELIA 8).* Veterinary Medicines Directorate, Addlestone, Surrey

Woodford MH (2001) *Quarantine and Health Screening Protocols for Wildlife Prior to Translocation and Release into the Wild.* Office International des Epizooties, Paris; Veterinary Specialist Group/ Species Survival Commission of the World Conservation Union (IUCN), Gland; Care for the Wild International, Rusper; and European Association of Zoo and Wildlife Veterinarians, Liebefeld-Berne

The Journal of Wildlife Rehabilitation. International Wildlife Rehabilitation Council, Suisun

6

Hedgehogs

Steve Bexton and Ian Robinson

Introduction

Only one wild species of hedgehog is native to the British Isles: *Erinaceus europaeus*, the (western) European hedgehog. It is unmistakable as the only indigenous British mammal to have spines.

Hedgehogs are found widely distributed throughout mainland Britain and Ireland and are absent from only a few Scottish islands. Their ability to thrive in close proximity with humans, their relative abundance and their comparatively easy capture make them one of the most common wildlife patients.

Reasons for their presentation to veterinary practices and wildlife hospitals show a marked seasonality. Springtime sees a propensity towards trauma cases, especially road accidents, as hedgehogs emerge from hibernation and begin to disperse for the breeding season. Males account for most of these casualties, as they range further in search of mates. Gardening activities also contribute to their hazards, especially strimming and mowing, and the warmer weather predisposes wounds to fly strike. True orphans can be seen at this time due to nest disturbance or mortality of the mother hedgehog. Most of the cases encountered in the latter half of the year are autumn juveniles and subadults trying to build up enough body reserves to survive the winter hibernation. Such individuals are often forced to forage during the daytime as well as the night, as food supplies become scarcer. Most of these hedgehogs also carry significant parasite burdens, with parasitic bronchopneumonia being especially prevalent. Hibernation is the major mortality factor in the species as a whole and up to 70% of young hedgehogs can die in their first winter.

Ecology and biology

Hedgehogs are common in many habitats, including parks, gardens, cemeteries, waste ground and farmland, generally preferring woodland edges, shrubland, grassland and hedgerows. They tend not to inhabit wetlands or large pine forests, and are not common on intensively farmed arable land or on moorlands and mountains.

They are solitary for most of the year and have a social structure based on mutual avoidance, except during courtship and breeding or when exploiting a particularly rich food source (Morris, 1969, cited in Reeve, 1994). Each hedgehog occupies a 'home range', which is usually established when youngsters first disperse. Home ranges vary in size depending on the type of habitat and availability of food, but generally cover about 10–30 ha. Males tend to have larger ranges than females, and rural home ranges tend to be larger than urban ones (Reeve, 1982; Morris, 1986). Hedgehogs are not territorial and the home ranges of different individuals often overlap. In the wild, aggression is rare, even between males, and fight wounds are rarely sustained.

Hedgehogs are nocturnal and activity during daylight hours is usually a sign of ill health or reduced ability to find enough food during the night. However, nursing mothers can sometimes be seen naturally foraging in the daytime and should be left undisturbed. Otherwise hedgehogs rest during the day, in nests constructed from vegetation (especially leaf litter) under the cover of hedges or shrubs. Their choice of nesting site can expose them to hazards such as the lighting of bonfires, or compost heaps being forked through.

During the night they forage for food, mainly using their keen sense of smell to find beetles, caterpillars, earthworms, slugs and other invertebrates. They are primarily insectivorous but are opportunistic omnivores and will occasionally eat small vertebrates and carrion. Activity continues throughout the night as they meander around sniffing for prey, sometimes travelling a mile or two in the process.

Biological data are given in Figure 6.1.

Hibernation

In the UK, the hibernation period is typically January to March but occasionally starts earlier in cold winters. The main trigger for hibernation is prolonged ambient temperatures below 8°C but other factors such as photoperiod, food availability and accumulation of sufficient reserves of body fat are probably also involved (Reeve, 1994). A specialized sturdy nest called a hibernaculum is constructed. During hibernation, the hedgehog's body temperature falls to below 10°C but hibernation is rarely continuous; hedgehogs will become active for periods throughout the winter and may change to other hibernacula.

Weight	Average adult 800–1200 g (fluctuates seasonally) Peak weight by 3 years of age Males generally larger than females
Sexing	Male: preputial opening usually mid-belly Female: vulva and anus short distance apart
Teats	5 pairs
Oestrus	Normally polyoestrous
Breeding season	April/May to September/October (Litters can be as late as October)
Gestation	35 ± 4 days (Reeve, 1984)
Litter size	3–5
No. of litters	1 or 2
Birthweight	8–25 g
Sexual maturity	8–10 months
Lifespan	Average 2 years (Morris, 1983) (Maximum 6–8 years in wild, 10 years in captivity) (Reeve, 1994)
Diet	Primarily insectivorous (beetles, caterpillars, slugs and other invertebrates) Also opportunistic omnivore (small vertebrates, carrion)
Respiration	Normal rate 20–25 breaths/min
Temperature	Normal rectal temperature about 35°C

6.1 Biological data for hedgehogs.

Anatomy and physiology

The spines, which cover the dorsum, are in fact modified hairs and number about 5000 on an adult (Morris, 1983). Their internal structure makes them efficient shock-absorbers, cushioning the impact when a hedgehog falls, and their sharp pointed tips deter most predators. The hedgehog's peculiar ability to roll up as a defence mechanism presents the would-be attacker with a tight ball of spines, each spine made to bristle by its own erector muscle. Strong muscles, the orbicularis and panniculus carnosus, control the actual rolling mechanism. The panniculus muscle covers the dorsum and flanks; the orbicularis is a circular 'purse-string' muscle all the way round the body.

The rest of the hedgehog's body, including the head, limbs and ventrum, is covered in normal hair. The hairs and spines are shed continuously and re-grow throughout the year.

The hedgehog has seven cervical vertebrae in a short strong neck. Each foot has five toes.

Dentition

There are 36 teeth in the adult (temporary dentition in parentheses):

$$2 \times \left\{ I\ \frac{3\,(3)}{2\,(1)}\ C\ \frac{1\,(1)}{1\,(1)}\ P\ \frac{3\,(3)}{2\,(2)}\ M\ \frac{3\,(0)}{3\,(0)} \right\} = 36\ (22)$$

The molars are cusped for crushing insects and the first upper premolar is four-sided. The timing of tooth eruption is variable and is therefore an unreliable means of ageing hedgehogs (Reeve, 1994).

Senses

The hedgehog's primary sense is that of smell, used for prey detection. Hearing is also very sensitive but the whiskers are of secondary importance. Eyesight is considered to be rather poor and blind hedgehogs kept in sheltered environments generally survive well.

Hedgehogs possess a vomeronasal organ used for sensory perception. They sometimes flick saliva with the tongue over their bodies in response to certain tastes and smells. This so-called self-anointing behaviour is still not fully understood but is perfectly normal.

Reproduction

Sex determination in adults is relatively straightforward in an unrolled individual (Figure 6.2). The breeding season starts shortly after arousal from hibernation and courtship is often long and noisy.

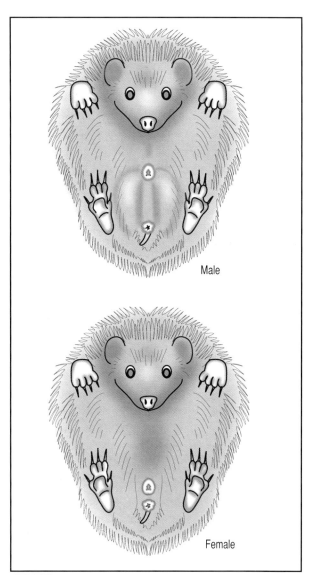

Male

Female

6.2 Male and female hedgehogs.

Age	Spines	Eyes and ears	Teeth	Rolling-up ability	Natural weaning	Forefoot epiphyses (radiographically)
At birth	Hairless with small pink pimples along back; umbilical remnant	Closed	Absent			
24 hours	First spines appear from pimples: white, bristly but flexible					
2 days	First appearance of second-generation spines, stouter and brown					
2 weeks	White and brown spines of equal length	Begin to open (complete by 17 days)	Deciduous begin to erupt	Partial		
3 weeks	White spines completely obscured by brown				Begin to follow mother on short foraging trips	
4 weeks				Full		
5–6 weeks					Weaned, fully independent	
2–3 months						Metacarpal and phalangeal epiphyses visible
3–4 months			Deciduous replaced by adult			
12 months			Full adult dentition (Morris, 1983)			
18 months						Only distal radius and ulna epiphyses incompletely fused; sesamoids radio-dense (Morris, 1971)

6.3 Development of hoglets.

Figure 6.3 gives details of the development of young hogs ('hoglets') from birth to weaning. Lactation in the hedgehog is thought to be specialized in that the transmission of some maternal antibodies continues throughout the suckling period (Morris and Steel, 1964). After weaning, the young hogs disperse to new areas to feed and gain enough weight to hibernate. This is an especially difficult time, with newly weaned youngsters succumbing to accidents, illness and predation (Reeve, 1994). Late litters are under the most pressure as they have less time to build up enough reserves for hibernation.

Ageing

Age determination in living hedgehogs is not straightforward. The timing of tooth eruption is variable and thus unreliable as a means of estimating age (Reeve, 1994). Tooth wear and tartar build-up in adults give only a rough estimate of age, as they are so dependent on other factors (mainly dietary). As bodyweight fluctuates seasonally, it can only be used to give an approximate age. In the young, the timing of spine emergence, opening of eyes and ears, and the ability to roll up are all good guides to age (see Figure 6.3).

Hedgehogs that are less than 18 months old can be aged with the help of forelimb orthopaedic changes seen radiographically (see Figure 6.3).

Capture, handling and transportation

Because their defence tactics are passive, hedgehogs are easy to capture and no special equipment is needed. Although they can bite, this is very unusual. They will sometimes make jerky upward jumps, in a bid to stab with their spines, and the wearing of a pair of sturdy gloves (e.g. gardening gloves) is recommended before picking up a hedgehog, to protect the hands from the spines and reduce the risks of disease transmission. Slight injuries to the hands caused by hedgehog spines can become septic, and hedgehogs can carry a number of zoonoses, including ringworm and salmonellosis.

Some hedgehogs will emit a warning snort, which can be mistaken for respiratory distress. Occasionally, to deter its captor, a hedgehog will emit a shrill warning cry, often misinterpreted as a sign of pain. Young orphan hoglets may emit high-pitched 'peeping' sounds to call for their mother; again, these are sometimes misinterpreted as a sign of pain.

The captured hedgehog is simply placed into a strong box, such as a pet carrier, with a secure lid so it does not escape, and with some leaves, newspaper or a towel for insulation.

Examination and assessment for rehabilitation

On initial presentation, it is important to ascertain the reason for intervention and to derive as much history as possible.

The most common reason for presentation of hedgehogs is because they were active during daylight, which is almost always a sign of ill health or injury. The only exceptions are when a sleeping animal is disturbed, when food is scarce, or when a nursing mother makes a foraging excursion in the day. If a hibernating hedgehog is accidentally disturbed it should be left alone, as long as the nest has not been destroyed and the weather is not too extreme. Otherwise it is probably best to keep the animal warm in captivity and provide food, until the next mild spell.

Clinical examination

It is advisable to wear latex examination gloves when handling hedgehogs, because of the risk of zoonoses.

Before a full examination, each patient should be observed in a quiet environment. Normally it will be curled up and should be checked to see whether any limbs or the head are protruding. Reluctance or inability to roll up when touched is usually a sign of ill health. Generalized weakness and debility cause hedgehogs to stagger and shake. General body condition should be estimated: thin hedgehogs have sunken flanks and a bony pelvis.

Attention should be paid to the respiratory system as disorders are very common, especially lungworm bronchopneumonia. The normal respiratory rate should be 20–25 breaths/min. Hyperpnoea and increased respiratory effort are usually obvious. Dyspnoea and open-mouth breathing always carry a grave prognosis, as they indicate severe damage to the respiratory system. Abnormal respiratory noises and coughing are also common findings, but a mild serous nasal discharge is usually normal.

In many instances, it is necessary to administer first aid and then to make a reassessment, or more detailed examination, once the patient is more stable. A moderate ectoparasite burden is normal in hedgehogs but massive numbers of ticks or fleas can indicate other problems. Hedgehogs should always be thoroughly checked for fly strike, which is extremely common in the warmer months. The most common sites are within orifices (the anus, the genitals, in and around the pinnae, under the eyelids, in the mouth) and associated with any wounds.

The buccal cavity should receive special attention to assess the condition of the teeth and palate. Tartar build-up and periodontal disease are common in both wild and captive hedgehogs. Traumatic fractures are common in this region, especially across the palate.

Uncurling a hedgehog

A more thorough examination involves uncurling the hedgehog (Figure 6.4). There are many techniques for uncurling the conscious hedgehog but generally it is important to avoid noise, clumsy handling, or touching the face or whiskers. An unsuitable method

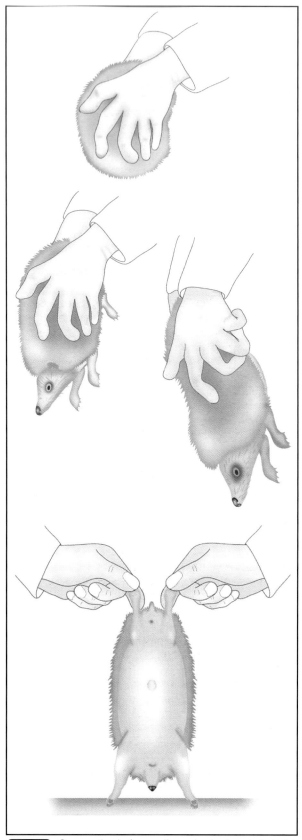

6.4 One method of uncurling a hedgehog is to hold it head-downwards over a flat surface. The hedgehog usually unrolls cautiously and tries to reach the surface. The back legs can then be grasped gently and the animal examined at leisure while it strives to reach the ground. (Redrawn after the *BSAVA Manual of Exotic Pets*, 1991.)

for uncurling hedgehogs is immersion in water: the risks of water inhalation are unacceptable. Some hedgehogs will unroll spontaneously if just left alone for a few minutes. Some workers bounce a rolled-up hedgehog gently between cupped hands. Another simple but effective method is to stroke the spines firmly from the neck to the rump.

Once uncurled, the hedgehog's hindlimbs can be grasped by sliding the fingers underneath its back end. The animal can then be kept uncurled by raising its back legs in the air in a 'wheelbarrow' position (see Figure 6.4). This permits a more detailed examination, especially of the ventrum and limbs. Smaller hedgehogs can be gently scruffed to prevent them from rolling up. A full and thorough clinical examination necessitates the use of general anaesthesia, which should be delayed until the patient is stabilized.

Sampling

Faecal examination for the presence of endoparasites is a useful procedure. Because endoparasites (especially lungworm) are so common, many workers worm all hedgehog patients routinely.

Radiography is often helpful. Blood sampling can be performed to aid diagnosis: the jugular vein is less accessible than in other species, due to the short neck and coverage with fat and fascia, but the lateral or medial saphenous vein can be considered instead. For haematology and biochemistry reference ranges, see Figure 6.5.

Pre-release considerations

Particular considerations to be borne in mind before releasing hedgehogs include the possibility of pregnancy, especially when examining adult female hedgehogs between April and October. Pregnant hedgehogs should be released as soon as possible, since litters born in captivity are often cannibalized.

The likelihood of survival back in the wild is the prime consideration for each hedgehog:

- The ability to roll up fully is essential in predator avoidance; in particular, obesity should be avoided, as this can reduce the ability to curl up tightly
- Olfaction is the primary sense and hedgehogs with severe nasal damage are unlikely to be able to forage for food effectively
- Eyesight is of lesser importance; blind hedgehogs can cope well but thrive better in a sheltered garden
- Hindlimb amputees can survive but should only be released in sheltered gardens, since their foraging ability may be affected.

Euthanasia

Hedgehogs that are deemed to be too ill or too badly injured to recover, or that would be unsuitable candidates for eventual release, should be euthanased using injectable pentobarbital. The intrahepatic route is usually used but intracardiac injection after first inducing general anaesthesia is also possible.

Parameter	Range
Haematology	
PCV	0.30–0.45
RBC (10⁶/mm³)	4.49–6.41
Haemoglobin (mg/dl)	9.9–16.3
MCH (pg)	16.8–18.2
MCV (fl)	49.1–53.2
MCHC (g/dl)	33.3–35.2
WBC (10⁹/l)	5.5–17.1
Neutrophils (%)	1.43–11.7
Lymphocytes (%)	2.3–5.1
Eosinophils (%)	0.47–1.87
Monocytes (%)	0.06–0.58
Basophils (%)	0.07–0.69
Reticulocytes (10⁹/l)	< 0.8
Thrombocytes (10⁹/l)	230–430
Biochemistry	
Total protein (g/l)	44–62
Albumin (g/l)	21–31
Globulin (g/l)	16–32
Glucose (mmol/l)	1.3–5.9
Urea (mmol/l)	2.9–12.7
Creatinine (μmol/l)	0–71
Bilirubin, total (μmol/l)	< 7
Cholesterol (mmol/l)	2.7–3.9
Calcium (mmol/l)	1.45–2.55
Phosphorus (mmol/l)	1.07–2.17
Sodium (mmol/l)	121–141
Potassium (mmol/l)	3.0–6.0
Chloride (mmol/l)	90–106
Alkaline phosphatase (IU/l)	20–80
AST (IU/l)	1.0–79.0
ALT (IU/l)	22–70
Amylase (IU/l)	< 1500
CK (IU/l)	< 360
LDH (IU/l)	< 490

6.5 Normal reference ranges for haematology and blood biochemistry in the European hedgehog (courtesy of MedLab, Tarporley, Cheshire).

First aid procedures

Hypothermia

Many patients will be hypothermic and feel cold to the touch (the normal rectal temperature of the hedgehog is about 35°C). Most hedgehogs will benefit from the immediate provision of additional warmth, using a heat mat or heat lamp.

Fluid therapy

Some degree of dehydration is usually present, detectable by skin tenting along the dorsum as in other species. Fluid therapy is given by the subcutaneous route, as the most readily accessible site. Hedgehogs have a large subcutaneous space along the dorsum (especially around the scruff) and skirt. The skin may need to be raised with fingers or soft forceps before the injection is given between the spines.

Injection sites

- The intravenous route is not easily accessible in hedgehogs. Intravenous fluid therapy is not an option, due to poor vein availability and difficulty in keeping cannulae in place
- The intraosseous route can be used for rapid absorption of fluids into the circulation. The proximal femur is suitable for cannulation
- Intraperitoneal administration also gives rapid absorption
- Intramuscular injections can be given into the orbicularis muscle, which is deep in the skirt, as this is accessible even in a rolled-up hedgehog, or into the gluteal mass of the hindlimb.

Anaesthesia and analgesia

Volatile inhalational anaesthetics offer the most convenient and effective means of anaesthetizing the hedgehog. Administration can be via a facemask or anaesthetic chamber. Maintenance can be with the facemask, or via an endotracheal tube, placement of which is greatly facilitated by using a stylette. Injectable agents can also been used (Figure 6.6).

Analgesia, if required, should be given as early as possible. Opiates or NSAIDs can be used (Figure 6.6).

Specific conditions

Trauma

Entrapment
Hedgehogs quite commonly become trapped in various hazards, including garden netting or barbed wire, down drains, in cattle grids and by plastic ring binders and tin cans. Once trapped they often instinctively roll up, making matters worse. Many can be freed without any long-term harmful effects but it is always advisable to monitor them for a few days, because lesions can develop as a result of ischaemia or pressure necrosis, and any minor wounds sustained can become infected. General anaesthesia is essential to check for injuries.

Skin wounds
Wounds are very common in hedgehogs and can be sustained by encounters with garden machinery, such as strimmers and mowers, or garden forks and spades. Road accidents and dog attacks often result in skin wounds.

Fresh wounds can be cleaned and sutured, after clipping away the surrounding fur or spines with scissors, but many wounds are already old and contaminated when first presented. It is important to check thoroughly for contamination with fly eggs or maggots (see 'Myiasis', below).

Drug	Dosage commonly used	Some indications
Anaesthetics and sedatives		
Isoflurane	Induction at 5% in oxygen and maintenance at 1–3%	Routine general anaesthesia
Halothane	Induction at 5% in oxygen and maintenance at 1–3%	Routine general anaesthesia
Medetomidine	100 µg/kg i.m.	In combination with ketamine for general anaesthesia. Variable effect, sometimes prolonged recovery
Ketamine	10–20 mg/kg i.m.	In combination with medetomidine for general anaesthesia. Variable effect, sometimes prolonged recovery
Atipamezole	300–500 µg/kg	To reverse effects of medetomidine
Diazepam	1–3 mg/kg i.m., i.v.	To control seizures in cases of poisoning (higher dose). Also can be used as sedative at lower dose
Fentanyl/fluanisone	0.5–1.0 ml/kg i.m.	Sedation and analgesia for minor work (e.g. suturing)
Analgesics and anti-inflammatories		
Buprenorphine	20–30 µg/kg i.m. tid	For severe pain associated especially with trauma, or for post-operative analgesia
Carprofen	5–10 mg/kg s.c. sid, orally bid	Analgesia and reduction of inflammation. Generally restricted to 3 days of therapy
Flunixin	2 mg/kg s.c., orally sid	For analgesia and anti-inflammatory effects; especially with toxaemia, severe lung inflammation or fly myiasis

6.6 Anaesthetics and analgesics for hedgehogs. (Note that no drugs are specifically licensed in the UK for use in hedgehogs. All doses quoted are widely accepted and based on experience of the authors and other hedgehog practitioners.)

Wounds are best cleaned with a solution that cleanses and removes necrotic tissue (e.g. Dermisol Multicleanse, Pfizer; Aserbine, Forley), then debrided and allowed to heal by second intention, with a hydrogel product to aid granulation. Infection, abscessation and cellulitis following skin wounds are more likely in hedgehogs than other species.

The most troublesome wounds tend to occur on the spined skin of the dorsum, which is loose-fitting and so predisposed to flaps and tears; it is also less vascular than furred skin (to reduce heat loss) and so heals relatively slowly. Consideration should be given to the effects on rolling up if deep wounds affect the underlying muscles.

Road traffic accidents

Road traffic accidents (RTAs) are very common. Hedgehogs with non-fatal injuries often manage to drag themselves around for some time before being found and thus injuries are often old, dirty and infected, and, in the summer, contaminated by fly eggs or maggots.

- Bone fractures are often compound. Hedgehogs are particularly prone to crushed feet, which they continue to drag around until infected and unable to be salvaged
- Pelvic fractures are especially important in female hedgehogs, which should be euthanased if there is any reduction of the pelvic canal, or kept in permanent captivity to avoid pregnancy and dystocia. Sciatic nerve damage often accompanies pelvic injury
- Spinal fractures and distal denervation can be detected by the panniculus reflex cut-off, whereby the bristling and erection of spines is absent caudal to the lesion. Often the hindlimbs are left protruding when the animal tries to curl. Radiography is needed for confirmation (Figure 6.7)
- Rupture and herniation of the abdominal muscles are not unusual with RTAs. Rupture of the diaphragm and traumatic rectal prolapse can also occur.

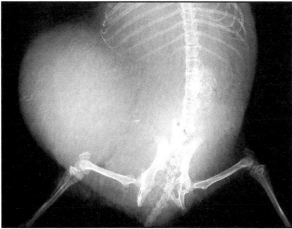

6.7 Dorsoventral radiograph of RTA casualty with fractured spine and ruptured abdominal muscle. (© Andrew Routh)

Limb fractures

The management of fractures in hedgehogs is similar to that in other small mammals, except in two important respects:

- The hedgehog's mechanism of rolling up, with the limbs tucked inside, means that fixators and dressings are more likely to become dislodged or loosened
- Many fractures are compound, contaminated, or infected by the time the hedgehog is found and so internal fixation techniques are often contraindicated.

Coaption splints and casts can be used on distal limb fractures, especially of the radius, ulna, tibia, metarsals and metacarpals. Plaster of Paris, synthetic casting material and rigid splints can all be used but special attention should be paid to keeping the dressings as dry and clean as possible. Intramedullary pinning is suitable for some fractures of the femur and humerus.

Naturally healed fractures are quite commonly found in hedgehogs admitted for other reasons. Sometimes these are malunions with distortion of the affected limb.

Limb amputation and the subsequent maintenance of the hedgehog in a sheltered walled garden is an option if the facilities exist, but three-legged individuals should not be released into the wild. Generally, only hindlimb amputees thrive.

Orbicularis muscle prolapse

A condition peculiar to the hedgehog because of its curling defence mechanism is 'popping off'. This often follows a severe struggle, which has caused the orbicularis (or purse-string muscle) to slip over the pelvis. The muscle then goes into spasm and remains in this position, causing the hedgehog to appear very peculiar, with the hindlimbs and pelvis visible and the spined skin of the back in a twisted shape. General anaesthesia causes the muscle to relax and it is then easily slipped back into place. Post-operative analgesia is indicated.

Subcutaneous emphysema

Another peculiar presentation is 'balloon syndrome', where the hedgehog is inflated with subcutaneous emphysema to up to twice its normal size (Figure 6.8). This usually follows some trauma to the anterior mediastinum, usually because of an RTA, but could also occur as a sequel to a gas-producing infection following a deep wound, or damage to some other part of the respiratory system (e.g. fracture of a rib). Because of the hedgehog's ability to roll up, the subcutaneous space over the dorsum is comparatively large and loosely attached. This means that there is a tremendous capacity for gas build-up, hence the striking appearance of such cases.

Treatment involves deflation with a simple incision or with a needle and a three-way tap. This procedure may need to be repeated several times if the gas reappears. Broad-spectrum antibiotics are advisable. The prognosis depends on the aetiology, size of mediastinal injury, and any concurrent injuries, especially pulmonary haemorrhage and emphysema.

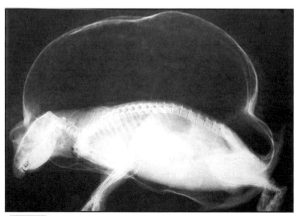

6.8 Lateral radiograph of 'balloon syndrome'. (© Andrew Routh)

Injuries to the snout

As hedgehogs are prone to snout injuries, any suspected trauma case (especially RTAs and dog attacks) should be anaesthetized for a thorough examination. In particular the maxilla and palate are often fractured, usually causing dyspnoea and open-mouth breathing. Damage to the turbinate bones within the nasal cavity can impair olfaction and affect foraging ability in the long term. Such fractures always carry a grave prognosis. Some fractures can be stabilized by stainless-steel wiring but many hedgehogs with traumatic maxillo-palatine fractures require euthanasia.

Burns

The hedgehog habit of nesting in bonfires is well known and they risk being burnt when the fire is lit. Affected hedgehogs have charred spines and skin burns (skin can slough many days later) and often smoke inhalation as well. Topical skin treatment is best achieved using a silver sulfadiazine cream; broad-spectrum parenteral antibiotics are also warranted. Oxygen therapy and supportive fluids are given in the early stages of treatment.

Poisoning

Close proximity to human environments, especially gardens, exposes hedgehogs to many potential poisons. Cases of poisoning may be underdiagnosed, because of the difficulty and expense of laboratory confirmation, unless a known exposure has occurred.

There is little specific information on the effects of many toxins in the hedgehog. The long-term effects of poisons, or the effects of chronic exposure, such as changes in behaviour, fertility, growth and immunity, are little known (Reeve, 1994). For general information on poisoning, see Chapter 2.

Metaldehyde

Although widely considered to be a major hazard to hedgehogs, metaldehyde poisoning is probably overdiagnosed in many instances. Toxicity is unlikely to occur from eating poisoned slugs but hedgehogs will ingest the slug pellets themselves (Keymer *et al.*, 1991). Approximately 5 g of pellets (equivalent to a heaped teaspoonful) contains enough metaldehyde to poison an adult hedgehog (Best, 2001). Metaldehyde

is rapidly broken down in the stomach to acetaldehyde, and values in the stomach contents of over 40 mg/kg bodyweight are considered toxic. At post-mortem examination there may be blue deposits within the gut and a smell of acetaldehyde in the stomach contents.

Clinical signs of poisoning include hyperaesthesia (especially to sound), tachycardia, anxiety, salivation, ataxia, dysmetria, tremors, occasionally bluish faeces or vomit, and death.

Treatment should include: diazepam injections at 2–3 mg/kg for sedation to reduce muscle fasciculations and resultant hyperthermia; Hartmann's fluid therapy to correct acidosis; and attempts to flush the stomach with milk, sodium bicarbonate or charcoal. Oxygen therapy is sometimes needed and injectable vitamin B_{12} may aid recovery.

Warfarin and other coumarin derivatives

Occasionally ingested by hedgehogs, coumarins interfere with vitamin K activity, causing a coagulopathy. Clinical signs are the same as in other species and can include pallor, epistaxis and haemorrhagic diarrhoea. The toxic effects of warfarin are more severe if chronic ingestion occurs, rather than a single dose.

Treatment involves very careful handling, soft bedding and the administration of vitamin K injection (5–7 mg/kg).

Post-mortem findings are of multiple haemorrhages; traces of the toxin may be found in the gastrointestinal tract.

Paraquat

Poisoning can occur immediately following herbicide spraying but the clinical picture in the hedgehog is exactly like that of severe lungworm infestation, bronchopneumonia or nasal trauma, and these conditions should always be considered first. Clinical signs include dyspnoea, open-mouth breathing, foaming at the mouth and cyanosis.

Treatment can be attempted with doxapram (5 mg/kg) and the provision of oxygen-enriched air but the prognosis is poor. Multivitamins may also help with recovery.

Post-mortem examination reveals congested lungs that appear purple/red and there may be hepatomegaly.

Pesticides

Methiocarb and other carbamates, organophosphates and polychlorinated biphenyls (PCBs) all inhibit acetylcholinesterase and can cause paresis, paralysis, salivation, seizures, abdominal pain, vomiting and diarrhoea. Terminally, there may be cyanosis, with death from respiratory failure.

The antidote is atropine (0.2 mg/kg) and oxygen therapy. Pralidoxime could be useful in cases of confirmed exposure, if given within 24 hours of organophosphate ingestion.

Alphachloralose

Poisoning is possible in hedgehogs that have scavenged from an alphachloralose-laced carcass (especially rabbits) but appears to be extremely rare. Variable clinical signs are possible, related to stimulation or depression of the central nervous system.

Treatment of known exposure would probably consist of injectable diazepam and the provision of adequate warmth and supportive therapy.

Ethylene glycol

Poisoning with antifreeze is possible in the hedgehog because ethylene glycol tastes sweet. Clinical signs are non-specific and include ataxia, progressive incoordination, depression, renal failure and death. Fluid therapy and other supportive measures could be attempted.

Viral diseases

Foot-and-mouth disease (FMD)

Natural infection of hedgehogs with FMD virus was reported in a cattle outbreak in 1947 (McLaughlan and Henderson, 1947). Some hedgehogs were asymptomatic but in others the disease was fatal. It seemed that hedgehogs were very susceptible to infection. Clinical signs included daytime activity, anorexia, sneezing, hypersalivation, and erythema and vesicles on the feet, tongue, snout, lip margins and perineum.

It is theoretically possible for the virus to overwinter in hedgehogs during hibernation and be reintroduced to livestock the following spring, but the role of hedgehogs in the spread of FMD is probably insignificant (Hulse and Edwards, 1937). To reduce disease spread during the 2001 FMD outbreak, movement restrictions on susceptible species were extended to include captive hedgehogs; as a result no hedgehogs could be taken to veterinary practices or wildlife centres until the restrictions were lifted.

Morbillivirus

Infection with morbillivirus is possibly not uncommon in free-living wild hedgehogs. Viruses have been isolated from healthy individuals, as well as from the faeces and lungs of sick ones (Visozo and Thomas, 1981). Most of the clinical signs are associated with the nervous system, including circling, running, hypermetria, incoordination, hindlimb paresis or paralysis, inappetence and weight loss. There may be an oculonasal discharge and sometimes blindness. The footpads may be swollen and ulcerated, or hyperkeratotic. Affected hedgehogs are usually awake during the daytime and do not curl up fully.

Treatment should involve supportive fluid therapy and the provision of broad-spectrum antibacterials to control secondary infections. Supplementary B vitamins may also help.

Post-mortem examination usually reveals bronchopneumonia and neurohistopathological lesions that resemble those of canine distemper.

Bacterial diseases

Salmonellosis

With salmonellosis, the most common clinical picture presents as a sudden outbreak of green diarrhoea in hand-reared hedgehogs at around weaning age.

Transmission is by the faeco-oral route. Asymptomatic carriers act as the most likely source of infection, though transmission can occur via carrion and associated invertebrates (e.g. carabid beetles and maggots). The species most often isolated is *Salmonella enteriditis* (PT 11) but *S. brancaster* and *S. typhimurium* are occasionally recovered (Keymer *et al.*, 1991). *Klebsiella* spp. can cause similar clinical signs. All such infections are potentially zoonotic.

Symptoms and diagnosis: Clinical signs can include dyspnoea, anorexia, weight loss, dehydration and diarrhoea (which may be mucoid or blood-flecked). There may be rectal prolapse from tenesmus, intussusception, and occasionally nervous signs due to meningitis. Peracute cases present as sudden death.

Direct faecal culture is often unremarkable. Diagnosis relies on the submission of whole fresh carcasses to a suitable laboratory for culture from the gut and liver.

Post-mortem examination usually reveals a mucohaemorrhagic enteritis, with congestion of the intestinal mucosa. There is often concurrent focal pneumonia, which may be catarrhal or purulent, and sometimes hepatomegaly, focal hepatic necrosis and signs of septicaemia.

Treatment: Treatment involves fluid therapy and provision of adequate warmth. Antidiarrhoeals such as kaolin sometimes help. Antibacterials, based on culture and sensitivity, can be used but may promote carrier status or prolonged shedding of bacteria. The prognosis is usually grave and mortality rates are high, especially in cases of septicaemia. Strict barrier nursing is essential to prevent disease transfer and extra precautions are necessary due to the risk of transfer to humans. Severely ill hedgehogs rarely recover and should be euthanased immediately to reduce suffering and disease transmission.

Bordetellosis

Bordetella bronchiseptica causes a contagious respiratory disease leading to tracheitis and catarrhal rhinitis, which may progress to bronchopneumonia. *Bordetella* infections often accompany lungworm infestations, commonly causing pneumonia (though *B. bronchiseptica* can also be recovered from healthy respiratory tracts). Other pathogens (e.g. *Pasteurella multocida*, other pasteurellae and haemolytic streptococci) are often found as opportunistic invaders (Saupe and Poduschka, 1995).

Clinical signs include dyspnoea, hyperpnoea, wheezy respiratory noises, nasal discharge and epistaxis. The prognosis depends on the extent of damage to the respiratory apparatus.

Suitable antibacterials include oxytetracycline, amoxicillin, enrofloxacin or cefalexin. NSAIDs are usually warranted, and mucolytics and bronchodilators are also often helpful. Severely dyspnoeic patients require oxygen therapy or nebulization but some cases are so severe as to warrant immediate euthanasia.

Leptospirosis

Leptospirosis is probably of little clinical significance in hedgehogs but is an important consideration for hedgehog workers because it is zoonotic. *Leptospira interrogans* sv. *bratislava* has been isolated from hedgehogs, which seem to act as a reservoir in the wild (Twigg *et al.*, 1968).

Yersiniosis

This usually affects juvenile hedgehogs, causing hindlimb weakness, chronic weight loss and sometimes diarrhoea. Affected individuals may die and on post-mortem examination display pathology consistent with pseudotuberculosis, namely white–grey caseous foci in liver or spleen and in mesentery, with mesenteric lymphadenopathy (Keymer *et al.*, 1991; Saupe and Poduschka, 1995). *Mycobacterium avium* and other mycobacteria have also been isolated from the mesenteric lymph nodes of hedgehogs (Smith, 1968; Matthews and McDiarmid, 1977).

Pyoderma and abscessation

Exudative dermatitis is occasionally encountered, especially of the ventral skin, and is usually associated with staphylococci, especially coagulase-positive *Staphylococcus aureus*.

Abscesses are extremely common anywhere on the body, with many possible pathogens isolated but especially staphylococci, *Escherichia coli* and sometimes *Pseudomonas* species.

Neonatal enteritis

Pale green sticky diarrhoea (leading to dehydration and death) occurs, especially in hoglets. *E. coli*, notably types 078 and 055, is often implicated (Smith, 1968). *Proteus* spp. can cause similar signs. Haemolytic *E. coli* infection causes the faeces to be streaked with mucus and blood, or to contain lumps of bright green jelly or occasionally pus.

Control of neonatal enteritis involves strict hygiene, isolation, and sterilization of equipment.

Tick-borne diseases

Q fever, a rickettsial disease caused by *Coxiella burnetti*, has been reported in hedgehogs but its clinical importance is unknown. In other species, it can cause an influenza-like disease. It is a zoonosis and can be transmitted by inhalation of dust or droplets of urine or faeces containing rickettsiae (Smith, 1968).

Borrelia burghdorferi, which can cause Lyme disease, has also been isolated from hedgehogs, but there have been no reports of clinical signs associated with infection. Transmission can be via the ticks *Ixodes ricinus* or *I. hexagonus*, and hedgehogs may act as a minor local wildlife reservoir of infection.

Fungal diseases

Ringworm

The only significant fungal infection of hedgehogs is ringworm. It is usually caused by *Trichophyton erinacei* (*T. mentagrophytes* var. *erinacei*), which is carried by up to 25% of hedgehogs but is often a subclinical infection (Morris and English, 1969).

T. erinacei is only mildly pathogenic to hedgehogs; there is little apparent irritation, even when comparatively severe skin lesions are present, and the hedgehogs continue to thrive well. Other dermatophyte species can also infect hedgehogs, including *Microsporum canis* and *M. gypseum*.

Symptoms and diagnosis: Severe ringworm infections can cause cracked crusty lesions and hair loss, especially of the face and head (Figure 6.9). The disease is generally non-pruritic and results in scab formation, typically on the snout and the crown of the head. Lesions invariably bleed when the scabs are removed. Other areas of the body can be affected (including ventral alopecia) and loss of spines can occur, with characteristic crusts of scale around the base. Chronic ringworm infections cause the pinnae to become thickened and crusted.

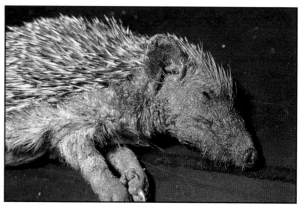

6.9 Severe ringworm lesions (*Trichophyton erinacei*) with concurrent *Caparinia tripilis* mite infestation. (© Andrew Routh)

There is often concurrent bacterial infection or mite infestation. Mites, especially *Caparinia tripilis*, have been implicated in the transmission of *T. erinacei*, because fungi have been recovered from their faeces (Smith and Marples, 1963).

Confirmation of ringworm is by culture on Sabouraud's agar, or demonstration of fungi on skin biopsy, and is essential since many other skin disorders resemble dermatophytosis and the clinical appearance is rarely pathognomonic. Direct microscopy is less reliable and *T. erinacei* does not fluoresce under a Wood's lamp.

Transmission: Transmission may be direct, as ringworm is more common in suburban hedgehogs with a greater population density and also more prevalent in males, who have more social interactions. The fungal spores persist well in dry nests (English and Morris, 1969) and so transmission may also occur by nest sharing. Male hedgehogs tend to use more nests (Morris and English, 1969, 1973).

T. erinacei is zoonotic and can affect hedgehog workers, in whom it causes an atypical lesion not easily recognized as ringworm (Figure 6.10). It tends to form a rapidly spreading, intensely pruritic and scaly lesion, initially vesicular, beneath a thickened epidermis. It is perhaps the most common zoonosis amongst wildlife rehabilitators.

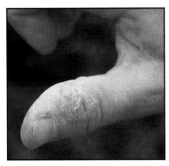

6.10 Hedgehog ringworm (*Trichophyton erinacei*) on human hands. (© Andrew Routh)

Dogs are also occasionally presented with ringworm due to *T. erinacei*, with lesions on the lips or muzzle from investigating hedgehogs.

Treatment: Spontaneous recovery of hedgehogs from ringworm has not been recorded but the widespread occurrence in the hedgehog population, and the low pathogenicity of the infection, calls into question whether treatment should be attempted. Chronic infestation in older hedgehogs with just thickened pinnae may be regarded as an incidental finding. However, the high zoonotic potential may justify treatment. More severe or widespread lesions are best treated with a prolonged course of an antifungal agent, such as griseofulvin or enilconazole. Recovery, and regeneration of hair and spines, is often a long process, depending on the severity of the initial lesions. Resolution of the skin lesions is an adequate basis to cease therapy but negative fungal cultures are considered confirmatory.

Ectoparasites

Fleas
Fleas are very common on all hedgehogs and easily visible, due to the hedgehog's sparse hair and spines. Most hedgehogs have fleas, especially during the summer, when there are often over 100 fleas per animal. Clinically, they cause little problem to the host and even pruritus seems minimal. Heavy flea burdens can indicate more serious problems. Severe infestations, often accompanied by other parasites, can cause anaemia.

The most common species is the hedgehog flea, *Archaeopsylla erinacei*. Flea eggs are laid in the nest, where the hatched larvae feed on detritus. These then infest other hedgehogs visiting the nest, or nestlings if it is a breeding nest.

Various treatments have been successful, especially pyrethrum, permethrin and fipronil, but generally only heavy burdens need treating.

Ticks
Ticks are commonly found on hedgehogs, especially around the pinnae and on the hindlimbs and skirt. The most common species to affect the hedgehog is *Ixodes hexagonus* but *I. ricinus* and *I. trianguliceps* have also been recorded.

Large burdens can cause anaemia but heavy infestations can also be indicative of other more serious problems. Tick bites occasionally cause local reactions and inflammation and they are potential vectors for Lyme disease, Q fever and tick paralysis. The incidence of tick-borne diseases in hedgehogs is largely unstudied.

Treatment: Tick removal is best performed using a commercial tick remover but in many cases it is probably unnecessary to extract every tick. Unlike tick removal in domestic species, the mouthparts are hardly ever left behind in the skin of a hedgehog. Some of the topical acaricides are also effective, including fipronil and ivermectin.

Mites
The commonest mite to be encountered on hedgehogs is the non-burrowing *Caparinia tripilis*. Up to 40% of hedgehogs may be infested but only severe infestations combined with other problems are life-threatening. Capariniosis often occurs synergistically with dermatophytosis (see Figure 6.9).

The mites are just visible to the naked eye as motile powdery deposits, especially around the eyes, ears and cheeks. Sometimes they are more generalized all over the body. Skin lesions consist of scurf and scale, with some hair and spine loss, and sometimes pruritis.

Capariniosis itself is often of little clinical significance, except that accumulations of skin debris and serum can predispose to fly strike and the mites may be a vector for dermatophytes.

Diagnosis is based on the clinical appearance of the skin, with detection of the mites, aided by a hand lens if necessary. Hair plucks and brushings can be examined microscopically. Topical avermectins are the treatment of choice.

Sarcoptes spp. are sometimes seen, especially in young hedgehogs, causing generalized erythema and alopecia, which can be fatal. Diagnosis is by deep skin scrapes from several sites. Treatment is with injectable ivermectin or amitraz washes.

Demodex erinacei causes follicular mange with raised papules and crusty skin lesions. Mites may be seen microscopically on deep skin scrapes within the sebaceous glands of haired skin. Demodicosis appears to be rare in hedgehogs. Treatment with amitraz can be successful.

Notoedres cati has occasionally been recovered from hedgehogs with encrustations on the head and ears, and *Otodectes cynotis* has been recorded as causing otitis externa. Presumably both parasites are acquired from contact with cats. Topical ivermectin, repeated every 7 days, is usually effective.

Harvest (trombiculid) mites are not uncommon in hedgehogs, appearing as tiny orange specks, often in the axillae, pinnae, ventrum and interdigital area. They are probably of little clinical significance.

Myiasis
Fly strike is very common in hedgehogs, especially on weak and debilitated individuals, predisposed by their inactivity during the day and their relaxed attitude to personal hygiene. Eggs are usually laid near wounds or other skin lesions, or around orifices (eyes, ears, mouth, nares, anus and genitals). A thorough inspection of these sites is important in all hedgehogs examined, especially in the warmer months of the year. Affected individuals often have a characteristic rotten odour.

Fly strike is most commonly caused by *Lucilia* spp. but also *Calliphora* spp. Both primary fly strike and secondary wound infestation occur.

Treatment: Maggots can kill their host rapidly, due to toxin formation, and treatment involves the physical removal of all maggots and eggs, wound cleansing, and therapy with ivermectin. Dental irrigators are useful for flushing out small maggots. Eggs adhering to fur are removed easily by clipping off the fur, or brushing with a toothbrush. Maggots under the eyelids can be squeezed out, then the lids can be wiped with a small soft paintbrush. The eyes should be treated with a viscous eye ointment (e.g. chloramphenicol eye ointment) to smother any remaining maggots. The ears can be gently wiped with a cotton bud, then instilled with insecticidal ear drops. Severe cases need antibacterial cover and NSAID therapy, for its antitoxic and analgesic effects. Fly strike in hedgehogs is often a very serious condition and many individuals will warrant immediate euthanasia on humane grounds.

Endoparasites

Crenosoma striatum
Adults and larvae of this nematode are commonly present in the lumen of the trachea, bronchi, bronchioles and alveolar ducts (Majeed *et al.*, 1989). Infestation is so common, especially in first-year hedgehogs, that treatment should be undertaken routinely. Some immunity seems to develop in older animals.

First-stage larvae are coughed up from the respiratory tract, swallowed and passed in the faeces. They subsequently enter the intermediate hosts – usually slugs and snails – where they develop to the infective stage. These molluscs are then ingested by a hedgehog and the infective larvae migrate to the airways. Direct transmission may also occur, since worms are sometimes found in the lungs of pre-weaned animals (Majeed *et al.*, 1989).

Symptoms and diagnosis: The clinical signs are mainly due to bronchitis and lung consolidation, with secondary bacterial bronchopneumonia (especially due to *Bordetella bronchiseptica*). There is a moist chesty cough, rattling breathing, weight loss, weakness, dyspnoea and sometimes a nasal discharge. Severe cases may be cyanotic, with open-mouth breathing, possibly leading to emphysema and circulatory failure.

Diagnosis is by detection of motile larvae (about 300 μm long) on preparations of direct faecal smears. As larvae are not passed continuously in faeces, one-off examination may pick up only about a quarter of cases.

Treatment: Waiting for a positive diagnosis may delay treatment too long. The morbidity rate of verminous pneumonia in first-year hedgehogs in the autumn approaches 100% and the mortality rate can be high. It is wise, therefore, to treat all such individuals as a matter of routine; levamisole is the most effective treatment. A suitable broad-spectrum antibiotic is used concurrently to control secondary bacterial bronchopneumonia.

Treatment in general involves the use of anthelmintics and antibacterials. The risk of anaphylaxis caused by worm die-off can be reduced by the concurrent use of a steroid, or NSAIDs may be used to reduce lung inflammation. Millophylline and clenbuterol can be added to aid expulsion of the worms. Mucolytics are useful when there is thick, tracheobronchial mucus present. Other useful therapies include oxygen and nebulization.

Nebulization: Nebulization is a useful adjunct to other therapy in hedgehogs with respiratory disorders and is relatively easy to perform, using a human asthma nebulizer or a custom-built chamber. Bronchodilators (e.g. salbutamol), mucolytics (e.g. acetylcysteine, carbocisteine) and antibacterials (especially gentamicin) are all suitable for nebulization. Health and safety considerations apply to avoid inhalation by operators.

Capillaria aerophila
Adult lungworms 10–13 mm long are commonly found in the epithelium of the respiratory tract, especially the bronchi. Nematodes may also be found in the epithelium of the bronchioles and the trachea, where they can occasionally cause tracheitis and tracheal granulomas. *Capillaria* is often found as a mixed lung infestation along with *Crenosoma*.

Eggs are shed in faeces and ingested by the transport hosts, which are chiefly earthworms and possibly also beetles. Direct transmission is also likely (Majeed *et al.*, 1989).

Diagnosis is by demonstrating the oval bipolar eggs in faeces but repeat examinations may be necessary, as they are not shed continually. The eggs resemble those of *Trichuris*. Treatment is the same as for *Crenosoma* (see above).

Intestinal *Capillaria*
Intestinal *Capillaria* spp. also occur, and differentiation of the eggs of different species is difficult without measurement techniques. They include *C. erinacei* and *C. ovoreticulata*, both of which are occasionally encountered in hedgehogs. They seem to be of low pathogenicity, even when present as heavy burdens, but may cause green mucoid diarrhoea, lethargy and weight loss. The bipolar eggs, passed in faeces, are difficult to distinguish from those of the lungworm *C. aerophila*. The intermediate host is the earthworm.

Most of the commonly used anthelmintics are effective (e.g. levamisole, fenbendazole, mebendazole).

Brachylaemus erinacei
This intestinal trematode (fluke) can cause lethal haemorrhagic enteritis in severe cases. Currently, the incidence is low and only in certain regions of the UK, but infestation is possibly becoming more common and widespread. Hedgehogs with flukes usually have burdens of other endoparasites as well, especially *Capillaria* spp.

The adult fluke is 5–10 mm long, 1–2 mm across and lancet-shaped. Unipolar eggs, which are slightly asymmetrical and measure approximately 20 μm x 30 μm, are demonstrable on direct faecal smears but are small and easily missed. The chances of detection are improved by flotation techniques. The metacercariae develop in the slug and snail intermediate hosts (Keymer *et al.*, 1991; Saupe and Poduschka, 1995).

Adult flukes can occur in the intestines and bile ducts of hedgehogs of all ages, causing weight loss, restlessness, scratching, climbing, inappetence and melaena, or mucoid slimy faeces. *Brachylaemus* infestation can be fatal if there is severe diarrhoea, or if the flukes enter the bile ducts.

Treatment is with praziquantel or niclosamide.

Cestodes

Hymenolepis erinacei is an uncommon and usually asymptomatic tapeworm infestation of hedgehogs. Similar to the incidence of hedgehog flukes, there may be some geographical variations in the abundance of cestodes in hedgehogs in the UK. Adult tapeworms, up to 80 mm long, may be found in the intestines, where they can cause weight loss and diarrhoea.

The proglottides (3 mm x 1 mm) are shed in the faeces and enter the intermediate hosts, which are arthropods (chiefly beetles). Eggs, with characteristic internal hooks, are occasionally visible on faecal smears. Treatment is with praziquantel.

Acanthocephala

Thorny-headed worms are often found in the intestines and mesentery of hedgehogs at post-mortem examination. Extreme cases can cause ulceration of the gut wall and can be fatal but most cases are symptomless. The most commonly isolated species are *Moniliformis erinacei* and *Prosthorhyncus* spp. (Smith, 1968; Keymer *et al.*, 1991). The intermediate hosts are probably insects. Praziquantel can be used as treatment.

Coccidiosis

It is not unusual to find coccidial oocysts in the faeces of hedgehogs but most seem to be asymptomatic. Occasionally, coccidiosis can cause inappetence, emaciation and haemorrhagic diarrhoea. The pathogenic species are *Isospora rastegaiev* and *I. erinacei*, and possibly some species of *Eimeria* (Saupe and Poduschka, 1995).

Treatment is rarely necessary but the sulphonamides are effective, especially sulfadimidine.

Other endoparasites

Toxoplasma gondii has been recorded but the severity and clinical significance of infection are unknown (Smith, 1968). *Giardia* and other species of intestinal protozoans may be encountered. Other nematodes recorded seem to be rare, and of little significance, but include *Physaloptera clausa* (from the oesophagus and stomach), *Gongylonema mucronatum*, ascarids, *Strongyloides* and *Trichinella* spp. (Saupe and Poduschka, 1995).

Other diseases

Dental disease

Dental disease is common in captive hedgehogs that are fed exclusively on soft foods but also surprisingly common in free-living wild hedgehogs. Tartar aggregations lead to gingivitis and bacterial infections, gum recession and periodontal disease. Treatment involves general anaesthesia, with endotracheal intubation recommended. Tooth extraction, descaling and polishing are the same as in domestic species. Antibacterials such as metronidazole/spiramycin or clindamycin are effective. The addition of hard foods

to the diet, such as dry catfood or insect chitin exoskeleton, may help to reduce tartar formation further.

Nutritional disease

Obesity: Most nutritional diseases are associated with the feeding of incorrect diets to hedgehogs in captivity. The most common likely problem is obesity. Overfeeding can have serious health effects, including cardiovascular compromise and fatty liver degeneration. Overfat hedgehogs also lose the ability to curl up fully and so, if released, are at increased risk from predation.

Dietary deficiencies: Vitamin or trace-element deficiency (e.g. zinc) can cause spine loss. Rickets (osteomalacia) can occur on low calcium diets. Nutritional secondary hyperparathyroidism and hypervitaminosis A and D should also be considered, as in other species.

Hindlimb paresis and paralysis and splayed legs in hand-reared orphaned hedgehogs of less than 4 weeks old can occur. Some respond to vitamin B_1 therapy and in these cases the condition is presumed to be caused by reduced thiamine absorption secondary to digestive disturbances.

Underweight autumn juveniles: Late litters born in August, September or even October, due to late conception in repeat breeders or (rarely) second litters, often have insufficient time to lay down the necessary body reserves to survive hibernation. To have sufficient fat reserves and therefore a favourable chance of surviving the winter, hedgehogs should have a minimum bodyweight of 550 g by November (Morris, 1984).

As autumnal temperatures drop, the amount of natural forage prey declines and the young hedgehogs are forced to forage in the daytime, when they are often found wandering around and presented for attention. The majority of these hedgehogs have significant endoparasite burdens, especially of lungworm, and routine anthelmintic treatment is essential. Otherwise, they should be kept in captivity until they have sufficient fat reserves to be released. Sometimes this involves keeping them over the whole winter and keeping them warm, with plenty of food, so that they do not go into hibernation. Once over 550 g bodyweight, they can be returned to the wild, even during winter, as long as the weather is not too cold and they have sufficient resources to build a winter nest. This is a viable alternative to keeping animals for the whole winter, thereby reducing the time they spend in captivity.

Other conditions

- Otitis externa is not uncommon, especially as a sequel to blowfly contamination of the ear canal. Treatment is with routine antibacterial ear drops, but daily application is more difficult in hedgehogs because they tend to roll up once the ears are touched
- Eye prolapse and globe rupture can occur after sharp trauma. Enucleation is usually necessary but end-stage eyes often shrink and fibrose, causing no problems. Blind or partially sighted

hedgehogs cope very well but are best maintained in sheltered environments with supplementary feeding provided

- Paraphimosis can occur in mature males, usually following trauma.

Therapeutics

A drug formulary for hedgehogs is given in Figure 6.11. Injection sites are described under 'First aid procedures' (above).

Drug	Dosage commonly used	Some indications
Antibacterials		
Enrofloxacin	10–20 mg/kg i.m., s.c. bid	Broad-spectrum, especially useful for respiratory tract infections and wounds
Amoxicillin/clavulanate	30–50 mg/kg i.m., s.c., orally bid	Broad-spectrum, useful for respiratory tract infections, skin and soft tissue infections (including abscesses) and enteritis
Clindamycin	10–20 mg/kg orally bid	Infected wounds, abcesses and dental infections
Oxytetracycline	50 mg/kg orally bid	Broad-spectrum bacteriostatic used especially for respiratory tract infections
Ampicillin	20 mg/kg orally, s.c.	Broad-spectrum bactericidal antibacterial
Amoxicillin LA	50–150 mg/kg every other day	Broad-spectrum bactericidal
Cefalexin	30 mg/kg i.m., s.c., orally sid or bid	Broad-spectrum bactericidal, may be particularly useful for skin and soft tissue infections, especially pyoderma, abcessation and infected wounds
Metronidazole/spiramycin (Stomorgyl, Merial)	¹/₂ tablet/kg orally	Dental infections
Antifungals		
Griseofulvin	30–50 mg/kg orally sid	Ringworm: treat for at least 4 weeks
Enilconazole	0.2% dilution made up, topical treatment every 3 days for 4–6 applications	Ringworm
Endoparasiticides		
Ivermectin	0.2–3 mg/kg s.c.	Gastrointestinal parasites. Has been used to treat lungworm infestation in hedgehogs, but onset of activity slower than levamisole and severe infestations not successfully treated
Levamisole	27 mg/kg 3 injections s.c. at 48 h intervals, i.e. every other day	Treatment of choice for lungworm. Other dose regimes can be employed
Fenbendazole	100 mg/kg orally sid for 5 days	Useful as in-feed treatment against gastrointestinal roundworms and lungworms. May have some effect on hedgehog tapeworms
Mebendazole	50–100 mg/kg orally sid for 5 days	Roundworms and tapeworms
Praziquantel	10–20 mg/kg i.m., s.c.	Tapeworms and *Brachylaemus* flukes
Sulfadoxine/trimethoprim	50 mg/kg s.c., i.m.	Coccidiosis
Sulfadimidine	200 mg/kg s.c. for 3 days	Coccidiosis
Ectoparasiticides		
Pyrethrum	Apply dusting of powder to skin	Widely used to treat external parasite problems, especially fleas
Permethrin	Apply dusting of powder to skin	Useful for treating fleas
Fipronil	Spray sparingly	For flea and tick infestation. **Always ensure good ventilation during and after treatment**
Amitraz	Apply 1:400 dilution as wash to skin every 3 days	For demodicosis and sarcoptic mange. Also essential to change bedding and clean out cage during treatment
Ivermectin	Dilute 1:9 with propylene glycol, apply 1–3 drops topically on to skin; repeat at intervals of 7–10 days	Useful to treat ticks, fleas and mites
Ivermectin	0.2–3 mg/kg s.c.	To treat mange and as adjunct to therapy for fly strike

6.11 Drug formulary for the hedgehog. (Note that no drugs are specifically licensed in the UK for use in the hedgehog; all doses quoted are widely accepted and based on experience of the authors and other hedgehog practitioners.) (continues)

Drug	Dosage commonly used	Some indications
Miscellaneous		
Methylprednisolone	1–6 mg/kg i.m. (single dose)	Long-acting corticosteroid
Betamethasone	0.5 mg/kg i.m.	Corticosteroid, may be of benefit in shock and circulatory collapse
Bromhexine (Bisolvon powder, Boehringer Ingelheim)	1 pinch on food bid	Mucolytic to aid expectoration of mucus, especially in cases of bronchopneumonia secondary to lungworm
Etamiphylline	30 mg/kg i.m., s.c. bid–tid	Cardiorespiratory stimulant, may aid when respiratory infection present
Clenbuterol (Ventipulmin, Boehringer Ingelheim)	1 pinch on food twice daily	Bronchodilator, to relieve bronchospasm and assist mucociliary clearance in hedgehogs with respiratory disease, including lungworm

6.11 (continued) Drug formulary for the hedgehog. (Note that no drugs are specifically licensed in the UK for use in the hedgehog; all doses quoted are widely accepted and based on experience of the authors and other hedgehog practitioners.)

Management in captivity

Housing

Hedgehogs in captivity can be housed singly or in small groups. Although not naturally gregarious, they rarely display any intolerance of one another, the only exception being that when unnaturally large groups are overwintered together they may fight in the early spring.

They can be kept in cardboard boxes or plastic tubs, allowing approximately 0.5 m² per individual for the purposes of hospitalization. Larger accommodation is better if they are in captivity for any length of time, allowing 1 m² per hedgehog in communal housing.

There should be no bars or wire mesh, as hedgehogs tend to scratch at surfaces and can easily injure their feet. They can climb and dig and so a secure lid or door is required to prevent escape. Newspaper or shavings can be used as bedding, which should be changed regularly as it becomes rapidly soiled with food, water and excreta. Hay and shredded paper are unsuitable as bedding materials, due to the risk of the material becoming wrapped round a limb, producing a ligature effect.

Feeding

Adult hedgehogs are relatively easy to feed in captivity and will readily consume a variety of suitable (and unsuitable) foods.

- Tinned cat food or dog food is satisfactory: approximately 80 g per hedgehog per feed, depending on the nutritional content of the brand offered. A vitamin/mineral supplement can be added if necessary
- Addition of pancreatic enzyme supplements will aid digestion, allowing more rapid build-up of body reserves in underweight juveniles
- Food for insectivorous birds or proprietary hedgehog foods (e.g. Spike's Dinner, Spike's Place) are suitable alternatives
- Invertebrates such as mealworms (*Tenebrio molitor* larvae) are also eaten and can be used as environmental enrichment. Natural foods such as beetles and earthworms can be given as treats, though some workers argue that they are unsuitable because they act as the intermediate hosts for so many hedgehog parasites
- Dried pelleted dog food or cat food can be incorporated into the diet to reduce the risks of tartar build-up and obesity
- The traditional bread-and-milk diet is nutritionally unsuitable and also tends to cause diarrhoea, due to lactose intolerance.

It is important not to feed *ad libitum*, as hedgehogs will overeat and become too fat. As they are nocturnal, it is more natural to feed in the evenings, but sick or underweight animals should be fed twice daily.

Drinking water should be provided in a shallow bowl. Drip drinkers can be used but are messier.

General points

- If kept in a warm environment (18–22°C) and well fed, overwintered hedgehogs will not hibernate. This is crucial for those that are underweight
- Regular handling should be discouraged, as the hedgehog will become accustomed to contact and will roll up less readily, putting it at greater risk of predation once released
- The claws should be checked, as they can become overgrown when hedgehogs are in captivity.

Rearing of orphans

Litters may be born at any time from May to October. If nests are disturbed, the mother hedgehog will often abandon her young or cannibalize them. This occasionally occurs when breeding nests are disturbed during gardening or building work. Also the mother may be killed, especially on the road, or die of some other cause. Deserted hoglets will often make a whistling or peeping sound. A thorough search must always be made of the surrounding area to ensure that no hoglets are left behind.

All orphans should be thoroughly checked for fly strike and first aid should be provided. Hoglets should be stimulated to defecate and urinate immediately on arrival and after each feed, by gently massaging from the belly to the anus with a damp cotton bud. The droppings of neonates are naturally bright green, becoming paler with time, until at weaning they turn brown.

Fostering hoglets on to other nursing females has occasionally been successful but is generally not advisable, due to the risk that the foster mother might kill and eat the youngsters. Hand-rearing (Figure 6.12) can be a time-consuming and difficult task and should not be undertaken lightly. Ageing techniques are described in Figure 6.3.

Age	Weight (g)	Feeding (milk replacer)
Newborn	12–20	2 ml every 2 h
Birth to 1 week	30–50	2 ml every 2–3 h
1–2 weeks	50–80	3–5 ml every 3–4 h
2–3 weeks	80–100	6–10 ml every 4 h
3–4 weeks	110–170	6 ml every 4 h Wean on to puppyfood Encourage to lap milk from dish
5 weeks	190–220	Weaned on to solid foods

6.12 Summary of feeding regime for orphan hoglets. Note that this table is intended as a guide for rearing by hand; there are many different regimes and each worker has their own preferred method. (See also Figure 6.3 for development of hoglets.)

The minimum ambient temperature should be about 25°C. This can be provided by a heat pad, heat lamp or incubator. A temperature gradient is needed, so that the hoglets can move away from the heat if they get too hot, as thermoregulation is not well developed (especially in neonates). Newspaper, plus a towel, is a suitable bedding substrate.

Strict hygiene and barrier nursing are essential to prevent cross-contamination of infections, especially when large numbers are being reared. Mixing hoglets from different litters should be avoided, as should mixing animals of different ages, and overcrowding. The quarters should be regularly cleaned out and a different set of equipment used for each litter group. All feeding utensils should be sterilized between feeds. Young hoglets seem to have poorly developed immunity and rely on a constant supply of maternal antibodies in their dam's milk for the whole lactation (Morris and Steel, 1964), which is difficult to mimic when they are artificially reared. In order to monitor progress, it is important to weigh the hoglets daily, before the first morning feed.

After arrival, the first feed should be a rehydrating solution (e.g. Lectade, Pfizer), with a gradual change to milk substitute over the subsequent few feeds. Many milk substitutes have been used with success, including goat's colostrum, goat's milk and many proprietary milk replacers. Ready-made liquid milk formula (e.g.

Esbilac, PetAg) is better than powdered versions, because inconsistencies in preparation and mixing are avoided. The milk is warmed and fed via a plastic pipette and kitten-size teat (some workers make small teats for very small hoglets by building up layers of modelling latex over a blunted hypodermic needle).

Individuals that are too weak, or reluctant to suckle, can be fed via an orogastric tube but the technique requires some experience to avoid aspiration pneumonia. Alternatively, they can be given a drop at a time into the mouth and allowed to swallow, until the sucking reflex becomes stronger.

The ability to self-feed from a dish varies greatly between individuals but they should always be encouraged to lap milk from a shallow dish. Once they are doing so, solid food (e.g. puppy food; see also adult feeding, above) can be added gradually.

Release

Most studies indicate that hedgehogs released back into the wild, generally adapt and survive well. Even artificially reared hedgehogs seem instinctively to thrive, forage, orientate themselves and build nests (Morris *et al.*, 1990, 1993; Morris and Warwick, 1994; Reeve, 1998). It should be noted that fully fit hedgehogs rarely return for supplementary feeding after release. Post-release weight loss generally occurs but this merely represents the excess weight acquired whilst in captivity (Reeve, 1998).

Choice of release site
It is best to choose an area where a wild population of hedgehogs already exists, because if hedgehogs are absent from an area there is a reason for it. Generally they favour 'edge habitats', i.e. areas between open land and dense vegetation (Reeve, 1994) (see 'Ecology and biology'). Gardens can be ideal release sites, especially if they contain shrubs, leaf piles, compost heaps and overgrown areas, but the problem of garden hazards must be borne in mind before hedgehogs are released. Walled gardens (especially where human residents are keen to provide additional feeding) are ideal for the release of disabled hedgehogs.

Sites near main roads should be avoided as far as possible, but this may be difficult as hedgehogs commonly travel more than 1 km in a night. Habitat type and the proximity of roads are more important considerations than the avoidance of predation.

Areas with ground-nesting birds should not be used as release sites, since hedgehogs occasionally eat eggs or nestlings. Such locations include bird reserves (especially with gulls and terns) and land managed for gamebirds.

Release techniques
Hedgehogs should not be released during extremes of weather; they need an opportunity to build a nest. Soft release (see Chapter 3) may reduce dispersal and enhance survival chances, but most rehabilitators find that hard release is simpler and comparatively successful.

Radio-tracking can be used to follow a hedgehog's movements for a short time. PVC ear tags, clipping particular spines, glue-on spine tags and colour marking with paint have all been used to identify released individuals.

Legal aspects

Hedgehogs have no special legislation but are covered by Schedule 6 of the Wildlife and Countryside Act 1981 (amended 1987), which makes it illegal to catch, trap or kill them without a licence. The Wild Mammals (Protection) Act 1996 protects them from cruelty.

Specialist organizations

The British Hedgehog Preservation Society
Knowbury House, Knowbury, Ludlow, Shropshire SY8 3LQ

St Tiggywinkles, The Wildlife Hospital Trust
Aston Road, Haddenham, Aylesbury, Bucks HP17 8AF

European Hedgehog Research Group
Website: www.ngo.grida.no/ngo/hedgehog

References and further reading

Best JR (2001) Diagnosis and treatment of poisoning in wildlife – a practical guide for rehabilitators. *Rehabilitator* **31**, 2–7

English MP and Morris PA (1969) *Trichophyton mentagrophytes* var. *erinacei* in hedgehog nests. *Sabouraudia* **7**, 118–121

Hulse EC and Edwards JT (1937) Foot and mouth disease in hibernating hedgehogs. *Journal of Comparative Pathology and Therapeutics* **50**, 421–430

Isenbugel E and Baumgartner RA (1993) Diseases of the hedgehog. In: *Zoo and Wild Animal Medicine – Current Therapy, 3rd edn*, ed. ME Fowler. WB Saunders, Philadelphia

Keymer IF, Gibson EA and Reynolds DJ (1991) Zoonoses and other findings in hedgehogs (*Erinaceus europaeus*): a survey of mortality and review of the literature. *Veterinary Record* **128**, 245–249

Majeed SK, Morris PA and Cooper JE (1989) Occurrence of the lungworms *Capillaria* and *Cremosoma* species in British hedgehogs (*Erinaceus europaeus*). *Journal of Comparative Pathology* **100**, 27–36

Matthews PRJ and McDiarmid A (1977) *Mycobacterium avium* infection in freeliving hedgehogs (*Erinaceus europaeus*). *Research in Veterinary Science* **22**, 388

McLaughlan JD and Henderson WM (1947) The occurrence of foot and mouth disease in the hedgehog under natural conditions. *Journal of Hygiene (Cambridge)* **45**, 474–479

Morris B and Steel ED (1964) The absorption of antibody by young hedgehogs after treatment with cortisone acetate. *Journal of Endocrinology* **30**, 195–203

Morris P and English MP (1969) *Trichophyton mentagrophytes* var. *erinacei* in British hedgehogs. *Sabouraudia* **7**, 122–128

Morris P and English MP (1973) Transmission and course of *Trichophyton erinacei* infections in British hedgehogs. *Sabouraudia* **11**, 42–47

Morris PA (1971) Epiphyseal fusion in the forefoot as a means of age determination in the hedgehog (*Erinaceus europaeus*). *Journal of Zoology (London)* **164**, 254–259

Morris PA (1983) *Hedgehogs*. Whittet Books, Weybridge

Morris PA (1984) An estimate of the minimum body weight necessary for hedgehogs (*Erinaceus europaeus*) to survive hibernation. *Journal of Zoology (London)* **203**, 291–294

Morris PA (1986) Nightly movements of hedgehogs (*Erinaceus europaeus*) in forest edge habitat. *Mammalia* **50**, 395–398

Morris PA and Warwick H (1994) A study of rehabilitated juvenile hedgehogs after release into the wild. *Animal Welfare* **3**, 163–177

Morris PA, Munn S and Craig-Wood S (1990) Released hedgehogs – can they cope? In: *Proceedings of the Third Symposium of the British Wildlife Rehabilitation Council*, ed. T Thomas. BWRC, Horsham

Morris PA, Meakin K and Sharafi S (1993) The behaviour and survival of rehabilitated hedgehogs. *Animal Welfare* **2**, 53–66

Parkes J (1975) Some aspects of the biology of the hedgehog (*Erinaceus europaeus*) in the Manawatu, New Zealand. *New Zealand Journal of Zoology* **2**, 463–472

Reeve NJ (1982) The home range of the hedgehog as revealed by a radiotracking study. *Symposium of the Zoological Society of London* **49**, 207–230

Reeve N (1994) *Hedgehogs*. T & AD Poyser, London

Reeve NJ (1998) The survival and welfare of hedgehogs after release back into the wild. *Animal Welfare* **7**, 189–202

Reeve NJ and Huijser MP (1999) Mortality factors affecting wild hedgehogs: a study of records from wildlife rescue centres. *Lutra* **42**, 7–23

Robinson I and Routh A (1999) Veterinary care of the hedgehog. *In Practice*, March, 128-137

Saupe E and Poduschka W (1995) Igel. In: *Krankheiten der Heimtiere, 3rd edn*, eds K Gabrisch and P Zwart. Schlutessche, Hannover, Germany

Smith JMB (1968) Diseases of hedgehogs. *Veterinary Bulletin* **38**, 425–430

Smith JMB and Marples MJ (1963) *Trichophyton mentagrophytes* var. *erinacei*. *Sabouraudia* **3**, 1–10

Stack MJ, Higgins RJ, Challoner DJ and Gregory MW (1990) Herpesvirus in the liver of a hedgehog (*Erinaceus europaeus*). *Veterinary Record* **127**, 620–621

Twigg GI, Cuerden CM and Hughes DM (1968) Leptospirosis in British wild mammals. *Symposium of the Zoological Society of London* **24**, 75–98

Visozo AD and Thomas WE (1981) Paramyxoviruses of the *Morbilli* group in the wild hedgehog (*Erinaceus europaeus*). *British Journal of Experimental Pathology* **62**, 79–86

7

Squirrels

Anthony W. Sainsbury

Introduction

There are two species of squirrel in the British Isles: the red squirrel, *Sciurus vulgaris*, and the grey squirrel, *Sciurus carolinensis*. Both are diurnal tree squirrels (Order Rodentia; Subfamily Sciurinae).

The red squirrel (see Figure 7.3) was previously widespread throughout the British Isles but it has now disappeared from much of the southern and central parts of mainland England, most of Wales, and parts of Ireland and Scotland. The loss of the red squirrel coincides with the spread of the American grey squirrel (Figure 7.1), which was introduced several times between 1876 and 1910 to different parks and estates throughout the country, and which is now widespread in England, Wales and Scotland. The red squirrel continues to decline in numbers and is likely to disappear completely from central and southern England and from Wales by 2030.

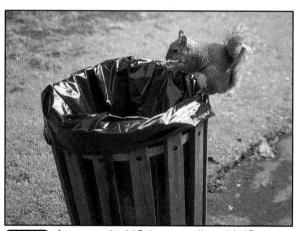

7.1 A grey squirrel (*Sciurus carolinensis*). (Courtesy of ME Cooper.)

The precise causes of red squirrel decline remain uncertain (Gurnell and Pepper, 1993; Gurnell and Lurz, 1997) but recent research suggests that red squirrel juvenile recruitment is lower when grey squirrels are present, and that this is influenced by habitat and tree seed availability (Wauters and Gurnell, 1999; Wauters *et al.*, 2000, 2001). There is increasing evidence that an infectious disease, parapoxvirus infection, has produced significant mortality of red squirrels. Also, it appears that the grey squirrel acts as a reservoir host for the virus

and so the alien species is implicated in the emergence of the disease as a threat to red squirrel populations (Rushton *et al.*, 2000; Sainsbury *et al.*, 2000). It is an offence to keep grey squirrels in captivity without a licence or to release them from captivity (see 'Legal aspects').

Ecology and biology

Both species inhabit conifer and broadleaved forests, and also urban parks and gardens with mature trees. They are solitary for much of the time but communal nesting may occur during winter and spring. Dominance hierarchies are not dependent on gender; larger and older animals are more dominant (Gurnell, 1991). Red squirrel densities are lower (0.3–1.0 squirrels/ha) than those of grey squirrels in broadleaved woods (2–8/ha) but tend to be similar in coniferous woods (0.03–1.3/ha). Aggressive encounters within species are rare but may result in bites to the ears, dorsum, rump or tail. Encounters between red and grey squirrels are mainly amicable (Wauters and Gurnell, 1999).

Scent marking occurs on specific branches or tree trunks, using urine and possibly secretions from mouth glands by face-wiping behaviour. Dispersal of juveniles and some adults principally occurs during the autumn and occasionally at other times of the year. Squirrels do not hibernate and are active all year, though they may remain in their nest (drey) for two or more days during severe winter weather. There is an annual cycle of numbers with a peak after breeding in the autumn, overwinter losses and a low in spring prior to recruitment.

The diet of free-living red or grey squirrels consists principally of tree seeds, such as hazelnuts, beechmast, acorns and conifer seed, as well as fruits, berries and fungi. Other foods include buds, shoots, flowers, bark, invertebrates and lichen (Gurnell, 1991). There are reports of squirrels eating bones found in their environment (Allan, 1935; Carlson, 1940; Coventry, 1940) and in captivity (Dickinson, 1995). Feeding signs for squirrels include hazel nuts split open, leaving two pieces of shell with clean edges, characteristic 'cores' of conifer cones with associated piles of stripped scales with clean cut edges (rather than the ragged edges made by birds), and bark stripping (Gurnell, 1991).

Anatomy and physiology

Red squirrels weigh between 270 g and 320 g when adult; grey squirrels are heavier and will weigh between 500 g and 600 g. The bodyweight can increase in the autumn by as much as 10% in the red squirrel and 17–13% in grey squirrels (Gurnell, 1991).

The dorsal coat of red squirrels varies considerably in colour from sandy to bright red or from grey to brown or dark brown. Often the tail is darker than the rest of the coat. The underside is creamy white in colour. During the autumn red squirrels grow long tufts on their ears and these are at their best in mid-winter. The tufts tend to thin during the spring and by the summer they have largely disappeared. The sides, limbs and paws of grey squirrels are often reddish brown; the underside is white or pale grey. Grey squirrels do not have prominent ear tufts. In both species, black (melanistic) forms exist. The body fur moults twice a year, apart from the ear tufts and tail hairs, which moult only once a year with new hairs growing in late summer/autumn.

The scent glands are present at the commissure of the mouth and in the upper and lower lips. There are four pairs of nipples in females. As with many other rodents, the sexes can be differentiated by the distance between the genital opening and the anus, which is very short in females and about 10 mm in adult males. The reproductive tract regresses in the autumn and perhaps in the winter if food supplies and weather are poor (Gurnell, 1991).

The faeces are cylindrical or round, slightly smaller than those of rabbits (8 mm diameter) and dark grey to black in colour but vary according to the diet (Gurnell, 1991).

Dentition

The incisors of squirrels, like those of other rodents, grow continuously and the lower incisors in particular occupy long sockets. The incisors have an enamel coating on the full length of their labial surfaces, while at the buccal aspect only the softer dentine is present and so the incisors are worn to a chisel-shaped cutting edge. The dental formula in both species is as follows:

$$2 \times \left\{ I \frac{1}{1} C \frac{0}{0} P \frac{2}{1} M \frac{3}{3} \right\} = 22$$

The first upper premolar is rudimentary and vestigial (Gurnell, 1991). In red squirrels, the lower incisors erupt at 19–21 days of age and the upper incisors at 31–42 days (Gurnell, 1991). The cheek teeth (molars and premolars) erupt from 7 weeks of age onwards and by 10 weeks of age all the cheek teeth are present (Tittensor, 1980). Primary first lower and only the second upper premolars are shed at 16 weeks of age and are replaced by permanent teeth (Holm, 1987). There are no canine teeth and there is a diastema between the incisors and the cheek teeth (Gurnell, 1987). The cheek teeth are quadrate with rounded blunt, cone-shaped bunodont marginal cusps and a concave central area (fossa) on their occlusal surfaces. The occlusal surfaces of the upper cheek teeth are traversed by weak transverse ridges (Gurnell, 1991; Kertesz, 1993). A young squirrel has a layer of enamel covering the surface of each cheek tooth, including the cusps and ridges. As age progresses this layer gets worn, exposing the underlying dentine (Shorten, 1954). Squirrels, like all rodents, have a marked degree of rostrocaudal gliding movement in their temporomandibular articulations and can move their jaws backward and forward (Crossley, 1995). The incisors of the lower jaw can be moved either towards (closed) or away (open) from each other and can be used to seize and crack nuts (Holm, 1987).

Reproduction

The breeding season of squirrels is between December/January (when both males and females of 9–10 months of age and older become sexually active) and August/September (when summer litters are weaned). There are two peaks in breeding: the first litters are born between February and April and the second between May and August (Gurnell, 1991). Males are fecund for most of the breeding season. Females are polyoestrous and in heat for approximately 24 hours during each oestrous cycle. They possess twin uterine horns leading to paired ovaries. A summary of reproductive traits, development of the young and longevity is given in Figure 7.2. On average, 75–85% of red and grey squirrels disappear during their first winter; thereafter average year-to-year survival improves to approximately 50%, depending on food availability.

Trait	Both species	Red squirrel	Grey squirrel
Breeding season	December–September		
Gestation period		36–42 days	44 days
Litter size	Average 3	1–6	1–7
Age develop hair covering	20–21 days		
Age eyes open	28–30 days		
Age begin to leave nest	7 weeks		
Age at weaning	8–10 weeks		
Age capable of breeding	10–12 months		
Mean life expectation at 6 months		3 years	F 4–5 years, M 2–3 years
Maximum life span		6–7 years (Gurnell, 1991)	9 years in wild 15 years in captivity

7.2 Reproductive traits, development and longevity of red and grey squirrels.

Capture, handling and transportation

Red squirrels are prone to 'breath-hold' when handled and must be restrained gently, quietly, with speed and only for short periods. When breath-holding, the squirrel becomes immobile and has a fixed stare. Breath-holding may in turn cause the squirrel to develop hypoxia, hypercapnia and a bradycardia, and this appears to be fatal in some cases. If this response is encountered, the squirrel should be placed immediately in a dark box or bag and allowed to recover unaided.

Both red and grey squirrels can inflict deep bites with their incisor teeth and possibly transmit zoonotic agents (see below and Chapter 2) and so it is advisable to wear gloves when handling them. Although the bite can penetrate leather gauntlets, the use of greater protection may make handling difficult. Alternative methods for restraint include the use of a net, a 'squeeze' cage, a sack (see below), or a wire handling cone (Figure 7.3). A squeeze cage designed for cats may be used for this purpose; or, when a squirrel is admitted in a cat basket without a squeeze device, towels may be fed through the mesh basket lid to secure the squirrel against the side of the basket (A.D. Routh, personal communication).

Traps

Various live traps for squirrels are available. Red squirrels (for which a trapping licence from the relevant government department is required) are best captured in a single-capture trap, with a removable nest box attached (Gurnell and Pepper, 1994); the trap is pre-baited with apple, carrot, maize, peanuts, sunflower seeds and hazelnuts for up to a week before setting. Grey squirrels can be trapped in multi-capture cage traps (Gurnell, 1996), usually baited with whole maize.

One method to remove a squirrel from its trap is to encourage it to enter a hessian sack. For example, the mouth of the sack can be closed firmly around the nest box, with the lid of the box being removed at the same time. Most squirrels will enter the sack voluntarily and, once there, can be confined to a corner. The physical form of the squirrel can be detected through the sack and the squirrel can be safely restrained by placing downward pressure on the dorsum, using the thumb and forefinger to control the head and neck and the remainder of the hand to control the body. The sack's mouth can then be reflected to examine the squirrel and, if necessary, apply a malleable rubber facemask to induce anaesthesia. Alternatively, the squirrel can be transferred from a nest box to a suitably sized handling cone (230 mm long, 20 mm diameter at the mouth) constructed of wire mesh (Figure 7.3). The squirrel will voluntarily run into the cone and can then be prevented from reversing by placing a finger behind it so that it can then be examined, or anaesthetized using a facemask. A sack, cone or nest box can also be used to transfer animals between cages.

Zoonoses

Infectious agents harboured by squirrels and known to infect humans include *Salmonella* spp., *Campylobacter* spp. (Duff *et al.*, 2001), rabies virus, *Borrelia burgdorferi* (Brown and Burgess, 2001), *Toxoplasma gondii* (Duff *et al.*, 2001), *Capillaria* spp, *Hymenolepis nana*, *Yersinia pseudotuberculosis*, *Trichophyton* spp. (Keymer, 1983) and *Erysipelothrix rhusiopathiae*.

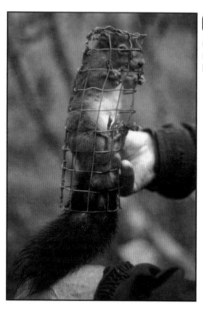

7.3 A red squirrel (*Sciurus vulgaris*) restrained in a handling cone.

Examination and assessment for rehabilitation

It is an offence to release grey squirrels into the wild in the UK (see 'Legal aspects' below and Chapter 5) and so only the red squirrel will be considered under this heading.

The potential for a successful rehabilitation and release of red squirrels must be established by a clinical examination using all relevant diagnostic methods. Body condition can be assessed as thin, good or fat by palpation of the soft tissues surrounding the femur. It is particularly important to ensure that the teeth are not overgrown and that they occlude satisfactorily. Findings that probably prevent successful rehabilitation and release, and therefore indicate that euthanasia is the best course of action, include incisor or molar overgrowth, malocclusion, an insufficiency of the organs of sight or hearing, and any disability that might permanently affect the squirrel's ability to climb or balance.

Blood can be collected from the femoral vein using a 2 ml syringe and 25 gauge needle (Figure 7.4). The technique is more easily carried out if the squirrel is sedated or anaethetized. The femoral vein is rarely visible and blind venepuncture is required. Figure 7.5 provides some reference values for haematology for

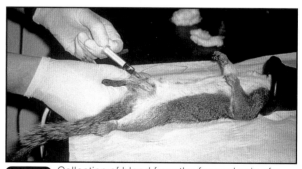

7.4 Collection of blood from the femoral vein of a squirrel. (Photograph by Terry Dennett.)

Variable	Range
Total haemoglobin (Hb) (g/dl)	9.90–17.41
Red blood cell count (RBC) (10^{12}/l)	4.92–8.29
Packed cell volume (PCV) (l/l)	30.29–52.62
Mean cell volume (MCV) (fl)	46.63–79.96
Mean cell haemoglobin (MCH) (pg)	14.11–27.76
Mean cell haemoglobin concentration (MCHC) (g/dl)	29.19–36.79
Reticulocytes (% RBC)	0.10–4.60
Heinz bodies (% RBC)	0.00–0.50
Total white cell count (WBC) (10^9/l)	0.00–12.28
Neutrophil count (10^9/l)	0.00–6.07
Lymphocyte count (10^9/l)	0.00–6.44
Monocyte count (10^9/l)	0.00–0.43
Eosinophil count (10^9/l)	0.00–0.58
Basophil count (10^9/l)	0.00–0.00
Platelet count [a] (10^9/l)	110.49–708.17
Erythrocyte sedimentation rate [b] (mm/h)	0.00–17.00
Fibrinogen [c] (g/l)	1.66–3.82

7.5 Haematology reference ranges for squirrels (n = 22) (Zoological Society of London Lynx Reference Database). [a] n = 15; [b] n = 11; [c] n = 12

the family Sciuridae. Sainsbury and Gurnell (1995) quoted some reference values for total protein, albumin, calcium, inorganic phosphate, alkaline phosphatase and alanine aminotransferase.

Euthanasia

Squirrels can be euthanased by dislocation of the neck or by intravenous or intraperitoneal injection of pentobarbital at a dose rate of 200 mg/kg bodyweight. The femoral vein is the author's preferred vein for intravenous injection. Dislocation of the neck is acceptable in conscious rodents of less than 150 g bodyweight but those of higher bodyweight must be sedated or anaesthetized prior to dislocation (Close *et al.*, 1997).

First aid procedures

Rehydration therapy is most easily administered by subcutaneous injection between the shoulder blades or lateral thorax. Intravenous administration will be required in a collapsed animal and the femoral vein is a possible route. Intraperitoneal administration is an alternative. It is important to keep collapsed squirrels warm and to administer analgesics.

Anaesthesia and analgesia

Like other rodents, squirrels do not vomit and so it is not necessary to starve them prior to anaesthesia. It may be valuable to administer fluids to squirrels under anaesthesia, by the subcutaneous route in well hydrated animals, to compensate for losses through respiration and urination. As for all small mammals with a high ratio of surface area to bodyweight, additional heat may be needed during anaesthesia to maintain body temperature.

Anaesthesia can be safely achieved by the use of isoflurane at 1–4% in oxygen, administered by a malleable facemask. Intubation is difficult but an intravenous catheter could be used as described for rats (Flecknell, 1996).

Ketamine at approximately 40 mg/kg bodyweight i.m. will provide sedation that wanes over a period of approximately 1 hour. Flecknell (1996) found that a combination of medetomidine (0.5 mg/kg) and ketamine (75 mg/kg) administered in the same syringe by intraperitoneal injection provided effective anaesthesia (though not necessarily for major surgery) in rats and this combination of agents has been used in grey squirrels by intramuscular injection (A.D. Routh, personal communication). Partial reversal of anaesthesia with atipamezole (1 mg/kg s.c.) is possible; in rats this should not be attempted until over 20 minutes after induction, due to the undesirable effects of ketamine.

On recovery, squirrels are best returned to a solid-sided wooden box with bedding material and an access port for monitoring the animal, which can be wrapped in kitchen foil or bubblewrap to reduce loss of body heat.

Analgesic use can be extrapolated from information available for rats (Flecknell, 1996), e.g. buprenophine (0.01–0.05 mg/kg s.c. or i.p. every 8 h) or carprofen (5 mg/kg s.c. once a day).

Specific conditions

Trauma

Traumatic injuries seen in squirrels include the results of road traffic accidents and bite wounds. The pathogenesis and treatment of these is similar to such injuries in other mammals.

Viral diseases

Parapoxvirus disease

Red squirrel parapoxvirus (RSPPV) is the aetiological agent of a disease known to cause high mortality in red squirrels (Sainsbury and Ward, 1996; Tompkins *et al.*, 2002). There is good evidence that the grey squirrel is a reservoir host of the RSPPV (Sainsbury *et al.*, 2001) and only a single case of disease associated with a parapox-like virus has been recorded in a grey squirrel (Duff *et al.*, 1996). It is unclear how the RSPPV is transmitted between squirrels but it is possible that direct or indirect skin-to-skin contact, or contact between body fluids and skin, is involved. The RSPPV produces characteristic skin lesions in red squirrels: erythematous exudative dermatitis and ulceration with some lesions covered by haemorrhagic crusts (Sainsbury and Gurnell, 1995) (Figure 7.6). These lesions are particularly located around the face, ventral skin surfaces of the body, medial skin of the legs and the genital region.

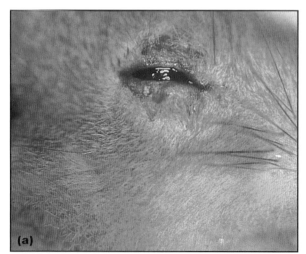

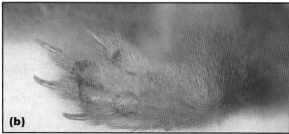

7.6 Parapoxvirus infection in red squirrel. (a) Lesions in facial area; (b) ulcerative lesions on toes. (Photographs by Terry Dennett.)

The disease can be diagnosed by electron microscopy of skin lesions. The clinical signs may be less severe in some cases and there is evidence that red squirrels show a variable immune response to the virus, and that some can survive the disease, despite showing the clinical signs for up to 4 weeks. These cases may benefit from supportive therapy such as antibiotics, antifungal agents, analgesics and fluids. Hand-feeding may be required if infections of the conjunctiva prevent vision. It might be possible to control the disease in the wild by preventing contact between red and grey squirrels, especially where grey squirrels may harbour the virus (i.e. all parts of England and Wales).

Adenovirus-associated disease

Diarrhoea is a common finding in sick squirrels. Diarrhoea, splenic necrosis and mortality have been associated with adenovirus infection of the intestine in captive and free-living red squirrels found dead (Sainsbury *et al.*, 2001; Couper, 2001). In most cases described, the large intestinal contents have a characteristic grey pasty appearance and adenovirus is detected by electron microscopy. The pathogenicity of adenovirus in red squirrels has not been confirmed and the distribution and prevalence of infection is unknown. Supportive therapy (fluids and antidiarrhoeal agents) should be administered.

Bacterial diseases

Bacterial enteritis can occur (Duff *et al.*, 2001) and it is likely that squirrels are susceptible to the same types of bacterial infections as are other rodents, e.g. by *Campylobacter* spp. and *Salmonella* spp. Antibiotic therapy should be used but it should be noted that

antibiotic toxicity due to disruption of the normal enteric microbial flora is likely to be as significant a problem as it is in other rodents. It would be wise to use antibiotic dose rates published for other rodents (see Chapter 8) and to choose an agent based upon sensitivity tests.

Ectoparasites

Fleas (*Monopsyllus sciurorum*), lice (*Neohaematopinus sciuri*) and sheep ticks (*Ixodes ricinus*) (Figure 7.7a) are found on red squirrels (Keymer, 1983), and in animals with concomitant disease the fleas and lice may increase to numbers at which it would be expected that they could cause additional debility. Keymer (1983) observed patchy alopecia in sick squirrels when heavily infested with lice and fleas. Grey squirrels are affected by the same species of lice and ticks as are red squirrels, but while *M. sciurorum* can infest grey squirrels the latter's pelage is more likely to be inhabited by the flea *Orchopeas howardii* (Keymer, 1983). Alopecia has been observed associated with infestation with larval harvest mites, *Neotrombicula* spp. (Figure 7.7b) but the clinical signs are usually mild. No other mites are known to infest squirrels in the UK.

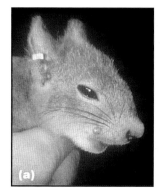
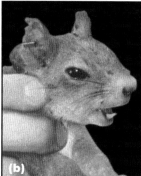

7.7 Ectoparasites on red squirrel. (a) Tick (*Ixodes ricinus*) on face. (b) Alopecia associated with infestation by larval harvest mites, *Neotrombicula* sp.

Fleas can be treated with fipronil. Tick infestations can be treated with ivermectin (200 µg of the 1% injectable solution/kg bodyweight, diluted in propylene glycol).

Endoparasites

Coccidiosis

The post-mortem findings from a survey of causes of mortality in red and grey squirrels in the UK suggested that coccidiosis could be a common cause of death in red squirrels (Keymer, 1983). Other authors have reported mortality due to coccidiosis: in red and grey squirrels in the UK (Tittensor, 1975, 1977) and red squirrels in Finland (Lampio, 1967). Several species of *Eimeria* have been described in red and grey squirrels and the pathogenicity of *E. sciurorum* has been confirmed experimentally (Pellérdy, 1974). However, although oocysts are frequently found in the intestine, coccidiosis has not been confirmed histologically in free-living squirrels in the cases reported above and there remains some doubt about the prevalence of this disease. It is possible that, as in other mammalian species, disease due to coccidia is precipitated by stressors or concomitant disease, or is secondary to poor management when in captivity (Radostits *et al.*, 1994).

Helminths
There is no evidence that helminths produce significant disease in red or grey squirrels (Keymer, 1983).

Other conditions

Malocclusion
Malocclusion occurs as a consequence of unaligned teeth, deviation of the mandible and maxilla from their usual position, or fractured teeth. Overgrowth of the incisors, which has been seen in free-living squirrels, can lead to difficulty in prehension and mastication, poor condition and eventually depression and starvation. In a survey of dental problems in free-living red squirrels (Kountouri *et al.*, in press) it was found that the most commonly encountered oral lesions were malocclusion of the incisor teeth (4 of 364 red squirrels) and attrition of the cheek teeth. The cause of malocclusion was unclear but was probably of degenerative, traumatic or nutritional origin. In some domesticated rodents there may be an inherited predisposition to develop the disease but there is no evidence to suggest this in squirrels.

Although it is possible to treat squirrels with malocclusion of the incisor teeth, the condition is likely to recur and therefore an animal with malocclusion is not suitable for rehabilitation.

Metabolic bone disease
Metabolic bone disease has been diagnosed in a wild red squirrel in the UK (Keymer and Hime, 1977) and in the reported case there appeared to be an association with supplementary feeding from bird tables. Affected red squirrels may show lethargy, weakness, loss of weight and a hunched posture due to curvature of the spine. A radiograph of an affected squirrel may show thin and uneven cortices of the long bones and coarse trabeculation. Captive rehabilitating squirrels may be prone to metabolic bone disease if their diet is not closely monitored. The only food source commonly fed to squirrels that contains a sufficient calcium/phosphorus ratio to prevent calcium deficiency is carrots (Gurnell *et al,*, 1990). Sunflower seeds and peanuts are high in unsaturated fatty acids which bind calcium in the gut and prevent absorption, thus tending to make the situation worse. To prevent metabolic bone disease see 'Feeding', below.

Cardiomyopathy
Robinson (1995) reported a cardiomyopathy in red squirrels examined after death. Sick squirrels in the same captive group appeared to respond to vitamin E and selenium therapy.

Encephalomyocarditis virus (a cardiovirus) has been isolated from red squirrels (Vizoso *et al.*, 1964).

Lens opacity
Opacity of the lens has been identified in dehydrated grey squirrels (A.D. Routh, personal communication). The lens clears after rehydration therapy (glucose saline) has been administered.

Therapeutics

The following injection techniques can be used in physically restrained or anaesthetized squirrels.

- **Subcutaneous injections** can be made under the skin overlying the neck or dorsal thorax, using a 25 gauge needle. Large volumes (up to 10 ml) can be administered.
- **Intramuscular injections** are best made into the quadriceps, using a 25 gauge needle. For rats, Flecknell (1996) recommended that no more than 0.2 ml should be injected in one site; red squirrels have a similar muscle size but grey squirrels are larger and greater volumes can be injected (0.5 ml).
- **Intraperitoneal injections** can be accomplished with the squirrel held with its ventrum uppermost, one hindlimb extended. The 25 gauge needle is introduced along the line of the leg into the centre of the caudal quadrant of the abdomen, to avoid the bladder and liver. Approximately 5 ml may be easily administered through this route.
- **Intravenous injection** is a difficult technique in squirrels. The femoral or ventral midline tail vein can be accessed.
- **Oral administration** may be possible by offering palatable medicines and fluids to be lapped from the end of a syringe. Medicines are difficult to administer to conscious squirrels by oesophageal or stomach tube because the restraint required to ensure that the catheter is properly placed may be too great a stressor. However, in certain cases, administration using a 20 gauge rodent catheter would be possible.

For dosage of some therapeutic agents, refer to those given in Chapter 8 for use in rats and mice.

Management in captivity

Housing
The housing of squirrels has been described in detail by Pepper (1998) and Davis (1998). Cages can be of galvanized weldmesh (25 mm) or stainless steel; squirrels are able to chew through softer materials such as aluminium. The cage should be elevated above 1 m because red squirrels, in particular, are arboreal. A nest box should be provided: suggestions include galvanized steel mesh boxes lined with plywood for insulation, which can be closed for capturing the squirrel, or cardboard boxes. Hessian sacking or paper should be used for bedding. Cage furniture usually includes a tree branch for the squirrel to chew.

Sick squirrels require warmth but temperatures should be gradually reduced to the ambient as the process of rehabilitation advances. Lighting too should ideally revert to natural levels as rehabilitation progresses. Prior to release, squirrels can be transferred to aviary-type caging with an outdoor run, which should be filled with plenty of branches to allow them to exercise and should have other cage furniture that they are likely to interact with in the wild, such as pine cones, logs, antlers and bones (Dickinson, 1995; Pepper, 1998).

Social grouping

Squirrels should generally be housed singly because they can be aggressive when in groups in cages. If a single-caged squirrel is housed within sight of another squirrel, screens should be erected between the two. It may be possible to group-house squirrels in large aviary-type outdoor enclosures in which there is at least one nest box available for each squirrel.

Behavioural problems

Squirrels housed in cages in captivity may develop stereotypic behaviour, such as to-and-fro movements or circling. It is not known whether this behaviour has any consequences for their welfare and survival in the wild but it is likely that the effects are minimal if the time in captivity is limited to a few weeks.

Feeding

Pepper (1998) fed a mixture of equal parts of whole-grain wheat, yellow whole maize and shelled peanuts to red and grey squirrels in captivity before gradually introducing them to a pelleted rodent diet. For squirrels that cannot be released, a rodent pellet (e.g. Mazuri Zoo Foods) provides a well balanced complete diet and is probably an ideal base, with small additional quantities of fruit and nuts to provide variety. It can take some time to wean squirrels on to pellet food and there may be initial weight loss; thus the transition from the previous diet must be carried out very gradually.

For animals that are to be released to the wild, it is advisable to use as natural a diet as possible, preferably comprising foods that will be found in the wild. In the USA, where grey squirrels are released, this might include acorns, pine nuts, walnuts, lichen, bark, various grasses, weeds, apples, plums and new growth from the tips of native trees and bushes (Davis, 1998). A diet fed to captive red squirrels by Dickinson (1995) included parrot mix, assorted nuts, Mazuri Zoo Food A (Mazuri Zoo Foods), Vitacraft Fruit Cocktail and Shaws Egg Biscuits (Shaws Pet Products, Aylesbury), supplemented by a variety of fruit and vegetables.

Many of the foods used to feed the squirrels in captivity have a low calcium:phosphorus ratio (e.g. nuts, maize and fruit). Squirrels are known to chew animal bones in the wild, probably partly as a means to ensure that their intake of calcium is sufficient. Therefore, it would be wise to give squirrels access to previously boiled porcine long bones (see 'Metabolic bone disease', above). As an additional safeguard to ensure that their calcium intake is adequate, calcium can be added to the drinking water (e.g. 1% Collo-Cal D, C-Vet).

Water should be provided *ad libitum* to squirrels in captivity and is usually offered in a water bottle or a secured dish. Wild-caught squirrels may not drink from a bottle initially and so water must be provided in a bowl until they are used to a bottle.

Rearing orphans

The dry matter of grey squirrel milk contains 39.6% solids, of which 67% is fat, 20% protein, 10% carbohydrates and 3% ash; it therefore has a high dry matter

and fat content (Kirkwood, 1989). Carnivore milk replacers have a higher percentage of fat than other replacers and can be used to raise orphan squirrels. Esbilac (Pet AG) and Cimicat (Hoechst) have been used by Davis (1998) and Dickinson (1995), respectively. Feeds will need to be given initially every 2 hours, starting with a total volume of approximately 3 ml/day for neonates. The anogenital area should be stimulated after each feed to induce urination and defecation. It may be valuable to feed Hartmann's (lactated Ringer's) or an electrolyte solution for the first one or two feeds to rehydrate the orphan and then gradually introduce the milk formula over the following three or four feeds and reduce the quantity of Hartmann's. If diarrhoea or bloat occurs, the volume of milk formula should be decreased. Weaning starts at approximately 4 weeks when grey squirrels weigh approximately 100 g. Apple, nuts, bark and pine cones can be offered. Davis (1998) gives further advice on hand-rearing.

Release

Pre-release assessment

If a squirrel has passed the assessment for rehabilitation, has been subsequently successfully treated and, following treatment, is believed to be healthy and shows no sign of behavioural abnormality, it should be considered fit for release. It is important that the squirrel's body condition is good and its bodyweight stable over a minimum of 7 days.

Release techniques

Site and time

Ideally the squirrel should be released in the same location as it was found. Davis (1998) recommended releasing orphaned grey squirrels at 12–14 weeks of age, before imprinting can occur. The best time of year for release is probably August to November, when squirrel populations have finished breeding and it is a normal time for dispersal and social reorganization. Furthermore, the weather is not cold or unduly wet in the UK and tree seed availability tends to be good at this time of year.

There do not seem to have been any studies that report on the success or failure of releases of rehabilitated squirrels but a few have reported on the release of captive-bred or translocated wild squirrels (Bertram and Moltu, 1986; Pritchard and Bruemmer, 1995; Venning et al., 1997; Wauters et al., 1997; Fornasari et al., 1997; Kenward and Hodder, 1998). These have been reviewed by Venning et al. (1997), who suggested that proximity to roads should be avoided when releasing squirrels due to the high probability that road traffic will kill dispersing squirrels. The presence of domestic dogs and cats in the release area may reduce the chances of successful releases. Red squirrels can be released successfully into both conifer and deciduous forests but should not be released into areas in which grey squirrels are present (even if there is a resident red squirrel population), because of the likelihood that the red squirrels will contract parapoxvirus infection.

Soft release

Kenward and Hodder (1998) carried out a soft release (see Chapter 3) of 14 red squirrels in Dorset from 3.4 m³ cages in which the animals were held for 3–6 days. Ten squirrels died within 45 days and all were dead by 126 days after release. In south-east Scotland, Pritchard and Bruemmer (1995) reported that 7 of 44 red squirrels in a release programme died prior to release, 9 died after release from cages measuring 4 m x 4 m x 2 m, in which the squirrels were housed for 10–20 days, and '2 or 3' had emigrated from the 280 ha woodland release site; the fate of the others was not known. Venning et al. (1997) reported the successful translocation of free-living red squirrels for conservation purposes, with better than 75% survival 2 weeks after release and better than 50% survival through to the following breeding season 6 months later.

The following soft release method was adopted by Venning et al. (1997) using a 1 ha pre-release pen in Thetford Chase, East Anglia. Each squirrel that had been translocated from elsewhere was placed on its own in a nest box, attached to a tree 3–4 m above ground level in the pre-release pen. Each box contained woodwool bedding and some food (apples, carrots, maize, peanuts, sunflower seeds, wheat and hazel nuts) and the entrance to each box was loosely plugged with woodwool to prevent the squirrel immediately bolting. Food and water, containing a calcium supplement (see 'Feeding') was placed on tables within the pen. The boxes were checked 6–9 hours later and if the woodwool plugs were still in place they were removed. Four hours later any squirrels remaining in their box were flushed out. The squirrels were housed in the pre-release pen for 4–6 weeks prior to release. Twenty food hoppers were available in the forest for squirrels to use within 400 m of the pen. After leaving the pen the squirrels were monitored by radio-tracking and live-trapping.

Usher-Smith (1995) found that 6 of 10 rehabilitated orphan red squirrels survived for a year after a soft release using portable release cages measuring 720 x 580 x 1350 mm high, wired to trees at approximately 0.7 m off the ground, and for 3¹/₂ months the squirrels could return to these release cages.

These examples illustrate how difficult the release of squirrels can be but show that it is more successful when the animals are given several weeks to acclimatize and pens in which to do so. Due to the work involved in a red squirrel release project, it may be better to release more than one animal at one time.

Hard release

Two hard-release (see Chapter 2) translocation studies have been carried out in continental Europe: one in an urban park in Antwerp, Belgium (Wauters et al., 1997) and one in woodland in Italy (Fornasari et al., 1997). In neither target area were red or grey squirrels present. Fornasari et al. (1997) released eight red squirrels, of which four remained alive after 2 months and a population of red squirrels was present 8 years later. In the Belgian study (Wauters et al., 1997), nest boxes were provided in the park and 19 red squirrels were released on the same day of capture from three different source areas. Of the 19 squirrels, 8 (3 males and 5 females) survived to breed.

Post-release monitoring

Released red squirrels should be marked. Subcutaneously implanted microchips or small tags (e.g. Dalton Mini Rototags) applied to both ears can be used (see Figure 7.7).

Legal aspects

It is important to note that it is an offence under the Grey Squirrel (Prohibition of Importation and Keeping) Order 1937 to keep grey squirrels without a licence, even if they are injured, and it is an offence to release them again under the Wildlife and Countryside Act (WCA) 1981. It is lawful to catch and euthanase a squirrel on welfare grounds.

Red squirrels are protected under the Wildlife and Countryside Act 1981 and it is illegal to disturb, capture or harm them without a licence from the relevant government department in the UK (e.g. Scottish Natural Heritage). It is also an offence to offer red squirrels for sale, or intentionally to kill them or intentionally to damage or destroy their shelters. The red squirrel is also listed on Appendix III of the 1979 Bern Convention (on the conservation of European wildlife and natural habitats), which regulates its exploitation. There is a clause in the WCA that allows for the capture and housing of red squirrels for veterinary treatment and rehabilitation purposes if they are not believed to be able to survive in the wild without intervention.

References and further reading

Allan PF (1935) Bone cache of a gray squirrel. Journal of Mammalogy **16**, 326

Bertram BC and Moltu DT (1986) Reintroducing red squirrels into Regent's Park. Mammal Review **16**, 81–89.

Brown RN and Burgess EC (2001) Lyme borreliosis. In: Infectious Diseases of Wild Mammals, eds ES Williams and IK Barker. Manson Publishing, London

Carlson AJ (1940) Eating of bone by the pregnant and lactating gray squirrel. Science **91**, 573

Close B, Banister K, Baumans V, Bernoth E-M, Bromage N, Bunyan J, Erhardt W, Flecknell P, Gregory N, Hackbarth H, Morton D and Warwick C (1997) Recommendations for euthanasia of experimental animals: Part 2. Laboratory Animals **31**, 1–32

Costa DL, Lehmann JR, Harold WM and Drew RT (1986) Transcoral tracheal intubation of rodents using a fibreoptic laryngoscope. Laboratory Animal Science **36**, 256–261

Couper D (2001) A study of the association between adenovirus and enteritis in free-living red squirrels, Sciurus vulgaris, in the United Kingdom. MSc Thesis, University of London

Coventry AF (1940) The eating of bone by squirrels. Science **92**, 128

Crossley DA (1995) Aspects of rodent dental anatomy. 1. Jaw movement in the rat. Journal of the British Veterinary Dental Association **4**, 1–2

Davis M (1998) The Western Gray Squirrel: Care in Captivity (revised edn). Wildlife Fawn Rescue, Kenwood, California

Dickinson P (1995) The maintenance of red squirrels in captivity. In: Rehabilitation of Red Squirrels, eds LM Collins et al., pp. 11–20. Zoological Society of Glasgow and West of Scotland, Glasgow

Duff JP, Scott A and Keymer IF (1996) Parapoxvirus infection of the grey squirrel. Veterinary Record **138**, 527

Duff JP, Higgins RJ, Sainsbury AW and Macgregor SK (2001) Zoonotic infections in red squirrels. Veterinary Record **148**, 123–124

Flecknell PA (1996) Laboratory Animal Anaesthesia, 2nd edn. Academic Press, London

Flecknell PA (1998) Developments in the veterinary care of rabbits and rodents. *In Practice* **20**(6), 286–295

Fornasari L, Casale P and Wauters L (1997) Red squirrel conservation: the assessment of an introduction experiment. *Italian Journal of Zoology* **64**, 163-167

Gurnell J (1987) *The Natural History of Squirrels*. Christopher Helm, London

Gurnell J (1991) Red squirrel (*Sciurus vulgaris*). In: *The Handbook of British Mammals*, eds GB Corbet and S Harris, pp. 177–186. Blackwell Scientific Publications, Oxford

Gurnell J (1996) The effects of food availability and winter weather on the dynamics of a grey squirrel population in southern England. *Journal of Applied Ecology* **33**, 325–328

Gurnell J and Lurz PWW (eds) (1997) *The Conservation of Red Squirrels*, Sciurus vulgaris L. People's Trust for Endangered Species, London

Gurnell J and Pepper, HW (1993) A critical look at conserving the British red squirrel, *Sciurus vulgaris*. *Mammal Review* **23**, 127–137

Gurnell J and Pepper H (1994) *Red Squirrel Conservation: Field Study Methods*. Research Information Note No. 255. Forestry Authority, Farnham

Gurnell J, Peck G, Pepper H and Davis J (1990) *Bone Disease in Captive Red Squirrels*. Forestry Commission, Wrecclesham

Holm J (1987) *Squirrels*. Whittet Books, London

Kenward RE and Hodder AH (1998) Red squirrels (*Sciurus vulgaris*) released into conifer woodland: the effect of source habitat, predation and interaction with grey squirrels (*Sciurus carolinensis*). *Journal of Zoology, London* **244**, 23–32

Kertesz P (1993) *A Colour Atlas of Veterinary Dentistry and Oral Surgery*. Wolfe Publishing, Aylesbury

Keymer IF (1983) Diseases of squirrels in Britain. *Mammal Review* **13**, 155–158

Keymer IF and Hime JM (1977) Nutritional osteodystrophy in a free-living red squirrel (*Sciurus vulgaris*). *Veterinary Record* **100**, 31–32

Kirkwood JK (1989) Artificially rearing young wild animals; rationale and techniques. In: *Proceedings of the Inaugural Symposium of the British Wildlife Rehabilitation Council, London, 19 November 1988*, eds S Harris and T Thomas, pp. 47–57. British Wildlife Council, c/o RSPCA, Horsham

Kountouri A, Sainsbury AW, du Boulay G and Kertesz P (in press) Oral disease in free-living red squirrels in the UK. *Journal of Wildlife Diseases*,

Lampio T (1967) Sex ratios and the factors contributing to them in the squirrel, *Sciurus vulgaris*, in Finland. *Finnish Game Research* **29**, 5–67

Pellérdy LR (1974) *Coccidia and Coccidiosis, 2nd edn*. Verlag Paul Parey, Berlin

Pepper HW (1998) *The Management of Squirrels in Captivity*. Forestry Commission Research, Alice Holt, Wrecclesham

Pritchard JS and Bruemmer C (1995) Investigation of methods to establish and subsequently manage a population of red squirrels in an isolated, commercially managed conifer plantation in South-East Scotland. In: *Proceedings of the Second NPI Red Alert for Red Squirrel Conservation*, eds DG Hughes and T Tew, pp. 67–71. Federation of Zoological Gardens of Great Britain and Ireland, Edinburgh

Radostits OM, Blood DC and Gay CC (1994) *Veterinary Medicine, 8th edn*. Baillière Tindall, London

Robinson I (1995) Red squirrels: disease and injuries. In: *Rehabilitation of Red Squirrels*, eds LM Collins *et al.*, pp. 21–27. Zoological Society of Glasgow and West of Scotland, Glasgow

Rushton SP, Lurz PWW and Gurnell J (2000) Modelling the spatial dynamics of parapoxvirus disease in red and grey squirrels: a possible cause of the decline in the red squirrel in the United Kingdom? *Journal of Applied Ecology* **37**, 1–18

Sainsbury AW and Gurnell J (1995) An investigation into the health and welfare of red squirrels, *Sciurus vulgaris*, involved in reintroduction studies. *Veterinary Record* **137**, 367–370

Sainsbury AW and Ward L (1996) Parapoxvirus infection in red squirrels. *Veterinary Record* **138**, 400

Sainsbury AW, Nettleton P, Gilray J and Gurnell J (2000) Grey squirrels have high seroprevalence to a parapoxvirus associated with deaths in red squirrels. *Animal Conservation* **3**, 229–233

Sainsbury AW, Adair B, Graham D, Gurnell J, Cunningham AA, Benko M and Papp T (2001) Isolation of a novel adenovirus associated with splenitis, diarrhoea and mortality in translocated red squirrels, *Sciurus vulgaris*. *Verhandlungsbericht des Erkrankungen der Zootiere* **40**, 265–270

Shorten M (1954) *Squirrels*. Collins, London

Tittensor AM (1975) *Red Squirrel*. Forestry Commission Forest Record 101. HMSO, London

Tittensor AM (1977) Red squirrel. Grey squirrel. In: *The Handbook of British Mammals, 2nd edn*, eds GB Corbet and HN Southern, pp. 153–172. Blackwell Scientific Publications, Oxford

Tittensor AM (1980) *The Red Squirrel*. Blandford Press, Poole

Tompkins DM, Sainsbury AW, Nettleton P, Buxton D and Gurnell J (2002) Parapoxvirus causes a deleterious disease in red squirrels associated with UK population declines. *Proceedings of the Royal Society, London, Series B*, **269**, 529–533

Usher-Smith J (1995) Rehabilitation and release of red squirrels. In: *Rehabilitation of Red Squirrels*, eds LM Collins *et al.*, pp. 29–32. Zoological Society of Glasgow and West of Scotland, Glasgow

Venning T, Sainsbury AW and Gurnell J (1997) Red squirrel translocation and population reinforcement as a conservation tactic. In: *The Conservation of Red Squirrels* Sciurus vulgaris L, eds J Gurnell and PWW Lurz, pp. 134–144. Peoples Trust for Endangered Species, London

Vizoso AD, Vizoso MR and Hay R (1964) Isolation of a virus resembling encephalomyocarditis from a red squirrel. *Nature* **201**, 849–850

Wauters LA and Gurnell J (1999) The mechanism of replacement of red squirrels by grey squirrels: a test of the interference competition hypothesis. *Ethology* **105**, 1053–1071

Wauters L, Somers L and Dondt AA (1997) Settlement behaviour and population dynamics of reintroduced red squirrels, *Sciurus vulgaris* in a park in Antwerp, Belgium. *Biological Conservation* **82**, 101–107

Wauters LA, Lurz PWW and Gurnell J (2000) The effects of interspecific competition by grey squirrels (*Sciurus carolinensis*) on the space use and population dynamics of red squirrels (*S. vulgaris*) in conifer plantations. *Ecological Research* **15**, 271–284

Wauters LA, Gurnell J, Martinoli A and Tosi G (2001) Does interspecific competition with grey squirrels affect the foraging behaviour and food choice of red squirrels? *Animal Behaviour* **61**, 1079—1091

Acknowledgements

The author would like to thank John Gurnell and Andrew Routh for their comments on an earlier draft of this chapter.

8

Other insectivores and rodents

Richard Saunders

Introduction

The species included in this chapter (Figure 8.1) are extremely common in terms of numbers but are presented relatively infrequently: out of 11,992 wild animal admissions to a wildlife facility in the east of England in the years 1999 and 2000, only 37 individuals of the species covered in this chapter were admitted – 12 voles, 2 moles, 11 shrews and 12 mice (A. Smith, personal communication). This is probably for the following reasons:

- Their small size makes them less noticeable
- They are usually nocturnal or crepuscular, or they live underground
- Most diseases or injuries prove rapidly fatal in these species
- Many people perceive some of the species to be vermin and would not present them for treatment.

However, they include species that are under threat or relatively rare due to habitat destruction or fragmentation (water vole, common dormouse) or are being actively reintroduced into areas of the UK in small numbers (common dormouse). Other, more numerous species are important indicators of environmental change (e.g. mice and voles) and are themselves an important food source for predatory species.

Reasons for admission

The main cause of injury and death in these species is predation. For example, of a year's production of field voles, 22% are taken by weasels and 13% by foxes; they are also the preferred prey of barn owls, especially in winter (Anon., 2001a), and fluctuations in vole populations can have effects on predator health (Appleby et al., 1999). Other predators include mink, otters and other mustelids, herons, other owl species, kestrels, buzzards, shrikes, corvids, predatory reptiles and fish. Victims of these predators are unlikely to be rescued and presented for treatment.

A major predator is the domestic cat. It is estimated that cats kill or bring into the house up to 200 million

Order and suborder	Family and subfamily	Species	Common name
Order Insectivora	Family Talpidae (moles and desmans)	*Talpa europaea*	European mole
	Family Soricidae (shrews)	*Sorex minutus* *Sorex araneus* *Neomys fodiens* *Crocidura suaveolens** *Crocidura russula**	Pygmy shrew Common shrew Water shrew Lesser white-toothed shrew Greater white-toothed shrew
Order Rodentia Suborder Myomorpha	Family Muridae Subfamily Microtinae (voles and lemmings)	*Clethrionomys glareolus* *Arvicola terrestris* *Microtus agrestis* *Microtus arvalis**	Bank vole Water vole Field or short-tailed vole Common vole
	Subfamily Murinae (rats and mice)	*Rattus norvegicus* *Rattus rattus* *Mus musculus* *Micromys minutus* *Apodemus sylvaticus* *Apodemus flavicollis*	Common or brown rat Ship or black rat House mouse Harvest mouse Wood mouse Yellow-necked mouse
	Family Gliridae (dormice)	*Muscardinus avellanarius* *Myoxus (Glis) glis*	Common dormouse Edible or fat dormouse
Suborder Sciuromorpha	Family Castoridae (beavers)	*Castor fiber*	European beaver

8.1 British insectivores and rodents discussed in this chapter. *Channel Islands only

small mammals per year, of which 65% are rodents and 19% are terrestrial insectivores (Woods *et al.*, unpublished data). These figures have been disputed by Nelson (2001) and Tabor (2001), with the latter claiming that the total was nearer 20 million mammals. Whilst some of these 'catted' prey are apparently undamaged and are immediately released, many are injured and some are presented for treatment.

Disturbance of nests by predators also leads to orphaned small mammals being discovered by the public. For example, the nests of common dormice, especially those that are near the ground, can be disturbed and the whole litter may be brought in by cats. Juvenile or hibernating dormice are often found after storms: the entire nest might be found blown out of a tree. Both common and edible dormice are accidentally disturbed in places such as lofts, haystacks, fruit stores and hedges, especially during hibernation (D. Woods, personal communication).

Juvenile animals have a peak incidence of injuries when dispersing from the nest environment. They may also suffer maladaptation problems from choosing unsuitable environments, such as moles selecting soil that is too dry or too waterlogged (Corbet and Harris, 1991).

Road traffic accidents are not infrequent (L. Garland, personal communication) but such small animals rarely survive to require treatment. Deliberate, accidental or malicious poisoning of most of these species usually results in rapid death (Anon., 2001a) or the animal dying below ground, so poisoning victims are rarely encountered, though populations may be adversely affected (Shore *et al.*, 1997). A further hazard is the increasing use of 'glue' traps, which can indiscriminately entrap small rodents and insectivores (Stocker, 2000).

Ecology, biology, anatomy and physiology

Insectivores

Moles

The European mole (*Talpa europaea*) is unpopular with groundsmen and gardeners, due to its soil spoil heaps (molehills). There is also potential for soil in molehills to contaminate silage production, and a mole's digging raises stones to the surface, which can damage machinery. Molehills covering 7% of the surface area of one field have been recorded (MacDonald, 1995). These are more common in the spring, when males are looking for females, or in times of food scarcity. Moles may legally be killed by approved traps placed in molehills, and by strychnine-laced earthworms (see Chapter 5).

However, moles are important aerators of soil and also eat large numbers of potentially harmful insect larvae. The tunnel systems form a food trap, which the mole patrols. Moles store food by killing and burying it when plentiful; when food is scarce, the tunnel system is extended in area and the moles tunnel deeper after earthworms (a major component of the diet). As an alternative to lethal mole control, the number of molehills can be decreased by encouraging increased earth-

worm numbers – for example, by not liming soil and by encouraging herb-rich swards (Edwards *et al.*, 1999).

Moles are born naked and blind in a spherical underground nest ('fortress') with vegetation for nesting material. There is no male parental care.

Shrews

There are two broad groups:

- Red-toothed shrews (*Sorex* and *Neomys* spp.) all have red-tipped teeth, due to iron deposition in the enamel. They include the pgymy, common and water shrews
- White-toothed shrews (*Crocidura* spp.) have no red tips to teeth.

In areas where one shrew species coexists with other shrew species, the different species are rarely found together at the same time. The common shrew (*Sorex araneus*) is the second most common mammal in Britain, with an estimated population of 41 million. Pygmy shrews (*Sorex minutus*; Figure 8.2) are the smallest mammals in Britain.

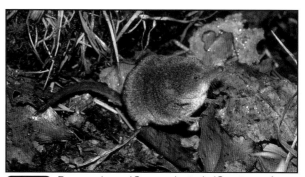

8.2 Pygmy shrew (*Sorex minutus*). (Courtesy of Andy Purcell/Conservation Education Consultants. © CEC.)

Bodies of shrews are frequently found inside discarded bottles, often in large numbers, as one corpse can attract others. They are unpalatable to predators because of their sebaceous secretions; thus they are rarely eaten once caught, especially by mammalian predators.

Shrews have a high metabolic rate and must feed regularly, consuming a high percentage of bodyweight in food daily; even more food is required during lactation. Their prey contains large amounts of water and indigestible chitin. White-toothed shrews add some plant material to the typical insectivore diet of shrews. The bodyweight of shrews varies markedly with season (Figure 8.3); this is not due solely to food availability, as it applies also to captive shrews.

Shrews are highly territorial, especially the males, and are generally solitary; the white-toothed shrews (*Crocidura suaveolens* and *C. russula*) are solitary but not as aggressive as other species. Shrew territories are marked with sebaceous scent glands and faeces. They are vocal animals, making a series of high, shrill squeaks. All species can swim but only the water shrew (*Neomys fodiens*; see Figure 8.17) hunts in water; it swims and dives well.

Parameter	Mole	Shrews	Water shrew	Pygmy shrew	Common shrew	White-toothed shrews
Distribution	Mainland Britain but not Ireland or Scottish islands		Sporadically throughout Britain; widespread but not numerous	Mainland Britain, fairly common and widely distributed; only shrew native to Ireland	Lowland mainland Britain but not in Ireland	Channel Islands only: lesser on Scilly Isles, Sark, Jersey; greater on Alderney, Guernsey, Herm
Habitat	Arable, pasture, grassland, woodland (mainly deciduous), gardens, golfcourses; avoid very heavy clay and acidic soils or areas liable to waterlogging		Close to water, living in tunnels along water's edge	Mainly in wooded areas (similar habitats to common shrew)	Rough pasture, woods, hedgerows, dunes, marshes	Wide variety but fairly dry, well vegetated
Active periods	Day and night, for periods of 4–4½ h interspersed with sleep periods of 3–4 h. No hibernation	Alternate between periods of activity and rest, approx. every 2–3 h. No hibernation	Alternate between periods of activity and rest, approx. every 2–3 h. No hibernation	Alternate between periods of activity and rest, approx. every 2–3 h. No hibernation	Alternate between periods of activity and rest, approx. every 2–3 h. No hibernation	Alternate between periods of activity and rest, approx. every 2–3 h. No hibernation
Food requirements per day (approx. % of bodyweight)	50%		Up to 50%	Over 100%	Up to 70%	Up to 55%
Appearance	Coat black velvety with coarse and fine hairs; moult three times a year. Long tapering mobile snout covered in vibrissae. Small deepset eyes, no external pinnae. Short furred tail held erect. Broad forelimbs, muscular shoulders, long strong claws; three antebrachial bones, elongated scapula. Testes in sac near tail base	Fur often short and velvety. Long pointed snouts, small pointed teeth	Fur dark brown/black dorsally (looks silvery in water), silver-grey underside, with sharp demarcation between the two; white patch above eyes; long hairs on toes; hairs on underside of tail form a keel. Fur often short and velvety. Long pointed snouts, small pointed teeth	Fur pale brown dorsal body, paler underside, fairly sharp dividing line between the two; no eye patch; short hairs fringe toes. Tail is thicker and hairier than common shrew, snout thicker and longer. Skull domed. Fur often short and velvety. Long pointed snouts, small pointed teeth	Fur dark brown dorsally, paler sides and grey-white belly fairly clearly demarcated; no eye patch; short hairs fringe toes. Ears short, covered in fur. Fur often short and velvety. Long pointed snouts, small pointed teeth	Fur reddish-brown. Large ears. Fur often short and velvety. Long pointed snouts, small pointed teeth
Weight	Male < 120 g spring/summer, > 95 g autumn/winter. Female < 110 g spring/summer, < 75 g autumn/winter		9–16 g	2.5–5 g	7–10 g	Lesser 3–7 g. Greater 4.5–14.5 g
Size	Male < 140 mm. Female < 130 mm		90 mm (+ 60 mm tail)	40–58 mm (+ 40 mm tail)	48–85 mm (+ 24–55 mm tail)	Lesser 50–75 mm (+ 24–44 mm tail). Greater 60–90 mm (+ 33–46 mm tail)

8.3 Characteristics and biological parameters of moles and shrews (continues).

Parameter	Mole	Shrews	Water shrew	Pygmy shrew	Common shrew	White-toothed shrews
No. of nipples	4 pairs		5 pairs	3 pairs	3 pairs	3 pairs
Senses	Eyesight poor, hearing only moderate, olfactory senses good Main method of food detection via touch and sensitivity to vibration (Eimers organs on vibrissae)	Eyesight poor Prey located by hearing, touch and smell	Eyesight poor Prey located by hearing, touch and smell	Eyesight poor Prey located by hearing, touch and smell	Eyesight poor Prey located by hearing, touch and smell	Eyesight poor Prey located by hearing, touch and smell
Dentition	$2 \times \left\{ I\frac{3}{3}\ C\frac{1}{1}\ P\frac{4}{4}\ M\frac{3}{3} \right\} = 44$		$2 \times \left\{ I\frac{3}{2}\ C\frac{1}{0}\ P\frac{2}{1}\ M\frac{3}{3} \right\} = 30$	$2 \times \left\{ I\frac{3}{1}\ C\frac{1}{1}\ P\frac{3}{1}\ M\frac{3}{3} \right\} = 32$	$2 \times \left\{ I\frac{3}{1}\ C\frac{1}{1}\ P\frac{3}{3}\ M\frac{3}{3} \right\} = 32$	$2 \times \left\{ I\frac{3}{1}\ C\frac{1}{0}\ P\frac{1}{2}\ M\frac{3}{3} \right\} = 28$
Breeding season	March–May		March–August	April–October	April–September	March–September
Oestrus	Cycle 3–4 days, duration < 24 h		Seasonally polyoestrous Post-partum oestrus seen	Lactational anoestrus sometimes seen	Post-partum oestrus (< 24 h) after first litter; later extended by lactation	Polyoestrous, post-partum oestrus; no delayed implantation reported
Gestation	28–30 days		20–24 days	20–21 days	13–19 days	Lesser 24–32 days Greater 27–33 days
No. of litters per year	Usually 1		2–3	2–3	2–3	Lesser 3–4 Greater multiple
Litter size	2–7 (usually 3–4)		3–9	4–7	5–7	Lesser 1–6 (mean 3) Greater 3–11 (mean 3–4)
Birthweight	3.5 g		< 1 g	0.25 g	0.5 g	Lesser 0.5–1 g Greater 0.8–1 g
Development of young	Furred at 14 days Weigh 60 g at 3 weeks Eyes open 22 days Leave nest at 35 days Share adult tunnels until 10 weeks	Born naked and blind	Dorsal pigments develop at 4 days Teeth start to erupt at 10 days Fur develops at 11 days First leave nest at 23–25 days Born naked and blind	Born naked and blind	Soft grey fur at 9 days Teeth red-tipped 11 days Weigh 5–7 g by 14 days Leave nest at 18 days Born naked and blind	Fur starts growing 7–9 days; fully furred 16 days Born naked and blind
Age at weaning	28–35 days		21–25 days	22–25 days	22–25 days	Lesser 17–22 days Greater 20–22 days
Lifespan	2½–3 years		< 19 months	< 1 year	< 1 year	18 months

8.3 (continued) Characteristics and biological parameters of moles and shrews.

Approximately 25% of the juvenile shrew population survive the winter to breed the following spring. Adult shrews usually die in the autumn after their breeding season; only water shrews, which can live for up to 19 months, breed for a second year.

The characteristics and biological parameters of the insectivores (moles and shrews) are outlined in Figure 8.3.

Rodents

Voles

Characteristics and biological parameters of voles are given in Figure 8.4. Voles, which are typically blunt-faced with small eyes, are amongst the most prevalent of British mammals, though the water vole (*Arvicola terrestris*; see Figure 2.4b) is relatively scarce and is rapidly declining due to loss and degradation of habitat, pollution and also predation by mink. Water voles swim and dive well; they dive into water if danger threatens and always have at least one underwater burrow entrance.

Lacking the shrews' noxious secretions, voles are eaten by many predators – including stoats, weasels, polecat, pine martens, wildcats, badgers, foxes, herons, kestrels, buzzards, eagles, harriers and owls. They are commonly brought in by domestic cats. The field or short-tailed vole (*Microtus agrestis*) is the most common British mammal, with an estimated population of 75 million, but is subject to population fluctuations on a cycle of 3–5 years.

Parameter	Bank vole	Field or short-tailed vole [a]	Water vole
Distribution	Mainland Britain and coastal islands	Widespread mainland Britain; absent Ireland, Scilly Isles and N Scotland	England, Wales and S. Scotland; absent Ireland
Habitat	Woodland, moist deforested areas, grassland, gardens, hedges	Grassland (creates runs in grass)	Near water; at least one burrow entrance under water
Active periods	Summer day and night. Winter mainly diurnal	Cycles (2–2½ h) of rest and activity; peak activity dawn and dusk. More nocturnal summer; more diurnal winter	Active every 2–4 h and for longer in the day than at night. Rarely outside in winter
Diet	Leaves, fruits, seeds, fungi, bark, berries	Predominantly grass	Waterside vegetation, 'lawns' of closely cropped grasses surrounding burrow entrances; also loose aquatic weeds
Appearance	Fur reddish-brown; blunt muzzle, small ears	Fur grey-brown; very short tail	Fur rich dark brown, occasionally black
Male weight	20–25 g	37 g (20–40 g)	150–300 g
Female weight	15–20 g	30 g (20–40 g)	150–300 g
Size (including tail)	100–110 mm (+ 35–70 mm tail)	100–120 mm	180–220 mm
Nipples	4 pairs	4 pairs	4 pairs
Breeding season	April–Sept.; can also breed in winter	April–Sept.	Spring/summer, starting earliest in warmer years
Oestrus	Induced ovulator	Induced ovulator	Induced ovulator
Gestation	17–22 days	18–20 days	20–22 days
No. litters per year	Multiple (at least 4)	5–6	1–4
Litter size	3–5	4–6	4–6
Birthweight	2 g (naked and blind)	2 g (naked and blind)	5 g (naked and blind)
Development	Dorsal skin darkens 3 days; coat develops 4–10 days. Eyes open 12 days. Weaned 17–18 days. Thermoregulatory ability develops 16–19 days. All molars erupted 28–30 days	21 g by September/October. Weaned 14–18 days	22 g within 14 days. Leave nest around 22 days. 160 g within 5 weeks of birth
Age at weaning	14–28 days	18 days	14 days
Sexual maturity	Spring following birth (male min. 1½ months, female min. 2 months)	6 weeks	From 5 weeks
Lifespan	Max. 18 months (mean 4 months)	Max. 18 months	5 months

8.4 Characteristics and biological parameters of voles. [a]Common vole is confined to Channel Islands and has characteristics and parameters very similar to those of the field vole.

Rats and mice

Characteristics and biological parameters of rats and mice are shown in Figures 8.5 to 8.7.

Rats and mice are found throughout the British Isles (though the yellow-necked mouse and the harvest mouse have more localized distributions), often in close association with human dwellings and agricultural land. All are largely nocturnal. Mice are important prey species for many animals.

Rats and mice have more pointed muzzles and longer tails than the voles, but shorter muzzles than the shrews. They are anatomically and physiologically similar to their domestic counterparts.

The common or brown rat (*Rattus norvegicus*; Figure 8.6a) and the ship or black rat (*Rattus rattus*; Figure 8.6b) swim well and are often found close to water. Both live in social groups. Brown rats burrow well; black rats are good climbers and rather shy.

Parameter	Common or brown rat	Ship or black rat
Distribution	Common and widespread	Patchy, now quite rare
Habitat	Towns and agricultural land (especially arable or near food stores); often close to water	Usually near water
Diet	Anything digestible	Omnivorous but more vegetarian than brown rat
Appearance	Fur brown; long naked tail	Fur dark brown to grey/black; slimmer than brown rat
Weight	100–600 g	150–200 g
Head and body length	220–280 mm	200 mm
Tail length	200–220 mm	260 mm
Nipples	6 pairs	5 pairs (variable)
Dentition	$2 \times \left\{ I \dfrac{1}{1} \ C \dfrac{0}{0} \ P \dfrac{0}{0} \ M \dfrac{3}{3} \right\} = 16$	$2 \times \left\{ I \dfrac{1}{1} \ C \dfrac{0}{0} \ P \dfrac{0}{0} \ M \dfrac{3}{3} \right\} = 16$
Breeding season	All year if food available	March–November
Oestrus	Post-partum oestrus within 18 h of birth; cycle 4–6 days; polyoestrous	Similar to brown rat
Gestation	21–24 days	21–22 days (23–29 if lactating)
No. of litters per year	Up to 5	3–5
Litter size	6–11 (depending on bodyweight of mother)	1–11 (usually 7–8)
Development	Born naked and blind Fully furred and eyes open 15 days	Born naked and blind
Age at weaning	21 days	About 21 days
Sexual maturity (female)	11 weeks; 115 g	3–5 months; 90 g
Lifespan	1–2 years	1 year

8.5 Characteristics and biological parameters of brown and black rats.

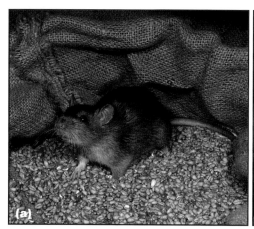
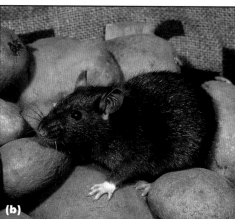

8.6 (a) Brown rat (*Rattus norvegicus*); (b) Black rat (*Rattus rattus*). (Courtesy of Andy Purcell/Conservation Education Consultants. © CEC.)

Parameter	House mouse	Wood mouse	Yellow-necked mouse	Harvest mouse
Distribution	Widespread	Throughout mainland Britain and islands	Patchy localized: found only in Wales, C and S England	Mainly S and C England; absent Ireland
Habitat	Usually in association with human habitation or arable land	Commonest mouse of woods, hedgerows, mature gardens; may come inside dwellings in colder weather	Woodland, especially ancient; may enter dwellings in colder months	Stalk zone of reeds, cereal crops, hedgerows, weeds
Nest	Vary from simple pallet to spherical. Any available material used	Underground burrows; nests of leaves, moss, grass (communal winter; females singly to breed)	Extensive burrows and nests	Nest size of tennis ball among plant stems
Diet	Seeds, vegetables, fruit, stored food	Seeds, seedlings, buds, fruit (pips only), nuts, snails, insects, spiders, woodlice, fungi, moss, bark, hips, haws, beetle larvae and adults, caterpillars, grain, grass flowers, weed seeds, earthworms, bulbs, beans, peas, tomatoes	Tree seeds (especially high-energy), fruits, some green plants, invertebrates (caterpillars, other insect larvae, worms)	Cereal grains, seeds, berries, insects, wheat aphids, nectar, moss, roots, fungi
Appearance	Fur greyish-brown dorsally, slightly paler underneath, normally quite greasy	Fur brown dorsally, pale underside	Similar to wood mouse (fur brown dorsally, white underside) but with yellowish collar around throat. Larger than wood mouse	Fur red to golden brown dorsally, pale underside. Blunt nose; small hairy ears
Weight	12–20 g	13–18 g winter 25–27g summer	14–45 g	4–6 g
Head and body length	75–100 mm	75–100 mm	95–120 mm	50–70mm
Tail length	75–100 mm	70–100 mm	75–120 mm	50–70 mm
Nipples	5 pairs	4 pairs		4 pairs
Dentition	$2 \times \left\{ I \dfrac{1}{1} \ C \dfrac{0}{0} \ P \dfrac{0}{0} \ M \dfrac{3}{3} \right\} = 16$	As house mouse (molar shape varies between species)	As house mouse (molar shape varies between species)	As house mouse (molar shape varies between species)
Breeding season	April–Sept.	Feb.–Oct.	Feb.–Oct.	May–Oct.
Oestrus	Cycle 4–6 days, post-partum oestrus within 24 h	Cycle 4–6 days, post-partum oestrus	Cycle 4–6 days, post-partum oestrus	Polyoestrous, post-partum oestrus
Gestation	19–20 days (up to 36 if lactating)	19–20 days (up to 26 when lactating)	23 days	17–19 days
No. of litters per year	Up to 10	Up to 6 (typically 1–2)	Successive Feb.–Oct.	2–3
Litter size	5–6	2–11 (typically 4–7)	2–11	3–8
Birthweight	1 g (naked and blind)	1–2.5 g (naked and blind)	2.8 g (naked and blind)	0.6–1 g (naked and blind)
Eyes open	2–3 days	16 days	13–16 days	8–9 days
Development	Skin darkens 5–7 days; hair half grown 8–10 days; hairgrowth complete and incisors erupted 14 days	Fur appears 6 days, starting on dorsum; incisors erupt 13 days; hindfeet darken 14 days; autumn-born young develop more slowly	Juvenile coat developed 14 days; yellow collar visible	Dorsal fur 4 days; ventral fur develops 8–9 days; juvenile grey/brown fur 14 days
Age at weaning	18 days	18–22 days (6–8 g)	21 days	15–16 days
Sexual maturity	5–6 weeks	2 months (male 15 g, female 12 g)	2–3 months (male 20 g, female 10 g)	35–45 days
Lifespan	1–2 years	< 1 year	1 year (av. 3–4 months)	< 18 months (generally 6 months)

8.7 Characteristics and biological parameters of mice.

House mice (*Mus musculus*) are less common than formerly, due to the improved protection of stored grain, and are less of a pest species than in the past.

Wood mice (*Apodemus sylvaticus*; see Figure 8.13) are the most common mouse of woods, hedgerows and mature gardens and are an important prey species. They cache food and live in underground burrows and nests of leaves, moss and grass, forming communal nests in winter but nesting singly to breed. Wood mice undergo torpor if subjected to food deprivation and cold weather.

The yellow-necked mouse (*Apodemus flavicollis*) was the last small mammal to be recognized as a separate species in Britain, in 1894. They are agile woodland mice and expert climbers. They enter dwellings mainly in autumn and winter months and this is not solely due to cold weather or decreased food availability, though the exact reasons are not fully understood (Anon., 2001b). They are a species of ancient woodland (their distribution is similar to that of mistletoe) and feed off tree seeds; they are therefore vulnerable to woodland loss and fragmentation (Anon., 2001a). They form extensive nests and burrows, some of which are used to cache food.

Harvest mice (*Micromys minutus*; Figure 8.8), Britain's smallest rodents, are preyed upon by weasels, stoats, foxes, cats, owls, hawks and crows, and their remains form 1% of barn owl pellets. They are excellent climbers, with prehensile tails almost as long as their bodies. They construct nests the size of tennis balls, among plant stems.

Dormice

Characteristics and biological parameters of dormice are given in Figure 8.9. Both species are largely nocturnal or crepuscular.

The preferred environment of the common or hazel dormouse (*Muscardinus avellanarius*; Figure 8.10) is coppiced hazel woodland, where it tends to live in trees at about 5 m above ground level. This habitat has been in decline, which both decreases the amount of available habitat and isolates small populations of dormice from each other. Dormice can live in commercial coppiced woods and recently much effort has been made to attempt to render these 'dormouse-friendly' and to release dormice into them, with some success (D. Woods, personal communication).

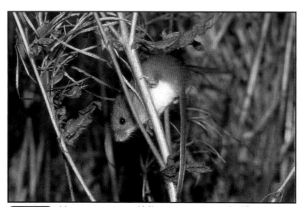

8.8 Harvest mouse (*Micromys minutus*). (Courtesy of Andy Purcell/Conservation Education Consultants. © CEC.)

Parameter	Common dormouse	Edible (fat) dormouse
Distribution	Scarce, localized and declining population; isolated colonies Wales and C and S England	Chilterns
Habitat	Preferably coppiced hazel woodland in trees at approx. 5 m above ground level	Preferably beech woods
Nest	Globular, 7.5 cm diameter (twice as big for breeding); hibernatory nests nearer or on ground	Arboreal, also rock clefts, old woodpecker holes, lofts
Hibernation	October–May	October–April
Diet	Flowers, nuts and fruits, especially honeysuckle and hazel; insects eaten in summer	Fruit and nuts, insects, birds' eggs and young birds, acorns, seeds, buds, bark, fungi
Appearance	Fur reddish; hamster-like appearance but well furred prehensile tail; male longer anogenital distance than female, and small dark-pigmented scrotum in breeding season	Greyish coat with pale underbelly; short muzzle, many whiskers, large eyes and small rounded ears; long furry tail
Weight	15–30 g (upper weight found only immediately prior to hibernation)	85–140 g (can be up to 250 g shortly before hibernation)
Size (head and body length)	80 mm (tail 60 mm)	120–150 mm
Nipples	4 pairs	4–6 pairs
Dentition	$2 \times \left\{ I \dfrac{1}{1} \, C \dfrac{0}{1} \, P \dfrac{1}{1} \, M \dfrac{3}{3} \right\} = 22$	$2 \times \left\{ I \dfrac{1}{1} \, C \dfrac{0}{0} \, P \dfrac{1}{1} \, M \dfrac{3}{3} \right\} = 20$
Breeding season	June to early August	June to early August

8.9 Characteristics and biological parameters of dormice. (continues) ▶

Parameter	Common dormouse	Edible (fat) dormouse
Gestation	21–24 days	30–32 days
No. of litters per year	1–2	1
Litter size (approx.)	4	5
Birthweight	Blind, naked	1–2 g; blind, naked
Development	Grey fur 7 days; coat well developed 13 days; leave nest 30 days	Fur developed 14–16 days
Eyes open	18 days	21–23 days
Age at weaning	Remains with mother until 6–8 weeks old	28–30 days, when leave nest
Sexual maturity	Spring of year after birth	Spring of year after birth (can be the following year in late-born young)
Lifespan	Max. 4 years in wild	Up to 6 years

8.9   (continued) Characteristics and biological parameters of dormice.

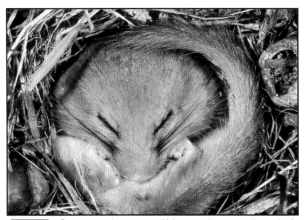

8.10   Common dormouse (*Muscardinus avellanarius*). (Courtesy of John Robinson/Conservation Education Consultants. © CEC.)

During hibernation, body temperature drops to 5°C or lower. For much of the rest of the year they are torpid during the day and predominantly active at night. They are very territorial in the breeding season.

The edible or fat dormouse (*Myoxus glis*; Figure 8.11) was introduced into Britain in Tring, Hertfordshire, in 1902. It is now established in the Chilterns and rarely seen elsewhere; it can be a pest in orchards and conifer plantations. Edible dormice are fairly sociable and largely arboreal. They can almost double their bodyweight before hibernation underground or in lofts during winter months.

European beaver

Characteristics and biological parameters of the European beaver (*Castor fiber*) are given in Figure 8.12.

This nocturnal species was once native to the British Isles but the last recorded sighting was near Loch Ness in 1527 (MacDonald, 1995). There are plans to reintroduce beavers to Scotland (Taylor, 1999) and there are also plans for their monitored release in south-east England as a conservation management species. There are captive groups elsewhere in the country. These animals may be presented to the veterinary surgeon for pre-release examination, or as wildlife casualties.

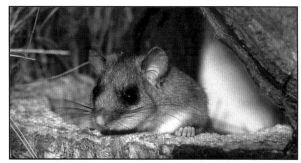

8.11   Edible dormouse (*Myoxus glis*). (Courtesy of Andy Purcell/Conservation Education Consultants. © CEC.)

Diet	Water plants, bark, roots, shoots and thistles
Weight	12–30 kg
Size (head and body length)	850–1300 mm
Nipples	4 pairs
Dentition	$2 \times \left\{ I\ \frac{1}{1}\ C\ \frac{0}{0}\ P\ \frac{1}{1}\ M\ \frac{3}{3} \right\} = 20$
Breeding season	October–November
Oestrus	2-week oestrous cycle; receptive for 10–12 h
Gestation	100–120 days
No. of litters per year	1
Litter size	2–4
Birthweight	230–630 g, born fully furred with open eyes
Development	Young not independent until 3 years of age; high juvenile survival rate
Age at weaning	3 months
Sexual maturity	2–2½ years
Lifespan	Approx. 10 years

8.12   Characteristics and biological parameters for European beaver.

Beavers are the second largest rodent species in the world (weights of up to 30 kg have been recorded for both the European and North American species) and have a large spatulate scaled tail, which is slapped on the water as an alarm signal. Scandinavian beavers are smaller and darker than the southern European ones. They have webbed hindfeet and smaller, more dextrous forefeet. Their adaptations to an underwater environment include eyes that are covered by a nictitating membrane under water, ears and nostrils that can close under water, and the ability to close off the throat with the base of the tongue, to enable them to carry sticks in their mouths under water.

Beavers pair for life. Sexing is difficult, as the urogenital and anal orifices open into a common cloaca. If manual palpation of the cloaca is equivocal, lateral radiography of the area can be used to demonstrate an os penis in the male.

Capture, handling and transportation

General handling techniques for these species are covered in greater detail in appropriate laboratory or domestic rodent texts (Flecknell, 1991, 1998; Fallon, 1996; Bauck and Bihun, 1997; Hrapkiewicz et al., 1998). However, they are much more liable to bite than equivalent domestic rodent species and are easily stressed, necessitating general anaesthesia for all but the most superficial examination (Fowler, 1993, 1995).

These animals should be handled or caught only when necessary. Indirect methods are less stressful – for example, catching in a net, box or tube and transporting them without direct handling.

Most small species are extremely fast and agile; some can jump and climb well; and most immediately head for cover – all exits and hiding places should be blocked up in advance. Mice are most likely to jump away, and voles and shrews to run away. Nets can be useful for initially trapping or recapturing the animals. The netting should be of solid material or very fine mesh, to avoid claws catching in the weave (Fowler, 1995), and the rims should be padded to avoid injury and escape.

Dim light should be used, to reduce activity levels and stress. Gloves increase the handler's confidence but severely reduce dexterity and control: the lightest gloves possible should be used, if at all. It is easy to grip smaller mammals too tightly and restrict breathing whilst wearing gloves (Fallon, 1996) and thick gloves only really have a place in the handling of the edible dormouse and the rat (A. Hudson, personal communication). Latex gloves may be used with the water shrew and with any individual suspected of carrying zoonotic infections; and as these infections are potentially present in all the species described here, it would be prudent to wear latex gloves in all cases. They may also be sufficient to prevent the bite of the smaller voles and shrews from breaking the skin.

Most species can be contained initially, and for medium-term accommodation, in small plastic pet boxes of the type sold for holding invertebrates, with a trapdoor opening in a removable top to allow the animal to be fed whilst minimizing the risk of escape (Stocker, 2000).

Moles
Moles can be held by the scruff of loose skin on the back of the neck and lifted very briefly by the tail, with the body supported (Bourne, 2001). It is important to avoid handling the sensitive nasal area (Lawson, 1999).

Mice, voles and shrews
These species can be caught in a net, then grasped by the head and neck and dropped into a suitable container (Bourne, 2002). They can be lifted briefly by the tail base only (to avoid sloughing); it is particularly important to avoid damaging the tail of harvest mice and common dormice (Poole, 1999). They can also be scruffed by the skin over the neck and back, with the tail held in the same hand (Bourne, 2002).

Dormice
To catch edible dormice, a net may be needed (Bourne, 2002), and robust housing and transport cages such as a cat basket are required (Stocker, 2000).

Common dormice are the only wild species described here that may routinely appear passive when they are handled (D. Woods, personal communication). Such behaviour in any other small wild mammal is abnormal and denotes illness, shock or stress. Interfering with common dormice requires a licence (see 'Legal aspects').

Beavers
Beavers are fairly passive, non-aggressive animals. Their main defence is to head for water if threatened. In water they are very agile and difficult to catch. On land they are slow-moving and easily caught. Whilst strong and powerful, they are tractable and can be guided towards a box for capture and transport. They do not tend to bite, but bites are potentially serious given their powerful teeth and jaws.

They do not need to be transported in water or hosed down, but should be offered food with a high water content, such as apples, during transport. Adequate ventilation and shade from the sun should be provided.

Zoonoses and other risks to humans
Most of the species covered in this chapter can inflict bites of varying severity. In addition, the saliva of water shrews contains venom from the submaxillary glands which is poisonous to vertebrate prey such as frogs and fish. Even if a bite does not break the skin, it will cause localized inflammation and pain in humans (Fowler, 1995).

Wild rats in particular are extremely vicious and must be handled with great care. They should not be cornered and they should not be handled directly unless absolutely unavoidable, when thick gloves should be worn. To minimize the risks of leptospiral infection, it is advisable to wear goggles and masks as well as impermeable gloves. Medical advice should be sought in the event of a bite from a wild rat, or suspected ingestion or inhalation of leptospiral infected material. Confirmation of leptospiral infection at post-mortem examination of the rat is advisable so that the need for human treatment can be assessed (A. Hudson, personal communication).

Actual incidences of zoonotic or domestic animal infection appear of generally minimal significance, with the exception of leptospirosis. *Yersinia pseudotuber-culosis* and *Campylobacter* have been isolated from British rodents (Pocock *et al.*, 2001). *Cryptosporidium parvum* and *C. muris* have been isolated from house mice, wood mice and voles (Bull *et al.*, 1998) and constitute a risk to humans, especially in immuno-suppressed individuals (Wells, 1937, cited in Rankin and McDiarmid, 1968), but the zoonotic potential of vole infection is unknown. *Mycobacterium bovis* was isolated from five rats and two moles in a study involving 5700 wild mammals, including badgers, from 1971 to 1978 (Evans and Thompson, 1981) but was not found in 875 voles in another study (Kirkwood, 1991, citing the 1987 study by the Ministry of Agriculture, Fisheries and Food). *M. tuberculosis* var. *muris* had an incidence of 1.4% in a study of 500 common shrews but its zoonotic potential is unknown. Beard *et al.* (2001) found *M. avium* subsp. *paratuberculosis* (the causative organism of paratuberculosis) in rats and wood mice.

Many zoonotic diseases are not currently present in the UK but could be introduced by the increasing numbers of people and animals moving around the world (Simpson, 1999). If introduced into the native rodent population, these infections (e.g. Omsk haemorrhagic fever, rabies, rat poxvirus, Boutonneuse fever, Q-fever and Rocky Mountain spotted fever) could conceivably achieve a foothold in the UK (Fraser *et al.*, 1991).

Examination and assessment for rehabilitation

If possible, the exact location where the animal was found should be recorded, particularly in the case of the common dormouse and water vole. This is in order to help in planning an effective release strategy. If beavers are found, it is worth contacting organizations in the area responsible for their release (currently only in Kent) and scanning the animal for an identifying microchip.

General anaesthesia is advisable for all but the most superficial examination (Fowler, 1993, 1995). Examination of the animal inside a transparent container (e.g. plastic box or glass jar), in dim light, is more productive than attempting to examine the animal in the hand and permits better inspection of the head, underside and extremities.

Anything more than very minimal limb damage, especially in climbing species, is likely to lead to an increased risk of predation. Damage to the tail, especially in the common dormouse and harvest mouse (which use tails for climbing) and water shrew (which uses them for swimming), may be significant, depending on the degree. Damage to the forelimbs of moles is likely to have an effect on digging and therefore on feeding capabilities. Visual defects in moles and shrews do not necessarily preclude release.

The treatment and release of pest species is controversial. The decision to euthanase or release such species is up to the individual veterinary surgeon, but the Wildlife and Countryside Act 1981 makes it an offence to release edible dormice and black rats.

Euthanasia

Euthanasia (see also Chapter 2) is best performed by intravenous or intraperitoneal barbiturate overdose, following gaseous anaesthetic induction if necessary. Cervical dislocation can be carried out as described in laboratory animal texts (Redfern and Rowe, 1987).

First aid procedures

Small mammals are prone to rapid heat loss and should be kept warm but care should be taken to avoid overheating them, especially if they are debilitated and unable to move away from a source of heat. An ambient temperature of 25–28°C should be provided for smaller casualty species in particular.

These species generally require almost constant food intake. Suitable food (see 'Rehabilitation'), in particular the more palatable and easily digestible items, should be provided at once. Immediate fluid therapy should be considered, especially if the casualty does not eat readily. Hypoglycaemia should be addressed if it is a concern.

Fluid therapy

For a full discussion of oral dosing, injection sites and amounts that can be given, see Fallon (1996), Bauck and Bihun (1997), Hrapkiewicz *et al.* (1998) and Orr (2002).

Intravenous injections and blood sampling

The jugular can be used in rats and larger species, but in most cases will be possible only under general anaesthesia as a cut-down procedure (Poole, 1999).

The lateral tail veins can be used in rats but are less useful in other species. Warming the tail dilates the vessels. In mice, the use of these veins is limited to the removal of small volumes of blood, but they are not suitable for injection purposes (Fallon, 1996). For blood sampling in voles, Poole (1999) suggested cutting 1 mm from the tail tip under general anaesthesia. Damage to the tail of species that require it for climbing (e.g. harvest mice) must be avoided.

In beavers, the ventral coccygeal vein is utilized. With the beaver in dorsal recumbency, the vein is located on the ventral aspect of the tail in the midline (S. Brown, personal communication).

Intramuscular injection

There is little difference in the rate of uptake from intramuscular and subcutaneous injections (McDiarmid, 1983). The intramuscular injection of irritant drugs or of excessive volumes can result in muscle necrosis and damage to adjacent nerves, in some cases resulting in self-mutilation (Hrapkiewicz *et al.*, 1998). Also, these species are easily stressed and fast-moving, and intraperitoneal and subcutaneous routes are generally quicker and easier to use. If intramuscular injections are to be given, no more than 0.05 ml should be given in any one site to a mouse-sized rodent (Flecknell, 1991).

Intraperitoneal injection

This is carried out with the animal well restrained or anaesthetized in dorsal recumbency. The needle is introduced at an angle of 20 degrees to the body, parallel to the midline, pointing cranially. The right caudal quadrant is used, to avoid perforating the caecum or the bladder. The syringe is aspirated before injection to check for visceral perforation (Hrapkiewicz *et al.*, 1998). Suggested volumes are up to 2 ml for a 30 g mouse and up to 5 ml for a 200 g rat (Flecknell, 1996).

Intraosseous injection

This gives similar rates of uptake to that of intravenous injection but is technically easier in these smaller species. The preferred sites are the proximal tibia or femur. Aseptic technique and local or general anaesthesia are required. Purpose-made intraosseous needles can be used. Alternatively, spinal or hypodermic needles of appropriate size can be used. The latter tend to become blocked with cortical bone unless the needle is attached to a syringe containing sterile saline (which is kept pressurized to maintain its patency) or a smaller needle or sterile stainless steel wire is used as a stylet.

Subcutaneous injection

Volumes similar to those for the intraperitoneal route can be given. Sites include the nape of the neck and dorsolaterally over the ribs (Bourne, 2002). The addition of hyaluronidase at 150 IU/litre of fluids increases the rate of uptake of subcutaneous fluids (Carpenter *et al.*, 2001).

Oral dosing

Oral administration of drugs or fluids is likely to prove immensely stressful for many of these species. In many cases it will not be practicable but in the case of debilitated individuals it may be a practical way of administering small quantities of fluids, especially if hypoglycaemia is a concern. Proprietary formulations such as Liquid Lectade (Pfizer), Duphalyte (Fort Dodge) or Critical Care Formula (VetArk), or intravenous formulations of glucose, may prove useful.

Anaesthesia and analgesia

Light anaesthesia is advantageous as an aid to rapid, complete examination of these species. The current anaesthetic of choice is isoflurane (Fowler, 1993) with induction taking place in a chamber at 4–5%, and maintenance by mask at 1.5–3%. A purpose-designed concentric mask is preferable (e.g. International Market Supply, Congleton, Cheshire), as it permits more efficient scavenging of waste gases. A snugly fitting mask with a rubber or latex edge can provide a sufficient seal to aid in ventilating the animal if required.

Small mammals have a high ratio of surface area to bodyweight and therefore require good insulation and an external source of gentle warmth to avoid hypothermia (Fowler, 1995; Flecknell, 1998). Conversely, it is important not to overheat them.

Most species do not require preoperative starving to avoid vomiting. Due to their high metabolic rates, especially in the shrews, even short periods of starvation are likely to be fatal.

Every effort to ensure a rapid return to consciousness and resumed food intake should be taken. The use of perioperative fluids by the oral, intraperitoneal, subcutaneous, intravenous or intraosseous route should be employed (see 'Fluid therapy' above). All fluids should be warmed to approximately 38°C before administration. Even with a short anaesthetic, the patient is often already in a state of dehydration and malnutrition and this should be addressed.

If any invasive procedure is carried out, the use of analgesics is warranted, both for welfare reasons and to ensure a rapid return to normal feeding behaviour. Self-trauma of the affected part may be seen if inadequate analgesia is employed. Carprofen at 4 mg/kg by a single subcutaneous injection and meloxicam at 4 mg/kg by oral administration have been widely used by this author in a number of these species. Buprenorphine (0.05 mg/kg) and butorphanol (2 mg/kg) can also be used at rat doses.

Moles

Moles have a relatively high urine volume and they excrete bicarbonate in their urine. This may be an excretory mechanism to cope with a hypercapnic environment (Haim *et al.*, 1987). It may be advisable to provide parenteral fluids perioperatively in this species even more so than others, to assist this mechanism and avoid acid–base balance disturbances. Intraperitoneal fluids have been given (Brash, personal communication).

Adaptation to a hypercapnic environment may also mean that the mole may not breathe spontaneously in a low carbon dioxide environment. Intermittent positive pressure ventilation (IPPV) or external chest compression during anaesthesia, and the use of carbon dioxide in inspired gases during the recovery period, might be required if apnoea occurs. However, no problems with recovery from isoflurane have been noted (M. Brash, personal communication). Neither were any problems noted in the case of 33 moles anaesthetized with a mixture of fentanyl/fluanisone, at 0.2 mg/ml fentanyl and 10 mg/ml fluanisone, with midazolam at 5 mg/ml and water for injection, mixed at a ratio of 1:1:2 and given by intraperitoneal injection at a rate of 0.2 ml per animal (S. Wolfensohn, personal communication). This combination gave 20–70 minutes of surgical anaesthesia, and all moles recovered without the use of opioid antagonists within 60–136 minutes.

Shrews

A combination of ketamine (20 mg/kg) and xylazine (1 mg/kg), given intramuscularly, has been reported to give 20–30 minutes of light anaesthesia in shrews (Fowler, 1993).

Voles

Alfaxalone/alfadolone has been used at a dose of 0.1 ml/kg i.p. to give approximately 30 minutes of anaesthetic time (Baker and Clarke, 1987). Pentobarbital has been used at a dose of 72 mg/kg i.p. It was considered less safe in stressed voles and a further 24 mg/kg was required for excited voles (Poole, 1999). Overdose is very easy and such agents require very precise weighing. They also tend to result in prolonged recoveries with poor analgesia.

Beavers

Adult beavers have been anaesthetized with a combination of medetomidine at 0.07 mg/kg and ketamine at 7.5 mg/kg given together by intramuscular injection. After 20 minutes, reversal was carried out using atipamezole at 0.3 mg/kg i.m. No problems were associated with this regime (S. Brown, personal communication).

Specific conditions

Injuries from predators can involve bites of varying degrees of severity, limb fractures (Figure 8.13), spinal damage or abdominal puncture and prolapsed intestines (Stocker, 2000). Even when only apparently minor injuries are noted, antibiotic therapy is warranted, as cat bites can commonly lead to *Pasteurella*-induced septicaemia (Korbel, 1990; Korbel *et al.*, 1992) (see also Chapter 9).

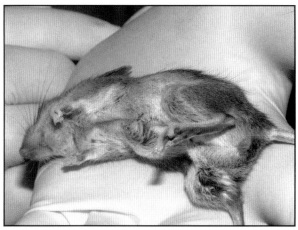

8.13 Wood mouse with a compound fracture of the tibia. Such fractures carry a poor prognosis, and euthanasia at an early stage is the best course of action. (Courtesy of G Cousquer.)

Moles

Juvenile moles spend more time above ground than adults when they first leave, increasing the risk of predation by birds of prey, foxes and cats. They may tunnel in unsuitable areas, leading to death by drowning. Non-fatally injured trapped moles may be seen, and it is possible (though unlikely) that non-fatal strychnine poisoning cases might be seen. Strychnine poisoning leads to death by asphyxiation following paralysis of the respiratory muscles; it can take as long as 2 hours for a mole to die and it cannot be considered to be humane, but such cases are rarely (if ever) noted as they tend to occur underground.

Intraspecific fighting is common, as moles are territorial and aggressive outside the breeding season. Non-fatally injured moles with fight wounds may be seen but they frequently die in the 24 hours following admission (Small, 1994). This may be due to a number of reasons, not necessarily pathological.

The host-specific fleas *Palaepsylla minor*, *P. kohauti* and *Ctenophthalmus bisoctodentatus* may be found (Lawson, 1999). The mites *Haemogamasus hirsutus*, *H. nidi* and *Eulaelaps stabularis* and an unnamed *Eimeria*-like coccidian, possibly *Elleipsisoma thomsoni*, have also been found on moles (Mohamed *et al.*, 1987). Their pathogenicity is unknown. Trematode species of the genus *Hyogonimus* have been found but their pathogenicity is unknown (Corbet and Southern, 1977).

Shrews

Endoparasites such as *Porrocaecum talpae*, which is found coiled subcutaneously in the common shrew, and *Hymenolepsis infirma* have been noted. These do not appear to have a significant effect on the host population but the former is transmissible to owls (Small, 1994). A number of helminth parasites were detected in common and pygmy shrews in a study (Roots, 1992) that concluded that no serious pathogenic effects were noted as a result of infestation. Fleas, ticks and mites are common. Water shrews have large endo- and ectoparasite burdens (Anon., 2001a).

Voles

External parasites recorded for voles include fleas, lice, ticks and mites (Blackmore and Owen, 1968; Corbet and Southern, 1977; Healing and Nowell, 1985). Internal parasites are also well documented in the above references but the significance of these parasitic infections on host health and population dynamics is largely unknown (Healing and Nowell, 1985).

Corynebacterium kutscheri infection has been reported in field voles. It may be more prevalent where there is a higher population density (Barrow, 1981).

Rats and mice

Kaplan *et al.* (1980) found a number of viral infections in experimentally immunosuppressed mice and voles, including pneumonia virus of mice (PVM), lymphocytic choriomeningitis virus, reovirus III, Theiler's mouse encephalomyelitis virus, ectromelia virus, mouse adenovirus, louping ill virus and encephalomyocarditis virus. Of these, only ectromelia and PVM were suspected of influencing population dynamics in wild mice and in general these diseases are of limited significance.

Heligmosomoides polygyrus was found in 98% of wood mice in one study and this parasite does have a negative effect on the survival ability of the host (Gregory, 1991). In another study, nine helminth species were detected in wood mice, with 92% of the mice having at least one species present (Behnke *et al.*, 1999). Several species of *Eimeria* can infect wood mice but their significance is uncertain (Nowell and Higgs, 1989).

Dormice

The nematodes *Rictularia cristata* and *Syphacia obvelata* have been recorded in the common dormouse (E.A. Harris, cited by Sainsbury *et al.*, 1996). This paper also described orbital infestation with *Rhabditis orbitalis*, the incidence of which is unknown but may be more of a problem at high population densities.

Therapeutics

Accurate weighing is important, for both drug administration and clinical assessment of these patients, and postal scales are particularly useful. However, even with reasonably accurate weighing, the animals' small body size and the relative uncertainty about dose rates suggest that drugs with a wide margin of safety should be used where possible.

Dose rates

Using dose rates and frequencies established by pharmacological studies in domestic rodents will give the most accurate dose rates, which can be found in Carpenter *et al.* (2001), Flecknell (1996, 1998), Fallon (1996), Bauck and Bihun (1997) and Hrapkiewicz *et al.* (1998). In the absence of established dose rates and frequencies, doses calculated by allometric scaling (based on metabolic rate) rather than bodyweight are more accurate (see Chapter 2); the method is described by Flecknell (1998). Doses extrapolated from larger domestic mammals are likely to be much too low for these species in most cases. Figure 8.14 gives dose rates for some parasiticides.

It may also be necessary to dose more frequently. Frequent medication of such animals, particularly orally, can be stressful and so the longest-acting preparation available should be used where possible. The addition of drugs to a highly palatable foodstuff may be useful (Flecknell, 1998). Sites of drug administration are noted above in 'First aid'.

Antibiotics

Some antibiotics can alter the normal gut flora of rodents and cause the development of fatal enterotoxaemias. Domestic rats and mice are rarely affected and wild ones are equally unlikely to have problems. Voles and dormice may be relatively more susceptible and it would be wise to avoid antibiotics that are particularly associated with such problems (e.g. penicillins, cephalosporins and especially lincosamides) unless there is a specific indication for their use. Parenteral antibiotics are generally safer in this regard than oral antibiotics. Fluoroquinolones and potentiated sulphonamides appear to be relatively safe to use both parenterally and orally. Concurrent and subsequent dosing with probiotics may be of use in avoiding problems. In the event of an enterotoxaemia developing, cholestyramine resin may be of value in binding toxins within the gut (Flecknell, 1998). Figure 8.15 lists doses for rats and mice.

Antibiotic treatment of species with zoonotic bacterial infections is not recommended, due to the risk of the animal resuming shedding of bacteria after release and the effects on bacterial resistance. Euthanasia is recommended in such cases.

Drug	Dose and application method	References	Notes
Flumethrin scab and tick dip	Animal totally immersed in dip for 10 s; repeated 2 weeks later	M. Brash (pers. comm.)	Avoids direct handling; group of animals (e.g. rats) can be treated *en masse*
Piperonyl butoxide	Used on substrate as directed	Poole (1999)	
Fipronil spray	Used to wet cotton wool or gloved hand and then applied at lower end of dose range (i.e. 3 ml/kg)	Personal observation	Care must be taken to avoid chilling animal with solution, especially under anaesthetic, or allowing it to succumb to fumes of alcohol used as carrier
Praziquantel	No dose given; suggestions as follows: 6–10 mg/kg orally 5 mg/kg s.c. or 10 mg/kg orally	Wagner (1987) cited by Lipman and Foltz (1996) Carpenter *et al.* (2001) suggested for gerbils, mice and rats Orr (2002)	Treatment of *Hymenolepis* spp. Zoonotic
Niclosamide	100 mg/kg orally at 7-day intervals	Fraser (1991)	Treatment of *Hymenolepis* spp. Zoonotic
Mebendazole	50 mg/kg orally	Fowler (1993)	
Ivermectin	Oral or subcutaneous; doses vary, 200–500 µg/kg. Appears to have wide margin of safety in these species; in view of their size, upper end of dose range should be used Percutaneous application of few drops after diluting 1:100 with 1:1 mixture of water and propylene glycol Topical spray made up of 5–10 mg ivermectin in 1 litre water	Fowler (1993) Tennant (1999) Carpenter *et al.* (2001) Orr (2002)	Effective against wide range of ecto- and endoparasites
Fenbendazole	50 mg/kg once daily for 5 consecutive days orally	M. Brash (pers. comm.) Tennant (1999)	

8.14 Parasiticides used in rats and mice.

Drug	Dose/comments
Amoxicillin	Rat: 150 mg/kg i.m. Mouse: 100 mg/kg s.c.
Ampicillin Injection, 15% w/v Oral preparations	50–150 mg/kg s.c. 200 mg/kg orally
Cephalosporins Cefalexin	60 mg/kg orally Rat: 15 mg/kg s.c. Mouse: 30 mg/kg s.c.
Chloramphenicol Injectable Oral preparations	Rat: 10 mg/kg i.m. bid Mouse: 50 mg/kg i.m., s.c. bid Rat: 20–50 mg/kg bid Mouse: 200 mg/kg tid
Clavulanate-potentiated amoxicillin	2 ml/kg orally (Synulox)
Enrofloxacin	10 mg/kg s.c., orally sid
Neomycin Oral preparations	Rat: 50 mg/kg s.c. Mouse: 2.5 g/l in drinking water Rat: 2.0 g/l in drinking water
Oxytetracycline, long-acting injection	60 mg/kg s.c., i.m. every 3 days
Potentiated sulphonamides (e.g. trimethoprim/ sulfadiazine)	120 mg/kg s.c., i.m. 24% solution = 240 mg/ml = 0.5 ml/kg
Sulfamerazine	0.02% in drinking water
Tetracycline Injectable tetracyclines Oral tetracycline	100 mg/kg s.c. (high dose used in respiratory disease) 5 mg/kg orally in drinking water
Tylosin	10 mg/kg s.c.

8.15 Antibacterial agents used in rats and mice. Note that streptomycin and procaine penicillin are toxic to rats and mice.

Management in captivity

Housing

Escape-proof housing is vitally important. Some general guidelines are as follows:

- Secure plastic or glass vivaria or aquaria are best for smaller species
- Ventilation must be good, to avoid potential high humidity (relative humidity should not exceed 50–60%)
- The ceiling should consist of close-gauge mesh, with a small door opening in it (Stocker, 2000)
- Wood is warmer and cheaper than plastic, glass or wire but difficult to clean and may be gnawed
- Wire cages are an option for species that gnaw

- Cages with walls at least partly of mesh rather than totally solid are another option but are less secure, more difficult to keep clean and will restrict normal nesting and burrowing behaviour
- Substrate options include sand, wood shavings, peat, hay, moss (Michalak, 1987), leaves, paper towel
- To reduce the stress of scent removal, avoid cleaning out too often (Poole, 1999) and leave some dirty bedding in place after each clean
- Water for swimming should be provided for aquatic species, e.g. water shrews (Figure 8.16).

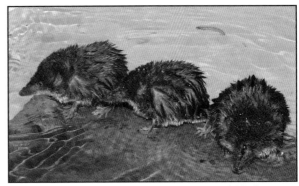

8.16 Hand-reared insectivores, such as this litter of water shrews, must be provided with a suitable environment during captivity in order that they can learn normal behaviour such as swimming. (Courtesy of G. Cousquer.)

For insectivores, further descriptions of husbandry can be found in Michalak (1987), Dryden (1975) and Rudge (1966). For rodents, accommodation requirements are well described in appropriate laboratory animal texts and by Michalak (1987) and Poole (1999). For common dormice, guidelines on long-term housing should be obtained from the Dormouse Captive Breeding Group (contacted via English Nature).

Wild species differ from laboratory animals in being more aggressive, more inclined to escape and more stressed by human contact. Therefore artefacts such as hide boxes, cardboard tubes, drainpipes and pots must be provided (especially for shrews), with adequate nesting material such as hay, leaves and moss. The substrate should be deep enough for burrowing but long-stranded material may entrap limbs and should be avoided (Bourne, 2002).

Details for different species are given in Figure 8.17.

Feeding

Drinking water

It should not be assumed that the smaller species can operate a rodent drinker bottle. Water should also be offered in a bird drinker or shallow bowl or jam jar lid, and drinkers should be positioned very close to the ground.

Feeding insectivores

Live food items should be adequately nourished for at least 48 hours before they are consumed;

Group	Structure	Nesting	Substrate	Humidity and water	Notes
Moles	Glass escape-proof vivarium No top required if container sufficiently tall (moles cannot climb)	Separate nesting boxes at each end	Layer of earth, peat and leaf litter deep enough to burrow into	Regular watering of soil necessary: moles require moderately high humidity May result in nasal lesions if soil too dry (M. Brash, pers. comm.)	'Collapse' the tunnels regularly to avoid stereotypy associated with lack of tunnelling opportunities in longer-term accommodation
Shrews	Escape-proof plastic or glass vivarium with lid Hide tubes or boxes	Hay, moss, leaves	Not shredded paper (rustling noise can upset them; Fowler, 1986; Dryden, 1975) Deep enough for burrowing	Can give water shrews some swimming water as part of enclosure but not essential (Henwood, 1985) (Figure 8.17)	Position food/water containers around edges of cage (shrews avoid exposed open centre of cage; Dryden, 1975) If swimming water provided, water shrews also need burrow in which to dry and groom themselves
Harvest mice	Cages at least 75 cm high	Dense vegetation (e.g. planting or by wedging entire tussock or bunches of oat/barley/wheat/ teasels tied together; Henwood, 1985) for climbing and nest building		Humidity < 50–60% Water in shallow containers at ground level	Fight if kept at high population densities
Wood mice	Escape-proof plastic or glass vivarium with lid Hide tubes or boxes	Hay, moss, leaves	Good depth of litter for burrowing	Humidity < 50–60% Water in shallow containers at ground level	
Dormice	Robust housing to deter escape by gnawing Agile and jump well	Nest boxes with vegetation above ground level	Vegetation and branches	Nest needs to be moistened occasionally during hibernation to avoid dehydration	Advice from dormouse captive breeders groups

8.17 Housing for insectivores and rodents in captivity.

otherwise they will be of dubious nutritional value, have an empty gut and can be dehydrated when they are eaten. It is advisable to improve their nutritional status by feeding them with sliced fruit and vegetables, powdered dog biscuits, flaked fish food and proprietary insect foods or 'gut-loading' formulae such as Grub Grub (for larvae) or Bug Grub (for adults) (both from VetArk).

The feeding requirements in captivity of some of the insectivores and rodents are shown in Figure 8.18. Commercial diets for a number of rodents exist and can be used as a basis for diets of rats and mice and as a supplementary diet for other small rodents. Additional ingredients for rodents include crushed oats, wheat, maize, fruit, vegetables and dog biscuits (broken or whole).

Group	Suitable foods	Notes and special needs
Moles	Earthworms, slugs, insects, waxworms, mealworms, diets for insectivorous birds, dogfood (preferably meat-in-jelly), chopped pinky mice	Place foods directly on substrate Water obtained mostly from food in wild but provide drinking water in shallow bowls in captivity (Small, 1994; Lawson, 1999)
Shrews	Maggots, fly pupae, mealworms, fresh meat, egg, food for insectivorous birds, crushed dried catfood (Dryden, 1975) Ideal prey size 6–10 mm	Food must always be available (high metabolic rate) Often discard unpalatable parts and sometimes cache their food (Bourne, 2002) Refection of milky white fluid from anus is normal; contains fat globules and partially digested food
Water shrews	Minced mixture of beef offal, fish, chicken (or rabbit or guinea pig), egg, sprouted wheat grains, mealworms (Michelak, 1987)	As for other shrews Have been given milk instead of drinking water (Michelak, 1987)
Voles	Whole oats, meadow hay, chopped carrots, rodent pellets (Baker and Clarke (1987) Chopped grasses, clover, garden flowers, seeds, dry oats, mouse food, crushed digestive biscuits, greens, leafy twigs with buds, hay	Field voles eat relatively more grass than other voles

8.18 Feeding captive insectivores and rodents. (continues) ▶

Group	Suitable foods	Notes and special needs
Bank voles	Prefer seeds, fresh vegetables (e.g. carrot, apple, cabbage), fresh grasses, hedgerow fruits	High water requirement: drinking water must be available at all times
Wood mice	Prefer seeds, berries, rosehips, green plants, insects	Tend to avoid root vegetables
Harvest mice	Birdseed, blowfly pupae, millet, rape, linseed, growing grasses, hedgerow flowers and fruits, insects, small qunatities of flaked fishfood	Immune to toxins of berries that are poisonous to humans (e.g. black bryony, *Tamus communis*)
Common dormice	Sunflower seeds and peanuts (in moderation), hazel nuts, rich tea biscuits, ripe fruit (e.g. grape, apple, banana, strawberry, other berries), corn, tomato, clumps of hazel or sycamore branches, canary eggfood, mynah birdfood (D. Woods, pers. comm.)	Also insectivorous in summer: moths, caterpillars On waking from hibernation, often eat pollen and nectar (D. Woods, pers. comm.)
Edible dormice	As for common dormice plus dry puppyfood, spinach, curly kale, pecan nuts (Stocker, 2000)	Will eat raw meat in captivity Drink large quantities

8.18 (continued) Feeding captive insectivores and rodents.

Rearing of young

Orphaned rodents and insectivores are generally altricial. Rearing them is extremely challenging and in many cases not possible unless they are sufficiently old (Spaulding and Spaulding, 1979). In some cases, euthanasia is likely to be the preferable course of action (Bourne, 2002). Age should be determined as accurately as possible at the outset.

Environmental temperature

These species exhibit poor thermoregulation and require well regulated temperatures of 35°C for a hairless infant and 32°C for one that is furred but has its eyes still closed. Once the eyes are open, the temperature can be dropped by 2.5°C weekly (Weber, 1978). A temperature gradient should be provided and soft, comfortable, disposable bedding is required.

Feeding

- The first feed should be of an oral rehydration solution (e.g. Lectade, Pfizer) followed by a gradual change to a milk substitute over several feeds

- A syringe, paintbrush, Pasteur pipette or piece of string as a 'wick' can be used for smaller rodents; a kitten-feeder can be used for larger ones
- Up to 35–40% of bodyweight can be fed daily, with no more than 25–50 ml/kg bodyweight given per feed
- Toileting should be performed on admission and after each feed (Bourne, 2002) by gently rubbing the anogenital region with a damp wisp of cotton wool until urination and defecation take place
- Records must be kept of weight, feeding amount, frequency, urination and defecation (Bourne, 2002).

The special feeding requirements of different species are outlined in Figure 8.19.

Release

In most cases of individual release of adults, hard release (see Chapter 3) into suitable environments is preferred. For species bred or raised in captivity, soft release is preferred. For species with exacting habitat requirements (e.g. common dormice, water voles),

Group	Milk replacers	How often	Time for weaning	Weaning foods
Moles and shrews	Esbilac or Zoological Milk Matrix 30/55 (PetAg) Mother's milk is concentrated high-fat	Hourly throughout day and night	As soon as possible	Live invertebrate food and finely chopped version of adult diet (Stocker, 2000)
Mice and voles	Goat's colostrum mixed 1:3 with milk replacer (e.g. Esbilac or Zoological Milk Matrix 30/44 (PetAg)	Every hour during daylight; every 2 hours overnight (a few drops per feed)	From 9 days of age	Mice: crumbled biscuits or rusks or cereal, soaked in milk replacer Voles: chickweed, dandelion, clover (Stocker, 2000)
Dormice	Goat's milk, or Lactol made up 1:3 with water Vitamin drops (e.g. Abidec) may be added	Four or five times daily, or every 2 hours from 6.30 a.m. to 11.00 p.m.	2–3 weeks	Rusks (Stocker, 2000), dry puppy food, Milupa babyfood, wholemeal bread, apple, raspberries, cherries, rosehips, sycamore seeds, hazelnuts in shell, acorns, hazel twigs, honeysuckle (French, 1989)

8.19 Feeding requirements of orphan insectivores and rodents.

liaison with experienced field workers is advised. Little research into the release or post-release success of other species has been carried out. The following release sites are recommended by Stocker (2000):

- Moles: deciduous woodland where there is no evidence of moles already present (to avoid territorial problems); they should be released in leaf litter and observed until underground
- Shrews, bank voles and field voles: hedgerows, gardens, verges and embankments
- Harvest mice: suitable fields of tall grasses or the hedgerows surrounding them
- Water voles: near small rivers and canals. The Mammal Society should be contacted before release, as there may be a release project in the area (Anon., 2001b).

Common dormice

A licence is required for any interference with common dormice and can be obtained from English Nature in England. Immediate release of uninjured adults is advised.

If a dormouse has been disturbed during hibernation, its nest should quickly be wrapped up again and covered over. If necessary, the nest and its occupant (with plenty of damp padding) may be transferred to a more secure ground location within 100 m of the original site, choosing a cool area out of direct sunlight. The nest can be covered with a flat stone to protect it from predators and to keep it moist and cool. If the dormouse is partially active, release nearby at dusk may be preferable (Bright et al., 1996).

The Dormouse Captive Breeding Group or English Nature should be contacted before release, which should be coordinated with release/reintroduction workers in the area. Any dormice not considered fit for release may be suitable for captive-breeding programmes.

Dormice are best released in pairs or small groups (D. Woods, personal communication) via a soft release (see Chapter 3) in early summer (French, 1989). A suitable environment without any existing dormice should be selected, as these animals live at much lower population densities than other rodents (Bright et al., 1996).

Legal aspects

Details of general legislation covering the species discussed in this chapter are given in Chapter 5. The following points are specific:

- Schedule 6 of the Wildlife and Countryside Act (WCA) prohibits the taking and killing of shrews by certain methods
- Schedule 2 of the WCA covers the place of rest or shelter of voles
- Control of the brown rat is permitted by certain approved methods (e.g. spring traps and poisons)
- Release of the black rat or the edible dormouse is illegal under Schedule 9 of the WCA

- Under Schedule 6 of the WCA, neither species of dormouse may be taken or killed by certain methods. Common dormice are also afforded considerable protection under Schedule 5 of the WCA, which makes it an offence to interfere with them except under licence (English Nature should be contacted if a licence is required). Additional protection is given by the EU Conservation (Natural Habitats) Regulations, which covers habitats rather than the animals themselves.

Specialist organizations

Dormouse Captive Breeding groups: contact English Nature

Mammal Society
15 The Cloisters, 8 Battersea Park Road, London SW8 4BG

Mammal Research Unit
School of Biological Sciences, Bristol University, Woodland Road, Bristol BS8 1UG

Beaver reintroduction:

Kent Wildlife Trust
Tyland Barn, Sandling, Maidstone, Kent ME14 3BD

References and further reading

Anon. (2001a) *Mammal Society Factsheets.* Mammal Society, London

Anon. (2001b) Mammal Society website, www.abdn.ac.uk/mammal

Appleby BM, Anwar MA and Petty SJ (1999) Short-term and long-term effects of food supply on parasite burdens in tawny owls, *Strix aluco. Functional Ecology* **13**, 315–321

Baker JP and Clark JR (1987) Voles. In: *UFAW Handbook on the Care and Management of Laboratory Animals, 6th edn*, ed. TB Poole. Longman, Harlow

Barrow PA (1981) *Corynebacterium kutscheri* infection in wild voles (*Microtus agrestis*). *British Veterinary Journal* **137**, 76–80

Bauck L and Bihun C (1997) Basic anatomy, physiology, husbandry and clinical techniques. In: *Ferrets, Rabbits and Rodents: Clinical Medicine and Surgery*, eds EV Hillyer and KE Quesenberry. pp. 291–306 WB Saunders, Philadelphia

Beard PM, Daniels MJ, Henderson D, Pirie A, Rudge K, Buxton D, Rhind S, Greig A, Hutchings MR, McKendrick I, Stevenson K and Sharp JM (2001) Paratuberculosis infection of nonruminant wildlife in Scotland. *Journal of Clinical Microbiology* **39**, 1517–1521

Behnke JM, Lewis JW, Zain SNM and Gilbert FS (1999) Helminth infections in *Apodemus sylvaticus* in southern England: interactive effects of host age, sex and year on the prevalence and abundance of infection. *Journal of Helminthology* **73**, 31–44

Ben Shauld, DM (1962) The composition of milk of wild animals. *International Zoo Yearbook* **4**, 333

Blackmore DK and Owen DG (1968) Ectoparasites: their significance in British wild rodents. *Symposium of the Zoological Society of London* **24**, 197

Bogne, GL (1979) Caring for wild orphans. *Defenders*, February, 30–44

Bourne D (2002) *UK Wildlife: First Aid and Care.* Wildlife Information Network, London (CD Rom)

Bright P and Morris P (1989) *A Practical Guide to Dormouse Conservation.* Mammal Society, London

Bright PW and Morris PA (1990) Habitat requirements of dormice (*Muscardinus avellanarius*) in relation to woodland management in Southwest England. *Biological Conservation* **54**, 307–326

Bright P and Morris P (1992a) *The Dormouse.* Mammal Society, London

Bright PW and Morris PA (1992b) Ranging and nesting behaviour of the dormouse (*Muscardinus avellanarius*) in coppice-with-standards woodland. *Journal of Zoology, London* **226**, 589–600

Bright P and Morris P (1993) Conservation of the dormouse. *British Wildlife* **4**, 154–162

Bright PW and Morris PA (1994) Animal translocation for conservation: performance of dormice in relation to release methods, origin and season. *Journal of Applied Ecology* **31**, 699–708

Bright PW and Morris PA (1996) Why are dormice rare? A case study in conservation biology. *Mammal Review* **26**, 157–187

Bright P, Morris P and Mitchell-Jones T (1996) *The Dormouse Conservation Handbook*. English Nature, Peterborough

Bull SA, Chalmers RM, Sturdee AP and Healing TD (1998) A survey of *Cryptosporidium* species in Skomer bank voles (*Clethrionomys glareolus skomerensis*). *Journal of Zoology* **244**, 119–122

Bullion S (1998) *Key to British Land Mammals*. Mammal Society/Field Studies Council, London

Carpenter JW, Mashima TY and Rupiper DJ (2001) *Exotic Animal Formulary, 2nd edn*. WB Saunders, Philadelphia

Chalmers RA, Sturdee AP, Bull SA, Miller A and Wright SE (1997) The prevalence of *Cryptosporidium parvum* and *C. muris* in *Mus domesticus*, *Apodemus sylvaticus* and *Clethrionomys glareolus* in an agricultural system. *Parasitology Research* **83**, 478–482

Churchfield S (1986) *Shrews*. Anthony Nelson, Oswestry

Churchfield S (1988) *Shrews of the British Isles*. Shire Natural History Series No. 30. Shire Publications, Princes Risborough

Churchfield S (1990) *The Natural History of Shrews*. Christopher Helm, London

Clark JD and Olfert ED (1986) Rodents. In: *Zoo and Wild Animal Medicine*, ed ME Fowler. WB Saunders, Philadelphia

Collen P (1995) The reintroduction of beaver (*Castor fiber* L.) to Scotland,: an opportunity to promote the development of suitable habitat. *Scottish Forestry* **49**, 206–216

Cooper ME (1987) *An Introduction to Animal Law*. Academic Press, London

Cooper ME and Sinclair DA (1989) Wildlife rehabilitation and the law: an introduction. Paper presented at the Second Symposium of the BWRC. British Wildlife Rehabilitation Council, London

Corbet GB and Harris S (1991) *The Handbook of British Mammals, 3rd edn*. Blackwell Scientific, Oxford

Corbet GB and Southern HN (eds) (1977) *The Handbook of British Mammals, 2nd edn*. Blackwell Scientific, Oxford

Cosgrove GE (1986) Insectivores. In: *Zoo and Wild Animal Medicine: Current Therapy 2*, ed ME Fowler. WB Saunders, Philadelphia

Crowcroft P (1957) *The Life of the Shrew*. Max Reinhardt, London

Dryden GL (1975) Establishment and maintenance of shrew colonies. *International Zoo Yearbook* **15**, 12

Edwards GR, Crawley MJ and Heard MS (1999) Factors influencing molehill distribution in grassland: implications for controlling the damage caused by molehills. *Journal of Applied Ecology* **36**, 434–443

Evans HTJ and Thompson HV (1981) Bovine tuberculosis in cattle in Great Britain. I. Eradication of the disease from cattle and the role of the badger (*Meles meles*) as a source of *Mycobacterium bovis* for cattle. *Animal Regulation Studies* **3**, 191–216

Fallon, MT (1996) Rats and mice. In: *Handbook of Rodent and Rabbit Medicine*, eds K Laber-Laird *et al.*, pp. 1–38. Elsevier Science, Oxford

Flecknell, P (1991) Rats and mice. In: *Manual of Exotic Pets, 3rd edn*, Eds PH Beynon and JE Cooper, pp. 83–96. BSAVA Publications, Cheltenham

Flecknell P (1996) Anaesthesia and analgesia for rodents and rabbits. In: *Handbook of Rodent and Rabbit Medicine*, eds K Laber-Laird *et al.*, pp. 219–238. Elsevier Science, Oxford

Flecknell P (1998) Developments in the veterinary care of rabbits and rodents. *In Practice* **20**, 6

Fowler ME (ed.) (1986) *Zoo and Wild Animal Medicine: Current Therapy 2*. WB Saunders, Philadelphia

Fowler ME (ed.) (1993) *Zoo and Wild Animal Medicine: Current Therapy 3*. WB Saunders, London

Fowler ME (1995) *Restraint and Handling of Wild and Domestic Animals, 2nd edn*. Iowa State University Press, Ames, Iowa

Fraser CM, Bergeron JA, Mays A and Aiello SE (eds) (1991) *Merck Veterinary Manual, 7th edn*. Merck and Co, Rahway, New Jersey

Flowerdew J (1984) *Woodmice*. Anthony Nelson, Oswestry

Flowerdew J (1993) *Mice and Voles*. Whittet Books, London

French HJ (1989) Hand rearing the common or hazel dormouse (*Muscardinus avellanarius*). *International Zoo Yearbook* **28**, 262

Gilot B, Quenin P and Joubert L (1981) Wildlife vectors of *Rickettsia conori* infection in the lower Rhone valley, France. *Bulletin de la Société des Sciences vétérinaires et de Médecine Comparée de Lyon* **83**, 91–103

Green C (1979) *Animal Anaesthesia*. Laboratory Animals Ltd, RMS Publishing, London

Gregory RD (1991) Parasite epidemiology and host population growth: *Heligmosomoides polygyrus* (Nematoda) in enclosed wood mouse populations. *Journal of Animal Ecology* **60**, 805–821

Gurnell J and Flowerdew JR (1994) *Live Trapping Small Mammals – a Practical Guide, 3rd edn*. Mammal Society, London

Haberl W (1995) *The Shrew Bibliography – a collection of more than 6000 references to research on the biology of Soricidae (Insectivora, Mammalia) and small mammal ecology. I*. CD-ROM Version 1995. Vienna

Haim A, van der Straelen E and Cooreman WM (1987) Urine analysis

of European moles (*Talpa europea*) and white rats (*Rattus norvegicus*) kept on a carnivore's diet. *Comparative Biochemistry and Physiology A: Comparative Physiology* **88**, 179–181

Harris S (1970) *The Secret Life of the Harvest Mouse*. Hamlyn, London

Harris S, Morris P, Wray S and Yalden D (1995) *A Review of British Mammals: Population Estimates and Conservation Status of British Mammals other than Cetaceans*. JNCC, Peterborough

Hathaway SC, Little TWA and Stevens AE (1982) Failure to demonstrate the maintenance of leptospires by house mice (*Mus musculus*) in the south east of England. *Research in Veterinary Science* **32**, 387–388

Hathaway SC, Little TWA and Stevens AE (1983a) Identification of a reservoir of *Leptospira interrogates* serovar *muenchen* in voles (*Microtus agrestis* and *Clethrionomys glareolus*) in England. *Zentralblatt fur Bakteriologie, Mikrobiologie und Hygiene* **254**, 123–128

Hathaway SC, Little TWA, Stevens AE, Ellis WA and Morgan J (1983b) Serovar identification of leptospires of the Australis serogroup isolated from free-living and domestic species in the United Kingdom. *Research in Veterinary Science* **35**, 64–68

Healing TD (1981) Infection with blood parasites in the small British rodents *Apodemus sylvaticus*, *Clethrionomys glareolus* and *Microtus agrestis*. *Parasitology* **83**, 179–189

Healing TD and Greenwood MH (1991) Frequency of isolation of *Campylobacter* spp., *Yersinia* spp. and *Salmonella* spp. from small mammals from two sites in southern Britain. *International Journal of Environmental Health Research* **1**, 54–62

Healing TD and Nowell F (1985) Diseases and parasites of woodland rodent populations. *Symposium of the Zoological Society of London* **55**, 193

Healing TD, Kaplan C and Prior A (1980) A note on some Enterobacteriaceae in the faeces of small wild British mammals. *Journal of Hygiene (London)* **85**, 343–345

Hellwing S (1973) Husbandry and breeding of white-toothed shrews (Crocidurinae) in the research zoo of the Tel-Aviv University. *International Zoo Yearbook* **13** 127–134

Henwood C (1985) *Rodents in Captivity*. Ian Henry Publications, Hornchurch, Essex

Hrapkiewicz K, Medina L and Holmes DD (1998) *Clinical Medicine of Small Mammals and Primates – an Introduction, 2nd edn*. Manson Publishing, London

Hubbard MJ, Baker AS and Cann KJ (1998) Distribution of *Borrelia burgdorferi sensu lato* spirochaete DNA in British ticks (Argasidae and Ixodidae) since the 19th Century, assessed by PCR. *Medical and Veterinary Entomology* **12**, 89–97

Jefferies DJ, Morris PA and Mullineux JE (1989) An inquiry into the changing status of the water vole (*Arvicola terrestris*) in Britain. *Mammal Review* **19**, 111–131

Kaplan C, Healing TD, Evans N, Healing L and Prior A (1980) Evidence of infection by viruses in small British field rodents. *Journal of Hygiene (London)* **84**, 285–294

Keymer I (1995) Some wildlife disease problems in Eastern England. *Journal of the British Veterinary Zoological Society* **1**, 2–6

Kharitonova NN, Leonov-Yu A and Hoogstraal H (1986) *Omsk Haemorrhagic Fever. Ecology of the Agent and Epizootiology*. Oxonian Press PVT, New Delhi

Kirkwood JK (1991) Wild mammals. In: *BSAVA Manual of Exotic Pets, 3rd edn*, eds PH Beynon and JE Cooper, pp. 122–149. BSAVA, Cheltenham

Korbel R (1990) Epizootiology, clinical aspects and therapy of *Pasteurella multocida* infection in bird patients after cat bites. *Tierarztliche Praxis* **18**, 365–376

Korbel R, Gerlach H, Bisgaard M and Hafez HM (1992) Further investigations on *Pasteurella multocida* infections in feral birds injured by cats. *Zentralblatt für Veterinarmedizin Reihe B* **39**, 10–18

Kozuch O, Nosek J, Lichard M and Grulich, I (1966) Transmission of tick-borne encephalitis virus by nymphs of *Ixodes ricinus* to the European mole (*Talpa europaea*). *Acta Virologica* **10**, 83 (English edn)

Lee WB and Houston DC (1993) The effect of diet quality on gut anatomy in British voles (Microtinae). *Journal of Comparative Physiology (B)* **163**, 337–339

Lipman NS and Foltz C (1996) Hamsters. In: *Handbook of Rodent and Rabbit Medicine*, eds K Laber-Laird *et al.*, pp. 59–90. Elsevier Science, Oxford

Little TW, Stevens AE and Hathaway SC (1986) Serological studies of British leptospiral isolates of the Sejroe serogroup. I. The identification of British isolates of the Sejroe serogroup by the cross agglutin absorption test. *Journal of Hygiene (London)* **97**, 123–131

Little TW, Stevens AE and Hathaway SC (1987) Serological studies of British leptospiral isolates of the Sejroe serogroup. III. The distribution of leptospires of the Sejroe serogroup in the British Isles. *Epidemiology and Infection* **99**, 117–126

MacDonald D (1984) *The Encyclopaedia of Mammals.* Andromeda, Oxford

MacDonald D (1995) *European Mammals: Evolution and Behaviour.* Collins, London

Marie NS (1968) Pseudotuberculosis in free living wild animals. *Symposium of the Zoological Society of London* **24**, 107

McCaughey WJ and Fairley JS (1971) Leptospirosis in Irish wildlife. *Veterinary Record* **89**, 447

McDevitt RM and Andrews JF (1994) The importance of nest utilisation as a behavioural thermoregulatory strategy in *Sorex minutus*, the pygmy shrew. *Journal of Thermal Biology* **19**, 97–102

McDiarmid A (1962) *Diseases of Free-living Wild Animals.* Food and Agriculture Organisation of the United Nations, Rome

McDiarmid SC (1983) The absorption of drugs from subcutaneous and intramuscular injection sites. *Veterinary Bulletin* **53**, 9–23

Meehan TP (1993) Insectivora, medical problems of shrews. In: *Zoo and Wild Animal Medicine: Current Therapy 3*, ed ME Fowler. WB Saunders, Philadelphia

Michalak I (1987) Keeping and breeding the Eurasian water shrew (*Neomys fodiens*) under laboratory conditions. *International Zoo Yearbook* **26**, 223

Michna SW (1967) Animal leptospirosis in the British Isles. A serological survey. *Veterinary Record* **80**, 394–401

Michna SW and Campbell RSF (1970) Leptospirosis in wild animals. *Journal of Comparative Pathology* **80**, 101–106

Mohamed HA, Molyneux DH and Wallbanks KR (1987) A coccidian in haemogamasid mites; possible vectors of *Elleipsisoma thomsoni* Franca, 1912. *Annales de Parasitologie Humaine et Comparée* **62**, 107–116

Moore D (1985) Meadow vole. In: *Infant Diet/Care Notebook*, eds S Taylor and A Bietz. American Association of Zoo Parks and Aquaria, Wheeling, W Virginia

Morris PA (1993) *A Red Data Book for British Mammals.* Mammal Society, London

Morris TH (1995) Antibiotic therapeutics in laboratory animals. *Laboratory Animal* **29**, 16–36

Munro R (1989) Zoonoses and wildlife. BWRC Symposium, Stoneleigh, Warwickshire

Nelson M (2001) Mammal society maligns 'murdering' moggies. *Veterinary Times*, April, p. 10

Nowell F and Higgs S (1989) *Eimeria* species infecting woodmice (genus *Apodemus*) and the transfer of two species to *Mus musculus. Parasitology* **98**, 329–336

Oftedal OT (1984) Milk composition, milk yield and energy output at peak lactation: a comparative review. *Symposium of the Zoological Society of London* **51**, 33–85

Orr HE (2002) Rats and Mice. In: *BSAVA Manual of Exotic Pets, 4th edn*, eds A Meredith and S Redrobe, pp. 13–25. BSAVA, Gloucester

Parker H, Rosell F and Holthe V (2000) A gross assessment of the suitability of selected Scottish riparian habitats for beaver. *Scottish Forestry* **54**, 25–31

Pocock MJO, Searle JB, Betts WB and White PCL (2001) Patterns of infection by *Salmonella* and *Yersinia* spp. in commensal house mouse (*Mus musculus domesticus*) populations. *Journal of Applied Microbiology* **90**, 755–760

Poole T (ed.) (1999) *The UFAW Handbook on the Care and Management of Laboratory Animals, 7th edn, Vol. 1.* Blackwell Scientific Publications, Oxford

Randolph SE (1995) Quantifying parameters in the transmission of *Babesia microti* by the tick *Ixodes trianguliceps* amongst voles (*Clethrionomys glareolus*). *Parasitology* **110**, 287–295

Rankin JD and McDiarmid A (1968) Mycobacterial infections in free living wild animals. *Symposium of the Zoological Society of London* **24**, 119

Redfern R and Rowe FP (1987) Wild rats and mice. In: *The UFAW Handbook on the Care and Management of Laboratory Mammals, 6th edn*, ed. TB Poole. Longman, Harlow

Roots CD (1992) Morphological and ecological studies on helminth parasites of the British shrews. *Journal of Helminthology* **683**, 247–254

Rudge AJB (1966) Catching and keeping live moles. *Journal of the Zoological Society of London* **149**, 42

Sainsbury AW, Bright PW, Morris PA and Harris EA (1996) Ocular disease associated with *Rhabditis orbitalis* nematodes in a common dormouse (*Muscardinus avellanarius*). *Veterinary Record* **139**, 192–193

Salt GFH and Little TWA (1977) Leptospires isolated from wild mammals caught in the south west of England. *Research in Veterinary Science* **22**, 126–127

Shore RF, Feber RE, Firbank LG, Fishwick SK, Macdonald DW and Norum U (1997) The impacts of molluscicide pellets on spring and autumn populations of wood mice *Apodemus sylvaticus. Agriculture, Ecosystems and Environment* **64**, 211–217

Simpson V (1999) *Potential Wildlife Zoonoses in Britain.* Proceedings of the BVA Congress

Small M (1994) *Wildlife Welfare (Mammals).* Intervet, Cambridge

Spaulding CE and Spaulding J (1979) *The Complete Care of Orphaned or Abandoned Baby Animals.* Rodale Press, Emmaus, Pennsylvania

Stocker LR (1995) Wild mammals seen in general practice. British Veterinary Zoological Society meeting, December 1993

Stocker L (2000) *Practical Wildlife Care.* Blackwell Science, Oxford

Strachan R and Jefferies D (1993) *The Water Vole (Arvicola terrestris) in Britain 1989–1990: Its Distribution and Changing Status.* Vincent Wildlife Trust, Ledbury

Stone D (1986) *Moles.* Mammal Society, London

Tabor R (2001) Cats are carnivores, not criminals. *The Cat*, May/June

Taylor K (1999) Scots eager for beavers. *BBC Wildlife*, January, p. 23

Tennant B (ed.) (2002) *BSAVA Small Animal Formulary, 4th edn.* BSAVA, Gloucester

Tickell O (1995) Exotic tastes: conservation: dormouse future depends on the sycamore tree. *BBC Wildlife*, December, p. 23

Twigg GI, Cuerden CM and Hughes DM (1968) Leptospirosis in British wild mammals. *Symposium of the Zoological Society of London* **24**, 75

Twigg GI, Hughes DM and McDiarmid A (1972) Leptospiral antibodies in dairy cattle: some ecological considerations. *Veterinary Record* **90**, 598–602

Watts CHS (1968) The diet eaten by wood mice (*Apodemus sylvaticus*) and bank voles (*Clethrionomys glareolus*) in Wytham woods, Berkshire. *Journal of Animal Ecology* **37**, 25–41

Weber WJ (1978) *Wild Orphan Babies, 2nd edn.* Holt, Rinehart and Wiston, New York

Webster JP, Ellis WA and MacDonald DW (1995) Prevalence of *Leptospira* spp in wild brown rats (*Rattus norvegicus*) on UK farms. *Epidemiology and Infection* **114**, 195–201

Yalden DW and Dyckowski J (1998) An estimate of the impact of predators on the British field vole (*M. agrestis*) population. *Mammal Review* **28**, 165–184

Acknowledgements

The author would like to thank Matt Brash for information on the captive husbandry of moles and voles, Anne Hudson for her comments on wild rats and mice, Doug Woods for his comments on common dormice, Andrea Smith for the admission figures for the species in this chapter, Derek Gow, Sarah Brown and John McAllister for their information on beavers, Tony Sainsbury for his comments on the dormice section, Debra Bourne and the Wildlife Information Network for information on a number of species covered here and Sian Peters for her general comments.

9

Bats

Andrew Routh

Introduction

The close association of bats with human habitation means that, when ill or injured, they are readily rescued and subsequently presented for veterinary attention and rehabilitation. Despite occurring in large numbers and being easily recognized as bats, the nocturnal nature of these animals means that many people know little about them and, as a result of superstition and misinformation, bats are often feared.

The Bat Conservation Trust, formed in the United Kingdom in the early 1990s, is an umbrella organization catering for all with interests in bats and their conservation. The membership is currently over 3500 and a significant proportion has interests relating to rescue and treatment of sick bats and their rehabilitation.

Bats are K-selected mammals, meaning that they are slow to mature and have high longevity (with individuals recorded as living in excess of 20 years) and low fecundity. In that all the other K-selected mammals are large, bats are fascinating subjects for study not only because they are such small K-selected mammals but also because they are outstandingly successful (Findley, 1993). UK populations of the rarer species number in their thousands and so, when coupled with their K-selected lifestyle, successful rehabilitation could benefit a local population.

UK species

Bats are currently subdivided into Microchiroptera and Megachiroptera (colloquially 'fruit bats'). All species found in the UK (Figure 9.1) are microchiropteran vespertilionids (vesper bats) or rhinolophids (horseshoe bats).

Decline in absolute numbers of bats was recorded throughout the 20th century but during that time the number of UK species remained steadfastly at 15, representing one quarter of the UK native mammal species. With the disappearance of the last known mouse-eared bat (*Myotis myotis*) from its hibernation site in the early 1990s, the species was presumed to be extinct in the UK, but the finding of an aged individual in 2001 in the south of the UK may indicate a small, relic population (Anon., 2001).

Species	Adult weight	Adult forearm length	Remarks
Greater horseshoe bat (*Rhinolophus ferrumequinum*)	13–34 g	51–60 mm	Horseshoe bat species are facially unmistakable and have unique echolocation sonograms
Lesser horseshoe bat (*Rhinolophus hipposideros*)	5–9 g	36–42 mm	
Mouse-eared bat (*Myotis myotis*)	28–45 g	54–68 mm	Very rare (if not extinct) in UK
Whiskered bat (*Myotis mystacinus*)	4–8 g	30–37 mm	Differentiation between these two species can be difficult
Brandt's bat (*Myotis brandtii*)	4.5–9.5 g	31–39 mm	
Natterer's bat (*Myotis nattereri*)	6.5–12 g	36–43 mm	Fine bristles on tail membrane
Bechstein's bat (*Myotis bechsteinii*)	7–13 g	38–47 mm	Rare, confined to southern central UK
Daubenton's bat (*Myotis daubentonii*)	6.0–12 g	33–40.5 mm	Common species, hunts over water
Pipistrelle bat (*Pipistrellus pipistrellus*)	4–8 g	28–35 mm	These figures are for both the 45 kHz (*P. pipistrellus*) and the 55 kHz (*P. pygmaeus*) phonic types; the latter is smaller but morphological differences are inadequate to differentiate species
Nathusius's pipistrelle (*Pipistrellus nathusii*)	6–15 g	32–40 mm	Only recently confirmed breeding in UK
Noctule bat (*Nyctalus noctula*)	18–40 g	47–58 mm	Both *Nyctalus* species emerge in the early evening; the body fur extends to the forearm and patagium

9.1 Resident bat species of the UK (after Greenaway and Hutson, 1990). (continues)

Species	Adult weight	Adult forearm length	Remarks
Leisler's bat (*Nyctalus leisleri*)	11–20 g	39–47 mm	
Serotine bat (*Eptesicus serotinus*)	15–35 g	47–57 mm	Very much a building-oriented species
Barbastelle bat (*Barbastella barbastellus*)	6–13 g	35–43 mm	Distinct species, unlike any other in Europe
Brown long-eared bat (*Plecotus auritus*)	6–12 g	34–42 mm	The genus is easy to identify by the ears but the grey long-eared bat is confined to Devon and the southern coast
Grey long-eared bat (*Plecotus austriacus*)	7–14 g	36–44 mm	

9.1 (continued) Resident bat species of the UK (after Greenaway and Hutson, 1990).

The pipistrelle (*Pipistrellus pipistrellus*), the UK's most numerous and widely distributed bat, was long regarded as a single species. Following identification of two 'phonic types' with differing echolocation signatures, and subsequent DNA analysis of individual bats, it is now considered that there are two separate species, *P. pipistrellus* and *P. pygmaeus* (see Figure 9.1).

On the European mainland, bats are known to migrate over some distance and some have been found resting on North Sea oilrigs, but the role of migration in the dynamics of the UK population has not been determined. Individuals from species not known to breed in the UK are found at intervals, but the previously presumed migrant or vagrant Nathusius' pipistrelle (*P. nathusii*) (Greenaway and Hutson, 1990) is now known to breed in the UK (P. Richardson, personal communication).

Ecology and biology

The UK Microchiroptera are nocturnal obligate aerial insectivores, with no alternative feeding strategies, focusing their hunting activities where prey insect species congregate. All species catch insects on the wing but some will also glean invertebrates from tree leaves. Their crepuscular habit, emerging from roosts around dusk, reduces the risk of predation by diurnal raptors (predation and starvation are the two greatest causes of natural death). It also reduces direct competition with the diurnal avian insect hunters, such as swallows. Hunting occurs mainly at dusk but lactating females have a bimodal activity curve and feed again just before dawn (Altringham, 1996).

The UK climate causes cyclical reductions in insect numbers, which obliges the avian aerial insectivores to migrate. The bats, to a greater or lesser degree, hibernate. Hibernation takes place in secluded environments where the temperature remains constantly low and humidity is high, but where freezing does not occur. Changes in ambient weather will lead to bats emerging to feed or to change hibernaculum if there is a risk of freezing.

Social, familial groups will often roost together – sometimes in their hundreds, as in the pipistrelle species. In contrast to hibernation sites, these roosts are above ground, dry and have fluctuating, often high, temperatures. Single-sex roosts form during the summer months. Females congregate to give birth and raise their almost invariably single young. These roosts may often be in human habitation. If the weather changes or if the food supply disappears, the females, with youngster attached, will move to another roost in the home range.

Anatomy and physiology

Bats are the only mammals that truly fly. This is achieved through modification of the forelimb, especially the distal bones, which form the mobile struts to support the wing. The webbing between the digits is specialized to form the wing membrane or patagium. The lifestyle of each species is reflected in wing shape but, as a unit, the wing shape can also be modified during flight to allow manoeuvrability (Altringham, 1996). The general anatomical features of bats are shown in Figure 9.2.

Contrary to superstition, bats are not blind but their occupation of the twilight zone renders sight a sense of low priority. Some bat species incorporate acute hearing in their hunting strategies and all UK bats use ultrasound echolocation in flight to catch their prey and to avoid static objects. Again individual species' lifestyle, environment and prey size leads to ultrasound emissions that differ in frequency and amplitude (Altringham, 1996).

Bats are heterotherms and adopt two strategies with body temperature (Ransome, 1990). They either maintain their core body temperature (regulate), or allow it to drop in parallel with ambient temperature (conform). Heterothermy is a specialized form of homeothermy, not a primitive one, and is the almost exclusive preserve of the temperate vesper bats and horseshoe bats (Altringham, 1996).

During periods of unseasonable cold weather bats will go into torpor. Body temperature drops, thereby reducing metabolic requirements. Torpor removes the imperative to hunt for limited prey, thereby saving the energy costs that would be incurred through the metabolically taxing effort of flying. The obligation to maintain a higher metabolic rate occurs in female bats from mid-pregnancy when they convert to homeothermy, but during lactation they revert back to heterothermy and daily torpor (Altringham, 1996).

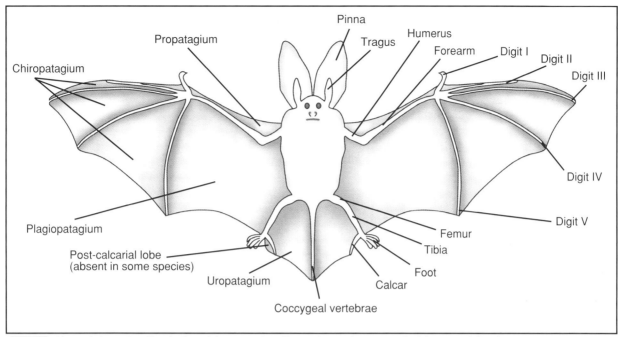

9.2 Ventral view of stylized microchiropteran bat illustrating major anatomical features (after Schober and Grimmberger, 1989).

Not only does seasonal fluctuation in temperature, and therefore prey availability, lead to changes in bat activity but a variation in metabolism is seen from day to day and on a circadian basis. During the day bats will rest and become heterothermic conformers, with a concurrent drop in metabolic rate. In the early evening, prior to leaving the roost to hunt, the bats will become more active as their metabolic rate increases to permit flying, thereby becoming heterotherm regulators.

Rapid arousal from torpor is a characteristic of the heterotherm conformer. The conformer will also arouse rapidly should ambient temperature fall to a critical level, usually freezing (Ransome, 1990) and this is the strategy employed by hibernating bats to avoid fatal exposure to sub-zero temperatures.

Capture, handling and transportation

Zoonotic risks

Whilst all concerned well-wishers and rehabilitators would prioritize the wellbeing of any bat perceived to be in trouble, their prime concern must be for their own safety. Although the risk must be put in context, in that it has only been reported on three occasions to date, European bat lyssavirus 2 – the virus isolated from a Swiss bat biologist who died from rabies in Finland and from the Scottish bat-worker who died in 2002 – has been detected in bats in the UK (Whitby *et al.*, 2000; Fooks *et al.*, 2002; Johnson *et al.*, 2002). Whereas the probability of encountering lyssavirus in a healthy bat is remote, the chances are much increased if the bat is ill. This is precisely the situation in which the rehabilitator and veterinary surgeon will encounter a bat.

Prophylactic rabies vaccination is available for those who work routinely with healthy bats, such as zoologists and conservationists. This has been extended to those who work within the field of bat rehabilitation (Done, 1998). Post-exposure vaccination is also available and is recommended for any unvaccinated individual who has been bitten. Even so, techniques used for the handling of bats must not only prevent injury to the bat but also preclude bite injury to handlers or ingress of saliva into any cut on their hands. The Veterinary Laboratories Agency (VLA) Rabies Diagnostic Unit continues to analyse fresh bat carcasses as an ongoing survey into rabies in bats in the UK (Mitchell-Jones, 1999a) (see 'Specific diseases').

Capture

For initial capture of a grounded bat, in particular by an unskilled person, intimate contact is not required and should be avoided. It will suffice to place a small clean cloth, such as a tea towel, over the bat and then transfer the cloth and the bat into an escape-proof container. A shoebox, with a few small air-holes made in the sides and the lid taped closed, will be adequate. If available, the small plastic tanks with clip-on lids as sold for small pets are more substantial and secure. For a short journey to a veterinary surgeon or rehabilitator, there is no need to provide food and water.

Handling

Handling for clinical examination does require intimate contact. As an absolute minimum safeguard, thin latex gloves should be worn when handling the smaller species. For the larger species, latex gloves will not provide adequate protection. A light pair of leather gloves (e.g. driving gloves) would be more appropriate. For specific handling techniques see 'Examination and assessment'.

At all times during handling, capture and transport attention should be paid to the prevention of escape. All species are small and have a very flat profile, enabling them to escape from all but the most secure containers.

Examination and assessment for rehabilitation

The initial part of the clinical examination must include thorough history-taking. If the bat is ultimately to be released back to the wild successfully, knowledge of the circumstances in which the bat was found, the exact place where it was found and the presence of nearby bat roosts is essential. All this information is useful for future reference, survey work and, in particular, in the event of legal action. Local bat groups, which can be contacted via the Bat Conservation Trust, will help to find roosts.

The species of bat should be ascertained, using a key or field guide (e.g. Greenaway and Hutson, 1990). Identification of an unusual or non-native species may indicate a migrant or accidentally imported individual, with potential zoonotic ramifications.

General examination

Before handling, it may be possible to determine general health through observation of the bat's posture and demeanour, and the nature of faeces or any fluids, such as blood, in the transport box.

The individual should be sexed (males have an obvious penis) and aged. It should be weighed and condition scored to at least a three-point system (i.e. good, moderate and thin). Thin, starved bats have an obviously 'tucked-in' abdomen (Figure 9.3).

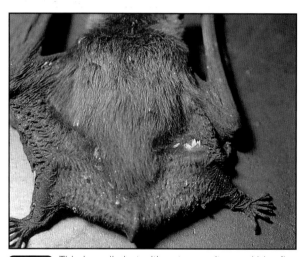

9.3 Thin juvenile bat with ectoparasites and blowfly eggs, showing 'tucked-in' abdomen.

Ageing

Very young, dependent bats are usually easy to identify through their relatively small size, underdeveloped wings and sparse pelage.

Ageing by gross inspection is more difficult with juvenile bats that have become independent. As with all mammal species, ossification of the growing bones takes place. Close scrutiny of the finger bones using transillumination will show bones that are still growing. Examination of the finger joints will reveal a terminal translucency of the phalanges in skeletally immature bats (Figure 9.4a); those with such lucencies are in their first summer (Racey, 1999).

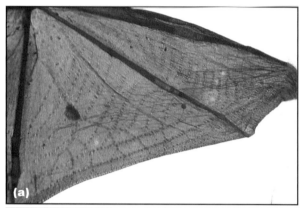

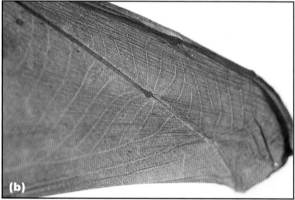

9.4 (a) Transilluminated juvenile finger joint, showing characteristic lucency. (b) Transilluminated adult finger joint. Note: Photographs are of dead specimens.

Clinical examination

Clinical examination should be systematic and ordered. Good light is essential and a hand lens or magnifying loupes advantageous. Examination is best facilitated by holding the bat dorsoventrally across the thorax, using the thumb and fingers in apposition – the 'palm grip' (Figure 9.5) (Racey, 1999). Restraint should be adequate to permit examination but not so much as to restrict breathing in what may be a compromised individual. Grasping the bat by the scruff is safe for the handler but appears to cause distress. A bat should never be restrained for examination solely by holding the extended wings.

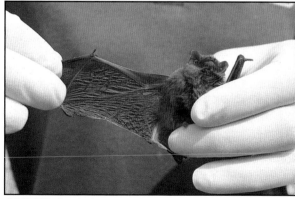

9.5 Bat held with wing extended, demonstrating 'palm grip'. Note: Photograph is of dead specimen.

A general appraisal should be made of the state of hydration, magnitude of any wounds and presence of ectoparasites. Specific attention should be paid to the mouth and jaw, eyes and ears. The ventral abdomen and body orifices should not be overlooked.

While supporting the body, each wing should be extended and examined in turn. The integrity of each long bone should be assessed and the mobility of each joint gauged. Comparison can be made with the contralateral wing. Any puncture or swelling, no matter how small, or area of unexpected mobility, should receive particular attention. The integrity of the wing membrane should be assessed and the size and situation of any holes or tears noted.

Each of the hindlimbs should be examined in a manner similar to that for the wings. The uropatagium, tail and calcar (see Figure 9.2) are important for flight in all species and integral to hunting in many.

Euthanasia

The severity of injuries found on initial presentation often indicates that immediate euthanasia should be performed. Euthanasia of a bat should be seen as a positive welfare action rather than a negative veterinary action. If a bat cannot fly it cannot hunt and cannot, therefore, be released back to the wild. Veterinary treatment of a bat that will become permanently disabled, and therefore unreleasable, must be done with the bat's welfare as the paramount concern.

The small size of the Microchiroptera means that euthanasia by physical means is both feasible and humane (Routh, 1991; Racey, 1999). Techniques described are generally limited to the breaking of the neck by placing a pencil across the cervical vertebrae with the bat held against a hard, flat surface and then pressure being applied to the pencil. The author is also aware of workers who have placed an injured bat in a limiting container, such as a cloth bag, and then delivered a blow to the cranium with a hammer. Both of these techniques achieve the required objective but the degree of trauma can reduce the value of the cadaver for post-mortem analysis (the latter technique precluding post-mortem investigation for rabies).

Many lay workers find such 'hands-on' techniques aesthetically unacceptable. An overdose of an anaesthetic agent is the only acceptable alternative and this can be through use of a volatile agent, or an injectable agent, or an injectable agent after induction of general anaesthesia (see Chapter 2).

Probably because it is completely 'hands off' and is uncomplicated, some lay workers advocate the use of low temperatures as a technique for euthanasia. Initially the bat is placed in a refrigerator and, when torpid, transferred to a freezer. This technique causes minimal distress to the human involved but is inhumane (Routh, 1991, citing R.E. Stebbings, personal communication), and euthanasia by hypothermia and subsequent freezing should not be performed under any circumstances. In a cold environment a bat will go into torpor. As the temperature approaches freezing its metabolic rate will increase and it becomes an active heterothermic regulator in an attempt to

avoid freezing to death. This is the physiological response that would occur in a similar situation in the hibernaculum. One must conclude that bats killed by freezing will have had a period when they were sentient, and subject to pain, as ice crystals were forming in their tissues.

First aid procedures

The rule of thumb for first aid must be 'cause no harm'. Thus, in the window of opportunity between rescue of a bat and its presentation to a veterinary surgeon, it may be well to advocate relative inactivity to the unskilled lay person. This would also minimize the risk to the finder of exposure to zoonotic disease.

Above and beyond this level of intervention, those familiar with the rescue of bats would probably wish to revive the bat. Provision of gentle heat to a torpid bat, either ambient or local, is beneficial. This requires placement in an escape-proof container in case the revived bat becomes active. The extra heat may produce rapid resolution in some instances. Any bat that revives may, in its heightened metabolic state, rapidly succumb to injuries that would anyway have inevitably proved fatal had it remained torpid.

Water may be provided in a very shallow container. In addition, lay rehabilitators may wish to administer electrolytes directly by mouth and some may also wish to administer fluids subcutaneously. Both require provision of materials and the latter technique requires training. Subcutaneous injection is most easily achieved using a 30 gauge needle to inject a small volume of warm crystalloid through a previously disinfected site on the dorsal thorax. Subcutaneous amino acid, electrolyte and dextrose solution (e.g. Duphalyte, Fort Dodge) or Hartmann's solution has been observed to work to good effect at a rate of 0.1 ml per 5 g bat. Its beneficial effect can be measured by anecdotal feedback indicating that subcutaneous fluids administered to a bat when rescued can have life-saving action and fluid therapy should be considered on its merit for all bats presented at the surgery. (For information regarding short-term housing and feeding, see 'Management in captivity and release'.)

Anaesthesia and analgesia

Analgesia

While acknowledging the need for analgesia to be a considered part of the therapeutic management plan for an injured bat, it is not easy in practice. The intention must be to achieve therapeutic levels without causing iatrogenic dose-related toxicity. It is difficult to advocate an analgesic agent that will safely accommodate both a bat's small size and its fluctuating metabolic pattern.

Pharmacologically, the opiates would act as analgesics. Lollar and Schmidt-French (1998) offered a postoperative protocol for butorphanol at 0.1 mg/kg, with administration by injection every 4 hours after dilution with saline. The author has used the non-steroidal anti-inflammatory drug carprofen at a dose rate of 2–4 mg/kg. This was titrated with water for injection and given by subcutaneous injection, to apparent good effect. Meloxicam, at a titrated canine dose rate diluted immediately pre-treatment with water, is another readily available agent that has been used in bats (E. Mullineaux, personal communication).

Anaesthesia

The use of general anaesthesia in bats has previously been opposed by a number of lay workers, due to what were perceived as unacceptably high levels of mortality. Hypothermia was advocated as an alternative 'safer' technique. For this the bat is placed overnight in the domestic refrigerator, conveyed to the operating theatre whilst torpid and operated on before arousal. Many bat workers now no longer promulgate the myth, but it does persist. Use of this technique by veterinary practitioners for anaesthesia is unacceptable. Over a decade ago it was suggested that surgery under hypothermic immobilization alone could constitute an offence under the Protection of Animals (Anaesthetics) Acts 1954 and 1964 (Routh, 1991, citing J.E. Cooper, personal communication).

The author has used, with minimal mortalities, the volatile agents halothane or isoflurane for both induction and maintenance. Both oxygen and nitrous oxide/oxygen mixtures have been utilized to deliver the volatile agent. Neither local anaesthetic agents nor injectable general anaesthetic agents can be advocated. Their narrow therapeutic ranges and long duration of action would be detrimental to the wellbeing of the patient and may cause mortality, making their use impracticable.

If basic principles are adopted (i.e. monitoring, provision of warmth, fluids and oxygen), general anaesthesia in bats is no more unsafe than general anaesthesia in other species. In all instances where surgery is to be carried out the bat must be adequately anaesthetized. Post-mortem examination of bats with relatively minor appendicular injuries, having died under general anaesthetic, often reveals severe internal injuries ('occult injuries') that would have led to death under anaesthetic irrespective of species or technique (Routh, 1991). The greater issue for consideration is not whether general anaesthesia is safe, but whether surgery is the appropriate course of action.

Specific conditions

Trauma

Cat attack

Bats, especially those species that roost in human habitation, frequently fall victim to domestic cats. Some bats may have pre-existing illness leading to their predation but cats have been observed waiting at roost entrances to catch healthy bats emerging at dusk to feed. Routh (1991) reported 50% of injured bats presented in a 2-year period as being victims of cat attack. In a survey of bats submitted for post-mortem examination, Simpson (1994) reported that 65% were due to traumatic injury and approximately 60% of these were directly attributable to cat attack. Daffner (2001), in her post-mortem survey, designated 15 of the 36 bats that had suffered trauma as being the known victims of cat attack. All injuries should be assessed and dealt with pragmatically. Many will be so severe as to warrant immediate euthanasia.

When Simpson (1994) carried out bacteriology on all fresh specimens in his survey, 25% had septicaemia from which *Pasteurella multocida* was isolated. All these bats had injuries consistent with their having been caught by cats. Daffner (2001), working with less fresh specimens where overgrowth from post-mortem invaders was common, was still able to isolate *P. multocida* from five individuals, including a pure culture from the heart blood of two. This would indicate that bats that have received non-fatal injuries have a high probability of succumbing to bacterial septicaemia. An abscess on the nose of a juvenile pipistrelle yielded *Pseudomonas aeruginosa*, and a non-haemolytic *Streptococcus* sp. was cultured from an abscess on an adult pipistrelle caught by a cat (Daffner, 2001).

Prophylactic antibiotic therapy is indicated for all suspected victims of cat attack. Unfortunately, the small size of bats limits the therapeutic options and precludes the use of piperacillin injections, the agent of choice for birds that have been 'catted'. A suitable alternative would be an oral clavulanate-potentiated amoxicillin.

Subcutaneous emphysema is a frequent sequel to cat attack. Deflation of the emphysema, sometimes on several occasions, and provision of antibiotic cover will often lead to successful resolution.

Fractures

As a presumed sequel to a cat attack, bats may present with fractures of the long bones, particularly the humerus and forearm. These can be repaired using splints or, in larger species, intramedullary pins (Lollar and Schmidt-French, 1998) or external fixators (E. Mullineaux, personal communication) with provision of antibiotic cover. However, all substantial fractures thus repaired carry a poor prognosis with respect to subsequent release. Post-operative activity is reduced and, although there may be good bony union, subsequent movement in the wing is often restricted, thereby rendering the bat incapable of sustained flight. Both extensive and 'salvage' orthopaedic surgery and, obviously, wing amputation (Routh, 1991) will produce permanently captive bats. Although several techniques for fracture repair have been described in depth by Lollar and Schmidt-French (1998), they too found that treated bats are almost invariably obliged to remain in captivity.

Greater success is likely with minor wing-tip and distal phalanges injuries. These can be tidied up with removal of non-viable tissue, through careful dissection under general anaesthesia. Deficits produced, in particular where non-viable bone fragments have been removed from digits, heal more quickly if the wound edges are coapted using an absorbable suture material with a swaged-on atraumatic needle, followed by judicious use of a protective spray (e.g. OpSite Spray, Smith & Nephew). Sustained flight is often possible after a short period of time but adequate flight must be determined before release is contemplated.

Fractures of the jaw have been observed in bats without other orthopaedic injury and are a possibility in an alert bat that steadfastly refuses to take solid food. These fractures cannot be repaired.

Wing tears and holes

Many bats, on presentation, have discrete holes in the patagium. These may be incidental findings. Bats in the wild incur minor injuries and their flight can be unimpeded by relatively large holes. Wing holes, however, may be the relatively minor, visible manifestation of a cat attack. Further thorough examination of the bat should be carried out. Holes heal very quickly (Figure 9.6). Once it is certain that there are no other injuries and that the bat is flying well, it can be released (Walsh and Stebbings, 1989).

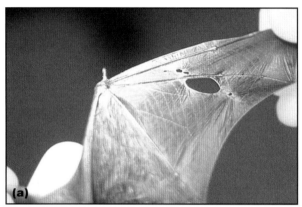

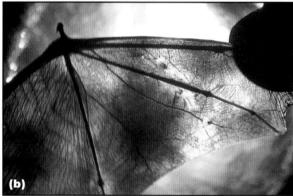

9.6 (a) Pipistrelle with numerous holes in wing membrane. (b) The same bat 10 days later. All the holes have healed without intervention.

Tears (i.e. holes that extend to and include the wing margin) have a far more guarded prognosis. They will heal given time but the resultant scar tissue, by restricting full extension of the wing, often prevents functional flight. Attempts to accelerate natural repair using fine sutures or surgical cyanomethacrylate glues, as described by Lollar and Schmidt-French (1998) and Stocker (2000), have proved unsuccessful in this author's hands. Furthermore, the cyanomethacrylate glues do not produce a tissue–tissue union (Routh, 1991) and apparent repair of the patagium may break down after release, with fatal consequences. Plastic membrane (e.g. OpSite Film, Smith & Nephew) can be used 'sandwich fashion', with or without surgical debridement (Stocker, 2000; E. Mullineaux, personal

communication) to support the wing membrane whilst it heals. Once healed, physiotherapeutic flying is essential and ability would have to be assessed before release is contemplated.

Entanglement and fishing-tackle injuries

Although the bat ultrasonic echolocation system is sensitive, it is not foolproof. Garden-frequenting species become entangled in monofilament netting used to protect fruit bushes. Entanglement in fishing line is the exclusive province of riparian (river-bank) Daubenton's bats caught up in discarded line hanging from foliage as they hunt close to the water's surface. This species may become hooked if a hook remains on the discarded line. Being hooked by the head or mouth occurs so often that it may be that the hook, suspended in mid-air by the line, is mistaken as a prey item.

Disentanglement and assessment of injuries may require a general anaesthetic. Depth of injuries and circulatory impairment should be assessed. The wound should be cleaned with antiseptic and may benefit from application of cleansing agents and repeated application of hydrogels (e.g. IntraSite Gel, Smith & Nephew). Antibiotic cover should be considered and regular exercise instigated to prevent scar tissue from restricting limb movement.

Oil contamination

Oil contamination of fur is a frequent presenting sign. Other contaminants include adhesives from fly-papers and cockroach traps. Water-soluble contaminants are most easily removed with a dilute solution of green household washing-up liquid (industrial degreasing agents are too severe). The fur is then rinsed thoroughly. This technique also works with oil but is often a more extensive procedure. With oil contamination the author has found sunflower-based margarine to be superior as a cleansing agent. It is worked into an area of fur and cleaned off using cotton buds. This procedure is repeated until no more oil is removed. Any residual margarine is groomed off by the bat, which remains active through not having been washed and rinsed. Oral kaolin and pectin gel will act as an adsorbent to minimize effects from previously ingested oil.

Poisoning

Agrochemicals, affecting both the bats and their insect prey, have contributed to the worldwide decline of bats (Stebbings, 1988).

Timber treatments

The use of timber treatments in house loft spaces represents a particular risk to bats that are using such areas to roost. Treatment of timbers and remedial building work are covered under the 1981 Wildlife and Countryside Act (see Chapter 5), thereby affording protection to bats and their roosts. In practical terms this gives the Statutory Nature Conservation Organizations (SNCOs) a statutory role in advising how damage to bats and to their roosts can reasonably be avoided or minimized (Mitchell-Jones, 1999b). Older timber treatments can remain toxic months after their application (Racey and Swift, 1986). Bats may be no more sensitive to these compounds than are other mammals, but stored liposoluble toxins may be released in fatal amounts when fat reserves are metabolized (Clark, 1988). Analysis of the liver of a pipistrelle bat from a roost where timbers had been treated with a compound containing dieldrin, pentochlorophenol (PCP) and tributyltin oxide (TBTO) showed a dieldrin concentration of 13.3 mg/g wet matter (Simpson, 1994). Newer, less toxic treatments are now available. Through enforcement of the law, public awareness, the replacement of the more toxic compounds (such as lindane) with permethrin, and the strict control of PCP, the number of future incidents should be minimized.

Algal toxins
Suspected poisoning from blue-green algal toxins has been recorded in the USA (Pybus *et al.*, 1986) and this could occur in the UK, especially in species such as the Daubenton's bat, which hunts over inland waters.

Viral diseases
The known virus burden in UK bats is low but consideration of bat viruses worldwide is worthwhile. Some occur elsewhere in species resident to the UK, species related to UK species or species that have been found as occasional vagrants in the UK (Greenaway and Hutson, 1990). Some viruses have insect vectors that may be inadvertently translocated, via the medium of modern rapid transport, to new countries (Simpson, 1999). Consideration of the viruses found in bats also demonstrates recent advances in the study of sylvatic disease and puts into perspective the relative zoonotic risks to which wildlife workers are exposed in different parts of the world.

Rabies (lyssaviruses)
The lyssaviruses, historically recognized and researched largely in the Northern Hemisphere, are the viruses in bats that have received the greatest attention. The European bat lyssavirus (EBL) has two subtypes, EBL1 and EBL2 (the lyssavirus serotypes 5 and 6), and more than 400 cases in bats have been recorded in Europe (Rupprecht *et al.*, 2001), including the three UK cases reported by Whitby *et al.* (2000), Johnson *et al.* (2002) and Fooks *et al.*, (2002). The reservoir for both subtypes is believed to be insectivorous bats and both have been responsible for human deaths. Should a bat be showing any behavioural or neurological signs leading one to suspect a case of rabies, it should be safely confined and the local Animal Health Office of DEFRA should be contacted for advice on how to proceed.

Others
Other potentially zoonotic viral diseases are known to affect bats outside the UK and there is potential for spread of disease through the migration of any sylvatic host species. It has been speculated that migrating birds or bats are the medium of reintroduction in the spring of the western equine encephalitis virus (WEEV) (Hayes and Wallace, 1977, cited in Yuill and Seymour, 2001).

Bacterial diseases
Other than invasive bacteria, the only bacteria recorded by Simpson (1994) were *Escherichia coli*, which were mostly associated with enteric disease. Culture of intestines of 36 bats in the same study proved negative for *Salmonella* spp., but Daffner (2001) isolated a *Salmonella* Group 4, 09, 12 sp. when heart blood and faeces were cultured following post-mortem examination of a whiskered bat (*Myotis mystacinus*). The bat had been in captivity for 3 days but the clinical significance of the *Salmonella* is not known. No *Campylobacter* species were isolated from any of the 73 bats in Daffner's survey.

Fungal diseases
Dermatophytes identified by Hill and Smith (1984, cited in Lollar and Schmidt-French, 1998) included *Trichophyton persicolor*, *T. mentagrophytes* and *Microsporum canis*. The survey by Simpson (1994) also identified ringworm but did not specify the species found. There is potential for zoonotic infection. Transmission is possible from infected humans, from conspecifics or from other species housed in a rehabilitation facility (see 'Diseases of the integument').

Histoplasma capsulatum has been reported from more than 30 countries (Sanger, 1981, cited in Burek, 2001) and is recognized as a cause of disease of bats in the USA (Barnard, 1995; Lollar and Schmidt-French, 1998). Infection, known as 'cave sickness', may be contracted by people working in caves through their contact with bat guano (Burek, 2001). The organism requires moist conditions and large amounts of guano for multiplication. In the UK, even in large roosts, droppings usually remain dry and the disease is not currently identified as a risk for bat workers (Mitchell-Jones, 1999a).

Parasites

Ectoparasites
Mites (*Steatonyssus* spp., *Dermanyssina* spp. and larvae of *Neotrombicula autumnalis*) (Simpson, 1994) are frequently seen. They are found in their greatest numbers on debilitated juveniles. This may reflect numbers acquired in the maternity roost and their persistence through weakness preventing grooming. The numbers may be so large as to contribute to the debility. On adult bats, mites – usually spinturnicids (Hutson and Racey, 1999) – are most apparent on the wings and may cause punctate damage to the patagium. To remove mites the use of sparing amounts of permethrin flea powder has been advocated (Anon., 2000b). Loller and Schmidt-French (1998) described the use of ivermectin injection (10 mg/ml) given orally immediately after diluting the solution in a ratio of 1:100 with water. A safer alternative used in orphan bats is to wipe the wing membranes with the rearing milk (a mixture of goat's milk, cream and live yoghurt) (G. Little, personal communication). Mites are lifted off and the remainder appears to be killed – probably through asphyxiation – by the non-toxic, greasy residue.

All bats are hosts to ischnopsyllid fleas. These are host species-specific and may allow indirect differentiation between closely related species, e.g. *P. pipistrellus* and *P. nathusii* (Hutson and Racey, 1999).

The soft tick *Argas vespertilionis* has been recorded (Simpson, 1994) and is presumed to be a vector of disease.

Other true ectoparasites include the cimicid bat-bugs and nycteribiid bat-flies, both of which feed on blood (Hutson and Racey, 1999). These, too, are presumed to be disease vectors. Infective forms of *Schizotrypanum* have been found in the gut of *Cimex pipistrelli* (Gardner, 1984, cited in Daffner, 2001) and stages of the haemoproteid *Polychromophilus murinus* were found in *Nycteribia kolenatti* collected from a Daubenton's bat (Gardner *et al*,, 1987, cited in Daffner, 2001).

Debilitated bats may become the victims of fly strike (myiasis), which can be a feature of terminal decline. Particular attention should be paid in the initial examination to back-grooming the fur, thereby avoiding blowfly eggs being overlooked. Diligent grooming, rather than the topical administration of potentially toxic drugs, is essential to ensure their removal.

Endoparasites

Lollar and Schmidt-French (1998), when reviewing the situation in the USA, stated broadly that bats may be parasitized by trematodes, nematodes and cestodes, but Daffner (2001) reported endoparasites in only one individual out of 73 bats examined in her UK survey. Roundworms, in particular, are described as infesting a number of sites in the body and some endoparasites are described as having complex life cycles. Lollar and Schmidt-French (1998) mentioned, anecdotally, treatment with pyrantel for nematodes and praziquantel for cestodes. Barnard (1995) advocated fenbendazole at 50 mg/kg daily for 3 days and Wilson (1988) mentioned thiabendazole for the treatment of ascarids, but none described clinical disease due to endoparasitism.

Protozoa

Babesia vesperuginis has been recorded in bats in south-west England and reported in bats in Cambridgeshire (Simpson, 1994). It is believed to be transmitted by the soft tick *Argas vespertilionis*. Splenomegaly was noted. Stained blood films of severely anaemic bats may demonstrate the parasite. Kunz and Nagy (1988) described collection of blood into a 70 µl heparinized capillary tube from the veins in the interfemoral membrane (uropatagium), or from the cardiac vein, which is prominent on the leading edge of the propatagium of the wing. Their technique was used on healthy bats weighing from 2 g to 15 g and therefore would be applicable to the species found in the UK.

Trypanosomes have been identified in blood samples of British bat species (Gardner, 1984, cited in Daffner, 2001). *Trypanosoma dionisii* and *T. vespertilionis* were isolated from five species of bat (*Pipistrellus pipistrellus*, *Nyctalus leisleri*, *N. noctula*, *Eptesicus serotinus* and *Myotis brandtii*) and were transmitted experimentally via *Cimex pipistrelli* (Gardner and Molyneux, 1988, cited in Daffner, 2001).

In a summary of enteric protozoans, Duszynski and Upton (2001) record 30 species of *Eimeria* in only 26 host species of bat and no records of *Isospora* or *Cyclospora*. With an estimated 925 bat species found worldwide, this figure is low when compared with over 400 eimerians found in rodents. The apparent lack of diversity is thought to be due to underinvestigation. When individual species are surveyed, the level of infection can vary markedly between species. Lifestyle may be the major contributory factor, with the species frequenting permanent (especially damp) roosts and the crevice-dwelling species that have more intimate contact with their faeces being most likely to be infected.

Gruber *et al.* (1996, cited in Duszynski and Upton, 2001) found renal coccidiosis with cystic tubular dilatation in one individual from each of the following species: *P. pipistrellus*, *M. mystacinus*, *M. nattereri* and *N. noctula*. All species are common in the UK (Schober and Grimmberger, 1989). Bernard (1995), without describing clinical signs, advocated treatment of coccidiosis with oral potentiated sulphonamides.

Suspected *Cryptosporidium* sp. was detected in heavy numbers in a faecal smear taken from a brown long-eared bat (*Plecotus auritus*) (Daffner, 2001).

Other conditions

Non-specific diarrhoea

Collapsed, dehydrated bats may void mucoid or watery diarrhoea. This may be the primary cause of the debility or may be the manifestation of scant gut contents following starvation. Many respond to symptomatic treatment including subcutaneous fluids, or rehydration with proprietary electrolyte solution, via a nasolacrimal duct cannula placed just on the tip of the tongue allowing oral adminstration, and judicious use of a kaolin and pectin gel (e.g. Kaogel V, Pharmacia & Upjohn).

Diseases of the integument

Bats spend a large amount of time grooming and keeping in good order the various membranes that are essential for flight. Care of the wing includes systematic licking of the patagium. Simpson (1994) reported both ringworm and staphylococcal dermatitis.

Bat carers have noted the occurrence of various necrotic conditions of the wing, particularly in long-term captives. Conditions seen by the author have included areas of wing membrane loss through dry or ischaemic necrosis, approximating to tissues supplied by an end artery, and an advancing wet necrosis, some 2 mm in width, occurring at the wing margin and causing progressive loss of the patagium. These differ in presentation from a moist, exudative lesion of the patagium causing areas of adhesion when the wing is folded in the natural resting position. Racey (1999) suggested that relative humidity is a key factor, with an ideal being around 80%. Too dry an environment is deleterious to the wing membrane and too wet an atmosphere leads to fungal and bacterial infection.

A noctule (*N. noctula*), presented as a recently rescued wild individual, showed changes that may allude to one possible aetiology. Initially there were a number of small, fluid-filled blisters on both wings distal to the carpus. As these settled, an oedema of the distal wing became apparent. Within a few days the wings underwent ischaemic changes, leading to dry gangrene, sloughing of each wing distal to the carpus and the bat's euthanasia. The uropatagium remained unaffected. This sequence of events has been observed by other rehabilitators (Stocker, 2000). The parallels between the observed lesions and wing-tip oedema in raptors (see Chapter 22) are remarkable and the bat had been found on the ground early in the spring following a few days of heavy frosts. Comparison of the conditions may suggest potential treatments, which could include agents to aid circulation such as the oral preparation isoxsuprine or topical nitric oxide cream (Tucker *et al.*, 1999).

The author has observed similar devitalizing changes to those seen in the patagium in the pinna of a brown long-eared bat. The individual was, through amputation of a wing, a long-term captive and the changes were restricted to the ipsilateral pinna. This species roosts with the pinnae folded under the wings. The inability of this individual to do so with the affected pinna would affect its microenvironment, which could lead to the production of the lesions and, ultimately, to the loss of the pinna.

Despite bacterial culture, fungal culture and histology, a definitive aetiology was not established in any of the cases seen by the author. All instances have also proved refractory to treatment with topical medication. The frequency of occurrence of lesions of the patagium indicates that this would be a fruitful area for research.

Lollar and Schmidt-French (1998) described ringworm as bald, circular patches within the fur or as pale iridescent areas where there is no hair. Scaly or yellowish crusting areas may also be ringworm. They recommended isolation, thorough cleansing of potentially infected housing and treatment of the bat with griseofulvin. As an alternative, topical natamycin wash can be used (E. Mullineaux, personal communication).

Fur loss occurs in some captive bats. Most frequently seen is a syndrome where the ventral head and neck are initially affected, but the alopecia may extend caudally to the ventral thorax and abdomen and cause skin erythema. One speculated cause of this is that the fluid expressed from decapitated mealworms, as they are fed by hand to the debilitated bat, has a corrosive or irritant action on the skin. Barnard (1995) believed that quinones, excreted by the mealworms, may contribute to this condition, in particular the fur loss.

Joint conditions

Infected abrasions of the carpus through poor housing on harsh, dirty surfaces are seen. Racey (1999) reported that horseshoe bats (*Rhinolophus* spp.) develop swollen carpal joints after even a few days in captivity, probably through restriction of movement.

Therapeutics

Since bats are heterotherms, and thus do not conform to allometric principles, and since they have circadian periods of torpor that may be accentuated through debility, it is difficult to propose a logical course of action when considering the dosage regime of therapeutic agents for bats. If one adheres to allometric principles, based on a metabolic weight, overdose would be likely in a bat that remained torpid. Conversely, allowance for torpor and appropriate reduction of drug dosage may mean that therapeutic levels are not achieved in the active bat. Dose rates (mg/kg) equivalent to those given to the domestic carnivores (with marked titration to allow for the small bodyweight of the bats) are used by the author.

Because of the requirement to combat infection, antibiotics are appropriate in injury, especially where cat attack may be suspected. Bacterial culture and antibiotic sensitivity tests should be carried out if at all possible. Routh (1991) advocated oral antibiotics for ease of administration, but offered no dose regimes. Antibiotics that appear to be well tolerated and that may, empirically, have had a beneficial effect include the synthetic penicillins and augmented derivatives, the cephalosporins, clindamycin and lincomycin. Potentially ototoxic compounds (e.g. the aminoglycosides gentamicin and neomycin) should not be used and the use of tetracyclines would be contraindicated in growing individuals.

The Bat Conservation Trust (Anon., 2000b) include enrofloxacin, which would be similarly contraindicated in growing individuals, as another antibiotic that may be beneficial. In addition, they give dose rates for four commercially available antibiotics. Lollar and Schmidt-French (1998), the apparent source of the dose rates for the previously mentioned antibiotics, also listed a tetracycline and advocated an oral combination of enrofloxacin and cefalexin for broad-spectrum therapy.

The author has not observed gastrointestinal disturbances indicating adverse effects from the action of antibiotics on the gut flora, but some workers will supplement the diet of a bat undergoing antibiotic therapy with preparations containing lactobacilli (Barnard, 1995).

Management in captivity

Housing

For initial housing and all but long-term captives, the most suitable accommodation is the clip-top plastic tank that can be purchased from most pet stores. These tanks are lightweight, can be easily cleaned and disinfected and are escape-proof. Substrate is provided in the form of paper towels, some of which should be trapped under the lid to provide a vertical surface behind which the bat can secrete itself. Heat, up to an ambient 32°C, should be provided at one end, thereby giving a temperature gradient. Water can be provided in a shallow dish or in a small bird hopper-type fountain. This set-up has served the author well and has much to commend it.

There are those who prefer wooden boxes on the grounds that they approximate more to the natural situation and are less acoustically harsh. These must be made from untreated timber. Plastic tanks have been blamed for the deaths of bats, due to the emission of toxic vapours. However, on post-mortem examination of such cases, this author has always found injuries that account for the deaths. Wooden boxes are heavy and can be difficult to clean thoroughly and to disinfect. The abrasive nature of the surfaces can cause erosions to the carpus, which may become infected, extend to the joint and prevent release.

Whichever system is used to house the bat for the bulk of the day, it is essential that flight is permitted on a regular and frequent basis (see 'Pre-release assessment'). Initial flight may be poor but it must be encouraged through persistence on the part of the rehabilitator. Failure of a bat to fly within a few days indicates undiagnosed injuries; it carries a poor prognosis and warrants further investigation.

Although social animals, there is no need to maintain bats in a social group while they are hospitalized. Individual care is needed and there is the risk of transmission of undiagnosed disease between individuals. This should be reviewed for long-term captives.

Feeding

The normal diet of bats in captivity is insects, bred primarily for use by aviculturalists and herpetologists. If these are not available, as an interim measure a commercial tinned cat food or convalescent diet (e.g. Hill's a/d, Hill's Pet Nutrition), offered on a toothpick, is well accepted.

Supplementation of the diet of an individual bat with some natural food is feasible (for example, moths caught in a moth trap can be fed to brown long-eared bats) but the nutritional demands of hospitalized bats cannot be met through the feeding of natural food. There is the additional risk that wild-caught food may be contaminated with agrochemicals.

The most common insect food offered is mealworms, the larvae of the beetle *Tenebrio molitor*, and these can be purchased from pet shops or by mail order. While representing a good source of calories and being readily accepted, they are *per se* nutritionally deficient, in particular with reference to the calcium:phosphorus ratio. The deficiency is increased when the mealworms are feeding in bran, which is low in calcium and contains the calcium-binding compound phytate. Using a proprietary complete dog kibble as the nutritional substrate for the mealworms is convenient, may augment their nutritional value and will gut-load them. Dusting the mealworms immediately pre-feeding with a proprietary vitamin and mineral supplement or using proprietary gut-loading supplements should also improve the mealworms' nutritional value. Bat workers dealing with large numbers of bats have their own husbandry protocols and diets for mealworms (Lollar and French-Schmidt, 1998) but these are labour-intensive.

Bats can readily be trained to take mealworms. The bat is restrained gently in the cupped hand and the abdominal contents of the mealworm are extruded, toothpaste-like, into the bat's mouth. Once the bat starts chewing, the empty exoskeleton can be gently pushed into its mouth. When the bat has adapted to mealworms offered in this manner, it can be offered decapitated mealworms with tweezers and should then progress to mealworms offered in a bowl. Progress is assessed through a combination of determination of weight gain (with reference to appetite and quantities eaten) and body condition score (subjectively looking at bony prominences such as the pelvic bones). Allowance has to be made when the bat changes from the sedentary, convalescing individual to the pre-release individual that is flying regularly.

Some people appear to be sensitive to mealworms. In a few severe cases respiratory signs may be seen but, more commonly, there is local skin irritation. Wiping the face after handling mealworms may cause an acute conjunctivitis. Due caution is advised and the use of latex gloves is prudent.

Barnard (1995) expressed concerns about quinones produced by beetles in the family Tenebrionidae. It is believed that these can accumulate in the feeding medium as older larvae, especially those approaching metamorphosis, excrete them. The quinones are implicated in illnesses, described as toxicities, in captive bats and Barnard (1995) described such a condition in a captive big brown bat (*Eptesicus fuscus*). Post-mortem analysis of the viscera was positive for hydroquinones at an estimated 10–20 parts per million. A lower grade of toxicity is thought to be one of the factors in fur loss. As a preventive measure, Barnard (1995) advocated feeding newly acquired mealworms on clean medium for 2 weeks before offering them to the bats, along with removal of any mealworms that are approaching metamorphosis. Keeping mealworms in a domestic refrigerator slows their development.

Some species of bat will eat waxworms (*Galleria mellonella*) and crickets (*Gryllus* spp.). These are commercially available and are inherently of greater nutritional value than mealworms, but tend to be more expensive.

Food intake, faecal quantity and quality, and bodyweight and condition should be monitored on a daily basis to gauge progress. Failure to eat after several days warrants further investigation and carries a guarded prognosis. Obesity has been recorded (Constantine, 1986; Stocker, 2000; Daffner, 2001).

Simpson (1994) reported a white liver syndrome, in particular in hospitalized pipistrelles. Due to its resemblance to a similar condition seen in lambs on low cobalt diets, he speculated that this could be dietary in origin.

Rearing of orphans

Maternity roosts are often close to or within residential dwellings; thus, a bat outside at an inappropriate time of the day is likely to be noticed. A drop in temperature may cause a roost to move, with individuals left behind. In cold weather semi-independent young may head towards the warmth of the house living area. On occasion, young bats may fall from a roost.

If an orphan appears healthy it should be looked after during the day, kept warm and hydrated using oral electrolyte, and returned to the roost at dusk in the hope that it will be picked up by its mother. This works in some cases and is the ideal conclusion.

If release does not take place, either the bat will have to be taken into captivity for rearing or euthanasia will have to be carried out (Barnard, 1995). The hand-rearing of orphans through to flight, whilst being difficult and time-consuming, is achievable. Housing, feeding and weaning are all well documented (Barnard, 1995; Lollar and Schmidt-French, 1998; Stocker, 2000), as are nutritional diseases manifesting themselves as deformity of the bones, in particular the finger bones (Simpson, 1994).

Release

Pre-release assessment

Because bats need to fly to catch prey items and use ultrasound echolocation in the process, it is vital to ensure that a bat is capable of sustained flight and that it is echolocating before its release is contemplated.

To assess flight a large, escape-proof room is needed. The smaller species are more manoeuvrable and can be assessed adequately in a room of average size, or perhaps a lightweight tent, but the larger species, especially if not completely fit, may need more extensive facilities. It is best to carry out the assessment in the evening when the bat will be more metabolically active.

The bat should be allowed to warm up thoroughly and become physically active before flight is attempted. Once active, it should be encouraged to launch itself from a height of around 1.5 m. It should then, after an initial drop, climb to above head height and circle the room's airspace. Bats that are unfit either fail to gain height, or fly poorly before descending to the ground, or keep inverting themselves to brush against surfaces, using their hindfeet to find a purchase on a wall or surface that will allow them to rest. Bats that are fit for release must fly vigorously for at least 10 minutes; those that show no signs of tiring (to the extent that one despairs of recatching them) are ready for release.

Conservationists and bat enthusiasts use commercially available electronic 'bat detectors' to observe bats and to study bat behaviour in the wild. These are tuned to pick up the ultrasound emissions through a microphone and then, in most versions, convert them down to 'real-time' sounds within the human auditory range. The converted sounds are listened to by means of an integral loudspeaker or headphones. While being flown in a confined space, the bat will use echolocation to prevent itself crashing into walls and static objects. A bat detector can be used to assess the use of echolocation; if possible, it should be tuned to the frequency that is characteristic of the species being flown. Ultrasound emissions should be audible whilst the bat is flying and they coincide with the successful negotiation of objects. It is unlikely that the characteristic 'feeding buzz', heard as wild bats home in on flying food items, will be heard during these trials.

At least one purpose-built 'bat flight' is being used for bats by a wildlife rehabilitator, to good effect (R. Jackson, personal communication). The flight has a fan at one end to push air gently in the manner of a wind-tunnel. The smooth plastic walls encourage flight by eliminating rest points. There is an observation window and an integral microphone is linked to a bat detector and speaker outside the flight area.

Release of adults

Release should be undertaken only when the bat is deemed fit for release, as judged by the parameters outlined above. A bat release is an 'all or nothing' event, as there is little chance of recapturing a bat that fails to perform adequately on release. If the exact site where the bat was found is known, the bat should be returned to that site. Even if the social group has changed roost site in the interim, it is presumed that this lies within the bat's home range and therefore it should readily orientate itself within the release area.

The release should take place at dusk and when weather conditions are favourable and conducive to flight. Heavy rain, wind, frost or snow preclude release. The presence of conspecifics in the area would indicate conditions that are inherently suitable. Ideally a feed and warm-up flight should have been carried out that evening at the rehabilitation facility. The warmed-up and active bat should be held in the hand and allowed to launch itself.

Post-release monitoring

Whereas wild bats are monitored to study population dynamics, there has been very little work published on post-release monitoring of rehabilitated bats. Any marking of a bat requires a licence to be issued by the statutory authorities (SNCOs). Whilst some techniques, such as clipping fur or gluing on small markers, are unlikely to be detrimental to the bat's survival, wing bands or radio transmitters are potentially life-threatening if used incorrectly.

An unpublished retrospective study of mark/recapture data, acquired incidental to other work, was carried out in the 1950s and 1960s. Healthy bats (*Myotis* spp., *Rhinolophus ferrumequinum* and *Barbestella barbestellus*) were taken from roosts for study, held in captivity, marked and released at intervals. The study put a limit on the time a bat should be hospitalized (Walsh and Stebbings, 1989): the failure to recapture marked bats with any regularity after they had been held beyond 3 weeks led to a ceiling of 20 days being proposed for the amount of time a bat could spend in captivity. Beyond that time in captivity it was deemed that the bat would be unable to survive subsequent release.

An extended time in captivity may be essential in order to release a bat with an optimal chance of survival and the 20-day limit is now promoted less vigorously (Richardson, 2000). Modern husbandry techniques and vigorous physiotherapeutic flying should allow the release of healthy bats well after 20 days in captivity.

As is the case in birds that have been ringed, returns of information on banded bats are low with reference to the numbers marked. Licensed post-release monitoring schemes are being carried out on both orphan and adult bats (P. Richardson, personal communication) but they are in their early stages and a valid study would have to be in the long term. Failure to find a bat in subsequent surveys – the criterion for survival in the original study (Walsh and Stebbings, 1989) – does not mean that it has failed to survive. The longest interval between a healthy Daubenton's bat being marked (with a wing band in an intensive population study) and its being found again, despite saturation local recapture of conspecifics, is 9 years (P. Richardson, personal communication). Its whereabouts in the interim are unknown, but this demonstrates that a lack of returns from wing-banding over the short term does not necessarily indicate poor post-release survival.

Release of orphans

Where debate arises is as to what should be done to release the hand-reared bats satisfactorily, as there is a considerable body of opinion that a large component of a bat's behaviour, including hunting skills, finding roost sites and behaviour with regard to conspecifics, is learnt.

Hand-reared bats will echolocate, hunt and catch insect prey in captivity (Barnard, 1995; G. Little, personal communication), indicating that this skill is innate, but whether this would translate into competent foraging behaviour in the wild in unknown. Worldwide studies on a number of species in the wild indicate taught behavioural components (Altringham, 1996). Ability to hunt is not the only behaviour required for successful survival. There needs to be successful interrelationship with conspecifics and information transfer is believed to occur, especially in communal roosts (Altringham, 1996).

Thus, the conventional train of argument follows that any bat that has been hand-reared without parental teaching and support will fail to survive after release (Walsh and Stebbings, 1989; Barnard, 1995; Anon., 2000a). There is always the possibility that, in the absence of proof of post-release survival, release of reared infants might constitute an offence under the Abandonment of Animals Act, 1969 (see Chapter 5).

However, Jones et al. (1995) radio-tracked the greater horseshoe bat (R. ferrumequinumm) and demonstrated that mother and offspring both leave the roost and forage separately. Adult bats cope with frequent, and often dramatic, changes in the local environment and so it may be reasonable to expect some flexibility in the behaviour of young bats.

An option, as yet poorly explored, would be to rehabilitate the bats by getting them fit enough to release with the aid of a naturalistic enclosure. Bat flights that allow the ingress of natural prey are simple to construct (Barnard, 1995; Lollar and Schmidt-French, 1998; Racey, 1999) but their success as pre-release environments has not been ascertained. It can be difficult, even through the use of insect-attracting lights, to encourage the bats to fly. One constraint on the stimulation of flight in captivity would be the observation that pipistrelle bats in the wild will only feed when insect density exceeds 300 per 1000 m^3 (Racey and Swift, 1985). If numbers are fewer, the bats will move on to forage elsewhere.

Stocker (2000) described a technique that he equated to 'hacking back' in raptors and that he has used to release hand-reared noctules (N. noctula) in a suitable environment. Soft release (see Chapter 3) immediately adjacent to a local roost of conspecifics is a further refinement of the technique. The fitness of the bats for release is determined. They are then taken to the release site at the roost and held in an enclosure. It is hoped that they will 'tune in' to the unrelated resident colony and have a degree of auditory liaison before being released, after a few days, at dusk (G. Little, personal communication). The success of this technique is, again, undetermined but, in the light of current knowledge, it represents the best chance to rehabilitate hand-reared orphan bats back to the wild if permanent captivity is to be avoided and if euthanasia of all orphans that fail to be retrieved by their parents is unacceptable.

Legal considerations

The Wildlife and Countryside Act 1981 affords full protection to wild bats, their roosts and hibernation sites. Section 10(3)(a) allows unlicensed persons to 'take' disabled bats, for the sole purpose of tending them, with the intention of releasing them when they are no longer disabled. Section 10(3)(b) permits the killing of bats that are so seriously disabled that no recovery is likely.

Within the Act there is no clear interpretation of the position regarding bats that fail to recover sufficiently to be released, nor those that have been rendered unfit for release through an act of commission, nor hand-reared orphans, nor captive-born bats.

Specialist organizations

Bat Conservation Trust
15 Cloisters House, 8 Battersea Park Road, London SW8 4BG
Tel.: 020 7627 2629
E-mail: enquiries@bats.org.uk
Website: www.bats.org.uk

Carcasses for rabies analysis

Bat carcasses are required for routine rabies screening. These do not need to be from suspected cases. They should be sent fresh, in a parcel that complies with current postal regulations, to:

Rabies Diagnostics Unit, Veterinary Laboratories Agency, Woodham Lane, New Haw, Addlestone, Surrey KT15 3NB

References and further reading

Altringham JD (1996) *Bats: Biology and Behaviour*. Oxford University Press, Oxford
Anon. (2000a) *Guidelines on Care of 'Grounded Bats'*. Bat Conservation Trust, London
Anon. (2000b) *Treatment of Bat Casualties for Veterinary Surgeons*. Professional Support Series. Bat Conservation Trust, London
Anon. (2001) Extinct bat returns – but all too briefly. *Bat News*, **60**, 5
Bernard SM (1995) *Bats in Captivity*. Wild Ones Animal Books, Springville, California

Burek K (2001) Mycotic diseases. In: *Infectious Diseases of Wild Mammals*, eds ES Williams and IK Barker, pp. 514–531. Manson Publishing, London

Clark DR Jr (1988) How sensitive are bats to insecticides? *Wildlife Society Bulletin* **16**, 399–403

Constantine DG (1986) Insectivorous bats. In: *Zoo and Wild Animal Medicine*, ed. ME Fowler, pp. 650–655. WB Saunders, Philadelphia

Daffner B (2001) *Causes of morbidity and mortality in British bat species and prevalence of selected zoonotic pathogens*. Thesis for MSc in Wild Animal Health, Institute of Zoology and Royal Veterinary College, London

Done J (1998) (correspondence) *Veterinary Times* **28**(7), 23

Duszynski DW and Upton SJ (2001) *Cyclospora, Eimeria, Isospora* and *Cryptosporidium* spp. In: *Parasitic Diseases of Wild Mammals*, eds WM Samuel *et al.*, pp. 424–427. Manson Publishing, London

Findley JS (1993) *Bats: a Community Perspective*. Cambridge University Press, Cambridge

Fooks AR, Finnegan C, Johnson N, Mansfield K, McElhinney L and Manser P (2002) Human case of EBL type 2 following exposure to bats in Angus, Scotland. *Veterinary Record* **151**, 679

Greenaway F and Hutson AM (1990) *A Field Guide to British Bats*. Bruce Coleman Books, Uxbridge

Hutson AM and Racey PA (1999) Examining bats. In: *Bat Workers' Manual*, eds AJ Mitchell-Jones and AP McLeish, pp. 39–45. Joint Nature Conservancy Committee, Peterborough

Johnson N, Selden D, Parson SG and Fooks AR (2002) European bat lyssavirus type 2 in a bat found in Lancashire. *Veterinary Record* **151**, 455–456

Jones G, Duverge L and Ransome RD (1995) Conservation biology of an endangered species: field studies of greater horseshoe bats. *Symposia of the Zoological Society of London* **67**, 309–324

Kunz TH and Nagy KA (1988) Methods of energy budget analysis. In: *Ecological and Behavioral Methods for the Study of Bats*, ed. TH Kunz, pp. 277–302. Smithsonian Institution Press, Washington DC

Lollar A and Schmidt-French B (1998) *Captive Care and Medical Reference for the Rehabilitation of Insectivorous Bats*. Bat World Publications, Mineral Wells, Texas

Mitchell-Jones AJ (1999a) Health and safety in bat work. In: *Bat Workers' Manual*, eds AJ Mitchell-Jones and AP McLeish, p. 20. Joint Nature Conservancy Committee, Peterborough

Mitchell-Jones AJ (1999b) Timber treatment, pest control and building work. In: *Bat Workers' Manual*, eds AJ Mitchell-Jones and AP McLeish, pp. 73–84. Joint Nature Conservancy Committee, Peterborough

Mitchell-Jones AJ and McLeish AP (eds) (1999) *Bat Workers' Manual*. Joint Nature Conservancy Committee, Peterborough

Pybus MJ, Hobson DP and Onderka DK (1986) Mass mortality of bats due to probable blue-green algal toxicity. *Journal of Wildlife Diseases* **22**, 449–450

Racey PA (1999) Handling, releasing and keeping bats. In: *Bat Workers' Manual*, eds AJ Mitchell-Jones and AP McLeish, pp. 51–56. Joint Nature Conservancy Committee, Peterborough

Racey PA and Swift SM (1985) Feeding ecology of *Pipistrellus pipistrellus* (Chiroptera: Vespertilionidae) during pregnancy and lactation. I. Foraging behaviour. *Journal of Animal Ecology* **54**, 205–215

Racey PA and Swift SM (1986) The residual effects of remedial timber treatment on bats. *Biological Conservation* **35**, 205

Ransome R (1990) *The Natural History of Hibernating Bats*. Christopher Helm, Bromley

Richardson P (2000) *Guidelines on Bats in Captivity*. Bat Conservation Trust, London

Routh A (1991) Bats in the surgery. *Veterinary Record* **128**, 316–318

Rupprecht CE, Stöhr K and Meredith C (2001) Rabies. In: *Infectious Diseases of Wild Mammals*, eds ES Williams and IK Barker, pp. 3–36. Manson Publishing, London

Schober W and Grimmberger E (1989) *A Guide to Bats of Britain and Europe*. Hamlyn, London

Simpson VR (1994) Pathological conditions in British bats. *Proceedings of Wildlife Diseases Association, First European Conference, November 22–24, 1994, Paris*, p. 47

Simpson VR (1999) Potential wildlife zoonoses in Britain. *Proceedings of BVA Seminar Day, Zoonotic Diseases of UK Wildlife, British Veterinary Association Congress, September 23, 1999, Bath*, pp. 1–8

Stallknecht DE and Howerth EW (2001) Pseudorabies (Aujeszky's disease). In: *Infectious Diseases of Wild Mammals*, eds ES Williams and IK Barker, p. 166. Manson Publishing, London

Stebbings RE (1988) *Conservation of European Bats*. Christopher Helm, Bromley

Stocker L (2000) *Practical Wildlife Care*. Blackwell Science, Oxford

Tucker AT, Pearson RM, Cooke ED and Benjamin NJ (1999) Effect of a nitric oxide generating system on microcirculatory blood flow in the skin of patients with severe Raynaud's syndrome. *Lancet* **354**, 1670–1675

Walsh ST and Stebbings RE (1989) Care and rehabilitation of wild bats. In: *Proceedings of the Inaugural Symposium of the British Wildlife Rehabilitation Council*, eds S Harris and T Thomas, pp. 64–72. British Wildlife Rehabilitation Council, c/o RSPCA, Horsham

Whitby JE, Heaton PR, Black EM, Wooldridge M, McElhinney LM and Johnstone P (2000) First isolation of a rabies-related virus from a Daubenton's bat in the United Kingdom. *Veterinary Record* **147**, 385–388

Wilson DE (1988) Maintaining bats for captive studies. In: *Ecological and Behavioral Methods for the Study of Bats*, ed. TH Kunz, pp. 247–264. Smithsonian Institution Press, Washington DC

Yuill TM and Seymour C (2001) Arbovirus infections. In: *Infectious Diseases of Wild Mammals*, eds ES Williams and IK Barker, pp. 98–118. Manson Publishing, London

Acknowledgements

The author is indebted to all bat workers, rehabilitators and veterinary surgeons who have freely discussed the subject matter of this chapter, not only in its preparation but also in over a decade of work with matters microchiropteran.

10

Rabbits and hares

Frances Harcourt-Brown and Katherine Whitwell

Introduction

In the British Isles there are three species of wild lagomorph: the European rabbit (*Oryctolagus cuniculus*), the brown hare (*Lepus europaeus*) and the blue (or mountain, Irish or varying) hare (*Lepus timidus*).

Distribution

The European rabbit can be found in all parts of the British Isles. The brown hare (Figure 10.1) is found throughout the UK, except for northern Scotland; it has been introduced into many Scottish islands, the Isle of Man, Anglesey and the Isle of Wight. It has also become naturalized in north-west Ireland. Population numbers fluctuate seasonally according to weather, food availability, farming methods, disease status, predation and culling. The blue hare is rare in the British Isles but may be found in Scotland and Ireland (Nowak, 1999). Scandinavian studies (Thulin, 1996) indicate that interspecific hybridization between female mountain hares and male brown hares occurs and that the hybrids are fertile.

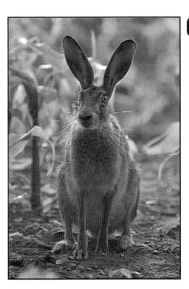

10.1 Brown hare. The hare is a larger animal than the rabbit, with longer limbs and ears and larger footprint. The coat is browner and the ears usually have black tips. (Courtesy of D Mason.)

Reasons for presentation

Wildlife lagomorph casualties tend to fall into four categories: orphans; juveniles that have been rescued from predators; individuals that have sustained a physical injury; and those that are suffering from some type of disease, such as myxomatosis or dysautonomia.

Orphan rabbits may come from nests that have been disturbed by dogs or by garden machinery. Young hares (leverets) may allow themselves to be picked up and are often erroneously assumed to be orphans; they tend to lie low and still in open fields and are thus susceptible to predation, injuries from farm machinery and direct spraying with toxic chemicals. Mature or juvenile hares that can be picked up by humans (or caught by domestic dogs) are almost certainly already compromised to some extent by injury, disease or blindness.

Ecology and biology

Habitat

The preferred habitat of the European wild rabbit is a sandy, hilly terrain with shrubs and woody plants, close to an area of cover, such as brambles, hedges or walls. In summer, rabbits graze on grass and selected plants. Repeated grazing of the areas close to their burrow results in a short turf or lawn. In the winter, when grass is scarce, they browse on leaves and shoots of trees and shrubs. They will strip bark and damage trees. They are not found at altitudes above 600 m.

Hares prefer a diversity of habitat. They thrive better in arable agricultural areas where cereals and root crops are grown, particularly if pasture is also available, than in a purely pastoral landscape. They like short open vegetation for feeding but need cover for resting (woods, hedges, uncultivated strips). Habitat quality is reduced by fragmentation (e.g. roads, developments). As a game animal they tend to be conserved in areas where big hare shoots are held and predators are controlled by gamekeeping. For these reasons, East Anglia has a large hare population. Livestock and the presence of humans are deterrents.

Social structure

Wild rabbits live in well defined social groups that inhabit complex burrows or warrens. They are essentially nocturnal but can also be seen grazing or basking during the day. Rabbits live in groups of two to eight adults, plus juveniles, with a defined social hierarchy (McBride, 1988). Young male rabbits are often driven from the group when they reach puberty, either to join another warren or to lead solitary lives in the hedgerows (Lockley, 1978).

Hares are mainly solitary in daytime, lying up in a shallow 'form', often in open countryside. They are active at dusk and nocturnally, and when feeding they congregate at favoured sites, such as where food is plentiful. They are not territorial and each has a home range (c. 20–40 ha). Social hierarchies may develop if food is scarce and in competition for females. In the breeding season (February to September), several males may cluster around one female, just before and during oestrus. The dramatic behaviour of females, which stand to repel the advances of males with their forepaws, is described as 'boxing'. Mating is rapid and there is no bonding; the males try to mate with as many females as possible.

Lifespan

The lifespan of wild lagomorphs is short and it is unusual to find a wild rabbit older than 2 years (McBride, 1988). Causes of death include predation, disease, starvation, exposure and drowning in the nest. In the wild, 75% of young rabbits die within their first 3 months. Free-ranging hares can (rarely) live for up to 7 years and those in captivity up to 12 years.

Anatomy and physiology

The coat of a rabbit is a mixture of black and light brown hairs, giving it an overall brown colour; entirely black rabbits are sometimes encountered. Hares have a browner coat than rabbits and are larger, with longer limbs and ears and usually black ear tips (see Figure 10.1). Rabbits and hares moult twice a year as adults, in spring and autumn; young hares have a juvenile moult.

Hare footprints are larger than those of rabbits, the hindfeet (with five toes) being placed ahead of the front (which have four toes visible). The average weights of adult hares in February are 3.23 kg (male) and 3.43 kg (female), compared with an average of 1.35–2.25 kg for rabbits.

Both hares and rabbits have anal, inguinal, sub-mandibular, lacrimal and Harderian scent glands. Much of the anatomy of wild lagomorphs, including that of the digestive system, follows the pattern of domestic rabbits and can be found in standard rabbit texts.

The dental formula for both rabbits and hares is:

$$2 \times \left\{ I \, \frac{2}{1} - C \, \frac{0}{0} - P \, \frac{3}{2} - M \, \frac{3}{3} \right\} = 28$$

The second upper incisors ('peg teeth') are vestigial and lie directly behind the first incisors.

Senses

Lagomorphs are prey for many species and have highly developed senses of vision, hearing and smell with which to detect predators. The ears are large (see Figure 10.1) and can be moved separately to detect sound from different directions. The large prominent eyes are positioned on the side of the head. In rabbits, the cornea occupies approximately 25% of the globe. These features give them a visual field of nearly 360

degrees. The retina of rabbits has a horizontal area of high photoreceptor density (the 'visual streak') that allows the animal to concentrate on all points of the horizon at one time, enabling it to be aware of a predator coming from any direction. Rods are the predominant photoreceptor cells and lagomorphs have good nocturnal vision.

If they detect danger, rabbits and hares thump their hindfeet, which transmits a sound that can be heard by other lagomorphs. They escape danger by running at high speeds over short distances and will emit a loud shrill scream when frightened, especially when captured. Hares (which have no burrows to which they can escape) may achieve speeds of 80 km/h (Nowak, 1999); they have proportionately larger hearts and are more muscular than rabbits, and are able to make sudden changes of direction to avoid predation.

Reproduction

Rabbits

Rabbits breed from February to September; they produce up to five litters per year, with five to eight young per litter. After a gestation period of 30–32 days, baby rabbits are born naked, blind and helpless and weigh 40–100 g at birth. They remain in the hidden, well insulated and secure nest and are suckled once (or occasionally twice) daily by a mother who spends very little time with them. The doe shows little maternal behaviour; she does not groom the young or keep them warm but remains in close vicinity to the nest. The babies drink sufficient milk in 2–5 minutes to last 24 hours, and it is possible for them to survive for more than 24 hours between feeds. Suckling normally takes place in the early morning; if the doe does return to the nest to feed the young for a second time, it is usually in the first few days after giving birth. Young rabbits are totally dependent on milk until day 10; they are usually eating small amounts of solid food by day 15 (Kraus et al., 1984) and start to leave the nest and be weaned at about 3 weeks of age. Figure 10.2a shows the features of a young rabbit.

Hares

Young hares are born in the open after a gestation period of 41–43 days; they weigh 80–130 g at birth. There are usually three litters per year, with one to four young per litter. In contrast to baby rabbits, leverets are precocious and are born fully furred, with their eyes open; they are able to run within a few minutes of birth. The doe goes away after eating the placenta and suckling and cleaning the leverets, only returning each evening to a location not far from the birth site to nurse and clean the leverets. The leverets disperse separately, initially a short distance from the birth site, and lie low and still in the grass through the day, regathering each evening shortly before the doe returns. She suckles them for 1–5 minutes whilst characteristically maintaining an erect surveillance posture. Post-suckling dispersal distances increase and suckling times decrease until the leverets become weaned after 4 weeks (McBride, 1988). Figure 10.2b shows the features of leverets.

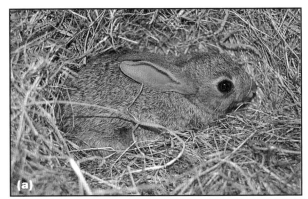

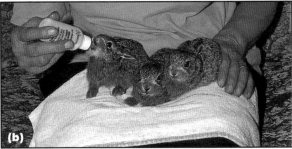

10.2 When presented with a baby lagomorph, it is important to distinguish a hare from a rabbit. Rabbits (a) are born underground without fur, blind and helpless. If found above ground, although they are of similar size to a leveret, they will be older, weaned and able to eat grass and other solid food. Leverets (b) are born fully furred with their eyes open and are mobile within minutes. If they permit themselves to be picked up they are probably still suckling and will require hand-rearing to survive. The coat texture and colour of leverets is variable, browner and less uniform than that of rabbits, which have a greyer tone. (Courtesy of D Mason.)

Capture, handling and transportation

Capture

Nets and cage traps can be used for the capture of wild rabbits and hares but capture, handling, transportation and caging are stressful experiences for them. There is a danger of spinal and other injury associated with attempts to escape. Loud noises, unfamiliar surroundings, transport, and the smell and presence of predators (including humans) add to the stress levels of a wild lagomorph that is already stressed by injury or disease.

In rabbits it is known that the effects of stress are significant and it is important to minimize stress during capture and transportation. Catecholamine release initiates a number of problems and in the short term it can cause heart failure or fatal oliguria (Kaplan and Smith, 1935). In the long term, stress affects many physiological functions. Stimulation of the sympathetic nervous system inhibits activity of the gastrointestinal tract. Reduced gut motility, in association with disruptions in carbohydrate metabolism, can have a potentially serious knock-on effect that results in hepatic lipidosis, liver failure and death. Reduced gut motility also affects the caecal microflora. Enterotoxaemia or gut stasis can result from any stressful situation.

Handling and transport

Wild rabbits and hares can be picked up by the scruff with a restraining hand under the hindquarters. They are unlikely to bite but may scratch with their hindfeet. Most will remain motionless unless they are given the opportunity to escape (for more information on handling see 'Examination and assessment'). They should be transported in small, dark containers that are ventilated and secure.

Zoonoses

There are several potential zoonotic infections of wild lagomorphs. An outbreak of verocytotoxigenic *Escherichia coli* O157 affecting visitors to an animal collection centre was traced to wild rabbits grazing the picnic area. The rabbits had carried the infection from a neighbouring cattle farm and their faeces had contaminated the ground (Pritchard *et al.*, 2001). *Giardia* (Johnson-Delaney, 1996) can affect both rabbits and humans but transmission between species does not appear to occur. *Toxoplasma gondii* affects a range of animals, including rabbits and humans; it can be transmitted by infected cat faeces or by eating undercooked meat. *Encephalitozoon cuniculi* is rare in wild rabbits but has caused illness in immunocompromised people, such as AIDS patients.

Tularaemia, caused by *Francisella tularensis*, can affect many vertebrate species and has zoonotic potential. Most human cases that have been linked to rabbits have followed exposure to the cottontail (*Sylvilagus floridanus*). According to Delong and Manning (1994), there have been no reported human cases of tularaemia acquired from *Oryctolagus cuniculus*.

Lagomorphs are a possible source of listeriosis, salmonellosis and leptospirosis, though no reports of human infection have been traced to wild rabbits or hares. In the UK, leptospirosis and toxoplasmosis have been diagnosed serologically in hares but evidence for clinical disease and pathology is absent. Hares are more susceptible than rabbits to brucellosis and pseudotuberculosis, both of which are potentially zoonotic (Broderson and Gluckstein, 1994). Lyme disease has been identified in hares in other European countries but not in the UK.

Examination and assessment for rehabilitation

During clinical examination, an assessment is required to decide whether to euthanase the animal, treat it with a view to releasing it, or treat it with a view to keeping it in captivity. Because lagomorphs serve as prey to so many species, any type of disability will compromise their survival in the wild. Injuries to the eyes or ears impair the detection of predators; limb injuries reduce the chances of escape; broken or abnormal teeth have long-term effects on the health of the individual and it is unlikely that the animal would survive. Therefore disabled lagomorphs should not be released. Euthanasia is indicated unless a secure, educated, permanent home is available. Because domestic rabbits are kept as pets, an increasing number of people wish to keep wild lagomorphs, especially rabbits, in captivity.

Restraint for examination

Careful restraint is necessary during clinical examination. The response of wild lagomorphs to danger is either to 'freeze' or to jump and flee. Wild rabbits will sit very still before making a sudden and often unexpected leap into the air. The consequences of jumping off the examination table might be broken bones or fractured teeth.

Wrapping the rabbit (or hare) in a towel can be a satisfactory method of restraint. Some individuals are susceptible to 'hypnosis' or 'trancing', an immobility response evoked by placing the animal on its back. The response is exhibited in many prey species under conditions that are stressful or threatening and is characterized by lack of spontaneous movement and failure to respond to external stimuli for several minutes. In rabbits, there is hypotonia of flexor and extensor musculature, abolition of the righting reflex, depression of spinal reflexes, miosis, and a drop in blood pressure, heart rate and respiratory rate. An awareness of external stimuli is maintained but there is a decreased response to noise and painful stimuli.

Clinical examination

Clinical examination follows the same principles as for other species.

- The sex of the individual can be determined by examining the external genitalia. The absence of palpable testicles does not necessarily mean that the animal is female. In lagomorphs, the testicles can be drawn into the abdominal cavity during periods of stress or poor nutrition. Eversion of the genital organ will reveal a penis or slit-like vulva
- Special attention should be given to the perineal area, the head and the limbs, and the abdomen palpated to screen for impactive illness
- Fly strike may be present, especially in rabbits with myxomatosis or open wounds
- If necessary, a blood sample can be taken from either the jugular, cephalic or marginal ear veins. Venepuncture is easier if the lagomorph has been sedated with a vasodilator such as fentanyl/fluanisone. Reference ranges for blood values in laboratory rabbits are given in Figure 10.3
- Radiography is indicated to screen for gun pellets or fractures.

Euthanasia

The method of choice for euthanasia is intravenous pentobarbital and the animal can be sedated prior to euthanasia. Alternatively, pentobarbital can be given intraperitoneally. If the injection is made intrahepatically or intrarenally, the onset of action is rapid. The topographical anatomy of the abdomen is illustrated in Figure 10.4.

Rabbits can also be killed by a blow on the back of the head or by dislocation of the neck (see Chapter 2) but these methods require experience and are inadvisable in the practice situation.

Parameter	Reference range
Haematology	
Erythrocytes[a] (10^{12}/l)	4–7
Haemoglobin (g/dl)	10–15
PCV (l/l)	0.33–0.48
MCV (fl)	60–75
MCH (pg)	19–23
MCHC (g/dl)	30–35
Reticulocytes (%)	2–4
Platelets (10^9/l)	250–600
White cells (10^9/l)	5–12
Neutrophils[b] (%)	30–50
Lymphocytes (%)	30–60
Eosinophils (%)	0–5
Basophils (%)	0–8
Monocytes (%)	2–10
Biochemistry	
Albumin (g/l)	27–50
Alkaline phosphatase (IU/l)	10–70
ALT (IU/l)	25–65
AST (IU/l)	10–98
Amylase (IU/l)	200–500
Bilirubin (μmol/l)	3.4–8.5
Bile acids (μmol/l)	< 40
Calcium (total) (mmol/l)	3.2–3.7 mmol/l
Calcium (ionized) (mmol/l)	1.71 (+ 0.11)
Cholesterol (mmol/l)	0.3–3.00
Creatinine (μmol/l)	44.2–229
Triglycerides (mmol/l)	1.4–1.76
Gamma GT (IU/l)	0–7.0
Globulin (g/l)	15–27
Glucose[c] (mmol/l)	4.2–7.8
Inorganic phosphate (mmol/l)	1.28–1.92
Potassium[d] (mmol/l)	3.2–7
Sodium (mmol/l)	138–150
Total protein (g/l)	54–75
Urea (mmol/l)	6.14–8.38

10.3 Blood values for rabbits, obtained from laboratory animals. Note that a fasting sample cannot be guaranteed by withholding food from rabbits as they ingest caecotrophs. (Sources: Harcourt-Brown, 2002; Gillett, 1994; Sanderson and Philips, 1981.) [a]Anisocytosis, polychromasia, small numbers of nucleated red blood cells and Howell Jolly bodies can be normal findings in rabbit blood films. [b]Neutrophil:lymphocyte ratio is approximately 1:1 in a healthy adult. [c]Stress can cause marked increase in glucose values. [d]Values can be affected by anaesthesia.

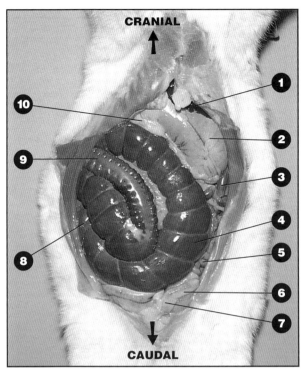

CRANIAL

CAUDAL

10.4 Topographical anatomy of the ventral abdomen of a female rabbit. Note the large ileocaecocolic complex that occupies most of the ventral abdomen. 1 = Liver; 2 = Stomach; 3 = Small intestine; 4 = Caecum; 5 = Small intestine; 6 = Uterus; 7 = Bicornuate cervix; 8 = Caecum; 9 = Proximal colon; 10 = Omentum.

First aid procedures

If the animal is to be treated, food and a quiet warm environment are needed. A quiet escape-proof cage away from loud noises, bright lights and the sight and smell of potential predators is necessary. Placing a blanket or towel over the cage gives the animal a sense of security. Heat pads or alternative heat sources are required for hypothermic animals but it should be borne in mind that rabbits are destructive and will chew through electric cables.

Analgesia is an essential part of any treatment protocol for lagomorphs (see below).

Reduced gut motility is a potential consequence of any painful or stressful situation and it is important to monitor appetite and faecal output. A source of fibre is required to maintain gut motility and optimal conditions in the caecum for bacterial fermentation. Fresh grass and a bed of good quality hay are essential.

Fluid therapy

The general principles of fluid therapy are covered in Chapter 2. Subcutaneous fluids (10–20 ml/kg as a single bolus) can be given into the scruff or the loose skin over the chest, but intravenous or intraosseous therapy is preferable for moribund patients.

Intravenous injection

The marginal ear vein or cephalic vein is the site of choice for intravenous fluid therapy. The intravenous catheter can be held in place with adhesive tape or a few drops of 'superglue'. A simple method is to cut one wing off a 21 or 23 gauge butterfly set before placing it in the marginal ear vein. The remaining wing can be superglued to the fur on the pinna to keep the needle in place. No bandaging is required to keep the needle in place in sedated or moribund patients, though a piece of bandage tied around the animal's neck can be used to hold the giving set out of the way.

Intraosseous injection

Intraosseous fluid therapy avoids the necessity of cannulating a small collapsed vein in moribund patients. In lagomorphs, the humerus is the preferred site for intraosseous fluids. Direct penetration of the marrow cavity is easier in the tibia or humerus than the femur. The anatomy of the head of the femur of lagomorphs requires penetration of the trochanteric fossa (Harcourt-Brown, 2002).

Intraperitoneal injection

Fluids can also be given intraperitoneally. The bladder should be empty and care is needed to avoid the thin-walled caecum that lies in the right ventral abdomen (see Figure 10.4). The injection should be given caudal to the umbilicus so that there is little chance of penetrating the liver, kidneys or spleen. It is important to draw back on the syringe to check for intestinal contents, blood or urine, in which case the syringe should be withdrawn and another attempt made.

Anaesthesia and analgesia

A summary of anaesthetic and sedative drugs for use in lagomorphs is given in Figure 10.5.

Drug	Dosage	Type of drug or indication	Comments
Acepromazine	0.1–0.5 mg/kg i.m., s.c.	Sedation	Not analgesic
Acepromazine + butorphanol	0.5 mg/kg + 0.5 mg/kg s.c., i.m.	Sedation	Can be mixed in same syringe Vasodilatory
Adrenaline	20 μg/kg s.c., i.v.	Cardiac arrest	Some products need diluting from 1:1000 (1 mg/ml) to 1:10,000 (100 μg/l) Can be given into the trachea
Aspirin	100 mg/kg orally	Analgesic	First aid pain relief

10.5 Anaesthesia and analgesia. (continues) ▶

Drug	Dosage	Type of drug or indication	Comments
Atipamezole	1 mg/kg s.c., i.m., i.v.		Reversal of medetomidene
Atropine	0.05 mg/kg (50 µg/kg) i.m.	Premedication	Atropinesterase, which metabolizes atropine, is produced by 40% of rabbits and so glycopyrrolate is preferable
Buprenorphine	0.01–0.05 mg/kg i.v., s.c.	Analgesia	Analgesic effects last 6–12 h
Butorphanol	0.1–0.5 mg/kg s.c., i.m., i.v.	Analgesic	Effects last 2–4 h
Carprofen	2–4 mg/kg s.c. sid	Analgesic	
Diazepam	1–2 mg/kg i.v., i.m.	Sedation	
Doxapram	5 mg/kg i.m., i.v.	Respiratory stimulant	
Fentanyl/fluanisone (Hypnorm, Janssen)	0.2–0.3 ml/kg i.m., s.c.		Premedication Analgesia Anaesthesia
Glycopyrrolate	0.01 mg/kg i.v. 0.2 mg/kg s.c., i.m.	Premedication Organophosphate poisoning	Does not cross blood–brain barrier and cause mydriasis
Ketamine	25–50 mg/kg i.m.	Sedation	Can be used in combination with other agents for anaesthesia
Ketoprofen	3 mg/kg orally bid	Analgesia	Care in hypotensive patients
Medetomidine + ketamine	0.2 mg/kg + 10 mg/kg i.m.	Anaesthesia	
Medetomidine + ketamine + butorphanol	0.2 mg/kg + 10 mg/kg + 0.5 mg/kg i.m.	Anaesthesia with pre-emptive analgesia	
Meloxicam	0.1–0.2 mg/kg orally sid	Analgesia	Palatable
Pethidine	5–10 mg/kg s.c. or i.m.	Analgesic	Lasts 2–3 h
Xylazine + ketamine	5 mg/kg + 35 mg/kg i.m.	Anaesthesia	

10.5 (continued) Anaesthesia and analgesia.

The anaesthetic combinations that are used in domestic rabbits (Flecknell, 2000) can be used in wild lagomorphs. Induction of anaesthesia with inhalational agents is unsatisfactory because it is stressful and many lagomorphs will hold their breath in response to the smell of an anaesthetic vapour. Induction with injectable agents is preferable. If induction with an inhalational agent is the only option, premedication with a sedative such as fentanyl/fluanisone or acepromazine is beneficial.

Injectable combinations of medetomidine or xylazine can be used with ketamine for anaesthesia (see Figure 10.5). Halothane or isoflurane is suitable for maintenance of anaesthesia and can be introduced by facemask. Endotracheal intubation is difficult.

Non-steroidal analgesics such as carprofen, meloxicam or ketoprofen are effective in lagomorphs. Even aspirin can be used as a first aid treatment. Narcotic analgesics such as buprenorphine are also effective.

Specific conditions

Trauma

Lagomorphs of any age can be injured by vehicles, farm machinery, gunshot, traps or predators. Injury compromises their ability to escape further predation, though recovery is possible in areas where predator numbers are low and food is plentiful. Injuries of the head or jaw can result in starvation. Coursing injuries by greyhounds or lurchers include deep crushing bites through the thorax and head, and skin lacerations, punctures and fractures of the hindlegs. All kinds of wounding can lead to secondary fly strike.

Fly strike

Fly strike is treated by clipping away soiled fur from the lesion and picking out the maggots. Sedation may be necessary. Drying the area with a hairdryer brings out the maggots, as they are attracted by the heat. A precautionary dose of ivermectin can be administered. Antibiotic therapy, supportive care and analgesia are required.

Surgical techniques

In some cases of trauma, surgical repair of wounds or fractures may be necessary. Lagomorph tissue is thin, delicate and friable in comparison with that of a dog or cat. The bones are brittle and liable to shatter. Orthopaedic repairs are similar to those in cats.

Rabbit blood clots very quickly. The blood volume is 55–65 ml/kg (Gillett, 1994) and up to 10% of this amount can be lost without untoward effect. Losses above 20–25% result in hypovolaemic shock.

Rabbits are also prone to the development of adhesions after surgery. The omentum is small and it is not always possible to omentalize viscera satisfactorily.

Foreign material such as talcum powder from gloves or lint from gauze swabs can induce adhesion formation. To minimize adhesion formation, it is important to use gentle surgical techniques with minimal tissue handling and fine suture material. Small gauge (3/0, 4/0 or 5/0) modern suture materials swaged on needles are satisfactory. Polydioxanone (PDS 11) or poliglecaprone can be used for most situations; 3/0 or 4/0 catgut is suitable to tie off blood vessels or ligaments. Skin closure with a continuous subcuticular suture with a buried Aberdeen knot is recommended (Flecknell, 1998). Additional skin sutures or tissue adhesive can be used, if necessary. Surgical staples can be used for skin closure but will need to be removed.

Viral diseases

Myxomatosis
Myxomatosis, caused by the myxomavirus introduced into Britain in 1953 from the South American forest rabbit (*Sylvilagus brasiliensis*), is a fatal disease of the European rabbit. Free-ranging hares rarely show clinical signs but they do show a limited serological response indicating infection. A rare transmissible nodular fibromatosis caused by a poxvirus occurs in the UK and in farmed hares in France and Italy. Lesions on ears, head and legs slightly resemble myxomatosis.

Myxomatosis in rabbits is characterized by subcutaneous swellings that exude a mucoid substance when sectioned. The disease is mainly spread by arthropods. In wild rabbits, outbreaks of myxomatosis wax and wane according to the virulence of the strain and the immune status of the native rabbit population. The life cycle of the insect vector affects the pattern of disease outbreaks and epidemiology of myxomatosis. In the UK, the European rabbit flea *Spilopsyllus cuniculi* is the major insect vector rather than mosquitoes, which are the vectors in other parts of the world. Fleas are an effective means of transmission because they can maintain infectivity throughout the winter and act as a reservoir of infection for the following year. Their life cycle is synchronized with the reproductive status of the doe, which results in heavy flea infestations of susceptible neonates (see 'Parasites').

Clinical signs: Myxomatosis starts with a skin lesion, typically 4–5 days after inoculation of the virus. The rabbit becomes viraemic. The eyelids become thickened and can become completely closed with a semipurulent ocular discharge (Figure 10.6). Secondary lesions develop throughout the body, typically on the nares, lips, eyelids and base of the ears, and on the external genitalia and anus. Aerosol infection can result in pneumonic signs. Highly virulent strains cause rapid death but low-virulence strains lead to inanition, secondary bacterial infection and predation. Very young rabbits are particularly susceptible to infection and die more rapidly than adult animals unless they have some passive immunity. Maternal transfer of antibodies gives passive immunity that lasts for 4–5 weeks. Some rabbits have a genetic resistance to infection (Fenner and Fantini, 1999).

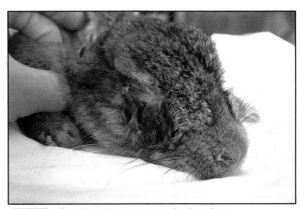

10.6 Rabbit with myxomatosis showing mucopurulent nasal and ocular discharges and typical swelling around the eyes. (Courtesy of G Cousquer.)

Prognosis and treatment: The prognosis for rabbits affected by myxomatosis is extremely poor, though the occasional individual will survive. The ambient temperature affects the course of the disease, with high environmental temperature (28°C) increasing recovery rates. Antibiotics, a warm environment and good nursing are required. The risk of secondary problems such as gastrointestinal stasis or pasteurellosis is ever present. Non-steroidal analgesics are useful but the use of corticosteroids is contraindicated due to their immunosuppressive effects. Opioid analgesics do not appear to be effective in ameliorating signs of pain (Robinson et al., 1999).

Viral haemorrhagic disease
Viral haemorrhagic disease (VHD) is a highly infectious lethal disease of rabbits, with a high mortality rate, and is now endemic in the UK. It is caused by a host-specific calicivirus that specifically affects the European rabbit, not cottontails or other small mammals.

VHD calicivirus can survive for long periods outside the host. It can remain viable for 22–35 days at 22°C but only for 3–7 days at 37°C, and can survive for several weeks in carcasses and skin – it is very stable in carcasses even after freezing and thawing (Lumeij, 1997). It is spread by oral, nasal and parenteral transmission and is present in urine and faeces from infected rabbits. Insects mechanically transmit the virus in viraemic blood from one animal to another, and fleas, blowflies and mosquitoes are known to spread the disease (Fenner and Fantini, 1999). It has also been demonstrated that domestic and wild carnivores can play an important role in the epidemiology of VHD, since virulent material can be collected from faecal material after experimental oral inoculation. Contaminated foods can be a source of infection.

When VHD is introduced into a susceptible population, the mortality rate is high and can be 90–100% in rabbits aged over 2 months. In wild rabbits, the disease appears to break out every other year. Infected young rabbits, of less than 4 weeks of age, remain unaffected; they survive and develop a lifelong immunity if they are exposed to the disease and so the morbidity and mortality rates fall when the disease becomes endemic. Unexposed rabbits become increasingly susceptible until

6–10 weeks of age, when physiological resistance to the virus disappears. The physiological age immunity of young rabbits has been ascribed to the increase in hepatic transaminase production that occurs after 5 weeks of age (Donnelly, 1997).

Clinical signs: VHD has an incubation period of 3–4 days. The calicivirus has a predilection for hepatocytes, and replicates within the cytoplasm of these cells. It is essentially a necrotizing hepatitis, often associated with necrosis of the spleen. Disseminated intravascular coagulation produces fibrinous thrombi within small blood vessels in most organs, notably the lungs, heart and kidneys, resulting in haemorrhages. Death is due to disseminated intravascular coagulopathy or to liver failure. The disease can be peracute, with animals being found dead within a few hours of eating and behaving normally. Acute cases are quiet, pyrexic with an increased respiratory rate and usually die within 12 hours. Dying rabbits are pallid, shocked and collapsed. Haematuria, haemorrhagic vaginal discharges or foamy exudate from the nostrils may be seen. Vascular infarcts can occur within the brain and occasionally convulsions or other neurological signs are seen just before death. Agonal vocalizing and cyanosis have been described (Donnelly, 1997). The 'classic' picture is a dead rabbit in opisthotonus with a haemorrhagic nasal discharge.

Prognosis: Adult rabbits invariably die from VHD and there is no treatment. The occasional rabbit can recover from the acute phase, only to develop jaundice and die a few days later.

European brown hare syndrome
European brown hare syndrome (EBHS) is caused by a calicivirus that is similar to but differs from the virus that causes VHD. Attempts to cross-infect rabbits and hares with heterologous virus have failed to induce disease. EBHS is highly contagious and in a susceptible population it can cause massive die-offs of hares of all ages, but in many years it causes only about 6% of deaths. EBHS causes a fatal characteristic hepatopathy that is so rapid that affected hares are in good bodily condition and often still have a full stomach when they die. Carcasses should be kept away from hares in captivity.

Bacterial diseases

Pasteurellosis
Although *Pasteurella multocida* is a common cause of disease in domestic rabbits, pasteurellosis is seldom encountered as a primary disease in wild rabbits. Disease occurs when predisposing factors give the bacteria the opportunity to multiply uncontrollably and overwhelm the physiological and immunological defences of the respiratory tract. After colonization of the upper respiratory tract, infection extends to the rest of the respiratory tract and tympanic bulla and can cause clinical rhinitis, conjunctivitis, pneumonia, tracheitis, dacryocystitis or otitis media. In wild lagomorphs, *P. multocida* can be found in wound infections and abscesses. Other bacteria such as *Staphylococcus*

aureus and *Escherichia coli* may also cause localized and generalized infections. Antibiotics and supportive care are used to treat these infections.

Treponematosis
Treponema cuniculi is a sexually transmitted spirochaete that causes crusty, inflammatory lesions on the face (lips, eyes, nose), perineum and external genitalia in both rabbits and hares (Lumeij *et al.*, 1994; Munro *et al.*, 1995). It is surprisingly common in wild hares and contributes to poor condition, increased chance of predation, and death from amyloidosis. Parenteral penicillin (40 mg/kg s.c., daily for 5 days) is the treatment of choice.

Paratuberculosis
Paratuberculosis, caused by *Mycobacterium avium* subsp. *paratuberculosis*, can affect rabbits. In Scotland, the high incidence of paratuberculosis in wild rabbits has been linked with a high prevalence of infection in cattle. Epidemiological studies found an association between the infection in wild rabbits and a history of Johne's disease on the farms where the rabbits were caught (Greig *et al.*, 1997). In the wild rabbits affected with paratuberculosis, general body condition was good although a proportion of them had thickened areas of intestinal mucosa with occasional granulomata. Large numbers of intracellular acid-fast bacilli were present in the lesions.

Other bacterial diseases
Yersinia pseudotuberculosis, which is widespread in the environment, causes internal abscesses and septicaemia in rabbits and hares. Affected rabbits exhibit a wasting disease, a dull coat and occasional diarrhoea.

Tularaemia is an acute septicaemic disease caused by *Francisella tularensis* that can affect wild rabbits and hares. Lice are known to be vectors.

Parasites
Wild rabbits and hares are host to a variety of endo- and ectoparasites (Hofing and Kraus, 1994).

Ectoparasites
Spilopsyllus cuniculi is the common flea that infests wild rabbits. The hare has no specific flea of its own but many hares carry rabbit, hedgehog or rat fleas. The predilection site for *S. cuniculi* is the ears, where fleas can be found in clusters along the edges of the pinnae. It is a small flea and its life cycle is influenced by the reproductive status of the host: egg maturation is dependent on female reproductive hormones, and successful reproduction of the flea requires contact with a rabbit in late pregnancy or with a newborn nestling. Increased blood corticosteroid concentrations in late pregnancy attract fleas, which attach firmly to the doe to feed. Within a few hours of parturition, fleas move from the doe to the newborn babies to feed, copulate and lay eggs in the nest. The eggs hatch and the larvae feed on flea dirt deposited in the nest by the adult fleas feeding on the pregnant doe. In this way, fleas are spread from one generation to the next and are an important vector of disease, especially myxomatosis.

Haemodipsus ventricosus is a sucking louse that affects wild rabbits and hares and may act as a vector for myxomatosis. It is a large louse, 1.5–2.5 mm in length (Owen, 1992), and can be present in large numbers.

Tick infestation (*Ixodes ricinus*) is frequent in some areas, with most of the ticks being attached around the head and neck. Small abscesses occasionally form at an adult tick attachment site.

A variety of mites (*Leporacus gibbus*, *Cheyletiella parasitovorax*, *Psoroptes cuniculi*) can affect rabbits. Skin lesions associated with mange mites are uncommon in free-living lagomorphs.

Endoparasites

Helminth parasites include *Graphidium strigosum* in the stomach, *Trichostrongylus* spp. in the small intestine and *Passalurus ambiguus*, an ascarid, in the large bowel (Allan *et al.*, 1999). The rabbit is the intermediate host for several tapeworms, such as *Taenia pisiformis*, *Taenia serialis* and *Echinococcus granulosus*, which affect dogs and cats. In most cases, infestation with tapeworm cysts does not produce disease, though heavy *T. pisiformis* infection can cause abdominal discomfort and distension. Lagomorphs are also the primary host for tapeworms. The cestode species varies in wild rabbits from different parts of the world. An example is *Cittotaenia ctenoides*, which has a free-living mite as its intermediate host. Cestode tapeworms are common in hares, sometimes in large numbers in the small bowel and fewer in the large bowel: orabatid mites are the intermediate hosts. It is believed that massive infections can cause clinical illness (Marcato and Rosmini, 1986). Verminous bronchopneumonia due to *Protostrongylus* spp. is recorded in hares in Europe (Marcato and Rosmini, 1986).

Protozoan parasites

Several protozoan parasites affect wild lagomorphs. For example, in common with all mammals, lagomorphs can be infected with *Toxoplasma gondii*, though infection is usually subclinical. The source of infection is grass contaminated by cat faeces. Sudden anorexia, pyrexia and death are the usual signs but central nervous system signs such as posterior paralysis or seizures can also occur (Leland *et al.*, 1992).

Although the microsporidian *Encephalitozoon cuniculi* commonly affects domestic rabbits, it appears to be rare in wild rabbits (Cox *et al.*, 1980; Cox and Ross, 1980). A single case of *E. cuniculi* was described in a wild rabbit in 1955 (Pakes and Gerrity, 1994).

Coccidiosis: Coccidiosis, caused by *Eimeria* spp., can be a major problem in rehabilitation centres. Good hygiene and prevention of cross-infection are necessary. Infected animals void oocysts that require oxygen and a period of a several days to become infective. Oocysts can survive for many years in the environment but do not survive in dry conditions. They are resistant to many disinfectants but a blowtorch can be used to flame hutches and kill oocysts, or a 10% solution of ammonia is effective (Pakes and Gerrity, 1994).

Eimeria spp. are host- and site-specific; as many as 14 species have been described in the rabbit and all but one are found in the small intestine, caecum or colon and cause intestinal coccidiosis. One species, *E. steidae*, inhabits the epithelial cells of the bile ducts, causing hepatic coccidiosis, and is a significant cause of mortality. Acute coccidiosis causes inappetence, weight loss, depression and diarrhoea that can be haemorrhagic. Clinical signs of hepatic coccidiosis are associated with the lesions in the liver and bile ducts and include weight loss, ascites, jaundice, diarrhoea and hepatomegaly. Weanling rabbits are most commonly affected by intestinal or hepatic coccidiosis.

It appears that all young hares in the UK become infected by *Eimeria* in their first year and in adverse conditions they are affected by clinical coccidiosis. In the UK, intestinal coccidiosis is the commonest cause of 'natural mortality' in young hares (Sargent, 1974; Whitwell, 1997). Most lesions are in the small intestine and perhaps for this reason diarrhoea is often not a feature. The large bowel is usually less severely affected. An age immunity develops and so in adult lagomorphs coccidiosis is not usually a cause of death.

Diagnosis of coccidiosis is made on clinical signs and evidence of coccidial oocysts in the faeces. Toltrazuril can be used to treat coccidiosis but is available only in large quantities. A paediatric suspension of trimethoprim/sulfamethoxazole (40 mg/kg) can be used to treat the individual patient.

Miscellaneous conditions

Plant toxicity

Actual proven cases of plant toxicity in lagomorphs are rare in the veterinary literature. Rabbits are known to be resistant to the toxic components of many plants, such as deadly nightshade and ragwort.

Amyloidosis

Many hares that have non-lethal chronic infections die from secondary amyloidosis. Heavy amyloid deposits can form in several organs: renal or hepatic failure is commonly the cause of death. This should be considered if treatment for a chronic infection is attempted.

Dental disease

A small number of adult lagomorphs suffer severe dental abnormalities, which are particularly serious when involving the cheek teeth. Septic sinus infections, traumatization or even piercing of the tongue by misaligned deviated teeth and consequent inability to swallow ropes of unchewed food lead to death.

Leporine dysautonomia

Since 1990 it has been recognized that hares suffer from a fatal dysautonomia that causes a severe chronic wasting illness (Figure 10.7), increased susceptibility to predation, and death (Whitwell, 1991). Although confirmation requires histological examination of ganglia, the clinical hallmarks are: approachability and lassitude, depression, marked weight loss, a palpable large bowel impaction, gastric distension, evidence of inability to swallow normally (grass protruding from the

117

sides of the mouth, perioral fur matting), inhalation pneumonia and bladder distension. It has been recorded as the second commonest cause of death in hares in Britain (Whitwell, 1997). The cause is uncertain but multiple cases can occur in one locality. Hares with dysautonomia are unlikely to recover even if treated, and those showing clinical signs suggestive of the condition (especially impaction and swallowing difficulties) should be euthanased to prevent further suffering. Too few have been seen alive to know whether they regularly also have dilated pupils. Dysautonomia has also been confirmed in a young wild rabbit (Whitwell, unpublished data).

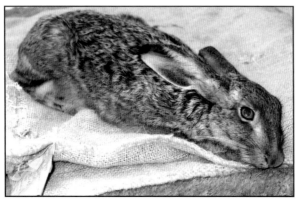

10.7 This moribund emaciated hare was so ill that it did not resist capture. After euthanasia, dysautonomia was confirmed histologically.

Other conditions

Although rare, internal neoplasia (e.g. lymphoma) will cause fatalities in hares. Hares also occasionally suffer from lesions such as uterine torsion or intestinal intussusception and are found dead.

Colitis causes diarrhoea and when severe, as in other species, can lead to prostration and death. The causes of colitis are often uncertain: sometimes crop sprays have been implicated but proof is lacking.

Environmental pollutants and pesticides

Although environmental pollutants and pesticides are blamed for declines in hare populations, there are few data from the UK. Tissue monitoring in Austrian hares has shown reductions in lead and mercury following restrictions of levels in fuels and seed dressings, but increases in cadmium, possibly associated with increased use of diesel fuel. Organochlorine levels have declined following control of pesticide and PCB use. Poisoning from illegal use of rodenticides is seen in hares (Tataruch, 2001). Organ and hair analysis in hares has been used for monitoring contamination by environmental pollutants and pesticides.

Therapeutics

A formulary for lagomorphs is given in Figure 10.8 (see also Figure 10.5 for anaesthetics and analgesics).

Drug	Dosage	Type of drug or indication	Comments
Antibacterials			
Cefalexin	15 mg/kg s.c. bid 20 mg/kg s.c. sid	Antibiotic	
Enrofloxacin	5 mg/kg s.c. bid 10 mg/kg s.c. sid 5–10 mg/kg orally bid	Antibiotic	Carries a product licence for use in domestic rabbits
Fusidic adic eye drops	1 drop/eye sid	Conjunctivitis	Carries a product licence for use in domestic rabbits
Fusidic ointment (Fuciderm, Leo)	Topical sid	Superficial pyoderma	
Gentamicin (Tiacil, Virbac)	1–2 drops/eye tid	Conjunctivitis	Give for 5–7 days
Metronidazole	20 mg/kg orally bid	Antibacterial	Treatment of enterotoxaemia
Oxytetracycline	15 mg/kg s.c., i.m., sid 30 mg/kg (depot) s.c. every 3 days 1 mg/ml in drinking water 50 mg/kg orally	Antibiotic	
Penicillin (Procaine)	40 mg/kg s.c. sid	Antibiotic	5–7 injections for *Treponema cuniculi*
Trimethoprim/ sulfadiazine	30 mg/kg orally bid 48 mg/kg s.c.	Antibiotic	
Trimethoprim/ sulfamethoxazole	40 mg/kg orally bid	Antibiotic Coccidiosis	'Co-trimoxazole' human formulation available as paediatric syrup Continue for 7 days

10.8 Drug formulary for rabbits and hares. Please note that the dosages given refer to domestic rabbits. (continues) ▶

Drug	Dosage	Type of drug or indication	Comments
Antiparasitic			
Albendazole	20 mg/kg orally sid	Anthelmintic	
Fenbendazole	20 mg/kg orally	Anthelmintic	
Imidacloprid	10 mg/kg topical	Fleas	Active against fleas but not mites Licensed for use in rabbits
Ivermectin	400 µg/kg s.c.	Mites	Treatment of choice for ear mites Repeat after 10–14 days
Praziquantel	6 mg/kg s.c.	Cestodes	Repeat after 10 days
Selamectin	12 mg/kg topical	Parasiticide	
Toltrazuril	25 ppm in drinking water Daily for 2 days; repeat after 5 days	Coccidiosis	
Miscellaneous			
Cisapride	0.5 mg/kg orally bid	Prokinetic	Product withdrawn – contact manufacturers
Dexamethasone	1–3 mg/kg i.m., i.v.	Anti-inflammatory	
Fluid therapy	10–20 ml/kg/h i.v.		Warm before use
	10–15 ml/kg s.c.		
Glucose 5%	10 ml/kg i.v., s.c.	Anorexia	Warm before use
Griseofulvin	25 mg/kg orally sid	Ringworm	Continue for at least 2 weeks
Metoclopramide	0.5 mg/kg s.c., orally, bid	Motility stimulant	May not be effective in young rabbits
Prednisolone	0.5–2 mg/kg orally, i.m., s.c.	Anti-inflammatory	

10.8 (continued) Drug formulary for rabbits and hares. Please note that the dosages given refer to domestic rabbits.

Routes of administration

- The **subcutaneous** route is suitable for the administration of most parenteral medications, with the loose skin over the scruff as the usual injection site
- For **intramuscular** injection, the cranial muscle mass (quadriceps) of the hindleg is the preferred site
- **Intravenous** injections can be given into the marginal ear vein, which is accessible and easily seen. A topical local anaesthetic cream can be applied over the vein before covering the site with a dressing or clingfilm. Full-thickness skin is anaesthetized after 45–60 minutes (Flecknell, 2000). An alternative site is the cephalic vein, as in the dog or cat. Other veins, including the jugular and femoral veins can also be used.

Antibiotic-associated diarrhoea

Some antibiotics have the potential to cause enteritis in lagomorphs by selectively killing certain bacteria and allowing pathogenic clostridial species to proliferate. *Clostridium* spp., in particular, can proliferate in the caecum or small intestine and cause rapid death due to the effects of enterotoxins. The choice of antibiotic and route of administration are important factors in the prevention of antibiotic-associated diarrhoea. Clindamycin, lincomycin and oral ampicillin carry a high risk of inducing diarrhoea, whereas enrofloxacin, tetracyclines and trimethoprim combinations are apparently safe. Oral antibiotics are more likely to induce diarrhoea than those given parenterally. There is conflicting information about the safety of penicillin for rabbits (Harcourt-Brown, 2002). Clinically, it appears to be a safe, effective antibiotic for rabbits as long as it is given parenterally. It is the most effective treatment for treponematosis.

Corticosteroids

Short-acting corticosteroids may be beneficial in cases of shock associated with trauma or blood loss, though there are potential hazards associated with the use of corticosteroids in lagomorphs. Their immunosuppressive properties may allow latent infections to flare up. As a general rule, non-steroidal anti-inflammatory drugs (NSAIDs) are preferable to corticosteroids for the non-specific treatment of pain and inflammation. NSAIDs are safe, effective and well tolerated.

Parasiticides

Fleas and external parasites can be killed with an avermectin such as ivermectin (400 µg/kg s.c.) or selamectin (12 mg/kg, topically). Imidacloprid carries a product licence for use in rabbits and is effective against fleas but not mites. Fipronil is not recommended for use in lagomorphs and the product carries a manufacturer's warning against its use in rabbits.

Management in captivity

Housing

Wild lagomorphs are fearful of humans and will make every attempt to escape. They can jump or scramble over heights of a metre or two and will squeeze through tiny spaces or burrow their way out. With hares, only leverets hand reared from a very young age are likely to adapt to permanent housing.

For long-term housing of rabbits, a secure wire-mesh enclosure is required (Figure 10.9). The floor should be meshed to prevent burrowing. It is very important to provide some sort of cover – drainpipes, boxes and rabbit hutches are suitable, though most rabbits prefer to live under a hutch than in it. Wild rabbits are very destructive and will chew through any wooden construction. Cardboard boxes or branches and twigs, especially from fruit trees, can be offered as alternatives for chewing.

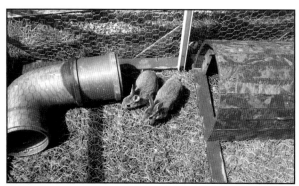

10.9 A secure enclosure is required for housing adult wild rabbits. Drainpipes or cloches in which the rabbits can hide make satisfactory alternatives to burrows.

Feeding

A balanced high-fibre diet of hay, grass, weeds and vegetables supplemented by a small amount of commercial rabbit food is satisfactory. Vegetables such as carrots, spring greens, broccoli, cabbage and kale are suitable for adult lagomorphs.

Rearing and release of young

Rabbits

Abandoned or orphaned wild rabbits can be reared by hand but the mortality rate is high. The glucose reserve of neonatal rabbits lasts approximately 6 hours *post partum*. Hypoglycaemia results in rapid ketosis and death (Kraus *et al.*, 1984). Hypothermic or moribund rabbits can be given fluids or milk replacers by stomach tube to correct hypoglycaemia. Passive immunity is obtained through the placenta and there is some evidence that neonates absorb antibodies from their intestine in the first few hours after birth (Brewer and Cruise, 1994).

Hares

Very young leverets, mistakenly presumed to have been abandoned, are sometimes removed inappropriately by members of the public and attempts are made, often disastrously, to rear them by hand. Removal of healthy leverets from the environs of their birth area is unwarranted intervention, unless there is unequivocal evidence to indicate that they will not survive if left where they are found. Only very young leverets (up to 1 week old) stand any chance of being reared successfully by hand and only rarely may they be able to adapt to permanent captivity as pets. They may be hyperactive in captivity but in a protected environment some have been known to achieve greater longevity than in the wild (almost 12 years in the case of tame hares kept by the 18th century poet William Cowper). These are the exceptions and preferably any healthy hand-reared orphan leveret should be released after weaning, at 6–12 weeks of age.

Housing

Young lagomorphs should be kept warm, dry and clean in a quiet place with suitable bedding material for burrowing. A towel or shredded tissue paper is satisfactory for making a nest, which can be put in a hay-lined cardboard box or basket and placed in a warm environment such as an airing cupboard. Alternatively, heat pads can be placed under the box to prevent hypothermia.

Feeding

Rabbits and hares suckle their young only once a day and their milk is very concentrated, of high nutritional value and with a low lactose content. The composition changes towards the end of lactation, when protein and fat levels increase.

Baby lagomorphs can be reared on powdered milk replacers (e.g. Esbilac, PetAg; Cimicat, Hoechst) or goat's milk. As milk replacers are a nutritional compromise, hand-reared lagomorphs need more than one feed a day and the milk replacer should not be too dilute (e.g. 2:1 powdered milk replacer to water).

In captivity, most young lagomorphs take two to four feeds a day, depending on their weight, appetite and general condition, and drink 2–30 ml of milk per feed, depending on their age. For example, hand-reared leverets usually begin with small feeds (1–5 ml per feed) three to six times a day, gradually reducing to once a day just prior to weaning at 4–6 weeks of age or older; volumes per feed increase gradually to 20–40 ml, with a maximum daily intake of perhaps 100 ml at the age of 2–3 weeks. Regular accurate weight recording of the animal is important for objectively monitoring progress and giving early warning of any problems (e.g. digestive disturbances, diarrhoea, coccidiosis, inhalation pneumonia or septicaemia, all of which require early therapy): the weight gain should be steady.

Mortality can occur from aspiration pneumonia due to inhalation of milk replacer or from enteritis. Rabbits are unusual among young animals in having very few microorganisms in the stomach and small intestine while suckling (Lang, 1981). An antimicrobial fatty acid or 'milk oil' is present in the stomach of a suckling rabbit. It is produced by an enzymatic reaction in the doe's milk (Brooks, 1997). This 'milk oil' gives some protection against enteric infection. Orphan rabbits that are fed on milk from other species do not develop this antimicrobial factor and are susceptible to bacterial infections introduced during feeding. It is important that only boiled water and sterile syringes and feeding tubes are used and that each feed is made up just prior to being given.

Most sucking animals are stimulated to urinate and defecate by the mother licking the perineum and lower abdomen. There is debate as to whether this is the case in all wild lagomorphs but it is recommended that such stimulation is given to hand-reared individuals. Between feeds, the young should be returned to the nest and left alone.

Weaning

For ages at natural weaning, see 'Reproduction', above. Baby rabbits start to leave the nest at about 18 days of age and at this stage small quantities of food suitable for rearing domestic rabbits (e.g. Burgess Excel Junior) can be offered, along with leafy vegetables and dandelions. Grass or hay must be freely available; hay is also used as bedding. If available, caecotrophs collected from healthy adults can be scattered in the hay or grass to colonize the intestinal tract of a young rabbit with healthy bacteria and protozoans. Alternatively, fresh caecotrophs can be liquidized and fed by syringe or mixed with the milk replacer. Probiotics can be used but they do not provide the bacteria that normally inhabit the hindgut of lagomorphs.

Leverets may be offered solids from the age of 1–2 weeks and these might include hay, grass, dandelion leaves, carrots, apples, clover and sow thistle.

Release

Adults

Only lagomorphs that are totally fit should be released into the wild. Until they are released, they should be handled only if necessary and must be encouraged to retain their fear of humans and predators such as dogs and cats. With rabbits, vaccination against VHD and myxomatosis is advisable to confer protection against these diseases.

It is important to choose the correct habitat for release. Hares, after a brief period of hospitalization, should be released to a site where wild hares are known to thrive and (importantly) where predators are controlled. If rabbits are released close to a warren, it is unlikely that they will be accepted by the resident rabbits (they may even be attacked by them) and so it is preferable to choose an uninhabited site. There should be an area of short grass for grazing and this feeding area should be close to cover into which the rabbit can bolt; undergrowth, brambles, hedges, boulders or walls are suitable. Dense woodland and long vegetation are not suitable, especially if the weather is wet. Follow-up monitoring is not possible once the animal has been released.

Young animals

At weaning, a choice has to be made whether to keep a baby lagomorph as a permanent pet or to release it at a later date. In the wild, the mother rabbit shows no maternal behaviour once the young have left the nest,

and the natural mortality rate of newly weaned rabbits is high. Because of this, many owners resist release at such a young age and wish to keep baby rabbits in captivity. Baby rabbits and leverets that are destined to be pets should be handled as much as possible as soon as they leave the nest.

On the other hand, if an animal is to be released later, it should not be handled but kept in an enclosure and released like an adult. For example, a healthy young leveret intended for release should not be 'petted' and should be replaced in its accommodation immediately after feeding and toileting. Same-age or sibling groups may be reared together.

Vaccination against myxomatosis can be given at 6 weeks and VHD at 10 weeks of age. At release, the box containing the 'nest' can be left open in a suitable release site. This mimics the situation in the wild and gives the animal somewhere to which it can return.

Legal aspects

For legal considerations relating to rabbits and hares, see Chapter 5.

References and further reading

Allan JC, Craig PS, Sherington J, Rogan MT, Storey DM, Heath S and Iball K (1999) Helminth parasites of the wild rabbit *Oryctolagus cuniculus* near Malham Tarn, Yorkshire, UK. *Journal of Helminthology* **73**, 289–294

Brewer NR and Cruise LJ (1994) Physiology. In: *The Biology of the Laboratory Rabbit, 2nd edn*, eds PJ Manning *et al.*, pp. 63–70. Academic Press, San Diego, California

Broderson JR and Gluckstein FP (1994) Zoonotic and occupational health considerations. In: *The Biology of the Laboratory Rabbit, 2nd edn*, eds PJ Manning *et al.*, pp. 356–366. Academic Press, San Diego, California

Brooks D (1997) Nutrition and gastrointestinal physiology. In: *Ferrets, Rabbits and Rodents. Clinical Medicine and Surgery*, eds EV Hillyer and KE Quesenberry, pp. 169–175. WB Saunders, Philadelphia

Corbet GB and Harris S (eds) (1991) *The Handbook of British Mammals*. Blackwell Scientific, Oxford

Cox JC and Ross J (1980) A serological survey of *Encephalitozoon cuniculi* infection in the wild rabbit in England and Scotland. *Research in Veterinary Science* **28**, 396 (abstract)

Cox JC, Pye D, Edmonds JW and Shepherd R (1980) An investigation of *Encephalitozoon cuniculi* in the rabbit *Oryctolagus cuniculus* in Victoria, Australia. *Journal of Hygiene* **84**, 295–300 (abstract)

Delong D and Manning PJ (1994) Bacterial diseases. In: *The Biology of the Laboratory Rabbit, 2nd edn*, eds PJ Manning *et al.*, pp. 131–170. Academic Press, San Diego, California

Donnelly TM (1997) Basic anatomy, physiology, and husbandry. In: *Ferrets, Rabbits and Rodents. Clinical Medicine and Surgery*, eds EV Hillyer and KE Quesenberry, pp. 147–159. WB Saunders, Philadelphia

Fenner F and Fantini B (1999) *Biological Control of Vertebrate Pests. The History of Myxomatosis – an Experiment in Evolution*. CABI Publishing, Oxford

Flecknell PA (1998) Developments in the veterinary care of rabbits and rodents. *In Practice* **20**, 286–295

Flecknell PA (2000) Anaesthesia. In: *Manual of Rabbit Medicine and Surgery*, ed. PA Flecknell, pp. 103–116. BSAVA, Gloucester

Gillett CS (1994) Selected drug dosages and clinical reference data. In: *The Biology of the Laboratory Rabbit, 2nd edn*, eds PJ Manning *et al.*, pp. 468–472. Academic Press, San Diego, California

Greig A, Stevenson K, Perez V, Pirie AA, Grant JM and Sharp JM (1997) Paratuberculosis in wild rabbits (*Oryctolagus cuniculus*). *Veterinary Record* **140**, 141–143

Harcourt-Brown FM (2002) *Textbook of Rabbit Medicine and Surgery*. Butterworth-Heinemann, Oxford

Harris S, Morris P, Wray S and Yalden D (1995) In: *A Review of British Mammals*. JNCC, Peterborough

Hofing GL and Kraus AL (1994) Arthropod and helminth parasites. In: *The Biology of the Laboratory Rabbit, 2nd edn*, eds PJ Manning *et al.*, pp. 231–258. Academic Press, San Diego, California

Johnson-Delaney CA (1996) Zoonotic parasites of selected exotic animals. *Seminars in Avian and Exotic Pet Medicine* **5**, 115–124

Kaplan BL and Smith HW (1935) Excretion of inulin, creatinine, xylose and urea in the normal rabbit. *American Journal of Physiology* **113**, 354–360

Kraus A, Weisbroth SH, Flatt RE and Brewer N (1984) Biology and diseases of rabbits. In: *Laboratory Animal Medicine*, pp. 207–237. Academic Press, San Diego, California

Lang J (1981) The nutrition of the commercial rabbit. Part 1. Physiology, digestibility and nutrient requirements. *Nutrition Abstracts and Reviews, Series B* **51**, 197–217

Leland MM, Hubbard CB and Dupey JP (1992) Clinical toxoplasmosis in domestic rabbits. *Laboratory Animal Science* **42**, 318–319

Lockley RM (1978) *The Private Life of the Rabbit*. Andre Deutsch, London

Lumeij JT (1997) Disease risks with translocations of rabbits and hares into, out of and within Europe. *Journal of the British Veterinary Zoological Society* **2**, 19–25

Lumeij JT, de Koning J, Bosma RB, van der Sluis JJ and Schellekens JFP (1994) Treponemal infections in hares in the Netherlands. *Journal of Clinical Microbiology* **32**, 543–546

Marcato PS and Rosmini R (1986) In: *Pathology of the Rabbit and Hare*. Societa Editrice Esculapio,

McBride A (1988) *Rabbits and Hares*. Whittet Books, London

Munro R, Wood A and Martin S (1995) Treponemal infection in wild hares. *Veterinary Record* **136**, 78–79

Nowak RM (1999) Order Lagomorpha. In: *Walker's Mammals of the World. Volume II, 6th edn*, pp. 1715–1738. The Johns Hopkins University Press, Baltimore

Owen DG (1992) Parasites of laboratory animals. In: *Laboratory Animal Handbooks No. 12*. Royal Society of Medicine Services, London

Pakes SP and Gerrity LW (1994) Protozoal diseases. In: *The Biology of the Laboratory Rabbit, 2nd edn*, eds PJ Manning *et al.*, pp. 205–224. Academic Press, San Diego, California

Philips CE (1981) Rabbits. In: *An Atlas of Laboratory Animal Haematology*, p.6. Oxford University Press, Oxford

Pritchard GC, Williamson S, Carson T, Bailey JR, Warner L, Willshaw G and Cheasty T (2001) Wild rabbits – a novel vector for verocytotoxigenic *Escherichia coli* 0157. *Veterinary Record* **149**, 567

Robinson AJ, Muller WJ, Braid AL and Kerr PJ (1999) The effect of buprenorphine on the course of disease in laboratory rabbits infected with myxoma virus. *Laboratory Animals* **33**, 252–257 (abstract)

Sanderson JH and Philips CE (1981) Rabbits. In: *An Atlas of Laboratory Animal Haematology*, p.6. Oxford University Press, Oxford

Sargent AP (1974) *A study of certain infectious diseases of the brown hare (*Lepus europaeus*) with specific reference to yersiniosis*. MPhil Thesis, ARC Compton, Berkshire

Stocker L (2000) *Practical Wildlife Care*. Blackwell Scientific, Oxford

Tataruch F (2001) Concentrations of environmental pollutants in European brown hares in Austria. In: *Proceedings, Symposium: The Decline of European Hares, Berlin*

Thulin C (1996) Introgression of mitochondrial DNA from *Lepus timidus* to *L. europaeus* in Scandinavia. In: *Proceedings XIIth Lagomorph workshop, Clermont-Ferrand, France*

Whitwell KE (1991) Do hares suffer from grass sickness? *Veterinary Record* **128**, 395–396

Whitwell K (1997) Natural causes of mortality in wild hares (*Lepus europaeus*) in Britain, 1993–95. *Gibier Faune Sauvage* **14**, 544–545

11

Badgers

Elizabeth Mullineaux

Introduction

The Eurasian badger (*Meles meles*) is the largest of Britain's carnivores. Badgers are found in most rural areas throughout Britain, at altitudes below 500 m, but are concentrated in south-west England and southern Wales. The most common reasons for veterinary attention are road traffic accidents (RTAs), injuries from baiting, snaring or poisoning, and territorial bite wounds from other badgers. Orphaned badger cubs are commonly presented in some areas and require veterinary involvement in their rehabilitation. Local badger groups, usually branches of the National Federation of Badger Groups (NFBG), are available nationally to assist with rehabilitation and release of casualties.

Ecology

Setts and social groups

Badgers live in setts – networks of underground tunnels and chambers with an area up to 1575 m^2 (Neal and Cheeseman, 1996). Setts have three to ten large entrances, which can be differentiated from those of foxes or rabbits by their large openings (30–60 cm) and heaps of earth with bedding material outside. No two setts are alike, their structure and size depending on the local soil type, presence of tree roots, and local availability of food and bedding. As a general rule, badgers prefer well drained soil in deciduous and mixed woodland and copses, where there is adequate food and bedding and an absence of human disturbance (Clements *et al.*, 1988). Sett chambers are lined with bedding, which prevents heat loss, particularly for cubs. Bedding consists of hay, coarse grass, straw or other vegetation that the badger can carry to the sett bundled between its chest and front legs. Unsuitable bedding material such as plastic and baler-twine can result in entangling of adults and deaths of cubs.

Each badger social group usually has one main sett within its territory but may also have a variety of additional setts. There are well marked paths between the different sett areas, main feeding areas and latrines. Latrines are often on territory boundaries; underground latrines at the end of chambers and side tunnels are also seen (Neal and Cheeseman, 1996). Territories vary from about 30 ha in high-density populations in optimal habitat, to 300 ha in less ideal environments (Cheeseman, 1979). Group and territory sizes are determined by the quality and distribution of food, respectively (Kruuk and Parish, 1982).

A typical social group consists of five animals, usually with a dominant male and a mixture of sexes and ages, but group size varies widely. Social groups of 2 to 35 animals and single-sex groups have been reported (Neal and Cheeseman, 1996). Communication between animals within social groups is mainly through scent marking, though vocalization and visual signs ('puffing up') are heard and seen, especially in cubs.

Periods of activity

Badgers are largely nocturnal, typically emerging from setts between sunset and dusk in the summer months and after dark in the winter. The time of emergence and the amount of time spent out of the sett depend on light intensity, weather conditions, food availability and social activities (Neal and Cheeseman, 1996). Night-time activities include foraging, marking of territory boundaries, digging, bedding collection, playing and mating, depending on the time of year. There is no true hibernation, though activity is greatly reduced between November and February.

Feeding

Badgers are omnivorous; they are largely opportunist foragers but their most important source of food in Britain is earthworms (Neal, 1988). Insects, small mammals, birds' eggs, invertebrates, cereals, fruit and seeds are all eaten. The exact composition of the diet depends on food availability, which is affected by locality and time of year. Water may be taken from streams, rain puddles and cattle troughs but most water is gained from the earthworm component of the diet.

When foraging, badgers usually amble along at a leisurely pace; they are, however, able to run fast, climb very well and swim if necessary (Neal and Cheeseman, 1996).

Suburban badgers

Badgers are very adaptable in suburban areas, with well documented populations in most large cities. Suburban badgers tend to emerge from setts later at night than their rural counterparts. Food is often taken from dustbins and gardens. Suburban badgers can become a nuisance and setts may cause subsidence. Literature is available to provide advice on such problems (Harris *et al.*, 1993), together with advice from local badger groups.

Anatomy and physiology

Badgers are powerful mammals, well adapted for digging and life underground. They have short strong limbs that are not unlike those of chondrodystrophoid dogs, exhibiting antebrachial characteristics such as cranial bowing of the distal radius, carpal valgus and external rotation of the distal limb, which are normal features. Hindlimbs and forelimbs are of a similar length, with five digits and long non-contractile claws. The back is relatively straight to support their weight and has less ability to arch than that of the domestic carnivores.

Dentition

The badger's skull has a pronounced sagittal crest in adults, supporting the well developed temporal muscles. Dentition reflects their omnivorous diet (temporary dentition in parentheses):

$$2 \times \left\{ I \; \frac{3\,(3)}{3\,(3)} \; C \; \frac{1\,(1)}{1\,(1)} \; P \; \frac{4\,(4)}{4\,(4)} \; M \; \frac{1\,(0)}{2\,(0)} \right\} = 38\,(32)$$

Incisors, canines and premolars are typical of a carnivore, whilst the last premolar and the molars are greatly modified for crushing and grinding, being broad and cusped like those of a herbivore. The first premolar is often vestigial or absent (Neal and Cheesman, 1996). Milk dentition erupts from the age of 4 to 6 weeks (canines, premolars, incisors – in that order) and permanent teeth from 10 to 16 weeks (incisors first).

Skin and coat

The skin is more mobile and tougher than that of dogs. There are long guard hairs and a dense underfur. The melanin band in the guard hairs gives the badger a greyish look from a distance, apart from its distinctive black-and-white striped head. Melanistic, albino and erythristic pelage types are recognized, with intermediate varieties (Neal and Cheeseman, 1996). There is no colour difference between the sexes.

Size

Size and weight depend on age, sex, food availability (Kruuk and Parish, 1983) and time of year. Population density has also been shown to have an influence on body condition and weight (Rogers *et al.*, 1997; Tuyttens *et al.*, 2000). Adult male badgers (boars) are usually heavier (9.1–16.4 kg) than females (sows) (6.5–13.9 kg) (Neal, 1977, 1986). Boars generally have broader heads than sows but the sexes are virtually impossible to tell apart at any distance in the field.

Normal parameters

Body temperature is around 37°C but can drop as low as 28°C in the winter months. Resting heart and respiratory rates in individuals familiar with human contact appear to be not unlike those of domestic dogs of a similar size (E. Mullineaux, unpublished data).

Senses

The badger has a highly developed sense of smell, which is used in social communication. Scent is produced from several sources:

- Sub-caudal glands under the tail above the anus (Figure 11.1)
- Anal glands much like those of dogs
- Sweat and sebaceous glands
- Urine.

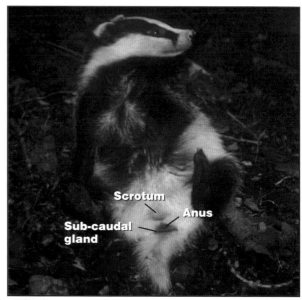

11.1 Male badger showing position of sub-caudal gland under the tail and dorsal to the anus. (Photograph: Colin Seddon.)

Interdigital scent glands may also be present, though these do not appear to have been anatomically described.

The sense of hearing is good and the ears are protected by the small pinnae during digging. The eyes are well adapted for night vision, with a predominance of retinal rods and a well developed tapetum. For this reason badgers are easily blinded by bright light. The eyes are not large for a nocturnal animal and the cubs in particular are very short-sighted.

Reproduction

Sexual maturity occurs at around 12–15 months of age. Badgers are induced ovulators. Mating can occur at any month of the year but is most frequent between February and March in the post-partum period and again in the autumn months. Badgers may delay implantation at the blastocyst stage for 2–10 months; implantation usually occurs in December and true gestation lasts about 7 weeks.

Cubs are born between mid-January and mid-March in Britain, with a peak in the first 3 weeks of February. Litter size varies from one to five, with an average of just under three, though this is reduced to an average of two by the time cubs are above ground (Neal, 1977); deaths in cubs are thought to be due in part to infanticide by dominant sows (Cresswell *et al.*, 1992). Growth rates rise rapidly between July and November and cubs reach an average of 8 kg in the first year and 10 kg in the second (Neal and Cheesman, 1996) (Figure 11.2).

Age of cub	Appearance	Eyes	Teeth	Size/Weight	Notes
At birth	Pink skin, sparse grey fur	Blind		Body 120 mm Tail 30–40 mm Total length 150–160 mm 75–132 g	
5 weeks	Full black and white coat	Eyes open	Milk teeth 4–6 weeks	800 g	
8 weeks				1500 g	Seen above ground close to sett
12 weeks			Permanent teeth 10–16 weeks	Approx. 3 kg	Weaning begins
15 weeks				Approx. 5 kg	Usually independent

11.2 Badger cub development (Data from Neal and Cheeseman, 1996 and P. Kidner, personal communication).

Population dynamics

In the wild it is unusual for badgers to reach more than 10 years of age, because of the high death rate in young animals. In studied populations, individuals of 14 and 15 years of age have been recorded and in captivity 19 years (Neal and Cheeseman, 1996).

Starvation is thought to be a major cause of death in both cubs and adult badgers. Increases in group size are followed by an increased mortality, reduced weight gain and reduced fertility within that group (Rogers *et al.*, 1997). Infectious disease is not thought to be a major factor in population regulation.

Historically, the major cause of reductions in badger populations has been direct action by humans. In the 1960s and 1970s digging, trapping, hunting and snaring kept badger numbers down. Legal protection from 1973 reduced these pursuits, though they still continue and can have a significant effect on numbers. Government operations to control tuberculosis in cattle by culling badgers can also have local and short-term effects (Cheeseman *et al.*, 1993; Tuyttens *et al.*, 2000). The greatest cause of identified badger deaths, even in TB-infected populations, is road accidents (Cheeseman *et al.*, 1988), which are estimated in tens of thousands annually. It is thought unlikely that even losses at such levels greatly influence population size (Neal and Cheeseman, 1996).

Capture, handling and transportation

Badgers are powerful animals with a dangerous bite and should be treated with respect at all times.

Capture and handling

In a field situation, a board can be used to encourage injured badgers into a cage or dustbin. Anglers' landing nets may assist with capture. Moribund animals can be gripped carefully, but firmly, by the scruff of the neck. In less debilitated individuals the scruff can be difficult to access and hold without danger to the handler and a more suitable option is use of a dog grasper. The hindquarters should be supported at all times if the animal is lifted by the scruff or with a grasper. Gloves tend to restrict grip and all but metal-enforced gauntlets offer little protection from bites.

Trapping cages

Trapping cages are available and organizations with frequent need to catch and transport badger casualties should use these or large crush cages. Cages should be of known weight, to allow easy calculation of bodyweight for sedation; they should also be free from blankets and bedding, to allow the crushing mechanism to work correctly.

Muzzles

Moribund animals must be treated carefully, as they can be unpredictable in their ability to move and bite, but may tolerate safe handling if muzzled. Baskerville-type muzzles (see Figure 11.4) are useful in allowing some normal jaw movement (for example, in panting or vomiting); in their absence, tape muzzles can be applied.

Transportation

Badgers are best transported in metal trapping or crush cages, which should be covered with blankets to minimize noise and disturbance. Prolonged periods in inappropriate cages should be avoided, as nose and limb injuries may occur.

Examination and assessment for rehabilitation

History-taking

A full history of the events leading to the presentation of a badger casualty, including its movement and behaviour during capture, should be obtained from the individuals involved. The *exact* location of where the animal was found must be recorded, since adult badgers must, as a general rule, be released back to the exact area where they were found (see 'Rehabilitation and release').

Restraint for examination

Whilst it may be necessary to administer immediate first aid to a casualty badger, care should be taken to ensure that this does not obscure the need for complete clinical assessment of the animal as soon as is practicable. Very young cubs and comatose or moribund adult animals will usually allow safe examination with minimal restraint, though a Baskerville muzzle (see Figure 11.4) is a useful precaution unless head injuries are severe. Most other casualties require some form of appropriate chemical restraint (see 'Anaesthesia and analgesia'). Clinical examination gloves should be worn and sensible hygiene precautions taken (see 'Tuberculosis').

Clinical examination

The clinical examination of a badger should in principle be no different from that for a dog or cat. Special attention should be paid to the animal's general condition (as evidence of chronic disease), mouth (tooth wear and jaw alignment), limbs and senses (especially vision). Underworn claws may be an indication of an animal that has failed to dig and live normally for some time. Full use should be made of available diagnostic facilities such as radiography, ultrasonography and laboratory tests (Figure 11.3). Due to the risk of tuberculosis, body cavities of badgers should not be drained until a reasonable assessment has been made, including auscultation, radiography or ultrasonography.

Parameter	Mean	Standard deviation
Haemoglobin (g/dl)	12.65	1.87
PCV (l/l)	0.371	0.070
RBC (10^{12}/l)	7.989	1.456
MCV (fl)	46.6	4.55
MCHC (g/dl)	34.49	3.32
MCH (pg)	16.01	1.76
WBC (10^9/l)	7.13	3.23
Neutrophils (%)	82.8	7.5
Band neutrophils (%)	0.1	0.4
Lymphocytes (%)	15.3	7.0
Monocytes (%)	1.7	2.0
Eosinophils (%)	0.1	0.5
Total protein (g/l)	78.996	10.412
Albumin (g/l)	34.272	6.087
Globulin (g/l)	44.723	11.510
Urea (mmol/l)	11.953	4.064
Creatinine (µmol/l)	63.32	20.85
Alkaline phosphatase (IU/l)	230.6	307.6

11.3 Values of common blood parameters in adult badgers (courtesy of Central Science Laboratory, Woodchester Park).

It should be remembered that sense organs (including vision) and the nervous system can only be assessed in the conscious animal and may require the assistance of someone with good knowledge of 'normal' badger behaviour.

Blood can easily be collected from the jugular vein of badgers (Figure 11.4). Urea levels may be

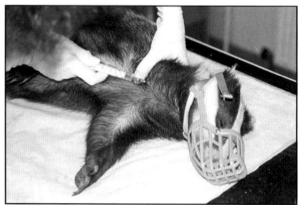

11.4 Badger sedated and muzzled with 'Baskerville' muzzle allowing blood collection from the jugular vein.

elevated in badgers consuming large numbers of earthworms, for example after a rainfall (M. Brash, personal communication).

Assessment for rehabilitation

The following questions should be asked before a treatment regime is decided:

1. *Is the animal at the end of its natural lifespan?*
   - Old animals can usually be easily identified by worn teeth and low bodyweight and condition
   - Animals with chronic disease will be in poor body condition and show specific signs of disease
   - Animals that have been displaced from setts because of age or disease may have territorial bite wounds, often at several stages of healing.

   Animals should be euthanased where old age or chronic debilitating disease is suspected. It may be argued that removal of such animals may cause unnecessary disruption of social groups but ethically it is difficult to justify the release of an animal that may shortly die.

2. *Would the healed injuries be expected to compromise the badger's life in the wild significantly?*
   This includes the ability to run, feed, defend territory and reproduce.

3. *Are veterinary skills and finance available to treat the animal adequately?*
   If skills, time and finance are not available to treat the badger casualty to high standards, especially if orthopaedic surgery is required, the animal should either be referred quickly to a veterinary surgeon with appropriate skills or be euthanased.

4. *Are suitable recovery and rehabilitation facilities available?*
   With the exception of a few minor casualties that can be released back to their site of capture within 24–48 hours, most casualties will need a period of recovery and suitable rehabilitation. In most cases

a wildlife hospital or private rescue centre should carry out this work and advice will be required from these sources or from local badger groups. If a place in a suitable centre is not available, treatment of the casualty should be reconsidered.

5. *Is a suitable release site available?*
   Adult badgers should be released at the exact spot where they were found. If this is not possible, euthanasia of these animals may be necessary (see 'Management in captivity and release'). Badger cubs need to be incorporated into release groups with other cubs; the sex of the cub and its TB status may determine its suitability for release (see 'Rearing of cubs') and this should be discussed with local rehabilitators at an early stage.

Euthanasia

Sedation or anaesthesia is usually required to examine badgers. Euthanasia is then most easily carried out using intravenous pentobarbital (150 mg/kg) into the cephalic, saphenous or jugular veins. If intravenous access is not possible, intracardiac or intraperitoneal injection may be used following anaesthesia.

First aid procedures

The principles of first aid treatment are broadly the same as in other species (see Chapter 2). Most of the injuries seen in badgers (RTAs, bites, snares) require intravenous fluid therapy (IVF) to treat circulatory shock or septicaemia. Intravenous access is easily carried out, usually via the cephalic vein, though saphenous and jugular veins are equally accessible. Fluid types and rates are as for domestic mammals and as described in Chapter 2. Mild sedation (diazepam, 0.25 mg/kg i.v. or i.m.) or the use of Baskerville muzzles prevents chewing of drip-lines, though most badgers requiring IVF are indifferent to drips and dressings.

Wounds should be dressed as necessary and limbs splinted as appropriate. Muzzles and Elizabethan collars may ensure that dressings remain in place in the short term but are rarely tolerated for long.

Analgesics must be provided (see 'Anaesthesia and analgesia'). Badgers showing neurological signs may be sedated safely with diazepam to effect. Short-acting steroids (e.g. Solu-medrone V, Pharmacia & Upjohn, 30 mg/kg i.v.) are appropriate in the early stages of nervous tissue damage.

Warmth should be provided for all casualties. Badger cubs are most easily managed in incubators. Adults can be placed in heated kennels or under heat lamps, or provided with other forms of external heat, but pads and wires that can be chewed should be avoided for all except the most seriously ill or sedated individuals.

Short-term hospitalization

Accommodation
Kennels for short-term accommodation should be of stainless steel; badgers are able to bite and dig through other kennel materials and so escape would be possible. Suitable bedding material needs to be insulating and absorbent (e.g. shredded paper, straw, blankets) and should be used in amounts sufficient to allow the animal to bury itself.

Badgers are largely nocturnal and are disturbed by excessive light and by the noise and smell of other mammal species (e.g. dogs); they are also susceptible to disease from domestic animals. For these reasons they should be kept isolated where possible; cage doors should be covered and the animals should spend the minimum time necessary in a veterinary practice before being moved to a specially equipped facility. The long-term care of badgers in captivity requires specially constructed facilities, details of which are available from local badger groups and the NFBG.

Feeding
The omnivorous nature of badgers means that they are able to eat a wide variety of foods. Suitable foods are given later (see 'Rearing of cubs' and Figure 11.10); in the short term, dog food (tinned or dried) can be offered. In reality many adult animals refuse to eat for several days in captivity but go on to make uneventful recoveries. Fresh water should be provided in a heavy bowl.

Anaesthesia and analgesia

Figure 11.5 gives doses of commonly used anaesthetic and analgesic products.

Drug	Dosage
Ketamine + medetomidine (Domitor)	5.0–7.5 mg/kg + 40 µg/kg i.m.
Ketamine + medetomidine + butorphanol	4 mg/kg + 20 µg/kg + 0.4 mg/kg i.m.
Atipamezole (Antisedan)	100–200 µg/kg i.m.
Diazepam	0.25–1.0 mg/kg i.v., i.m.
Propofol	4.0–6.5 mg/kg (depending on premedication) i.v.
Thiopental	5–20 mg/kg (depending on premedication) i.v.
Carprofen (Rimadyl injection)	4 mg/kg i.v., i.m., s.c.
Meloxicam (Metacam injection)	0.2 mg/kg s.c. single dose
Meloxicam (Metacam oral suspension)	0.1 mg/kg orally following injection
Buprenorphine (Vetergesic)	10 µg/kg i.m.
Pethidine	3 mg/kg i.m.
Morphine	0.25 mg/kg i.m.

11.5 Anaesthetic and analgesic drugs commonly used in badgers.

Intramuscular combinations
General anaesthesia with ketamine alone, as described for research sampling procedures (MacKintosh *et al.*, 1976), is very safe but produces poor muscle relaxation and hyperaesthesia in badgers, making it unsuitable

for most veterinary procedures. The addition of acepromazine, alpha-2 agonists or benzodiazepines improves the quality of surgical anaesthesia. The most common anaesthetic combinations used for minor procedures in badgers by veterinary surgeons in practice and for sampling in modern research facilities (de Leeuw *et al.*, in press) are ketamine with medetomidine, or ketamine with medetomidine plus butorphanol.

Where possible, the animal should be weighed prior to anaesthesia (pre-weighed cages assist with this procedure) and doses should be calculated accurately. The drugs are usually given by intramuscular injection into the quadriceps or lumbar muscles, through the bars of a crush cage. As with all species, medetomidine causes respiratory and circulatory depression in the badger and this author prefers to supply oxygen (mask or endotracheal tube) where possible to all badgers anaesthetized in this way and to monitor oxygen saturation levels and cardiac and respiratory functions throughout anaesthesia. Body temperature should be monitored and maintained at 37°C.

Medetomidine can be reversed with an equal volume of atipamezole given intramuscularly as soon as procedures have been completed. Badgers do not appear to suffer from the ketamine-induced hysteria sometimes seen in dogs when such anaesthetic combinations are reversed, but some veterinary surgeons prefer not to reverse medetomidine in short procedures (M. Brash, personal communication). The addition of butorphanol to the combination reduces the amount of medetomidine required and provides additional analgesia but prevents the use of other opioid analgesics that may be more suitable for major procedures.

These anaesthetic combinations appear safe in badgers provided that good anaesthetic and post-anaesthetic monitoring is carried out. Both combinations can be topped up with gaseous agents as required.

Intravenous agents

Propofol and thiopental can be used, with the same safety considerations as in domestic animals. Most badgers will require some form of deep premedication (e.g. medetomidine sedation) to allow intravenous access, though it is possible to minimize this in small cubs or animals with intravenous catheters already placed. Propofol followed by gaseous isoflurane maintenance would be the recommended combination for major surgical procedures.

Gaseous anaesthesia

Both isoflurane and halothane can be used safely but it is this author's preference to use isoflurane, because the health status of most badgers is unknown. Some form of premedication (e.g. medetomidine or acepromazine) or intravenous agent is usually required to allow safe masking or intubation. Anaesthesia can be induced in cubs by mask, with gentle restraint or a Baskerville-type muzzle for safety. Intubation may be a little more difficult than in dogs, due to more restricted jaw opening; a laryngoscope may help laryngeal visualization.

Analgesics

All injured badgers should receive appropriate analgesia both for welfare reasons and to ensure most rapid return to normal feeding and behaviour patterns. Most of the non-steroidal anti-inflammatory drugs (NSAIDs) that are common in small animal practice appear to have been used without significant problems in badgers. This author's preference is carprofen or meloxicam injections for short-term use (e.g. before surgery) and meloxicam in food for longer-term use (see Figure 11.5). This author's experience of using opioid analgesics such as buprenorphine, pethidine and morphine in badgers has been unproblematic. The use of these drugs is usually restricted to pre- and post-surgical cases.

Specific conditions

Territorial wounds

'Territorial' wounds are a common cause of natural death in badgers (Gallagher and Nelson, 1979) and one of the most common reasons for presentation of badgers at veterinary practices.

Territorial wounds are those injuries inflicted on individual badgers by other badgers. Generally they result from fighting over territory boundaries, especially in areas of high badger density (Neal and Cheeseman, 1996), or as a result of dominance battles within social groups. Bite wounds may be seen in both sexes at all times of year but there are seasonal trends: the peak prevalence in male animals is around mating time; in females, the overall incidence is lower, with peaks after the breeding season and in the early winter months (Neal and Cheeseman, 1996).

The wounds are usually around the rump (Figure 11.6), head and throat (Gallagher and Nelson, 1979; Lewis, 1997). Occasionally, bite wounds may penetrate the chest wall, resulting in pyothorax and pleurisy. There are reports that, rarely, the major vessels may be punctured, resulting in rapid death (Gallagher and Nelson, 1979).

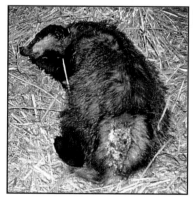

11.6 Typical 'territorial' bite wounds on the rump. (Photograph: Secret World.)

The most commonly seen wounds are around the rump and tail base. These vary from small fresh tears and punctures to significant loss of skin and musculature. There is often secondary bacterial infection (β-haemolytic *Streptococcus*, *Staphylococcus aureus* and coliforms) and, in the summer months, cutaneous myiasis. Although the wounds appears extensive, with significant secondary infection and contamination, they are generally straightforward to treat, and heal well with minimal or no intervention. More extensive wounds may take several weeks to heal.

Assessment
Animals with territorial wounds can be divided into two broad categories:

- Young animals (both sexes), usually in good condition, with no concurrent injuries. Wounds in these badgers should be treated as described below and the animals released quickly
- Older animals (usually male), often with evidence of several episodes of wounding (wounds at various stages of healing), underweight and with worn or broken teeth. These animals require careful assessment and all their problems treated if they are to be released.

The latter category is the more common and old male badgers with serial wounds present the veterinary surgeon with an ethical dilemma regarding treatment. Territorial disputes are a normal part of badger social interaction, and rapid release with minimal intervention is probably the most ecologically sound approach. Tattooing of badgers with treated bite wounds prior to release, allowing post-release monitoring, is a useful aid to assessing the success of intervention. The most severe cases, however, would either require a protracted period in captivity or be likely to die on release. These animals should be euthanased on welfare grounds.

Treatment

1. The badger must be anaesthetized (see 'Anaesthesia and analgesia') for full examination and assessed as to its suitability for rehabilitation.
2. Clipping of excessive amounts of hair from around wounds should be avoided, as this only prolongs the rehabilitation period.
3. Wounds should be flushed with sterile saline or cleaned with diluted chlorhexidine solution, as preferred.
4. Wounds should not generally be sutured. Larger wounds require major debridement prior to suturing and generally heal much better by secondary intention.
5. Topical treatments such as hydrogel products (e.g. Intrasite gel, Smith & Nephew) and semi-permeable dressing sprays (e.g. Opsite spray, Smith & Nephew) are also of benefit. Hydrocolloid dressings (Granuflex) sutured over the debrided wound have been used successfully by some authors (G. Cousquer, personal communication).
6. The short-term use of intravenous fluid therapy and NSAIDs may be needed. A course of broad-spectrum antibacterials should be started where bacteraemia or cellulitis is suspected; potentiated amoxicillin (8.75 mg/kg) and enrofloxacin (5 mg/kg) are both suitable in adult animals. Badgers often do not eat well in captivity and so injectable products rather than tablet medicine in food must be used. It should be noted that territorial bite wounds from other badgers, unlike bites from dogs, heal well with minimal intervention and rarely cause systemic signs; excessive medication is not normally required.
7. Daily topical cleaning and treatment should continue until wounds are healed. This is usually easily performed without sedation in the case of rump wounds: a thick blanket in the hands of an experienced carer is usually adequate to cover and restrain the animal's head. Head and neck wounds may require the animal to be sedated every few days for the wounds to be treated.

Digging and baiting injuries
Although badger baiting has been illegal since 1835, it was still legal to hunt, dig and kill badgers before the Badger Act of 1973. Despite now being illegal and the focus of concern for animal welfare groups, badger digging and baiting continues throughout Britain (Neal and Cheeseman, 1996).

Badgers subjected to baiting are generally dug from their setts, injured to prevent them from running away and then have dogs set upon them (Meyer, 1986). Such badgers may present as dirty and muddy from being dug. There may be limb or skull injuries as a result of shooting or being hit with a spade. Hindlimb fractures and dislocations may result from being pulled down by larger dogs. Typical dogfight bites and tears to limbs and face will also be present.

Treatment
Badgers with such injuries usually require emergency first aid, including intravenous fluid therapy at shock rates (15–30 ml/kg/h), analgesics (see 'Anaesthesia and analgesia') and broad-spectrum antibacterials (as for territorial wounds) before being anaesthetized for fuller examination and radiographs. Badgers with dog bites require much more intensive treatment than those with bite wounds from other badgers. The decision to treat baiting injuries must be made on clinical assessment and consideration of the requirements for successful release.

Legal procedures
Records of the badger's injuries (including photographs) and copies of radiographs should be kept in case prosecutions are possible. If dogs are presented that have been involved in baiting, they should be examined thoroughly and radiographs taken as appropriate. Dogs usually have injuries to the face, especially the lower lips and jaw, and forelimbs, some of which may be old injuries from previous episodes of damage (M. Brash, personal communication). Badger hairs found in a dog's mouth, faeces and vomit (induced as necessary) may be used as evidence in prosecution cases, as forensic laboratories are able to differentiate between hair types. Guidance in dealing with suspicious cases, with respect to client confidentiality, should be sought from the Royal College of Veterinary Surgeons.

Snares and trapping injuries

Although it is illegal to set snares intentionally to trap badgers, these animals do get caught in snares set illegally or intended for other species (Figure 11.7a). The size and power of the badger in its attempts to release itself from the snare often result in considerable injury (Figure 11.7b,c). Other traps and non-malicious materials such as netting may also prove hazardous to badgers. All such materials, traps and snares are best removed under general anaesthesia or sedation, preferably with the badger and trap brought to the veterinary surgery.

Careful examination of the whole badger for concurrent injuries must be carried out and radiographs taken where necessary. It is common to have injuries to the jaw and limbs caused by the badger's attempts to escape.

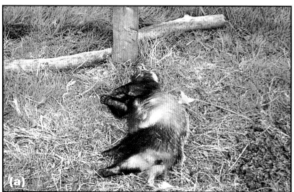

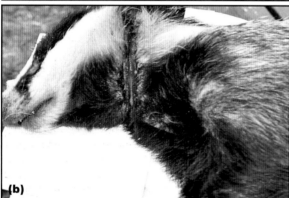

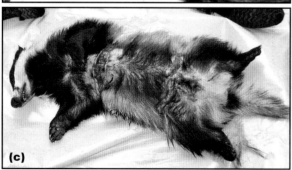

11.7 Snares. (a) Dead badger caught in a 'drag snare'. This type of snare is of dubious legality for any species, as the fact that it can be dragged limits its ability to be checked on a regular basis. In this case the snare has become trapped on a fence post. (b) Resulting wounds to the neck of the drag-snared badger. (c) Dead badger showing snare wounds around the chest and abdomen. (Photographs: M. Brash.)

Treatment

Intravenous fluid therapy, broad-spectrum antibiotics and analgesics are all usually required. It is not uncommon for there to be a delay in the development of tissue damage resulting from pressure necrosis around and distal to the site of snare or trap injuries and for this reason animals should be kept in captivity for at least a week prior to release (NFBG, 2002).

Road traffic accidents

RTAs account for at least half the badger deaths in monitored populations (Cheeseman *et al.*, 1987) and this is reflected in the frequency of their presentation to veterinary centres. The range of injuries seen are not dissimilar to those encountered in dogs involved in RTAs. Badgers will be shocked and require initial first aid treatment as described earlier. Once stable, sedation or anaesthesia is usually required to allow a complete clinical examination.

Fractures

Simple jaw fractures (mandibular symphysis or ramus) and closed long bone fractures clear of joints can be successfully repaired with a reasonable prognosis using appropriate orthopaedic implants. As in other species (see Chapter 2), fracture fixation planning should take into account the animal's tolerance of implants and the need to remove metalwork prior to release. Young badgers appear to tolerate dressings and external fixator systems much better than do adults. Badgers are robust animals and heal well but their lifestyle requires near-perfect healing for normal function. Surgical skills and finances must be available to ensure the best possible outcome. If the best possible care is not available, the animal should be euthanased for welfare reasons.

Compound fractures and those affecting joint movement carry a poor prognosis, as do fractures of the spine and pelvis. Animals with such injuries should be euthanased at an early stage.

Occasionally, badgers with healing or healed old fractures will be presented. These must be assessed on individual merit, taking into account the degree and success of healing and the normality of function. Old pelvic fractures in female animals can result in dystocia and these individuals should be euthanased if there is significant narrowing of the pelvic canal.

Thoracic trauma

Because of the risk of bovine tuberculosis, haemothorax or pneumothorax following RTAs in badgers must be treated with caution. Simple closed drainage on a single occasion should be carried out carefully under appropriate sedation or local anaesthesia, to allow diagnosis (together with radiography and ultrasonography) and treatment of minor problems. Placing of chest drains and repeat drainage are unlikely to be well tolerated and are anyway not recommended, for human health and safety reasons. Badgers requiring repeat chest drainage should be euthanased because of the zoonotic risks.

Ruptured diaphragms in badgers are generally straightforward to repair in the manner described in standard texts for small animals. Badgers are easily intubated for positive pressure ventilation during surgery, and needle drainage of the chest at the end of surgery is usually adequate. Assuming good post-surgical recovery and lack of concurrent injury, release is possible 7–10 days later.

Abdominal trauma
Abdominal trauma in a badger following an RTA requires careful asessment to ensure that the animal is not released with long-term problems. To allow full assessment and treatment, general anaesthesia and exploratory laparotomy are usually required. With the exception of simple abdominal wall injuries (without gut prolapse) and splenectomy, most abdominal injuries carry guarded or unknown prognoses, and euthanasia may be the best course of action. Splenectomy is straightforward where indicated but carries unknown risks of reduced immunity and should be considered carefully. Healed splenic and hepatic lesions from RTAs are incidental findings at post-mortem examination of badgers (Gallagher and Nelson, 1979).

Poisoning
As well as malicious intent (see Chapter 2), the varied omnivorous diet of badgers makes them susceptible to accidental pesticide or rodenticide poisoning. Poisoning cases should be treated symptomatically, as described in Chapter 2, or specific antidotes given if the causal agent is known. Cases that do not respond quickly to treatment should be euthanased.

Viral diseases

Distemper and rabies
Canine distemper has been found in badgers in continental Europe (van Moll *et al.*, 1995) but no serological evidence of the virus has been found in surveys in Britain (Delahay and Frolich, 2000). Rabies has been recorded in European badgers (Hancox, 1980) but they are not considered a primary host for the virus.

Parvovirus
Mustelids are known to be susceptible to several strains of parvovirus (Williams and Barker, 2001), though there are no records of infection in badgers in Britain. Clinical signs and histopathological findings consistent with parvovirus infection have been seen in groups of captive-reared badgers by this author and others (M. Butler, personal communication) but canine parvovirus could not be isolated in these cases. The possible susceptibility of cubs in rehabilitation facilities to parvovirus suggests that suitable precautions should be taken to prevent infection. An attenuated parvovirus vaccine (Kavak P69, Fort Dodge) has been used successfully by this author in cubs considered at risk. Vaccination of wildlife is discussed in Chapter 2.

Tuberculosis

History
Mycobacterium bovis is responsible for bovine tuberculosis but may also affect a wide range of mammals, including humans. From the early 20th century the disease was viewed as a problem in cattle, with zoonotic implications. Testing of cattle was introduced in the 1930s and by the 1960s compulsory testing had reduced the disease to a low level. Pockets of disease persisted in south-west England, preventing total eradication.

In 1971 *M. bovis* was isolated from a dead badger found on a Gloucestershire farm, where cattle were also infected (Muirhead *et al.*, 1974). Subsequently, badgers became a focus for the then Ministry of Agriculture Fisheries and Food (MAFF) investigation into the spread of TB. In 1973 the Badger Act was introduced to protect badgers from persecution, whilst at the same time authorizing agriculture ministers to issue licences for culling badgers to prevent possible disease transmission. Between 1975 and 1980, as a control method, badgers were gassed on confirmed TB-infected agricultural premises by MAFF. A government report (Zuckermann, 1980) ended gassing and introduced cage trapping and shooting of badgers in infected social groups around farm breakdowns in cattle ('Clean ring strategy'). The culling policy was reviewed a few years later ('Interim strategy') (Dunnet *et al.*, 1986). Live-badger diagnostic test trials were run from 1994 with limited success.

Despite badger culling, the incidence of TB in cattle has increased. Krebs (1997) recommended the development of a cattle vaccine, improved cattle husbandry methods and major research into the causes of TB, including studies into the contribution of badgers and other wildlife to the disease in cattle and a trial to test the effectiveness of badger-culling strategies. The culling trial is likely to run for 5–10 years. Current information is available on the website of the Department for Environment, Food and Rural Affairs (www.defra.gov.uk).

The disease in badgers
A large proportion of badgers infected with tuberculosis show no clinical signs, whereas apparently healthy badgers have excreted bacilli for up to 3 years (Clifton-Hadley *et al.*, 1993). Badgers without visible post-mortem lesions may have microscopic histopathological lesions and show evidence of early disease containment or latency of infections (Gallagher *et al.*, 1998).

Badgers with clinical tuberculosis show non-specific signs of weight loss and resultant poor condition (Clifton-Hadley *et al.*, 1993). Auscultation of the chest may suggest lung lesions or pleurisy. Clinical signs associated with renal disease may be evident, and superficial drainage lymph nodes associated with infected bite wounds may be palpably enlarged.

Post-mortem examination
Gross lesions of tuberculosis are most commonly found in the lungs and bronchiomediastinal lymph nodes (Gallagher and Nelson, 1979; Clifton-Hadley *et al.*, 1993). Lesions vary from miliary granulomatous tubercles to large abscesses with necrotic centres (Clifton-Hadley *et al.*, 1993; Gallagher *et al.*, 1998). Lung lesions due to tuberculosis may be difficult to differentiate from those related to helminth or fungal infections (Gallagher *et al.*, 1998). The presence

of lung lesions reflects both the main route of infection in badgers and a predilection site for *M. bovis* (Clifton-Hadley *et al.*, 1993). Haematogenous spread to the lungs from other sites of infection is also possible (Gallagher and Nelson, 1979).

As a result of haematogenous spread, renal lesions are the second most commonly seen gross lesions of tuberculosis infection (Gallagher and Nelson, 1979; Clifton-Hadley *et al.*, 1993). Lesions in the liver, spleen and gut may occur in a similar way. Infected bite wounds are not uncommon, especially in male animals, producing a particularly severe and rapid form of disease progression (Clifton-Hadley *et al.*, 1993; Wilkinson *et al.*, 2000).

Mortality rates

Although tuberculosis remains the most significant infectious cause of death in badgers, total losses are low, especially when compared with road deaths (Cheeseman *et al.*, 1988). In endemically infected badger populations tuberculosis accounts for less than 10% of badger deaths (Clifton-Hadley *et al.*, 1993). In medium/high-density badger populations, social structure appears to limit the spread of tuberculosis between animals (Delahay *et al.*, 2000). Disruption of social patterns (e.g. culling operations) could increase disease transmission (Cheeseman *et al.*, 1993; Tuyttens *et al.*, 2000) and therefore be counterproductive in bovine tuberculosis eradication.

Testing for tuberculosis in badgers

Bacterial culture: The most reliable method of identifying *M. bovis* infection in badgers is culture of tissue samples collected at post-mortem examination (Gallagher and Horwill, 1977). However, this is to be discouraged in veterinary practice because of the risk of zoonotic spread; suspect cases should be sent to an approved laboratory.

Samples for culture may be collected from live anaesthetized badgers and sent for standard culture and biological testing (Little *et al.*, 1982) at suitable laboratories. Sites for sampling are those used in current research programmes and reflect the sites of tuberculous lesions found in badgers (Figure 11.8).

Site of possible infection	Sample
Lung	Swab (pharyngeal/tracheal) or aspirate of sputum
Lung or gut	Swab (rectal/faecal) or sample of faeces
Kidney	Urine
Skin bite wound	Swab of skin wound/abscess

11.8 Sampling sites for bacterial culture for *M. bovis*.

The practical use of such tests in rehabilitation work is limited by the time necessary for cultures to yield mycobacteria (6–12 weeks) and the low sensitivity of testing, due to the intermittent excretion of bacilli.

Blood testing: Haematological values have been shown to vary with the course of disease in individual animals and may show anaemia, leucopenia and lowered haemoglobin concentrations in infected animals (Mahmood *et al.*, 1988). Biochemical parameters can reflect the location and extent of tuberculous lesions, most notably in increases in blood creatinine levels associated with renal lesions (Chambers *et al.*, 2000). Such changes are inconsistent and should not be used for the diagnosis of *M. bovis* infection.

The most useful diagnostic tool for rehabilitation programmes remains serological testing using the indirect ELISA for *M. bovis* in the live badger. Blood can be collected most easily from the jugular vein in a sedated adult animal (see Figure 11.4) or a well restrained cub. A 1 ml serum sample is necessary for testing through the Veterinary Laboratory Agency at Bristol (see 'Specialist organizations').

A single serological test in an individual animal has a low sensitivity (40.7%) but high specificity (94.3%) (Clifton-Hadley *et al.*, 1995). It is therefore of limited use for detecting individual infected animals but produces few false positives. As a result of the limitations of the test, adult badgers for rehabilitation are not normally tested for TB but are released back to where they were found to avoid any possible risk of spreading TB (see 'Management in captivity and release').

In situations such as cub rearing, where translocation of animals might be necessary, it is essential to minimize the risk of releasing infected animals. A 'triple testing' policy has been adopted by organizations dealing with large numbers of cubs (NFBG, 2002). Animals are classified as positive on the basis of a single positive result from blood tests taken on three occasions during rearing and are euthanased. By adopting this method, the overall sensitivity of the test is increased to 79.2% (Forrester *et al.*, 2001). If infection in the population is low, the probability that animals testing negative are truly negative is 99.8% at 1% prevalence (Forrester *et al.*, 2001). Unfortunately this is at some cost, since the number of false positives can be very high (95.5% at 1% prevalence) (Forrester *et al.*, 2001), resulting in negative animals being euthanased. In reality, few cubs test positive and the costs both financially and in terms of losses from false positives are considered to be worthwhile.

Dealing with TB in badgers in veterinary practice

Health and safety: Those dealing with badgers on a regular basis must be aware of the risk of TB and must ensure that suitable risk assessments are put in place for staff and rehabilitators working with badgers (see Chapter 5). Suggested precautions should include the following:

- Staff dealing with badgers must have a current Heaf skin test and BCG (Bacille Calmette-Guérin) vaccination
- Latex gloves must be worn when dealing with badgers. Avoid unnecessary contact with saliva, urine, faeces and open wounds

- Surfaces coming into contact with badgers should ideally be cleaned with Lysol (1 part to 39 parts water) with a contact time of 1 hour in order to kill mycobacteria (R. Delahay, personal communication)
- Post-mortem examinations must not be carried out on badgers suspected of being infected with TB; samples should be taken only from a closed carcass. Some external laboratories are able to carry out necropsies to culture for tuberculosis; whole closed carcasses should be sent for this purpose
- If post-mortem examinations of badgers not suspected of having tuberculosis are carried out, protective clothing (including masks) must be worn and the number of exposed staff kept to a minimum. Ideally, a closed area with extraction fans should be used
- Badgers suspected of having TB should be euthanased.

Release: The following precautions should be taken to avoid the risk of spreading *M. bovis* infection between areas (NFBG, 2002) (see also 'Release', below).

- All adult badgers should be returned to the exact site at which they were found. As a result of the limitations of available tests, testing for TB is not usually carried out
- If animals (mainly cubs) are to be released in a different area, triple testing for TB should be carried out (Forrester *et al.*, 2001)
- Badgers found in a TB-infected area should not be released into TB-free areas.

Other bacterial diseases

The bacteria involved in bovine tuberculosis and bite wounds are discussed above. Badgers have been recorded as carrying leptospires (*Leptospirus australis*, *L. javanica* and *L. hebdomadis*), possibly as a result of eating infected small rodents, but no clinical significance has been attached to this infection (Salt and Little, 1977; Gallagher and Nelson, 1979). *Salmonella* spp. are frequently cultured from badgers (Wray *et al.*, 1977) with *S. agama* being the principal isolate (Gallagher and Nelson, 1979). Limited clinical significance has been attached to these bacteria. Badgers are also susceptible to anthrax (Neal and Cheeseman, 1996).

Fungal diseases

Lung adiospiromycosis is a frequent post-mortem finding in badgers (Hancox, 1980) and may be confused histopathologically with tuberculosis lesions (Gallagher *et al.*, 1998). Animals showing clinical lung disease should be euthanased because of the risk of *M. bovis* infection. Histoplasmosis has been recorded in the lymphatics of badgers (Hancox, 1980). Dermatophytes have been isolated from badger setts (Hancox, 1980) but there appear to be no reports of clinical cases.

Parasites

There are many literature reviews of the badger's ectoparasites and endoparasites (e.g. Hancox, 1980; Jones *et al.*, 1980; Corbet and Harris, 1991).

Ectoparasites

The most common ectoparasites are the badger-specific biting louse *Trichodectes melis* and the badger flea *Paracercas melis*. Most other ectoparasites are opportunists found in other species, including ticks (*Ixodes* spp.) commonly found on the head and inner thigh areas of badgers. Mange in badgers, caused by *Sarcoptes scabiei,* has been reported in Britain (Neal, 1977) and in continental Europe (Samuel *et al.*, 2001) but there are no clinical studies to show the occurrence of this parasite in badgers in Britain.

Ectoparasites are rarely a clinical problem in badgers except in emaciated and debilitated individuals, where the number of lice in particular can become high. Ectoparasiticides should be used only where the burden is clinically significant or the animal requires a lot of human handling; this is especially the case in cubs. Fipronil has been used successfully for this purpose by this author for several years. It is likely that other ectoparaciticides for small animals could be used equally successfully.

Endoparasites

Most endoparasites of badgers occur infrequently, apparently as accidental infections from other species (Jones *et al.*, 1980). There appears to be little clinical significance attached to them.

Protozoal infections

Trypanosoma pestani (Peirce and Neal, 1974a) and a piroplasm (Peirce and Neal, 1974b) have been found in badgers in Britain. Parasitaemias recorded are low and tick vectors are likely (Gallagher and Nelson, 1979). No clinical significance has been attached to these infections.

Other diseases

A wide variety of diseases has been recorded from post-portem examinations of individual badgers, usually in aged animals. These include arteriosclerosis, polyarthritis, pyometritis, valvular endocarditis, liver haemangioma and cystic kidneys (Gallagher and Nelson, 1979). There appear to be few records of neoplasia in badgers. Individual badgers with specific conditions should be treated on their own merit, following the principles of assessment outlined above.

Dental disease

Older badgers frequently present with severe dental disease. In some post-mortem studies, excessive tooth wear and dental tartar have been the only significant findings in emaciated animals (Gallagher and Nelson, 1979). Teeth must always be examined in badger casualties as an indicator of age and to assist in decision-making for rehabilitation and release.

Teeth are frequently fractured or have pulp cavities exposed in road traffic accidents. An animal that is otherwise fit but has damaged teeth should have them treated or removed, as appropriate, before release. Animals with either severe dental disease or many teeth missing should be euthanased.

Therapeutics

Sites of injection

- The cephalic, saphenous and jugular veins are all accessible in badgers for the intravenous administration of fluids and medication
- The rump is usually the most accessible area when a badger is in a crush cage but intramuscular injection into this area often produces a slow and unreliable response to sedative or anaesthetic drugs, presumably as a result of inadvertent injection into fat rather than muscle. Where at all possible, therefore, intramuscular injections are best given into the quadriceps or lumbar muscles
- Subcutaneous injections can easily be given into the scruff of an already restrained individual.

Dosage

In the author's experience, the use of common veterinary drugs at the standard doses as for domestic dogs has been unproblematic. Suggested drugs have been given throughout this chapter for specific conditions as appropriate. Doses for anaesthetic and analgesic products are given in Figure 11.5.

Management in captivity

For short-term housing and feeding of adult badgers, see 'Short-term hospitalization', above. Adult badgers should generally be kept in isolation from other animals (including other badgers) during their captivity. Longer-term care of adults requires a specially constructed facility, details of which can be obtained from the NFBG.

Rearing of cubs

Most cubs brought into captivity are 8–10 weeks old, at an age when they first venture above ground. Younger cubs, from a few days old, may be presented as a result of interference in setts by dogs, or because cubs have come above ground early in response to hunger after the death or injury of their mother. For guidance on ageing a cub see Figure 11.2.

Feeding

The basic examination and assessment for rehabilitation of cubs are no different from those of adults. Badger cubs require the same care as other neonates (warmth, food and stimulation to pass faeces and urine) but will not wean until 8–10 weeks of age, which means that reasonably large cubs still require milk feeds. Most milk replacers suitable for puppies will be adequate for badger cubs, but Esbilac (PetAg) at half strength is preferred by many rehabilitators (P. Kidner, personal communication). Suggested frequencies and feeding volumes are given in Figure 11.9 (approximately 0.5 ml/g/24 h) but these vary greatly between individual cubs.

Approximate age	Weight	Total volume (24 h)	No. feeds (24 h)
1 week	280 g	140 ml	9
4 weeks	600 g	300 ml	5
8 weeks	1500 g	750 ml	4

11.9 Feeding times and volumes for badger cubs (P. Kidner, personal communication).

When feeding, cubs tend to push out their sub-caudal gland (see Figure 11.1). This is normal and should not be confused with straining for other reasons.

Older cubs (over 8 weeks of age) will take a variety of weaning foods, as suggested in Figure 11.10. Rehabilitators tend to use a wide variety of food to mimic the badger's varied and omnivorous diet but tinned puppy food will usually be accepted in the short term.

Stage	Age	Weaning foods
Stage 1	8—10 weeks	Milupa, Weetabix, scrambled eggs, yoghurt, porridge
Stage 2	10 weeks or more (and adults)	Minced meat, minced tripe, puppyfood, sausages, cooked chicken, dead day-old chicks, peanut butter sandwiches, grapes, sunflower seeds, cheese, kitchen scraps

11.10 Weaning foods for badger cubs (P. Kidner, personal communication; NFBG, 2002).

Pre-release management

In order to be released successfully, badger cubs need to be reared in social groups. Cubs kept as individuals tend to develop stereotypic behaviour and become unreleasable. Those dealing with individual cubs should contact local or national badger groups at an early stage to ensure that suitable rearing and release facilities are available. Good record-keeping will help those involved in a cub's subsequent management.

Cubs should be identified by microchip as soon as possible and tattooed (under licence) before release (Figure 11.11). Serological testing for tuberculosis should be carried out three times during rearing (see 'Tuberculosis'): the first test should be at 6–8 weeks of

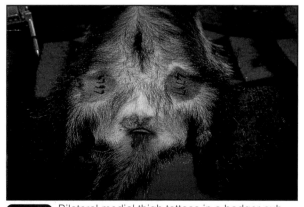

11.11 Bilateral medial thigh tattoos in a badger cub prior to release. (Photograph: Colin Seddon.)

age and ideally before the cub is mixed with others; a gap of at least 4 weeks should be left between subsequent tests and the last test should be carried out as close to release as possible (NFBG, 2002).

Release

Adults

Adult animals are not normally tested for tuberculosis prior to release. This is because of the limitations of a single serological test (Forrester *et al.*, 2001) and the time duration and cost implications of multiple testing (see 'Tuberculosis' and 'Rearing of cubs'). Any potential disease transmission risk is minimized by releasing the animal back where it was found.

Because of that risk, and because of the territorial nature of badgers, adults should be released at the *exact* site where they were found (NFBG, 2002). A good history is required for this to be possible. If there is no history of where the animal was found, the badger must either be euthanased or, if young, incorporated into a release group (see 'Rearing of cubs').

Badgers are best released from dusk onwards. To avoid further accidents where animals have been found at the roadside, it may be necessary to release them late at night when traffic is reduced.

There is some merit in tattooing adult animals (under licence) prior to release in order for post-release monitoring to be carried out (see Figure 11.11). Details of tattoo registers are available from the NFBG.

Cubs

Cubs are usually released via artificial setts at 6–8 months of age in groups of five to eight, with an appropriate sex ratio: there should be more females than males, and at least two males in the group (typically with four to six females). More information is available from the NFBG.

Legal aspects

Badgers are protected under the Protection of Animals Act 1911 and 1912 (Scotland) when captive, and under the Wild Mammals (Protection) Act 1996 in the wild. General aspects of this legislation are discussed in Chapter 5.

Badgers have been given protection against digging and baiting under various pieces of legislation over the years. These were brought together under the Protection of Badgers Act 1992. This legislation is unusual in that it protects both the badger and its sett. The main features of this Act are as follows (Neal and Cheeseman, 1996):

- It is illegal to:
  - kill, injure or take any badger or attempt to do so
  - dig for a badger
  - possess a dead badger, or any part of a dead badger, or an object derived from one if that badger was taken in contravention of the Act
  - sell, have in possession or under control a live badger

  - mark, ring or tag a badger (microchips are not considered an offence and licences are available for tattooing)
  - damage, destroy or prevent access to a badger sett
  - cause a dog to enter a sett or disturb a badger in a sett.

- It is not an offence to kill a badger provided that it can be shown that it happened accidentally.

- It is legal to:
  - damage a sett unwittingly during lawful action
  - euthanase an injured badger
  - take and treat an injured badger or rear a cub, provided that the individual is released as soon as it is no longer incapacitated.

Licences are issued by the nature conservation agencies (English Nature, Scottish Natural Heritage, Countryside Council for Wales) to allow for the keeping of badgers in zoos, the translocation of badgers, the marking (tattooing) of badgers, and interference with setts for research, land development, archaeological investigation or the gathering of evidence about an offence.

Licences are issued by the relevant government bodies (DEFRA in England, SERAD in Scotland, NAWAD in Wales) to allow badgers to be killed or setts interfered with for the prevention of spread of disease and to prevent damage to land, crops, poultry or property. They are also issued to allow interference with setts for agricultural and forestry work, or the maintenance or construction of watercourses, drainage or sea and tidal defences.

Specialist organizations

National Federation of Badger Groups (NFBG)
15 Cloisters Business Park, 8 Battersea Park Road, London SW8 4BG
Website: www.nfbg.org.uk

Scottish Badgers
8 Thornburn Grove, Edinburgh EH13 0BP
Website: www.scottishbadgers.org.uk

Secret World (Pauline Kidner)
New Road, East Huntspill, Somerset TA9 3PZ
Website: www.secretworld.co.uk

Dr Richard Delahay (*for advice on ecology and tuberculosis*)
Central Science Laboratory, Woodchester Park, Nympsfield, Gloucestershire GL10 3UJ
Website: www.csl.gov.uk/groups/cmg/cmg2/wpcontents.htm

Veterinary Laboratories Agency (*for TB ELISA blood testing*)
Langford House, Langford, Bristol BS40 5DX Tel.: 01934 852421

References and further reading

Chambers MA, Gavier-Widen D, Stanley PA and Hewinson RG (2000) Biochemical and haematological parameters associated with tuberculosis in European badgers. *Veterinary Record* **146**, 734–735
Cheeseman CL (1979) The behaviour of badgers. *Applied Animal Ethology* **5**, 193
Cheeseman CL, Wilesmith JW, Ryan J and Mallinson PJ (1987) Badger population dynamics in a high density area. *Symposia of the Zoological Society of London* **58**, 279–294

Cheeseman CL, Mallinson PJ, Ryan J and Wilesmith JW (1993) Recolonisation by badgers in Gloucestershire. In: *The Badger*, ed. TJ Hayden, pp. 78–93. Royal Irish Academy, Dublin

Cheeseman CL, Wilesmith JW, Stuart FH and Mallinson PJ (1988) Dynamics of tuberculosis in a naturally infected badger population. *Mammal Review* **18**, 61–72

Clements ED, Neal E and Yalden DW (1988) The national badger sett survey. *Mammal Review* **18**, 1–19

Clifton-Hadley RS, Wilesmith JW and Stuart FA (1993) *Mycobacterium bovis* in the European badger (*Meles meles*): epidemiological findings in tuberculous badgers from a naturally infected population. *Epidemiology and Infection* **111**, 9–19

Clifton-Hadley RS, Sayers AR and Stock MP (1995) Evaluation of an ELISA for *Mycobacterium bovis* infection in badgers (*Meles meles*). *Veterinary Record* **137**, 555–558

Corbet GB and Harris S (eds) (1991) *Handbook of British Mammals*, 3rd edn. Blackwell Science, Oxford

Cresswell P, Harris S and Jeffries J (1990) *The History, Distribution, Status and Habitat Requirements of the Badger in Britain*. Nature Conservancy Council, Peterborough

Cresswell WJ, Harris S, Cheeseman CL and Mallinson PJ (1992) To breed or not to breed: an analysis of the social and density-dependent constraints on the fecundity female badgers, *Meles meles*. *Philosophical Transaction of the Royal Society London* **338**, 393–407

de Leeuwe ANS, Forrester GJ, Spyvee PD, Brash MGI and Delahay RJ (in press) *Journal of Wildlife Diseases*

Delahay RJ and Frolich K (2000) Absence of antibodies against canine distemper virus in free-ranging populations of Eurasian badger in Great Britain. *Journal of Wildlife Diseases* **36**(3), 576–579

Delahay RJ, Langton S, Smith GC, Clifton-Hadley RS and Cheeseman CL (2000) The spatial-temporal distribution of *Mycobacterium bovis* (bovine tuberculosis) infection in a high density badger (*Meles meles*) population. *Journal of Animal Ecology* **69**, 1–15

Dunnet GM, Jones DM and McInerney JP (1986) *Badgers and Bovine Tuberculosis – Review of Policy*. HMSO, London

Forrester GJ, Delahay RJ and Clifton-Hadley RS (2001) Screening badgers (*Meles meles*) for *Mycobacterium bovis* infection using multiple applications of an ELISA test. *Veterinary Record* **149**, 169–172

Gallager J and Horwill DM (1977) A selective oleic acid albumin agar medium for the cultivation of *Mycobacterium bovis*. *Journal of Hygiene* **79**, 155–160

Gallagher J and Nelson J (1979) Causes of ill health and natural death in badgers in Gloucestershire. *Veterinary Record* **105**, 546–551

Gallagher J, Monies R, Gavier-Widen M and Rule B (1998) Role of infected, non-diseased badgers in the pathology of tuberculosis in the badger. *Veterinary Record* **142**, 710–714

Hancox M (1980) Parasites and infectious diseases of the Eurasian badger (*Meles meles* L.): a review. *Mammal Review* **10**(4), 151–162

Harris S, Jefferies D, Cheeseman C and Booty C (1993) *Problems with Badgers?* RSPCA Wildlife Department, Horsham

Jones GW, Neal C and Harris EA (1980) The helminth parasites of the badger (*Meles meles*) in Cornwall. *Mammal Review* **10**(4), 163–164

Krebs JR (1997) *Bovine Tuberculosis in Cattle and Badgers*. Report to the Rt Hon. Jack Cunningham MP. Ministry of Agriculture Fisheries and Food, London

Kruuk H and Parish T (1982) Factors affecting population size, group size and territory size of the European badger (*Meles meles*). *Journal of Zoology (London)* **196**, 31–39

Kruuk H and Parish T (1983) Seasonal and local differences in the weight of European badgers (*Meles meles*) in relation to food supply. *International Journal of Mammalian Biology* **48**, 45–50

Lewis JCM (1997) Badgers for vets. 2. Common problems. *UK Vet* **2**(3), 68

Little TWA, Naylor PF and Wilesmith JW (1982) A laboratory study of *M. bovis* infection in badgers and calves. *Veterinary Record* **111**, 550–557

Mackintosh CG, MacArthur JA, Little TWA and Stuart P (1976) The immobilization of the badger (*Meles meles*). *British Veterinary Journal* **132**, 609–614

Mahmood KH, Stanford JL, Machins S, Watts M, Stuart FA and Pritchard DG (1988) The haematological values of European badgers (*Meles meles*) in health and in the course of tuberculosis infection. *Epidemiology and Infection* **101**, 231–237

Meyer R (1986) *The Fate of the Badger*. Batsford, London

Muirhead RH, Gallagher J and Burn KJ (1974) Tuberculosis in wild badgers in Gloucestershire: epidemiology. *Veterinary Record* **95**, 552–555

NFBG (2002) *Protocol for the Rescue, Rehabilitation and Release of Badgers*. National Federation of Badger Groups, London

Neal EG (1977) *Badgers*. Blandford Press, Poole

Neal EG (1986) *The Natural History of Badgers*. Croom Helm, Beckenham

Neal EG (1988) The stomach contents of badgers. *Journal of Zoology (London)* **215**, 367–369

Neal EG and Cheeseman C (1996) *Badgers*. Poyser Natural History,

Peirce MA and Neal C (1974a) *Trypanosoma (megatryparum) pestania* in British badgers (*Meles meles*). *International Journal of Parasitology* **4**, 439–440

Peirce MA and Neal C (1974b) Piroplasmosis in British badgers (*Meles meles*). *Veterinary Record* **94**, 493–494

Rogers LM, Cheeseman CL and Langton S (1997) Body weight as an indicator of density-dependent population regulation in badgers (*Meles meles*) at Woodchester Park, Gloucestershire. *Journal of Zoology* **242**, 597–604

Roper TJ (1992) Badger *Meles meles* setts – architecture, internal environment and function. *Mammal Review* **22**, 43–53

Roper TJ, Conradt L, Butler J, Christian SE, Ostler J and Schmidt TK (1993) Territorial marking with faeces in badgers (*Meles meles*): a comparison of boundary and hinterland latrine use. *Behaviour* **127**, 289–307

Salt GFH and Little TWA (1977) Leptospires isolated from wild mammals caught in the south west of England. *Research in Veterinary Science* **22**, 126–127

Samuel WM, Pybus MJ and Kocan AA (eds) (2001) *Parasitic Diseases of Wild Mammals*. Manson, London

Tuyttens FAM, Macdonald DW, Rogers LM, Cheeseman CL and Roddam AW (2000) Comparative study on the consequences of culling badgers (*Meles meles*) on biometrics, population dynamics and movement. *Journal of Animal Ecology* **69**, 567–580

van Moll P, Alldinger S, Baumgartner W and Adami M (1995) Distemper in wild carnivores: an epidemiological, histological and immunocytochemical study. *Veterinary Microbiology* **44**, 193–199

Wilkinson D, Smith GC, Delahay RJ, Rogers LM, Cheeseman CL and Clifton-Hadley RS (2000) The effects of bovine tuberculosis (*Mycobacterium bovis*) on mortality in a badger (*Meles meles*) population in England. *Journal of Zoology* **250**, 389–395

Williams ES and Barker IK (eds) (2001) *Infectious Diseases of Mammals*. Manson, London

Wilson G, Harris S and McLaren G (1997) *Changes in the British Badger Population, 1998 to 1997*. People's Trust For Endangered Species, London

Wray C, Baker K, Gallagher J and Naylor P (1977) Salmonella infection in badgers in the South West of England. *British Veterinary Journal* **133**, 526–529

Zuckermann, Lord (1980) *Badgers, Cattle and Tuberculosis*. HMSO, London

Acknowledgements

The author would like to thank Pauline Kidner and the staff of Secret World wildlife rescue centre and Richard Delahay of the Central Science Laboratory for their assistance with this chapter and for their continued encouragement and sharing of expertise. Matthew Brash, Chris Cheeseman, Phil Scott and the co-editors of this book are thanked for their comments on earlier drafts of the chapter.

12

Otters

Victor R. Simpson and Michael A. King

Introduction

Otters belong to the subfamily Lutrinae in the family Mustelidae. There are 13 species in the world but the Eurasian otter (*Lutra lutra*) is the only species native to the British Isles (Figure 12.1). Two other species, the Asian small-clawed otter (*Aonyx cinerea*) and the American river otter (*Lutra canadensis*), are commonly kept in captivity in Britain and, as they occasionally escape, they too may be presented to the veterinary surgeon as a 'wild' animal.

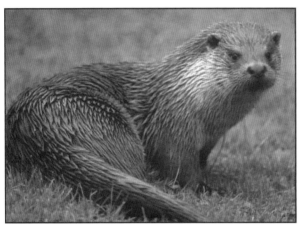

12.1 Adult Eurasian otter (*Lutra lutra*). The Asian small-clawed otter is smaller and has a more rounded face. (Courtesy of C Seddon.)

In the late 1950s and early 1960s the otter hunts in England and Wales observed a sudden and dramatic crash in the population of otters. This led to almost immediate curtailment of hunting, followed by a ban in 1977, but there was no apparent improvement. Later studies provided circumstantial evidence which suggested that the crash was due to organochlorine pesticides (Chanin and Jefferies, 1978) and/or polychlorinated biphenyls (PCBs) (Mason, 1989). These compounds were progressively banned or withdrawn and a recent study has demonstrated a marked decline in pesticide and PCB residues in otter tissues (Simpson *et al.*, 2000). At the same time there has been a strong population recovery, with otters spreading eastwards from their strongholds in south-west England and Wales, and otters are increasingly being submitted for veterinary attention.

Although the majority of otters submitted for postmortem examination are the result of road traffic accidents (Mason and O'Sullivan, 1992; Simpson, 1997), experience suggests that most otters submitted for veterinary treatment either have septic bite wounds, or are abandoned or orphaned cubs suffering from exposure, dehydration and starvation. Occasionally the bite wounds are due to attack by domestic dogs but the great majority are the result of intraspecific fighting (Simpson, 1997).

Ecology and biology

The Eurasian otter is essentially a solitary animal. An adult male (dog) may have a territory of up to 25 miles of waterway and within this area there may be two or three smaller territories occupied by breeding females (bitches) and their young (cubs). Otters mark their territory by depositing faeces (spraints) on prominent stones, tree roots, etc. and also by urine marking. The boundaries of male territories overlap and are continuously disputed, but conflicts between females are said to be uncommon (Erlinge, 1968). Studies from south-west England have shown evidence of intraspecific aggression in both sexes, with bite wounds present in around 22% of all males and 12.5% of females (Simpson and Coxon, 2000).

Otters are seldom seen, spending much of their time during the day resting up in a den, or holt, or under bankside vegetation. That they are usually shy and nocturnal is probably a reflection of persecution by humans; in some areas (e.g.the Western Isles) they may be diurnal and relatively confiding. As the otter population expands, they are also being reported with increasing frequency in busy towns and cities in England.

The otter is essentially a fish-eater and is therefore seldom found far from water. In England and Wales it is found mostly on freshwater systems but in some areas, notably the west of Scotland, it inhabits the coast and feeds on marine species. Although it comes into conflict with fishermen, particularly when it takes salmonids or valuable carp, the preferred prey are eels and (at certain times of the year) frogs. Otters occasionally eat birds and small mammals but they do not normally eat carrion.

Anatomy and physiology

The otter is a typical mustelid, with short legs, an elongated head and a muscular neck of almost equal thickness that runs smoothly into the long body. There is little free skin over the neck and this makes the animal difficult to 'scruff'. A mature dog will weigh around 7.5–10 kg, a bitch around 5–7 kg, with respective overall lengths of around 110–120 cm and 100–105 cm.

The eyes are set well forward in the skull and are small, possibly because otters do not rely as heavily on sight as on some of their other senses. There are groups of long sensory bristles, called vibrissae, on the muzzle and cheek, above the eye and on the elbows; they form an almost complete circle around the anterior part of the body and are believed to be important as tactile organs where visibility is bad, particularly in the location of prey. The ear pinnae are small and rounded.

The feet are well adapted for swimming, with webs between all five toes. The front feet are larger and have longer claws than those on the back. The coat is adapted for immersion, with a short outer coat and a dense undercoat that traps air. As with all mustelids, there are large scent glands on either side of the anus. The male has an os penis (or baculum) rather like a domestic dog. In the bitch there are usually four nipples but they tend to be very inconspicuous unless she is lactating; even then, it is often only the caudal pair that are active.

Dentition is as follows (Harris, 1968) (with temporary dentition in parentheses):

$$2 \times \left\{ I \ \frac{3\,(3)}{3\,(3)} \ C \ \frac{1\,(1)}{1\,(1)} \ P \ \frac{4\,(1)}{3\,(2)} \ M \ \frac{1\,(1)}{2\,(0)} \right\} = 36\ (24)$$

Eruption times are shown in Figure 12.3. The roots of the second lower incisors are set back, giving the impression of overcrowding, but this is normal (Figure 12.2).

Much of the internal anatomy is typical of carnivores and has been summarized elsewhere (Simpson,

1997). The mandibular salivary glands and lymph nodes lie at the angle of the jaw, whilst the retropharyngeal nodes lie dorsolateral and slightly caudal to the larynx. The thyroid glands are unlike those in other mustelids: they are long, flat and tapering, with no isthmus, and are closely applied to the trachea. There is normally a cardiac thymus but no cervical thymus. The heart is unusually globular, with a thick-walled left ventricle and a much thinner right ventricle. Care should be taken not to interpret this as ventricular hypertrophy. The lungs resemble those of a badger, with two lobes on the left, three on the right and an intermediate lobe, also served by the right bronchus. The seven-lobed liver is similar to a dog's but there are both common hepatic and cystic bile ducts, linked by a network of anastomoses, which join the duodenum adjacent to the pancreatic ducts. Unlike those of other British mustelids, the otter's kidneys are multilobular and more resemble those of a bovine or a cetacean.

Reproduction

Bitch otters do not breed until they are around 2 years of age and they produce no more than one litter a year. Cubs may be born during any month and it is thought that this is possible because, based on observations in captivity, otters appear to be continuously polyoestrous (Mason and Macdonald, 1986). However, studies on wild otters in Norway and also in south-west England suggest that they may be induced ovulators, or have periods of anoestrus (Heggberget and Christensen, 1994; Rivers, 1997). As far as is known, delayed implantation does not occur, though it does take place in the American river otter. Some data on reproduction and development are shown in Figure 12.3.

Oestrous cycle (captive)	45–50 days (Wayre, 1979)
Duration of oestrus	14 days (Wayre, 1979)
Gestation period	61–63 days (Stephens, 1957; Mason and Macdonald, 1986)
Litter size	2–3 mostly (Mason and Macdonald, 1986)
Birthweight (captive)	100 g approx. (Reuther, 1999)
Eyes open	30–35 days (Heggberget, 1996)
Permanent incisors erupt	13 weeks approx. (Heggberget, 1996)
Permanent canines erupt	15 weeks approx. (Heggberget, 1996)

12.3 Reproduction and development in the otter.

The cubs are born in a den, or holt, and are blind but with hair. They double their bodyweight every 10 days for the first 3 weeks and gain around 300 g every 10 days after that, weighing around 3 kg at 100 days (Reuther, 1999). They start to emerge from the holt at about 8–12 weeks of age, which coincides with weaning. An important feature, relevant to rehabilitation, is that the cubs then remain dependent on the bitch until they are 10–12 months of age. It is believed that the dog plays no part in their rearing.

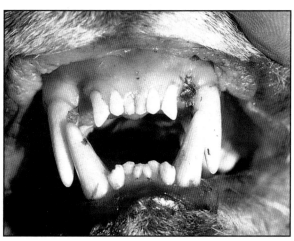

12.2 Staggered alignment of lower incisors. This is normal.

Life expectancy

Although otters in the wild may live as long as 15 years, this is unusual and most die in the first few years. A study in the Shetlands showed that the life expectancy for a 1-year-old otter was 3.14 years and a similar study on specimens from mainland Scotland and England gave a figure of around 2.75 years (Kruuk, 1995). For otters in south-west England the life expectancy may be even lower, as a study between 1988 and 1994 gave a mean age at death of 2 years (Simpson, 1997). These figures should be interpreted with care, as a high proportion of the otters examined in such studies are road traffic casualties and it is likely that immature animals are over-represented. There is little evidence of infectious disease in wild otters and the principal cause of natural mortality is intraspecific aggression (Simpson and Coxon, 2000).

Capture, handling and transportation

Otters are not easy to handle and capture can be difficult unless the animal is severely injured or debilitated. People experienced in dealing with otters try to avoid handling them and strongly advise against it. If necessary, they would prefer to persuade and guide the otter into a cage, ideally of crush design. If this is not possible, nets with padded rims (to avoid damaging the otter's teeth) are recommended, as is the use of thick gloves for personal protection. Graspers can be used but the anatomy of the otter is such that the neck is of equal thickness to the head and so it is recommended that the grasper should be positioned diagonally across the body, encircling one foreleg as well as the neck, or grasping just behind the forelegs.

If the veterinary surgeon assesses that the animal is fit enough, sedation may be administered whilst it is still in the net or grasper, thus enabling further examination or transport. Otters are quick to escape and it is essential to have a secure cage on hand at the time of capture and also for subsequent transport.

Otters in Britain do not normally carry any significant zoonotic infections. Apart from their ability to bite, they pose little threat to humans.

Examination and assessment for rehabilitation

When an otter is admitted, it is important to keep a record of where it came from so that, when it has recovered, it can be returned to that same location. However, if the animal was ill due to intraspecific fighting, there is a possibility that this problem will recur if it is put back in the same area.

Observations on factors such as mobility, coordination and feeding behaviour need to be carried out on the conscious animal, but for many conditions it is necessary to sedate or anaesthetize the otter (for anaesthesia and analgesia, see later).

The loss of an eye may not be as serious in an otter as in some species, as apparently healthy blind otters have been observed in the wild (Williams, 1989). The vibrissae, on the other hand, are probably very important, especially where the animal may be feeding in cloudy water. A full set of teeth may not be important but badly fractured or infected teeth should be removed.

Although a damaged tail tip could be amputated, it is doubtful whether an otter could hunt successfully without most of its tail. It might be able to hunt effectively following a limb amputation, especially a hindleg, but if so compromised it may not then be able to maintain its dominance and hence its territory. For the same reason, a male that has been castrated during a fight is probably best euthanased. Fractures to the os penis should be examined critically, as callus formation could obstruct urine flow.

In view of the foregoing, and also because of problems of managing otters in captivity, assessment needs to be relatively severe, particularly in the case of a weak or old specimen. Rehabilitation time can often be long, especially for cubs, and currently very few specialist otter rehabilitation centres are available. If there is one locally, it should be contacted as soon as the otter shows signs of improving. Most veterinary practices and 'broad-spectrum' wildlife sanctuaries are not suitable. At one time disabled otters might have been used in captive-breeding programmes but, in view of the natural recovery of the wild population, there is now little justification for such work and there are limited suitable placements for such animals.

Blood sampling

If blood is required for haematology or biochemistry it should be possible to obtain a sample from either the jugular vein or the vein in the midline ventral tail, or alternatively the femoral vein. The dense coat of the otter can make intravenous injections difficult for the inexperienced, but the jugular vein is readily visualized by having an assistant turn the otter on to its back, with its hindquarters held well above the level of the head, and then moistening the skin with spirit. The jugular vein runs from the point of the shoulder to the angle of the jaw. It is preferable not to clip the fur in case early release is possible. The haematological and biochemical characteristics of Eurasian otters in the wild have not been well studied but there is a comprehensive report of values in animals from a rehabilitation centre and this provides valuable data (Lewis *et al.*, 1998). Values for animals of all ages and both sexes in that study are shown in Figure 12.4 but it should be noted that there are differences related to age and sex (for details, see Lewis *et al.*, 1998).

Euthanasia

Where euthanasia is necessary it may be advisable to administer intramuscular sedation first (see later), followed by intravenous or intraperitoneal injection of pentobarbital.

Parameter	Mean (sd)	Range
Haemoglobin (g/dl)	15.7 (3.62)	7.6–20.5
RBC count (10^{12}/l)	7.01 (1.0)	4.8–9.11
PCV (l/l)	0.53 (0.12)	0.28–0.74
MCV (fl)	75.8 (13.1)	46.7–96.6
MCH (pg)	22.4 (4.2)	12.8–28.0
MCHC (g/dl)	29.4 (2.27)	25.2–33.8
Reticulocytes (% RBC)	1.77 (2.0)	0.2–9.8
Total WBC count (10^9/l)	6.44 (2.77)	3.03–13.9
Neutrophil count (10^9/l)	3.99 (2.62)	1.62–12.1
Lymphocyte count (10^9/l)	1.66 (0.84)	0.59–4.61
Monocyte count (10^9/l)	0.20 (0.16)	0.0–0.62
Eosinophil count (10^9/l)	0.57 (0.38)	0.07–1.73
Basophil count (10^9/l)	0.016 (0.04)	0.0–0.2
Platelet count (10^9/l)	676.89 (403)	43–1983
Fibrinogen (g/l)	2.61 (1.21)	0.0–5.7
Urea (mmol/l)	11.4 (2.79)	7.42–22.6
Creatinine (µmol/l)	67.5 (23.5)	33–128
Bicarbonate (mmol/l)	22.7 (3.93)	14.2–32.0
Sodium (mmol/l)	150.2 (2.75)	145–159.3
Potassium (mmol/l)	4.77 (0.44)	3.68–5.77
Total protein (g/l)	63.2 (6.41)	48–77
Albumin (g/l)	32.5 (2.44)	27.0–38.2
Globulin (g/l)	30.3 (5.15)	19–44
Calcium (mmol/l)	2.20 (0.13)	1.94–2.45
Inorganic phosphate (mmol/l)	2.51 (0.59)	1.58–4.50
Total bilirubin (µmol/l)	1.13 (1.51)	0.0–4.5
Cholesterol (mmol/l)	2.38 (0.47)	1.26–3.57
Creatinine kinase (IU/l)	434.7 (287.1)	183–1844
AST (IU/l)	132.9 (75.5)	45–459
Gamma GT (IU/l)	20.5 (9.02)	4–45
ALT (IU/l)	82.8 (46.6)	19–296
AP (IU/l)	43.2 (24.3)	10–104

12.4 Haematological and biochemical data from 41 and 47 otters, respectively, of both sexes and all ages (from Lewis *et al.*, 1998).

First aid procedures

Normal principles of first aid apply but due to difficulties in handling otters, and assuming the patient is not severely shocked, it is probably less stressful for both the otter and the clinician if the casualty is sedated for examination. Dosage should be adjusted according to initial assessment of the patient and an informed estimate of likely bodyweight. The first aid requirements of the patient can then be assessed more accurately by normal clinical examination.

Road traffic casualties may be in shock and corticosteroids in large doses have a part to play in the early treatment of such cases. Analgesics should be used during recovery from trauma and following surgery. NSAIDs, such as carprofen and meloxicam, should be well tolerated (see Figure 12.5).

Radiography is useful, especially in cases of road traffic injury or suspected shooting, but ultrasonography is rendered impossible by the air trapped in the dense coat. It would be preferable not to clip off hair. Fractures should be repaired by internal fixation methods, as the otter is likely to remove external supports rapidly. Repair should be attempted only if release is a confident expectation.

Bite wounds and abscesses should be treated routinely by cleansing, debridement and broad-spectrum antibiotic cover (long-acting preparations are useful in order to minimize further handling). Fresh wounds should be repaired by subcuticular suturing using absorbable suture material.

Abandoned cubs

Although cubs may be left unattended by parents for periods of time, they do not normally leave the holt until about 8 weeks old, by which time they should weigh around 1.5 kg. Therefore, any cubs found out in the open and weighing much less than this may well have been abandoned or orphaned. Such cubs are likely to be hypothermic and dehydrated. Warmth and electrolytes, initially by parenteral routes, should be provided.

Fluid therapy

It is unlikely that an otter would tolerate an intravenous drip once sedation wears off. Fluids are probably best given intraperitoneally or, in the collapsed or sedated patient, intraosseously.

Hospitalization

Short-term housing must be in escape-proof cages, preferably made from stainless steel and smooth inside, in a quiet location away from other animals. Thus a normal veterinary practice situation is not ideal other than for very short-term hospitalization. Fresh drinking water must be available and should be provided in a heavy unspillable bowl. Feeding will depend on the age of the patient (see 'Management in captivity and release').

Anaesthesia and analgesia

Severely injured patients can be masked down using isoflurane and oxygen (or halothane/oxygen if isoflurane is not available). Most otters require intramuscular administration of an anaesthetic or sedative agent before gaseous anaesthesia will be tolerated.

Otters may be immobilized with ketamine alone but there are several reports that this can cause hyperthermia (Reuther, 1983; Reuther and Brandes, 1984). It may also cause intense excitement during recovery and otters should therefore be allowed to recover in a quiet, dark place for at least 2 hours (Reuther, 1983). It is better to use ketamine in combination with other drugs, as described in Figure 12.5.

Drug	Dose rate	Notes
Anaesthetics		
Ketamine	7.8–16.0 mg/kg	Risk of hyperthermia and excitement on recovery (Reuther, 1983) No reversing agent
Ketamine + diazepam	18.0 mg/kg + 0.5 mg/kg	Good relaxation but risk of hyperthermia (Kuiken, 1988) No reversing agent
Ketamine + medetomidine	4–5 mg/kg + 100–120 µg/kg	Good relaxation Partial reversal by atipamezole (300–480 µg/kg) (Lewis, 1991)
Ketamine + medetomidine + butorphanol	5 mg/kg + 80 µg/kg + 0.4 mg/kg	Good relaxation, analgesia Can be mixed in one syringe Partial reversal by atipamezole (240 µg/kg)
Isoflurane	3–4% in oxygen	Good anaesthesia Safest method for debilitated and shocked patients Difficult to administer to otters without premedication as above
Halothane	2–4% in oxygen	As isoflurane but less safe
Analgesics		
Butorphanol	0.4 mg/kg	Usually as part of anaesthetic combination Short-acting
Carprofen	2–4 mg/kg	Effective NSAID Injectable or oral (tablet)
Meloxicam	0.2 mg/kg	Effective NSAID Injectable or oral (liquid)

12.5 Anaesthetics and analgesics for otters.

Intubation of the anaesthetized otter can be difficult due to the shape of the larynx but may be achieved with the help of a laryngoscope or an introducer to adjust the angle of the tube. Post-operative analgesia must be considered in injured patients at induction and continued post-operatively (Figure 12.5).

Specific conditions

Trauma

Bite wounds inflicted by other otters are mostly to the face (Figure 12.6) or anus and genitals. The feet are also often bitten and toes may be amputated (Simpson, 1997; Simpson and Coxon, 2000). Although many bites are obvious, they are not always easily seen and can be overlooked, particularly around the perineum. The wounds often become infected, usually with *Streptococcus* spp. Mixed infections with organisms such as *Escherichia coli* are common, and unidentified anaer-

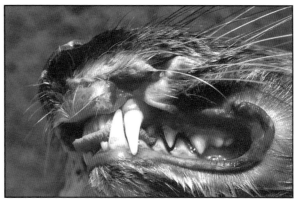

12.6 Intraspecific aggression: healing bite wounds to the face of a young adult otter. Note also the loss of incisors. The erosion of enamel on the anterior aspect of the lower canine is a common finding.

obes have been described in necrotic tissue (A. Patterson and G. Foster, personal communication). Infection often tracks subcutaneously or between muscle layers well away from the puncture wound. Bites inflicted by domestic dogs are normally much more extensive and where large dogs are involved there may be, for example, crushed ribs and internal haemorrhage.

Other injuries caused by intraspecific biting include fracture of the os penis (Stephens, 1957) and damage to eyes. Loss of incisors and fractured canines are commonly seen and many such cases also appear to be a result of fighting. Fractures of the cheek teeth, especially the carnassials (Figure 12.7), occur and may easily be missed on clinical examination. They often lead to root abscessation, osteomyelitis and septicaemia. As with septic bite wounds, these conditions often prove fatal.

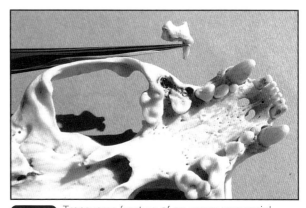

12.7 Transverse fracture of an upper carnassial tooth, with resulting root abscess. This lesion frequently results in a fatal septicaemia.

As well as bite wounds to the feet, severe cuts to the pads or webs (probably caused by broken glass in watercourses) are occasionally seen. Badly eroded foot pads, particularly on the hindfeet, are seen in animals that have been in prolonged conflict with another otter. These cases, mostly males, are usually in very poor physical condition and frequently have blackish, tarry material coming from the anus. This is quite distinct from normal spraints, which, although often soft, are formed.

Viral diseases

Viral infections of otters appear to be rare, though several potentially fatal ones have been recorded. A tentative diagnosis of Aleutian disease was made histologically on an otter from Norfolk (Wells *et al.*, 1989). Canine distemper has been recorded in captive otters in Germany (Geisel, 1979) but the condition does not seem to have been diagnosed in free-living ones. There is a single record of rabies in a free-living otter, also in Germany (Wilhelm and Vogt, 1981). Feline infectious peritonitis has been suspected in a captive Asian small-clawed otter (Van de Grift, 1976).

Bacterial diseases

There is little evidence of significant bacterial disease in wild otters. Stephens (1957) referred to a case of tuberculosis in Cornwall but the organism was not typed. More recently, *Mycobacterium avium* subsp. *avium* was shown to be the cause of massive lesions involving the mesenteric lymph nodes in an otter in Scotland (A. Patterson, personal communication). Other bacterial infections occasionally recorded are pseudotuberculosis, caused by *Yersinia pseudotuberculosis* (Keymer, 1992), and salmonellosis. Keymer (1992) recovered *Salmonella binza* from the gut of an otter in Norfolk and considered that it could have derived from day-old poultry chicks. Similarly, day-old chicks were thought to be the source of *S. enteritidis* phage type 6 which caused fatal gastroenteritis in a captive Asian small-clawed otter (V.R. Simpson, unpublished data). *S. enteritidis* has also been isolated from a free-living otter in Russia (Benkovskii *et al.*, 1973).

Aeromonas hydrophila was isolated from the heart and lungs of an otter that died from severe adiaspiromycosis (Simpson and Gavier-Widen, 2000). The same organism was isolated from the haemorrhagic lungs of an otter that had apparently died after eating toads (V. Simpson and M. Rule, unpublished data). These infections were thought to be opportunistic, as the organism is ubiquitous in freshwater systems.

Keymer (1992) reported jaundice in otters and suggested leptospirosis as a possible cause. Histological examination of a large number of livers and kidneys from south-west England showed no lesions suggestive of leptospirosis (Simpson, 1998) and there is as yet no supporting evidence for this condition in otters.

An unnamed *Brucella* sp. has been isolated from otters in Scotland, as well as from various pinnipeds and cetaceans, but the pathological significance of this isolate is currently uncertain (Foster *et al.*, 1996). *Plesiomonas shigelloides* was implicated as a probable cause of abortion in an otter fetus in Scotland (Weber and Roberts, 1989).

With the exception of salmonellosis, it is unlikely that any of these infections would be diagnosed in the live animal. The choice of antibiotic in a case of salmonellosis would depend on the results of *in vitro* sensitivity tests.

Fungal diseases

Small greyish granulomas, which, especially when mineralized, may resemble those of tuberculosis (Figure 12.8), are commonly seen in otters' lungs. They are due to inhaled spores of the fungus *Emmonsia* sp. and the condition is referred to as adiaspiromycosis. Although severe infections may prove fatal (Simpson and Gavier-Widen, 2000), the condition is normally of little clinical significance and there is no accepted form of treatment.

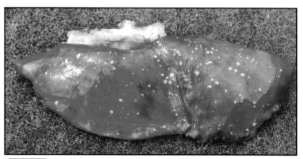

12.8 Left lung of an otter showing numerous lesions suggestive of tuberculosis. Histopathological examination showed that they are partially mineralized granulomata due to adiaspiromycosis.

Parasites

Although various metazoan parasites have been recorded in otters, there is little evidence that they cause disease. Small numbers of ixodid ticks are sometimes present, mostly in debilitated animals. In North America infection of *Lutra canadensis* with the kidney worm *Dioctophyme renale* is not uncommon and the parasite has been recorded in *L. lutra* in the UK (Corbet and Harris, 1991), but the authors are not aware of any records in recent years. In a study in Denmark, *Angiostrongylus vasorum* larvae were identified in the lungs of a single otter (Madsen *et al.*, 1999) but this parasite has not been seen in otters in Britain, despite the fact that the infection is common in foxes and domestic dogs (Simpson, 1996).

Significant metazoan parasite infections appear to be very uncommon but, should treatment be needed, fenbendazole in feed or ivermectins by injection are thought to be safe and effective (see Figure 12.12).

There is little evidence of protozoal diseases. An otter from south-west England had *Sarcocystis* sp. in the external eye muscles but there was no obvious pathology associated with the infection (Simpson, 1998).

Other diseases

Eye disease

Blindness was reported to be common in otters in England between 1957 and 1980. One or both eyes were affected, appearing white, but they were not examined by a pathologist and the precise nature of the lesion is uncertain (Williams, 1989). Lenticular cataracts were seen in a case of suspected Aleutian disease in Norfolk (Wells *et al.*, 1989). Recent investigations in south-west England have shown evidence of what appears to be retinal dysplasia in approximately 12% of cases and suspected lesions in a further 25% (Williams *et al.*, 1998). These findings merit further investigation.

Incoordination

Otters have been observed showing signs of incoordination or disorientation and possibly blindness in Ireland and England (Mason and O'Sullivan, 1992; Wells *et al.*, 1989) but histopathological examinations on brains were either not carried out or no lesions were seen. The aetiology is obscure and the prognosis is poor. Lesions of leucoencephalopathy affecting cerebrum, cerebellum and medulla were seen in a blind and ataxic otter in Cornwall. In this case the lesions were considered to be a consequence of a blow to the head, as it had been submitted after being hit by a lorry (S. Scholes, M. King and V. Simpson, unpublished data).

Mercury poisoning

Chronic mercury poisoning may cause brain damage and has been suspected in otters in Shetland (Kruuk and Conroy, 1991). High tissue levels of mercury have also been recorded in England (Mason *et al.*, 1986). Unfortunately, brains were not examined histologically in either case.

Hydrocephalus

Cubs showing signs of incoordination should be examined carefully for evidence of hydrocephalus, including radiographic examination (Green and Green, 1998). The cranium may be visibly rounded (Figure 12.9) and on post-mortem examination there is marked thinning of the cerebral hemispheres, flattening of the sulci and prolapse of the cerebellum through the foramen magnum (V. Simpson, unpublished data). The prognosis in these cases is bad and euthanasia is recommended.

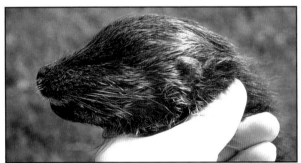

12.9 Hydrocephalus in an otter cub; the cranium is markedly domed. The animal also showed signs of ataxia.

Renal calculi

Renal calculi may be diagnosed during radiography or post-mortem examination (Figure 12.10). In most cases they are confined to the renal pelvis but small calculi may sometimes be seen in medullary papillae. It would appear that they have never been described in ureters or bladder. The prevalence varies greatly according to geographical region; for example, around 32% positive in Scotland, 16% in Denmark but less than 1% in south-west England (Simpson, 1998; Weber, 2001). Although urolithiasis is common in captive otters, especially in Asian small-clawed, the calculi in these animals are normally calcium oxalate whereas in wild otters they are mostly ammonium

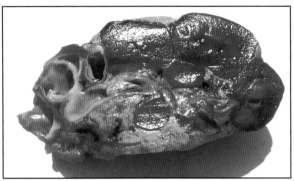

12.10 Sagittal section through a kidney affected by urolithiasis. One calculus has been left *in situ* in the grossly thickened pelvis. Note the cystic degeneration of several lobules and the extensive replacement fibrosis.

urate (Keymer *et al.*, 1981; Weber, 2001). Keymer *et al.* (1981) suggested vitamin A deficiency as a possible cause but Simpson (1998) found no evidence to support this hypothesis. The aetiology remains unknown but in wild otters it may be related to the high-purine diet (Weber, 2001). Despite the size of some of these calculi, and secondary cystic degeneration of kidney lobules, there is little evidence that they are of clinical significance in free-living otters. There is no accepted form of treatment.

Oil pollution

As with waterfowl, otters are vulnerable to oil spills. Post-mortem examinations performed on 13 otters that died following one incident in Shetland showed that five were suffering from haemorrhagic gastroenteritis, believed to be due to ingestion of oil (Baker *et al.*, 1981). Ulceration of the mucosa of the stomach, with dark, haemorrhagic, mucoid material in the intestine and blackish tarry material around the anus, is also a common finding in otters with extensive bite wounds (Figure 12.11). These animals are usually males in very poor physical condition (Simpson, 1997). Similar mucosal ulceration may be seen in orphaned cubs that have died during attempted hand-rearing and it is possible that the lesions in both cases could be the result of extreme stress (Simpson and King, unpublished data).

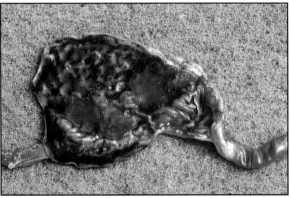

12.11 Opened stomach of an otter, showing masses of blackish mucoid material that also extended through much of the intestine. These changes are often seen in severely debilitated individuals, especially bitten males.

Adrenal hyperplasia

The adrenal glands in bitten, emaciated males, and also in females that are lactating or in late pregnancy, are often greatly enlarged and nodular, especially the left adrenal. Although adrenal hyperplasia may result from prolonged stress, a positive correlation between adrenal size and the hepatic concentration of some PCB congeners has also been demonstrated (Simpson, 1998). Adrenal aplasia, together with renal aplasia, has been reported in *Lutra canadensis* in the USA and appears to be linked to levels of polyhalogenated hydrocarbons in the environment (Henny *et al.*, 1996).

Reproductive disorders

Evidence for reproductive disorders is uncommon but there was considerable concern during the 1980s that PCBs might be interfering with breeding, particularly in females (Mason, 1989). Heggberget (1988) described an unusual cystic uterus in Norway and several possibly similar cases were recorded in south-west England between 1988 and 1996 (Simpson, 1997). Further cystic and convoluted uteri have been seen in Denmark (Elmeros and Madsen, 1999). The aetiology and significance of these changes is uncertain; they could simply represent a normal stage of uterine development during early pregnancy and further studies are needed. Leiomyomas of the uterus have been described on several occasions in sea otters (*Enhydra lutris*) (Williams and Pulley, 1981) and also in an otter in Norfolk (Keymer *et al.*, 1988). A single case of pyometra was seen in an otter from south-west England (Rivers, 1997).

Therapeutics

Many common drugs can safely be used to treat otters and these are shown in Figure 12.12. All the normal antibiotics can be used in otters. Broad-spectrum drugs with efficacy against anaerobes are preferable but long-acting preparations of other antibiotics are also useful to minimize handling. It seems that otters will accept palatable preparations of antibiotics such as amoxicillin/clavulanic acid in their feed and this is widely used.

Routes of administration

- **Oral**: this is the least stressful route but is dependent on the patient eating and on drug palatability
- **Subcutaneous injection**: the usual site is the dorsum between the shoulder blades
- **Intramuscular injection**: this is useful for anaesthetic/analgesic and initial antibiotic administration; the quadriceps femoris is the commonly preferred muscle
- **Intravenous injection**: this is only practical in anaesthetized or very sick otters; the jugular vein is normally used
- **Intraperitoneal injection**: the usual site is posterior to the umbilicus with the needle angled cranially; this route is useful for administration of fluids to dehydrated and shocked patients
- **Intraosseous injection**: either the tibial crest or trochanteric fossa can be used; these sites are

Drug	Dosage
Antibiotics	
Amoxicillin	15 mg/kg sid to bid
Ampicillin (long-acting)	15–25 mg/kg
Amoxicillin/clavulanate	8.75–20mg/kg i.m. or s.c. sid 12.5–25 mg/kg orally bid or tid
Clindamycin	11 mg/kg orally sid 11 mg/kg orally bid for osteomyelitis
Corticosteroids	
Dexamethasone	0.2 mg/kg i.v., i.m. sid anti-inflammatory dose 5.0 mg/kg i.v. for shock
Parasiticides	
Fenbendazole	50 mg/kg sid for 3 days
Ivermectin	0.2 mg/kg s.c. once
Selamectin	6 mg/kg cutaneously
Fipronil	7.5–15 mg/kg cutaneously
Vitamins	
Multiple vitamins (Multivitamin Injection, Arnolds)	1 ml/5 kg i.m., s.c. every 14 days
Minerals and vitamins (SA37, Intervet)	1–4 g per day suggested
Multiple vitamins (Fish Eaters tablets, Mazuri)	1–2 per day suggested

12.12 Chemotherapeutics for otters.

good for fluid administration in shocked and dehydrated patients
- **Cutaneous application**: sprays or 'spot-on' preparations – usually parasiticides – are often applied to the skin.

Management in captivity

Accommodation

Initially, casualty animals must have accommodation that offers security, warmth, quiet and no bright lighting. In the longer term, wild otters are difficult to manage in captivity and they are renowned for their ability to escape. The pen should be constructed of chain-link or welded mesh and must extend 0.75 m below ground to prevent them from digging out. It must either be covered or be at least 1.8 m high and have inward-facing overhangs at the top of the sides to prevent the otters from climbing out.

The animals must have access to sufficient water of good quality to allow development of swimming skills and they should also have clean drinking water. They need sufficient space to exercise on land, and enclosures must be in a quiet location to minimize stress and offer secluded areas for rest. The site should have the facilities needed to maintain hygiene and to allow for capture and handling.

Feeding

The diets of captive otters often contain a lot of frozen fish. To compensate for losses during storage and also possible thiaminase-induced problems, it is wise to add vitamin supplements (e.g. Fish Eaters tablets).

Rearing of cubs

It is quite possible to rear otter cubs by hand but it should be remembered that they are normally dependent on their mother until they are 10–12 months old and will need expert and lengthy rehabilitation if they are to survive in the wild. Young cubs need anogenital stimulation after every feed in order to urinate and defecate.

Otter's milk is rich in fat and protein but very low in lactose – 24% fat, 11% protein, 0.1% lactose, 0.8% ash (Ben Shaul, 1962). The following is a recipe for replacement milk:

  1 part Esbilac (Kruuse)
  2 parts water
  1 part Multimilk (Vetripharm)
  1 part whipping cream
  Fish Eaters tablet (Mazuri) and cod liver oil.

This can be offered in a cat's feeding bottle every 3–4 hours, including at night. Cubs can then be weaned on to a mixture of Esbilac and liquidized white fish. The Otter Trust uses commercial replacement milks for puppies or kittens but once the cubs' eyes are fully open they are given finely chopped fish (especially eels), minced beef, egg yolks and, when bigger, chopped-up day-old chicks (Wayre and Wayre, 1999).

Minimal handling and human contact as they grow older will ease rehabilitation to the wild. Cubs may need rehabilitation until they are over 12 months old yet should not develop dependence on or familiarity with humans. They will also need to develop hunting skills.

Release

The Otter Trust recommends that, prior to being released back into the wild, otters should be held in a release pen in their intended new location for about two weeks (though some workers suggest that such a long period may not be necessary). Food must continue to be provided after their release until they fail to return for it – typically only a few days. Release into the wild requires specialist knowledge of suitable habitats with a view to food sources, water quality, etc. and also existing otter populations: some areas are now well populated with wild otters and new releases into such locations are likely to suffer intraspecific aggression – and may end up being rescued again. There are organizations that have expertise in these fields and it is strongly recommended that they be consulted.

It is highly desirable to microchip any otters that are going to be returned to the wild and although there is no government organization with responsibility for keeping records, details can be passed to the RSPCA Wildlife Rehabilitation Coordinator.

Legal aspects

Otters are covered under the Wildlife and Countryside Act 1981 and are listed in Schedules 5 and 6 (see Chapter 5). This makes it an offence to capture an otter except in the case of a disabled animal taken solely for the purpose of tending and then releasing it when it has recovered. Various methods of capture are prohibited, including snares, traps and any net.

Specialist organizations

Most county wildlife trusts have an Otters and Rivers Project Officer who will be able to provide valuable local knowledge. Other useful contacts are:

The Otter Trust
Earsham, Bungay, Suffolk NR35 2AF
Tel.: 01986 893470
Fax: 01986 892461
Website: www.ottertrust.org.uk

International Otter Survival Fund
Broadford, Isle of Skye, Scotland IV49 9AQ
Tel. and fax: 01471 822 487
E-mail: iosf@otter.org
Website: www.otter.org

Wildlife Rehabilitation Coordinator, RSPCA Headquarters
Wilberforce Way, Southwater, Horsham, West Sussex RH13 WN
Tel.: 0870 555999

The Vincent Wildlife Trust
10 Lovat Lane, London EC3R 8DT

References and further reading

Baker JR, Jones AM, Jones TP and Watson HC (1981) Otter *Lutra lutra* mortality and marine oil pollution. *Biological Conservation* **20**, 311–321

Benkovskii LM, Golovina TI and Scherbina RD (1973) Studying the diseases and parasites of the otter from Sakhalin Island. *Vestnik Zoologie* **7**, 21–24

Ben Shaul DM (1962) The composition of milk of wild animals. *International Zoo Yearbook* **4**, 333–342

Chanin P and Jefferies D (1978) The decline of the otter *Lutra lutra* L. in Britain: an analysis of hunting records and discussion of causes. *Biological Journal of the Linnaean Society* **10**, 305–328

Conroy J, Yoxon P and Gutleb A (eds) (2000) *Proceedings of the 1st Otter Toxicology Conference, Isle of Skye, September 2000.* IOSF, Broadford, Isle of Skye

Corbet GB and Harris S (1991) *The Handbook of British Mammals.* Blackwell Scientific, Oxford

Elmeros M and Madsen AB (1999) On the reproductive biology of otters (*Lutra lutra*) from Denmark. *Zeitschrift fur Saugetierkunde* **64**, 193–200

Erlinge S (1968) Territoriality of the otter *Lutra lutra* L. *Oikos* **19**, 81–98

Foster G, Jahans KL, Reid RJ and Ross HM (1996) Isolation of *Brucella* species from cetaceans, seals and an otter. *Veterinary Record* **138**, 158–586

Geisel O (1979) Staupe bei Fischottern (*Lutra lutra*). *Berliner und Munchener Tierarztliche Wochenschrift* **92**, 304

Green R and Green J (1998) Disease and health problems in British otters (*Lutra lutra*) at a rehabilitation centre. *Proceedings of the VIIth International Otter Colloquium, Trabon, Czech Republic, March 14–19, 1998*

Harris CJ (1968) *Otters: a Study of the Recent Lutrinae.* Weidenfeld and Nicholson, London

Heggberget TM (1988) Reproduction in the female European otter in central and northern Norway. *Journal of Mammalogy* **69**, 164–167

Heggberget TM (1996) Age determination of Eurasian otter (*Lutra lutra* L.) cubs. *Fauna norvegica Serie A* **17**, 30–32

Heggberget TM and Christensen H (1994) Reproductive timing in Eurasian otters on the coast of Norway. *Ecography* **17**, 339–348

Henny CJ, Grove RA and Hedstrom OR (1996) *A field evaluation of mink and river otter on the Lower Columbia River and the influence of environmental contaminants.* Final report to The

Lower Columbia River Bi-State Water Quality Program, USA, February 12, 1996. National Biological Services, Northwest Research Station, Corvallis, Oregon

Keymer I (1992) Diseases of the otter (*Lutra lutra*). *Proceedings of the National Otter Conference, Cambridge, September 1992,* pp. 30–33

Keymer IF, Lewis G and Don P (1981) Urolithiasis in otters (Family Mustelidae, Subfamily Lutrinae) and other species. *Sonderdruck aus Verhandlungsbericht des XXII Internationalen Symposiums uber die Erkrankungen der Zootier, Halle/Saale,* 391–401

Keymer I, Wells G, Mason C and Macdonald S (1988) Pathological changes and organochlorine residues in tissues of wild otters (*Lutra lutra*). *Veterinary Record* **122**, 153–155

Kruuk H (1995) *Wild Otters: Predations and Populations.* Oxford University Press, Oxford

Kruuk H and Conroy J (1991) Mortality of otters (*Lutra lutra*) in Shetland. *Journal of Applied Ecology* **28**, 83–94

Kuiken T (1988) Anaesthesia in the European otter. *Veterinary Record* **123**, 59

Lewis JCM (1991) Reversible immobilisation of Asian small-clawed otters with medetomidine and ketamine. *Veterinary Record* **128**, 86–87

Lewis JCM, Pagan L, Hart M and Green R (1998) Normal haematological and serum biochemical values of Eurasian otters (*Lutra lutra*) from a Scottish rehabilitation centre. *Veterinary Record* **143**, 676–679

Madsen AB, Dietz HH, Henriksen P and Clausen B (1999) Survey of free-living otters (*Lutra lutra*) – a consecutive collection and necropsy of dead bodies. *IUCN Otter Specialist Group Bulletin* **16**(2), 65–75

Mason C (1989) Water pollution and otter distribution: a review. *Lutra* **32**, 97–131

Mason CF and Macdonald SM (1986) *Otters: Ecology and Conservation.* Cambridge University Press, Cambridge

Mason CF and O'Sullivan WM (1992) Organochlorine pesticide residues and PCBs in otters (*Lutra lutra*) from Ireland. *Bulletin of Environmental Contamination and Toxicology* **48**, 387–393

Mason C, Last N and Macdonald S (1986) Mercury, cadmium and lead in British otters. *Bulletin of Environmental Contamination and Toxicology* **37**, 844–849

Reuther C (1983) Immobilisation of European otter with ketamine hydrochloride. *Berliner-und-Munchener Tierarztliche Wochenschrift* **96**, 401–405

Reuther C (1999) Development of weight and length of Eurasian otter (*Lutra lutra*) cubs. *IUCN Otter Specialist Group Bulletin* **16**, 11–25

Reuther C and Brandes B (1984) Occurrence of hyperthermia during immobilisation of European otter (*Lutra lutra*) with ketamine hydrochloride. *Deutsche Tierarztliche Wochenschrift* **91**, 66–68

Rivers SA (1997) *Histology of the ovaries and uterine horns of the European otter (*Lutra lutra*).* Project report, MSc in Veterinary Pathology, University of London

Simpson VR (1996) *Angiostrongylus vasorum* infection in foxes (*Vulpes vulpes*) in Cornwall. *Veterinary Record* **139**, 443–445

Simpson VR (1997) Health status of otters (*Lutra lutra*) in south-west England based on postmortem findings. *Veterinary Record* **141**, 191–197

Simpson VR (1998) *A post mortem study of otters (*Lutra lutra*) found dead in south west England.* R&D Technical Report W148. Environment Agency, Bristol

Simpson VR and Coxon KE (2000) Intraspecific aggression, cannibalism and suspected infanticide in otters. *British Wildlife* **11**, 423–426

Simpson V R and Gavier-Widen D (2000) Fatal adiaspiromycosis in a wild European otter (*Lutra lutra*). *Veterinary Record* **147**, 239–241

Simpson V, Bain M, Brown R, Brown B, and Lacey R (2000) A long-term study of vitamin A and polychlorinated hydrocarbon levels in otters (*Lutra lutra*) in south west England. *Environmental Pollution* **110**, 267–275

Stephens MM (1957) *The Otter Report.* Universities Federation for Animal Welfare, Potters Bar

Strachan R and Jefferies DJ (1996) *Otter Survey of England 1991–1994.* Vincent Wildlife Trust, London

Van de Grift ER (1976) Possible feline infectious peritonitis in short clawed otters, *A. cinerea. Journal of Zoo Animal Medicine* **7**, 18

Wayre P (1979) *The Private Life of the Otter.* Book Club Associates, London

Wayre P and Wayre J (1999) The rescuing, rearing and rehabilitation of orphaned otters. *Journal of the Otter Trust* **III**(3), 81–86

Weber HB (2001) *Untersuchungen zur Urolithiasis beim Eurasischen Fischotter,* Lutra lutra. Inaugural Dissertation, Institut für Zoologie der Tierarztlichen Hochschule, Hannover

Weber JM and Roberts L (1989) A bacterial infection as a cause of abortion in the European otter, *Lutra lutra. Journal of Zoology* **219**, 688–690

Wells G, Keymer I and Barnett K (1989) Suspected Aleutian disease in a wild otter (*Lutra lutra*). *Veterinary Record* **125**, 232–235

Wildlife Information Network WILDPro Modules. Royal Veterinary College, London. www.wildlifeinformation.org

Wilhelm A and Vogt D (1981) Rabies in an otter, *Lutra lutra. Monatshefte für veterinarmedizin* **36**, 361

Williams DW, Flindall A and Simpson VR (1998) Retinal dysplasia in wild otters: a pathological survey. In: *Abstracts of the 3rd European Wildlife Disease Association Conference, Edinburgh, 1998,* p. 11

Williams J (1989) Blindness in otters. *IUCN Otter Specialist Group Bulletin* **4**, 29–30

Williams TD and Pulley LT (1981) Leiomyomas in two sea otters (*Enhydra lutris*). *Journal of Wildlife Diseases* **17**, 401–404

Acknowledgement

The editors would like to thank Grace Yoxon for her comments on an earlier draft of this chapter.

13

Other mustelids

John E. Cooper

Introduction

Although the badger and the otter are the members of the Mustelidae that are most frequently presented as casualties, perhaps partly on account of their size and popularity, there are other members of the family found in Britain that may from time to time need attention. These are the stoat (*Mustela erminea*), weasel (*Mustela nivalis*; Figure 13.1), polecat (*Mustela putorius*; Figure 13.2), pine marten (*Martes martes*) and the (introduced) American mink (*Mustela vison*; Figure 13.3). The polecat and pine marten have limited distribution but the others are widespread. The mink is a non-indigenous 'pest' and it is therefore not legal to possess or to release a mink, unless authorized to do so by licence (see later and Chapter 5).

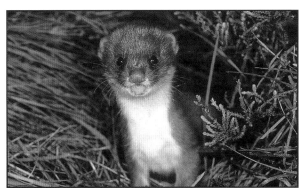

13.1 A weasel (*Mustela nivalis*), Britain's smallest mustelid, illustrating the inquisitive but cautious nature of this species. (Courtesy of Andy Purcell/ Conservation Education Consultants. © CEC)

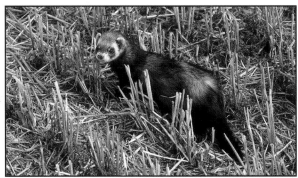

13.2 The polecat (*Mustela putorius*) is a medium-sized mustelid that hunts in woodland and open grassland. (Courtesy of Andy Purcell/Conservation Education Consultants. © CEC)

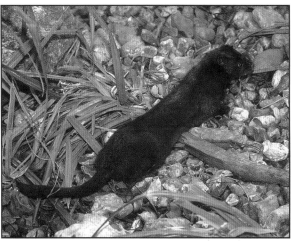

13.3 The American mink (*Mustela vison*), an attractive but highly destructive introduced species, is active both on land and in the water. (Courtesy of Andy Purcell/Conservation Education Consultants. © CEC)

It is important to distinguish between polecats and ferrets. The ferret is generally accepted to be an albino form of the European polecat which has been domesticated for over 2000 years (Owen, 1984). The ferret was developed for catching rabbits and rats and continues to be used for such purposes, as well as being widely kept as a pet and for scientific study. Hybridization of escaped ferrets with wild (free-living) polecats occurs and as a result a whole range of colours may be seen (Birks and Kitchener, 1999). Such animals, often called 'polecat-ferrets', may vary considerably in terms of their temperament, especially docility, and a 'polecat' submitted as a casualty may well be an escaped captive animal – which carries with it the legal and ethical dilemmas that are inherent in giving treatment to (or euthanasing) an animal that has an owner (see Chapter 5).

Ecology and biology

The smaller mustelids are similar in many respects in so far as their anatomy, physiology and behaviour are concerned. They are a family of animals characterized by agility, an inquisitive nature, carnivorous feeding and a variety of other anatomical characteristics. Biological data are listed in Figure 13.4.

Species	Weight[a] (mass) (g)	Moult	Teats	Gestation (post implantation)	Litter size	Life expectancy
Stoat	200–300 g	Twice a year	4–5 pairs	30–35 days	6–12	Rarely > 5 years
Weasel	50–200 g	Twice a year	3–4 pairs	34–37 days (no delayed implantation)	4–8	Rarely > 5 years
Polecat	500–1700 g (seasonal variation in males)	Twice a year	4–5 pairs	42 days	5–10	Up to 8–10 years
Pine marten	1200–1800 g	Twice a year	2 pairs	30 days	1–5	Up to 8–10 years
Mink	500–1500 g	Twice a year	2–4 pairs	28–30 days	4–6	Up to 10 years

13.4 Biological data for mustelids. [a] Can vary (in most mustelids) between different sexes and at different times of year.

An important difference between members of the family relates to habitat. The stoat, weasel and polecat are essentially terrestrial animals, hunting in woodland, grass verges or rough country. The pine marten, on the other hand, is largely arboreal (certainly when denning but it forages on the ground), while the mink is essentially semi-aquatic. Territories vary considerably and are influenced by such factors as time of year, breeding status and food availability.

Anatomy and physiology

As detailed above, the basic morphology of the mustelids is very similar. Relatively little detailed information is available on their physiology, with the exception of laboratory studies that have been carried out on the ferret and the mink.

Dentition
The dental formula for the genus *Mustela* is characterized by pronounced canines and reduced premolar teeth:

$$2 \times \left\{ I\ \frac{3}{3}\ -\ C\ \frac{1}{1}\ -\ P\ \frac{3}{3}\ -\ M\ \frac{1}{2} \right\} = 32$$

Dental abnormalities, including asymmetry and supernumerary incisors, are a feature of some polecats and it has been suggested that this might be attributable to ferret genes.

The pine marten (*Martes martes*) has a different formula from that of the genus *Mustela* and this extra dentition is reflected in its longer mandible, maxilla and facial appearance:

$$2 \times \left\{ I\ \frac{3}{3}\ -\ C\ \frac{2}{1}\ -\ P\ \frac{4}{4}\ -\ M\ \frac{1}{2} \right\} = 40$$

Sexing
Sexing of mustelids is not difficult. The male has a pronounced anogenital distance and the os penis is usually palpable. The testes may or may not be apparent: this is seasonal. Male mustelids tend to be larger than females and may have a more pronounced odour.

Handling, capture and transportation

All mustelids can bite and have a tendency to retain their grip, thus often causing tissue damage and considerable pain. This has to be borne in mind when handling these animals – especially if they are injured and frightened, when the tendency to bite can be even more marked. The majority will also produce a strong odour from their scent glands, which will quickly pervade the environment and leave its mark on clothing and equipment. Stocker (2000) advocated placing a polythene sheet under any basket used to move mustelids, in order to minimize spread of scent gland secretions.

Capture
The capture of a sick or injured mustelid may be possible by hand, with gloves, but usually only if the animal is very weak or incapacitated. More often the animal will need to be trapped and this in itself may require specific authority, either under the law (see Chapter 5) or by obtaining relevant permission from the landowner. A trap baited with meat (preferably dead chicks or mice) is usually needed.

Transportation
Mustelids should be transported in a darkened box in which the air-holes are small and thus will not allow a sharp nose or teeth to protrude. The design of box used by ferreters – made of wood with a sliding lid and air-holes low down at ankle level – is ideal. Newspaper and other bedding should be placed inside, partly to protect the animal and partly to minimize soiling of the box. Mustelids are generally bright, active animals that respond rapidly to stimuli such as light, sound and movement; therefore, the box should be carried gently. The animals must always be transported carefully, especially when they have been exposed to stressors, such as injury and close contact with humans.

Examination and assessment for rehabilitation

The preliminary examination of a mustelid can be superficial (i.e. observation with minimal handling) and this may be necessary initially before a full clinical examination can be carried out. Full examination is likely to require anaesthesia (see later).

As in other species, assessment for rehabilitation or euthanasia depends on the clinical findings. It is generally true that mustelids are sturdy animals that in captivity appear to tolerate injuries remarkably well. Whether they thrive in the wild with, say, a missing foot or amputated end of tail is another matter and much work is needed on this aspect.

The same general rules apply to mustelids as to other species, i.e. that an animal which is severely injured and unlikely to regain substantial normal function should not be released. Nor should a mustelid that is blind or has greatly compromised dentition. The absence of functional scent glands is also a reason for not returning a mustelid to the wild, since these glands play an important part in defence and marking of territory.

Pre-release assessment of the smaller mustelids has not been properly documented but should include a full clinical examination with blood tests, if practicable, and a check that ectoparasite and endoparasite numbers are not excessive. Most free-living mustelids harbour parasites (see later) and it may be unwise to attempt to eliminate these before release, as they might confer some degree of protection in the wild.

Euthanasia

The question of whether or not an animal that is unsuitable for release should be euthanased or retained in captivity is a perennial one and applies no less to mustelids than to other species. It should be pointed out that relatively few British mustelids are kept in captivity and therefore retention of some individuals for educational purposes may be justifiable. Some may reproduce in captivity (the first recorded instances of captive-breeding of weasels were by Frances Pitt many years ago) but there is probably little justification for releasing captive-bred mustelids into the wild other than pine martens, which are very restricted in numbers (Corbet and Harris, 1991).

One indication for euthanasia is likely to relate to the species that has been presented. The mink is a non-indigenous 'pest' and as such may not by law (see Chapter 5) be either kept or returned to the wild without specific authority.

Euthanasia of mustelids is best performed by the administration of an overdose of anaesthetic agent. Work on mink – for instance, using carbon dioxide and other gases (Hansen *et al.*, 1991) – provides useful guidelines on possible methods for these and other mustelids and also on the possible effect of using such techniques in terms of the animal's welfare.

First aid procedures

Immediate first aid for mustelids falls into the same categories as that for other species (see Chapter 2).

Haemorrhage needs to be controlled, as do convulsions and other serious clinical signs. Administration of fluids is not easy, as it can prove difficult to gain access to a vein: the subcutaneous, intraperitoneal or intraosseous routes may well prove easier. Dextrose should be included in fluids, as the smaller mustelids have a high metabolic rate. Likewise, their long lean shape makes them vulnerable to rapid loss of heat. Nursing must include warmth, and oxygen (in an incubator) can prove valuable.

Treatment of these animals is not easy. They do not tolerate dressings and bandages very readily and other techniques, such as the administration of fluids, are often far from simple.

Anaesthesia and analgesia

Anaesthesia

Correct anaesthesia is probably best achieved, in all species, by the use of isoflurane but other agents can also be employed.

If the animal can be handled, it may be masked down with isoflurane. Alternatively, an anaesthetic chamber can be used; the animal (or the animal in its travelling box) is placed inside the chamber while isoflurane and oxygen are pumped through. The addition of nitrous oxide has much to commend it; it is a good muscle relaxant (and will enhance that provided by isoflurane) and has an important analgesic effect. However, it must be remembered that analgesia ceases when the nitrous oxide is switched off.

Where isoflurane is not available, halothane can be used, or an injectable agent. The injectable agent of choice is usually ketamine but some other compounds, including alfaxalone/alfadolone, can prove useful. Ketamine may be given by the intramuscular or subcutaneous routes: in an emergency it can be sprayed on the animal's mucous membranes. Small doses may be taken orally but only if heavily disguised in solid or liquid food.

Mustelids are generally good patients in so far as anaesthesia is concerned, but an animal that is badly damaged or shocked, and stressed as a result of coming into captivity, may be more easily overdosed by agents that would normally be considered safe. This is another reason for using nitrous oxide; it reduces the amount of isoflurane/halothane that needs to be used.

Likewise, there is merit in combining with ketamine another agent such as midazolam: muscle relaxation is improved and the midazolam may make the procedure safer, by reducing the amount of the dissociative agent that is needed.

Analgesia

Knowledge of analgesia in mustelids is very limited and is based almost entirely on experience with the domestic ferret. There is no doubt that all mustelids respond adversely to pain and that this can be an important factor in how they fare in captivity. If in doubt, standard analgesics (such as carprofen) should be given, using the dosages recommended for rodents and lagomorphs (see Chapters 8 and 10). It is better to risk killing the patient with an analgesic than for it to suffer unnecessarily.

Specific conditions

Non-infectious conditions

Non-infectious conditions are likely to include trauma (the most prevalent), hyperthermia, hypothermia, burning or electrocution and (rarely) drowning. Although mustelids are physically strong and generally robust, their enquiring nature and boldness often result in their being hit by motor vehicles or injured by a fall or in encounters with other species and so they may present with fractures, internal injury and severe soft tissue wounds. They also sometimes fall into water containers; all are able to swim but if they cannot escape they become progressively more wet, cold and tired. Each of these situations requires prompt attention – initially first aid and stabilization, followed by specific medical or surgical intervention as appropriate.

Hyperthemia and hypothermia

Hyperthermia (overheating) is well recognized in working ferrets and can occur occasionally in free-living animals. Hypothermia (often followed by hypoglycaemia) may result when a mustelid is exposed to extremely cold weather or is trapped in cold water and is unable to warm itself rapidly.

Burning and electrocution

Burning can occur if an animal is trapped in a forest or heath fire or because it has made its home in or near a bonfire. Electrocution occasionally occurs when a mustelid climbs an electrified security fence, especially if the animal is already wet from dew or rain.

Dental conditions

Attrition of the teeth is one of a number of dental conditions that have been reported in free-living polecats, as well as in ferrets, and it may contribute to loss of condition and accidents.

Infectious conditions

Although described by Stocker (2000) as 'comparatively free of recognisable diseases', British mustelids may be presented with a range of clinical and subclinical infectious conditions such as salmonellosis, tuberculosis, other bacterial diseases, Aleutian disease and ecto- and endoparasitism (see Chapters 11 and 12). Corbet and Harris (1991) provided a useful resumé of diseases of the family Mustelidae, and Cooper and Sainsbury (1995) depicted some examples of clinical cases.

The diseases and pathology of mustelids, with particular reference to the stoat, were discussed by McDonald and Larivière (2001) and McDonald et al. (2001), based on studies in New Zealand and Britain, respectively. These two papers provided useful information on some of the pathogenic organisms, including metazoan parasites, that may be significant in terms of morbidity and mortality in these species; they also included extensive bibliographies, which offer a valuable database for those who may have to deal with mustelid casualties.

Techniques

Surgical techniques in mustelids are essentially similar to those used in other small mammals and can often be extrapolated from work with ferrets – or even cats. The smallest of the British mustelids, the weasel, presents particular problems on account of its size; microsurgical techniques may be needed and the patient will be very susceptible to hypothermia and hypoglycaemia.

Endoscopy can be carried out with relative ease in mustelids, using techniques similar to those that are routine in ferrets (Brearley et al., 1991).

Therapeutics

Substantial data exist on the treatment of working, pet and laboratory ferrets (Oxenham, 1991; Cooper and Sainsbury, 1995; Lewington, 2000) but most of the agents recommended are not licensed for use in this species. Care must therefore be taken in assuming that they might also be of value in other animals of the same family. Nevertheless, in the absence of reliable data, it is suggested that mustelid casualties should be treated with the same spectrum of medicines, at comparable doses, as is the domestic ferret. It is likely that the data on medicines given for the otter (see Chapter 12) can be extrapolated to other mustelids.

Management in captivity

Housing

The principles of housing the smaller mustelids ('expert escapologists') were outlined by Porter (1989), who advocated modifying a standard ferret hutch. The accommodation must take into account the desire of these animals to be able to hide when sleeping and the tendency of some species to live in groups, within which there is intense social activity. A solitary young stoat or weasel may fail to thrive because of lack of company. It may even be worth (cautiously) introducing another species in order to encourage normal behaviour patterns. A ferret is the best choice but there are anecdotal records that a kitten can be used, with apparent success.

Feeding

Although all mustelids are evolutionarily adapted to an animal diet, most will take a certain amount of plant food. The badger is essentially omnivorous and the stoat largely carnivorous but other species vary in the extent to which they will take vegetable material. Meat is always a useful dietary item to encourage animals to feed (see below). Feeding of bread and milk to ferrets has often been strongly criticised, but the willingness of this species to take this diet and others that contain milk can prove to be a life-saver if a ferret is dehydrated or needs emergency sustenance. Other mustelids have similar tastes and therefore milk-containing diets are usually worth trying, for a short time only.

Otherwise, the staple diet offered should be based on meat. Casualty animals may find it difficult to cope with hair, feathers and bones and so removal of these, or provision of butcher's meat, may be wise initially. Sometimes the casualty animal may not immediately recognize plain meat as acceptable food and therefore may reject it: palatability can then be enhanced by the addition of small amounts of skin or viscera. Tinned dog foods and cat foods also sometimes prove acceptable.

Very sick mustelids should be given liquid food with a syringe (they readily take items that are placed in the mouth or on the back of the tongue) and an oesophageal/stomach tube is usually easily passed. Once an animal is taking solid food voluntarily, this should be offered several times a day – especially to weasels, which, on account of their size, have a high metabolic rate.

Rearing of orphans

There is substantial information about the rearing of young polecats and ferrets dating back many years (Pitt, 1921). Some data are available on weasels and stoats (Pitt, 1921) and also on pine martens, largely as a result of studies by the late HG Hurrell (Hurrell, 1968a,b, 1981). For many years the Zoological Society of London successfully bred weasels (Shaw and Fisher, 1963) and this also yielded useful information on the care of youngsters.

Various milks have been used (cow's, goat's) as well as a range of products for human babies. In recent years successful rearing of most *Mustela* and *Martes* species has been achieved using 'ferret formulae', consisting of commercial dried milk products (e.g. Esbilac or Lactol) mixed with three times their weight of water.

Release

Behavioural problems are likely to occur in mustelids for the reasons outlined above. As a general rule, the shorter the time in captivity, the more likelihood there is of success in returning the animal to the wild.

Pre-release health 'screening' is advisable and protocols prior to translocation or release for this group of animals are suggested in Woodford (2001). Recommendations for prophylaxis include the administration of vaccines, including distemper (not of ferret or canine cell-line origin), killed feline panleucopenia and – if it is considered a risk – leptospirosis bacterin.

The ability of the animal to fend for itself is important; thus, an adult that is already capturing prey before becoming a casualty is more likely to be able to survive than is a youngster that may not have learned how to hunt effectively. Habituation to humans can be distinctly disadvantageous.

Site assessment
The success of release also depends upon the habitat. Research on pine martens by Bright and Smithson (2001) indicated that reintroduction into some areas of England would be more likely to result in death from predator control, traffic accidents and being killed by foxes. Such studies could assist in determining where release of this and other species should or should not be attempted following rehabilitation.

Mustelids that are released in inappropriate sites may cause problems because they compete with established animals of the same species or kill domestic animals (e.g. chickens, rabbits) or wild species (e.g. voles). Careful assessment must first be carried out and the advice of local naturalists, familiar with the area, is often invaluable. In particular, locations where there is a high density of traffic or where there is gamekeeping are usually unsuitable.

Legal aspects

There are no specific legal considerations relating to the taking into captivity and tending of mustelids, other than that both the pine marten and the polecat are protected under the Wildlife and Countryside Act 1981 (WCA) and that mink may not be kept in captivity (Destructive Imported Animals Act 1932) or released (WCA) without specific authority. Other general legislative considerations are covered in Chapter 5.

References and further reading

Birks JDS and Kitchener AC (eds) (1999) *The Distribution and Status of the Polecat* Mustela putorius *in Britain in the 1990s*. Vincent Wildlife Trust, London

Brearley MJ, Cooper JE and Sullivan M (1991) *A Colour Atlas of Small Animal Endoscopy*. Wolfe, London

Bright PW and Smithson TJ (2001) Biological invasions provide a framework for reintroductions: selecting areas in England for pine marten releases. *Biodiversity and Conservation* **10**, 1247–1265

Cooper JE (1990) Skin diseases of ferrets. In: *The Veterinary Annual*, eds CSG Grunsell *et al*. Butterworths, London

Cooper JE and Sainsbury AW (1995) *Exotic Species*. Mosby-Wolfe, London

Corbet GB and Harris S (eds) (1991) *The Handbook of British Mammals*. Blackwell, Oxford

Hansen NE, Creutzberg A and Simonsen HB (1991) Euthanasia of mink (*Mustela vison*) by means of carbon dioxide (CO_2), carbon monoxide (CO) and nitrogen (N_2). *British Veterinary Journal* **147**, 140–146

Hartup BK, Kollias GV, Jacobsen MC, Valentine BA and Kimber KR (1999) Exertional myopathy in translocated river otters from New York. *Journal of Wildlife Diseases* **35**, 542–547

Hurrell HG (1968a) *Pine Martens*. HMSO, London

Hurrell HG (1968b) *Wildlife: Tame but Free*. David and Charles, Newton Abbot

Hurrell HG (1981) *Fling, the Pine Marten*. Westway, Plymouth

Lewington JH (2000) *Ferret Husbandry, Medicine and Surgery*. Butterworth-Heinemann, Oxford

McDonald RA and Larivière S (2001) Diseases and pathogens of *Mustela* spp., with special reference to the biological control of introduced stoat *Mustela erminea* populations in New Zealand. *Journal of the Royal Society of New Zealand* **31**, 721–744

McDonald RA, Day MJ and Birtles RJ (2001) Histological evidence of disease in wild stoats (*Mustela erminea*) in England. *Veterinary Record* **149**, 671–675

Owen C (1984) Ferret. In: *Evolution of Domesticated Animals*, ed. IL Mason. Longman, Harlow

Oxenham M (1991) Ferrets. In: *Manual of Exotic Pets*, eds PH Beynon and JE Cooper. BSAVA, Cheltenham

Pitt F (1921) Notes on the genetic behaviour of certain characters in the polecat, ferret and polecat-ferret hybrids. *Journal of Genetics* **II**, 99–115

Porter V (1989) *Animal Rescue*. Ashford, Southampton

Shaw M and Fisher J (1963) *Animals as Friends and How to Keep Them*. JM Dent, London

Stocker L (2000) *Practical Wildlife Care*. Blackwell Science, Oxford

Woodford MH (ed.) (2001) *Quarantine and Health Screening Protocols for Wildlife Prior to Translocation and Release into the Wild*. OIE, VSG/IUCN, Care for the Wild International and EAZWV, Paris

Acknowledgement

I am grateful to Dr J.D.S. Birks for helpful comments on an early draft of this chapter.

14

Wildcats

Dick Best

Introduction

The wildcat (*Felis silvestris*) is confined to the mainland of the north of Scotland. It is a very shy animal, being largely crepuscular and nocturnal and preferring to inhabit moorland edges, scrub and forests, where it feeds mainly on rabbits and hares but also on a variety of birds and smaller mammals. The wild population is at threat from persecution and by interbreeding with feral domestic cats, since hybrids may be fertile.

Persecution is probably the major cause of death in wildcats but starvation, predation on kittens and road traffic accidents are also important.

They are solitary animals, with the females holding a territory and the males roaming over a larger area. Mating occurs in the late winter and spring and the peak time for kittens to be born is May. Dens are used in the winter and for breeding and are usually in rocky crevices, hollow trees or old badger setts or rabbit holes.

Anatomy and physiology

The anatomy and physiology of wildcats is similar to those of the domestic cat except that wildcats are more robust than a typical tabby domestic cat. They have stripes on the coat but not blotches. The tail is distinctly more bushy than that of a domestic cat; it has three to five broad black rings and a black, rounded tip (Figure 14.1).

Hybrids with domestic cats, and subsequent generations, can be difficult to distinguish from wildcats, although hybrids do tend to retain the thinner tails of domestic cats and to lack the broad, black tail rings of the wildcat. Hybrids can be distinguished with a degree of accuracy from the measurements of their skulls (Corbet and Harris, 1991). Identification of hybrids is important to ensure that only pure wildcats are released into the threatened, free-living populations.

Capture, handling and transportation

Adult wildcats are extremely aggressive and dangerous animals and should be handled only by those with suitable experience and proper equipment. If an animal requires prolonged hospitalization and treatment, it should be referred to a centre with the necessary facilities.

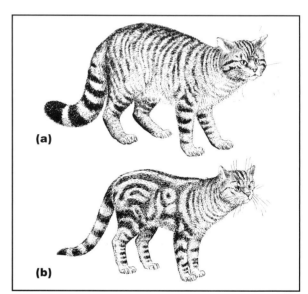

14.1 Wildcat (a) and domestic cat (b). Note the bushy, truncated tail of the wildcat. Reproduced from Corbet and Harris (1991) with the permission of Blackwell Science.

Once an adult wildcat has been restrained in a trap, dog grasper, anglers' landing net or equivalent, it should be sedated (unless it is in an extremely debilitated or comatose state) before being transported in a suitable cage and examined. Kittens may be restrained and lifted by the scruff of the neck.

Examination and assessment for rehabilitation

Examination and assessment of a sedated wildcat casualty follows the routine for clinical examination of a domestic cat. The criteria for assessment for rehabilitation are the general ones outlined in Chapters 2 and 3. Euthanasia, if required, would be performed as for the domestic cat.

First aid

Techniques for wound management and stabilization follow standard techniques used in small animal practice and as detailed in Chapter 2.

A large crush cage would be suitable for immediate emergency accommodation. Short-term hospitalization requires a strong cage (preferably a metal one), designed so that the cage can be divided to allow cleaning without disturbing the animal.

Anaesthesia and analgesia

Intramuscular injections of combinations of medetomidine and ketamine at dose rates suggested for domestic cats are suitable for sedation and induction of anaesthesia, which can then be prolonged with standard methods of intubation and inhalation anaesthesia using halothane or isoflurane.

Analgesia can be achieved using medications as recommended for domestic cats.

Specific conditions

The majority of wildcat casualties appear to be traumatic injuries associated with shooting, trapping or road traffic accidents, or the abandonment of dependent kittens.

Trauma

Apart from the problems associated with handling a fractious patient, as outlined above, the clinical aspects of treatment of injuries follow those applicable to domestic cats.

Infectious diseases

Very little information is available on the incidence of infectious diseases in wildcats but it is safe to assume that they will be susceptible to pathogens infecting domestic cats. To ensure that rehabilitated wildcat casualties do not introduce infections into the wild population, it is essential that precautions are taken to prevent any direct or indirect contact between wildcats in captivity and domestic cats.

Evidence is available that wildcat populations in France are infected with feline retroviruses (Froment *et al.*, 1998). Although the origin of the infection has not been established, the source is likely to be from contact with domestic cats in the field.

Therapeutics

Standard dosages and routes of administration as recommended for domestic cats can be used in wildcats.

Management in captivity

The medium- and long-term care of a wildcat casualty requires secure accommodation and special handling facilities and such a patient should be passed to a unit that can meet these requirements.

As a member of the Felidae, the wildcat is highly susceptible to any pathogen affecting domestic cats. It is essential that every care is taken whilst the animal is in captivity (especially within a veterinary practice) to keep it in strict isolation from any contact, direct or indirect, with domestic cats. This is important not only to prevent the wildcat from contracting an infectious

disease but also to prevent it carrying a previously unencountered pathogen back to the wild population when it is released. Pre-release screening of casualties, especially long-term ones or those that have been close to domestic cats, for certain pathogens (e.g. feline leukaemia virus, feline panleucopenia, feline calicivirus and rhinotracheitis, feline corona virus) would be prudent. In captivity, a wildcat should be fed a diet that is as close to its natural diet as possible, i.e. whole carcasses of poultry, rabbits and other rodents. In emergencies, day-old chicks may be offered, as well as proprietary cat food.

Rearing of young

Wildcat kittens can be reared using milk replacement powders as prepared for rearing domestic kittens. Whenever possible, the kittens should be reared in conspecific groups. Before being considered for release into the wild, kittens should first of all be positively identified as wildcats by those suitably qualified to do so. Their release, and preparation for release, should be supervised by experienced groups.

Release

A casualty that has been captive for only a short period is most appropriately released at the location where it was found. Long-term captivity poses the potential problem of placing a released animal within the existing territory of another wildcat. This would require a soft release method (see Chapter 3) and the assistance of naturalists, such as staff of Scottish Natural Heritage, with local knowledge of wildcat populations.

Care should be taken with identification so that wildcat/domestic cat hybrids are not released.

Legal aspects

Wildcats are one of the species covered by the Dangerous Wild Animals Act (see Chapter 5). Holding them in captivity requires a licence from the local authority.

Specialist organizations

Scottish Natural Heritage
2–5 Anderson Place, Edinburgh EH6 5NP

Hessilhead Wildlife Rescue Centre Trust
Gateside, Beith, Ayrshire KA15 1HT

References and further reading

Corbet GB and Harris S (1991) *Handbook of British Mammals, 3rd edn.* Blackwell Science, Oxford
Fromont E *et al.* (1998) Prevalence and pathogenicity of retroviruses in wildcats *Felis silvestris* in France. Summary of paper presented at Conference of European Association of Zoo and Wildlife Veterinarians, Edinburgh, September 1998

Acknowledgements

Acknowledgements are due to Gay and Andy Christie, Grace Yoxon and Sandra Bonor for their helpful comments on this chapter.

15

Foxes

Matthew G.I. Brash

Introduction

The red fox (*Vulpes vulpes*) is found almost throughout the British Isles. As well as on the mainland, it is present on the Isle of Wight, Anglesey and Skye, but not on the Orkneys, Shetlands or the Isle of Man. It was introduced only recently to the Isle of Wight by terrier men for sport.

Post-mortem examinations have shown that the most common causes of mortality are traumatic injuries (mainly from road traffic accidents, hunting, shooting, snaring and trapping), septic bite wounds and malicious poisoning (Simpson, 1996), and these are the most likely reasons for foxes being presented to the veterinary surgery. Relatively little is known of the diseases of foxes in Britain; there have been numerous case reports of diseases, parasites and other pathological conditions but only small numbers of individuals have been studied. There is also a particular bias in the literature towards diseases that are of economic or zoonotic importance to humans but may be of little importance to the fox (e.g. the tapeworm *Echinococcus*).

Ecology and biology

Habitat

The British red fox can be subdivided into urban/suburban foxes and rural foxes, displaying very differing feeding and hunting patterns. The home range of the urban/suburban fox is often only 30 ha whilst that of a fox inhabiting a truly agricultural area can be as much as 200 ha, or even up to 1000 ha on the fell tops of Cumbria (Doncaster and Macdonald, 1991a,b). Populations can also fall into two broad categories; the 'residents' that patrol the same home range night after night, and the 'itinerant' foxes that travel across much larger tracts of land, presumably searching for a territory. Residents may attack itinerant foxes as they pass through their territory.

In an undisturbed area, the resident foxes live in family groups of up to six adults, containing one dog and several vixens. It is not known what effect fox control (e.g. hunting) has on this stable system. Foxes live in an earth, which may be a single-entrance hole, a badger sett that they have taken over or, in urban areas, any quiet area that provides a suitable denning place. They generally only use the earth when the cubs are young or go to ground in it when they are threatened or in bad weather conditions.

The fox is an alert, elusive and mainly nocturnal animal, most commonly active at dawn and dusk but frequently seen during daytime. Communication between foxes is by barking (screaming) and 'coughing', as well as by marking with urine and faeces and expelling the contents of the anal sacs.

Feeding

Generalizations can be made about the fox's diet, the major items being voles, rabbits, hares, birds, fruit and carrion, depending upon seasonal availability. They supplement their diet with items such as berries, worms and insects, and feed mainly at night. The diet also depends on the availability of particular foods where the fox lives: obviously the diet of the urban dustbin fox is different from that of the moorland fox. One reason for the fox's success in such diverse habitats is its ability to hunt or scavenge without developing dependency on any specific food source. Surplus food will be cached and this habit often starts in cubs when they are only 8 weeks of age.

Cubs will eat solid food from the age of 3–4 weeks, beginning with regurgitated material delivered by the vixen. The dog will help, as will non-breeding sisters from the previous year's litter.

The development of hunting and prey-eating techniques by juvenile foxes is of paramount importance to their survival, particularly for rural foxes. It is most commonly movement of prey that prompts pursuit amongst young fox cubs, but sound stimuli will often produce a rapid hunt for the source of the noise. These biological factors are important to remember when foxes are kept in captivity in the long term.

Anatomy and physiology

Biological data for foxes are given in Figure 15.1. Anatomically, foxes are very similar to domesticated dogs. There are five toes on the forelimbs and four on the hindfeet. The first digit (dewclaw) on the forelimb is rudimentary and does not make contact with the ground. The lengths of the forelimbs and hindlimbs relative to the length of the spine are greater than in most species, suggesting swiftness and endurance.

Weight	Variable according to season (heavier in winter), diet and sex Means: adult male (dog) 6.5 kg, female (vixen) 5.5 kg
Life expectancy	Av. 18–24 months in wild Up to 14 years in captivity
Breeding season	Female: January/February Male: fertile November to early March
Oestrus	Monoestrous; 1–6 days (av. 3 days) Mild vaginal swelling, no pre-oestrous bleeding
Ovulation	Spontaneous
Gestation	53 days Young usually born late March (January–April)
Sexual maturity	10 months

15.1 Biological data for foxes.

Coat

Foxes have a marked individual variation in coat colour, even between littermates. The most common colour impression is that of a reddish-brown with grey-white underparts (Figure 15.2). There is seasonal variation in coat colour and it has also been reported that older foxes are lighter in colour; however, coat colour cannot be reliably used in ageing foxes. Variations of coat colour exist and there have been reports of true albinos and white foxes (Talbot, 1906), but melanistic variants do not appear to have been reported in Britain. Young cubs are brown to black in colour (Figure 15.3).

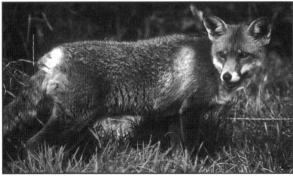

15.2 Red fox (*Vulpes vulpes*) showing typical coat colour. (Courtesy of C. Seddon)

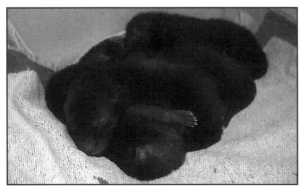

15.3 Fox cubs may have a very dark chocolate brown coat colour, making them easy to confuse with domestic puppies.

There is a dense underfur and the guard hairs are of variable length, grey or black proximally and brown distally. The tail is a thick quiver-shaped brush, up to 130 mm in diameter and about two-fifths of the length of the animal. The tip of the tail often contains some white fibres. The ventral fur changes colour around parturition and will fall out totally in lactating vixens (this should not be confused with mange).

Moulting occurs once a year. The coat is at its thickest in winter and is shed in April/May, starting at the feet and working dorsally and cranially. Underfur is shed before the guard hairs. By July the coat is at its sparsest, with a thin incipient covering of underfur and a sparse covering of the old guard hairs. Again, it is important not to confuse this natural moult with mange.

Glands

Both sebaceous and apocrine glands are present throughout the coat. The heavily cornified skin of the feet contain merocrine sweat glands. There is a supra-caudal tail gland (known colloquially as the 'violet gland', as it smells of violets), approximately 5 cm from the base of the tail. It is located by the presence of black hairs that overlap this area; the gland is oval and devoid of underfur. A thick, yellowish waxy secretion is produced from tubular apocrine glands and it has been hypothesized that this secretion is used in communication (Lloyd, 1980). The paired anal glands produce a secretion used for scent-marking, which can be expelled under voluntary control on to whatever object is being scent-marked. There are no glands on the nasal planum, which is usually dry.

Dentition and digestive system

The fox is dolichocephalic. The dental formula (with temporary dentition in parentheses) is as follows:

$$2 \times \left\{ I \ \frac{3\,(3)}{3\,(3)} \ C \ \frac{1\,(1)}{1\,(1)} \ P \ \frac{4\,(3)}{4\,(3)} \ M \ \frac{2\,(0)}{3\,(0)} \right\} = 42\,(28)$$

The long, sharp canine teeth are situated well forward, diminishing the pressure that they can apply; their main function is to catch and kill prey. The loss of the upper molars compared with a dog is notable: the third molar is vestigial and often absent; the fourth premolar in the upper jaw is larger and with the first molar tooth in the lower jaw forms the main flesh-shearing carnassial teeth. Age can be determined by examination of wear on the teeth.

The articulation of the jaw offers little movement other than opening and closing. Lateral movement is also hindered by the prominent canine teeth.

As the fox is a carnivore, its intestines are short. The stomach has a capacity of 900 ml. The short small intestine is approximately 1.1 m long; there is a vestigial caecum, and the large intestine is 50 cm long (Lloyd, 1980).

Senses

Hearing is the best developed sense; the fox, being a predator of small mammals, needs to be able to detect and locate sounds accurately. The fox uses movement of its head and ears to locate sounds (e.g. voles underneath leaves) to a high level of accuracy.

Vision is short range but well adapted to the fox's way of life. It has a crucial role in finding food in daylight but is subordinate to sound stimuli in sunlight and plays little part in darkness (Osterholm, 1964). The eyes are placed frontally and have a large round pupil in poor light conditions, which is reduced to a vertical slit in bright light. The good short-range vision is used to judge short distances accurately, with good limb and eye coordination. Visually, movement is important: if an object remains static, it will not be noticed.

The central area of the retina has a higher proportion of cones than of rods, whilst peripherally there are more rods. A nictitating membrane is present but only moves when the eye is closed.

Smell is also integral in hunting. As vision is impaired in the dark, hearing and smell both assume greater importance in hunting and particularly scavenging. The sense of smell is also important as a means of communication. The vibrissae on the muzzle are highly developed as a tactile sense.

Reproduction

The vixen has four pairs of teats, each of which has eight to 20 lactiferous glands. These are pale in nulliparous females and darker in parous females. The uterus is a narrow elongated bifurcated organ, more similar in appearance to a cat's than a dog's.

The dog has a small scrotum, held tightly to the ventral abdomen and covered in whitish fur. The penis is held tightly to the ventral wall in the prepuce. Extrusion is easily performed manually for examination. There is a small prostate and a small glandular vesicle associated with the vas deferens where it joins the urethra.

If a vixen is unmated, or if mating is unsuccessful, pseudopregnancy can occur, lasting about 40 days, but without milk production. Food availability plays an important part in reproductive success, so much so that in very bad years a vixen may not even come into season. It has also been shown that fox numbers can fluctuate in relation to vole numbers, lagging behind by approximately 12 months (Chirkova, 1955).

Two vixens may share an earth, denning together and rearing the cubs as a single group; the same dog will be the father. The young are usually born in a dry hole, or a den with a single hole and no bedding. Suburban foxes will choose any cover (e.g. beneath a garden shed) and so it is young suburban cubs that are predominantly presented to the veterinary surgery. The cubs are unable to thermoregulate for the first 2 weeks; thus they sleep one on top of each other to conserve heat. In captivity, an incubator is useful to provide warmth.

Cub development is outlined in Figure 15.4. Male cubs grow faster than females.

At birth	Birthweight 70–100 g Blind and deaf Short dark grey or black fur
11–14 days	Eyes open (initially blue) Fur around feet begins to darken; erect sparse juvenile guard hairs ('fuzzy' appearance) Short muzzle begins to elongate
21–28 days	Deciduous teeth begin to erupt Begin to eat solid food regurgitated by parents
6 weeks	Fully moulted (coat reddish-brown) Deciduous teeth fully erupted Weaned Start to play outside den; adults continue to bring food
July/August	Begin to gain independence
September	Independence usually complete; peak time for dispersal and casualties
6 months	All adult teeth erupted; retention of deciduous teeth common for a time

15.4 Development of fox cubs.

Capture, handling and transportation

Foxes should be treated in the same way as a fractious cat: they will snap and bite whilst trying to escape and can easily move in three dimensions, leaping upwards whilst trying to escape. Injured foxes can be caught by a net or herded into a box. Once in a net, they can be pinned using a soft-headed broom and then scruffed. As a last resort a quick-release dog grasper can be used – preferably one with a rubber end as a fox can damage its teeth or mouth whilst attempting to bite the end of the pole.

It is important to keep handling of a conscious fox to a minimum so as to minimize stress. Gauntlets or gloves can be helpful whilst handling but they do interfere with scruffing. When lifting a fox by the scruff, its body should always be supported under the rump. A fox should never be held by its tail.

Once the animal is scruffed, a muzzle or tape muzzle can be put on with care to prevent biting (Figure 15.5). Wrapping the body in a large towel will

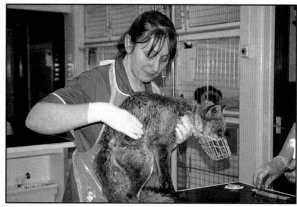

15.5 Debilitated foxes can be handled safely following placement of a muzzle, allowing administration of a drip. (Photograph: Secret World.)

help to subdue the fox, as will covering its head and eyes with a blanket. Occasionally difficult foxes may be presented and in these cases it is sensible to use a crush cage, followed by intramuscular sedation or anaesthesia.

Foxes should be transported in a large dog cage or crush cage, covered with a blanket to minimize stress. In emergencies any suitable container will suffice, such as a dustbin.

Zoonoses

It is important to be aware of the quick nature of foxes and of the fact they have very sharp needle-like canine teeth and sharp claws. Care must be taken when handling them, with particular thought being given to the risks of being bitten or scratched. As foxes are becoming more established in urban areas, they may form a reservoir for zoonoses (Figure 15.6 and Chapter 2). They not only hunt but also scavenge, consuming other mammalian corpses and thus further spreading certain diseases. In addition they act as a reservoir of disease that can spread to domestic dogs.

Examination and assessment for rehabilitation

As most foxes are presented for trauma (RTA or wounded), it is important to make a good assessment of the initial parameters prior to anaesthesia allowing complete examination (see 'Anaesthesia and analgesia'). This may only be possible by a visual examination through the wires of the cage, or by assessing the animal in a run.

Clinical examination

Full clinical examination is essential: it is critical to be able to determine the potential to rehabilitate a fox. Areas of greatest significance are those areas affecting the fox's ability to hunt: limbs, jaw, teeth, ears and eyes.

Damaged limbs, especially those that are fractured, are poor prognostic indicators, as the long time required for good orthopaedic repair means that successful release to the wild is unlikely. This is primarily because foxes are territorial and by the time it returns to the wild the injured fox will have been ousted from its niche. Foxes should be carefully examined for broken

Disease	Causal agent	Comments
Salmonellosis	*Salmonella*, various spp.	
Leptospirosis	*L. icterohaemorrhagica, L. canicola*	Ten of the 15 serotypes of leptospirosis have been identified in foxes
Ringworm	*Trichophyton* spp. (e.g. *T. equi*)	
Mange (scabies)	*Sarcoptes scabies* var. *canis*	Also spreads to dogs
Toxoplasmosis	*Toxoplasma gondii*	
Tuberculosis	*Mycobacterium bovis*	
Lyme disease	*Borrelia burgdorferi*	Transmission via tick *Ixodes dammini*
Colibacillosis	*Escherichia coli*	
Staphylococcus	*Staphylococcus* spp.	
Actinobacillosis	*Pseudomonas mallei*	Not in British Isles
Q fever	*Coxiella burnettii*	Especially from animals with large number of ticks
Cryptosporidiosis	*Cryptosporidium parvum*	Especially urban areas
Giardiasis	*Giardia* spp.	
Trichinosis	*Trichinella spiralis*	
Capillariasis	*Capillaria hepatica, C. aerophilia*	
Campylobacteriosis	*Campylobacter jejuni*	
Rabies	Lyssavirus	Not reported in foxes in UK at present
Leishmaniasis	*Leishmania infantum*	Intermediate agent sandfly, has been recorded in Jersey; not in UK at present
Rickettsial zoonoses	E.g. *Rickettsia conori* Vector: *Rhipicephalus sanguineus*	Transmission via arthropod vectors (usually fleas, ticks)
Parasitism	*Echinococcus granulosis, E. multilocularis*	Not in UK at present
Septic bite wounds	General bacteria, especially *Streptococcus* spp.	Foxes have very sharp, needle-like teeth

15.6 Potential zoonoses from foxes.

limbs or pelvis, and radiographs taken where appropriate. A fox should be euthanased if such injuries are present. In juvenile female foxes the effect of fractures on parturition should be considered.

Chronic conditions, such as severe mange or anorexia, are also a reason for immediate euthanasia as these are usually secondary to a more severe underlying problem.

Blood collection

Blood samples may be needed for routine haematology and biochemistry (Figure 15.7) or serological tests. The cephalic vein is readily accessible, even in a conscious scruffed or muzzled fox. Other available blood vessels include the jugular and saphenous veins.

Parameter	Range
Haemoglobin (g/dl)	13.4–17.8
PCV (%)	36–55
Red blood cells (10^{12}/l)	8.6–10.6
MCV (fl)	34–49
MCHC (g/dl)	33–37
MCH (pg)	14–18
White blood cells (10^9/l)	3.7–7.9
Neutrophils, segmented (10^9/l)	1.8–4.8
Lymphocytes (10^9/l)	0.9–2.8
Monocytes (10^9/l)	0.04–0.3
Eosinophils (10^9/l)	0.04–1.12
Basophils (10^9/l)	<0.06
Total protein (g/l)	47–65
Albumin (g/l)	29–37
Globulin (g/l)	23–35
Urea (mmol/l)	5.3–13.2
Creatinine (µmol/l)	61–115
ALP (IU/l)	11–157
ALT (IU/l)	< 117
Cholesterol (mmol/l)	3.35–6.79
CK (IU/l)	22–242
LDH (IU/l)	< 178
AST (IU/l)	24–96
GGT (IU/l)	3–15
Total bilirubin (µmol/l)	7–17
Calcium (mmol/l)	2.01–2.65
Phosphorus (mmol/l)	0.81–2.23
Sodium (mol/l)	135–151
Potassium (mmol/l)	4.0–4.8
Chloride (mmol/l)	111–117
Magnesium (mmol/l)	0.5–0.71
Glucose (mmol/l)	4.84–8.91

15.7 Normal haematological and biochemical parameters of foxes (data courtesy of Med Lab, Cheshire).

First aid

If the fox passes an initial clinical examination, pre-anaesthetic treatment should involve the administration of analgesics and antibiotics, with administration of fluids either orally or intravenously (see Figure 15.5), simple cleaning of wounds, and stabilization of fractures. Foxes are often in a state of near-fatal circulatory collapse (i.e. cardiovascular shock) by the time they allow themselves to be caught and this should be a paramount consideration at initial examination.

Diazepam at 1 mg/kg bodyweight can assist if placement of a drip is necessary. Treatment otherwise follows that for domestic dogs. Full anaesthesia is often a practical and sensible approach as it allows a thorough clinical examination, placement of an intravenous drip, radiography and other procedures without adding further to the animal's high degree of stress. In cases of severe infections or trauma, intravenous fluids should be given to provide support even if the patient is not clinically dehydrated. Heat should also be provided wherever practical.

Short-term housing and feeding

In the surgery, foxes should be kept away from the sight, sound and smell of domestic species to minimize stress and to avoid transmission of disease.

Foxes do not make good in-patients at a veterinary surgery and so the time for which they remain in the surgery should be kept to a minimum. However, there is a noticeable difference between urban and rural foxes: the former will often settle, provided that they feel secure.

For short-term, immediate and emergency care, an ordinary kennel with a blanket hung across the barred gate is sufficient and dog food is suitable. It is sensible to make use of private or specialist rehabilitation facilities rather than admitting a fox to the surgery for a prolonged period of time.

Anaesthesia and analgesia

Induction

Critical to the success of anaesthesia is a suitable period of peaceful induction, ideally by putting the cage or box containing the fox in a quiet darkened room for at least 10 minutes during induction. If no darkened room is available, the cage should be covered with a blanket.

Care should be taken when anaesthetizing debilitated foxes and it is important always to weigh them accurately where practical. Warmth should be provided, as many anaesthetic cases may be in a state of cardiovascular shock. Suitable sources of heat include heat mats, bubblewrap, electric blankets, or plastic gloves filled with hot water.

Choice of drug

Anaesthetic and analgesic drugs for use in foxes are listed in Figure 15.8.

Drug	Dosage	Notes
Anaesthetics		
Medetomidine + butorphanol + ketamine	0.02 mg/kg + 0.4 mg/kg + 4 mg/kg i.m.	Can reverse with atipamezole at 0.1 mg/kg
Tiletamine + zolazepam (Zoletil 20)	10 mg/kg i.m.	
Ketamine + xylazine	20 mg/kg + 1.0 mg/kg i.m.	
Propofol	4–6 mg/kg i.v.	Use cephalic vein
Analgesics		
Carprofen	4 mg/kg s.c.	
Buprenorphine	10–20 µg/kg i.m.	
Butorphanol	0.2 mg/kg	
Pethidine	3.3 mg/kg i.m.	

15.8 Anaesthetic and analgesic drugs for use in foxes.

Ketamine

Historically, research work involving anaesthetizing of foxes has often been carried out using ketamine on its own. This is safe and relatively cheap but the acidity of ketamine can cause muscle damage, a relatively large volume is required for adequate effect and it is non-reversible. Ketamine is therefore better combined with an alpha-2 agonist such as xylazine or medetomidine.

Medetomidine

Medetomidine alone induces an unsatisfactory sedation. Medetomidine/ketamine combinations, when used with an opiate (such as butorphanol), require a low volume and offer fast induction. The author has anaesthetized a considerable number of foxes for minor surgery or examination without any complications and with no deaths attributable to the combination. The injection should be mixed in one syringe and given intramuscularly, ideally into the quadriceps. Useful immobilization is achieved for 30–60 minutes.

If extended periods of anaesthesia are required, intubation followed by maintenance with a gaseous anaesthetic agent can be carried out. There are many variations on the triple combination but the one given in Figure 15.8 is that preferred by this author.

Other injectable agents

Tiletamine/zolazepam (Zoletil 20, Parke Davis) is a useful anaesthetic agent, given at a dose rate of 10 mg/kg, but it is unavailable in the British Isles without a Special Treatment Authorization from the Veterinary Medicines Directorate (further information on Zoletil can be found in Chapter 2 and obtained from the manufacturers). Propofol can be used where intravenous access is possible.

Gaseous anaesthesia

Once the fox is anaesthetized, intubation should be carried out. A 6 mm endotracheal tube, with the cuff inflated, works well. Foxes have very long jaws and so the larynx is positioned caudally. A laryngoscope can be helpful in locating the epiglottis. Anaesthesia can then be maintained in the normal manner, with isoflurane or halothane.

Specific conditions

Trauma

Most adult foxes presented to the surgery have traumatic injuries, usually from gunshot wounds, RTAs or snare injuries (bite wounds are considered under 'Bacterial infections'). Particular care should be taken at the primary examination to determine whether successful release to the wild is viable, each case being treated on its own merits. If release is not possible, immediate euthanasia is the best course of action and most cases fall into this category.

Even straightforward fractures make difficult long-term cases, due to the length of hospitalization during fracture fixation. It is important to be able to release a fully fit and healthy fox within 6 weeks, so that it has a reasonable chance of regaining its territory. If this is not possible, euthanasia should be considered.

Road traffic injuries

Initial assessment may be made with the fox controlled and muzzled. Compound fractures, multiple limb fractures and cranial or obvious spinal injuries are cases for immediate euthanasia. If none of these is apparent, the fox should be anaesthetized and the examination repeated. A radiographic examination is important to eliminate hidden or more subtle fractures, particularly of the caudal mandible and pelvis. This allows planning of fracture fixation, if it is to be carried out. Appropriate analgesia, fluid therapy and antibiotics should be provided at this point.

Of all the orthopaedic injuries presented, only basic fractures of the limbs should be considered as candidates for treatment. External skeletal fixation and intramedullary pins can be used to stabilize fractures. It is important to remove metalwork prior to release.

Gunshot injuries

Many foxes will tolerate minor gunshot injuries, particularly 'scatter' from shotgun pellets, without any clinical signs. There is no need to remove these pellets, unless they are causing complications. Appropriate antibiotics (see Figure 15.11) and analgesics (see Figure 15.8) should be administered. The wounds should be cleaned and, where appropriate, sutured closed. Foxes are good healers and most minor skin wounds will heal well, provided that contamination and infection are minimized.

More major wounds from gunshot injuries must be treated on their own merits but in most cases euthanasia will be the most appropriate course of action if the fox will have long-term debilitating injuries.

Snare injuries

Foxes, being inquisitive animals, often get caught in snares. These may have been laid for rabbits, with the fox being an accidental victim, or they may have been laid intentionally for foxes. Where practical, the snare should be removed under controlled circumstances at the surgery, under general anaesthetic. This avoids injuries to the handler, as well as allowing a better assessment of the injuries suffered by the fox.

The fox should be anaesthetized and given appropriate analgesic (see Figure 15.8) and antibiotic cover (see Figure 15.11). Aggressive fluid therapy should be given to prevent potential renal damage from the catabolites of muscle damage. The snare should be cut off, and the limb or appendage examined closely. All the other limbs and the head should be closely examined to check for injuries sustained whilst the fox was struggling to escape from the snare. Dental and jaw injuries are particularly common, especially chipped or fractured canine and molar teeth. Often apparently quite mild snare injuries cause marked tissue damage that may not be immediately visible.

The fox should be kept in captivity for at least a week to be assessed for longer-term damage, such as pressure necrosis due to the snare. Provided that there is no apparent long-term damage, these cases make good candidates for release.

Poisoning

It is illegal to place poisoned baits for the destruction of foxes except in a wildlife rabies emergency, at the discretion of the Home Office minister, but foxes are often the target of deliberate poisoning, particularly in rural areas. Rabbits or pheasants laced with strychnine (itself an illegal poison except for moles) are commonly used to get rid of target foxes that may be poaching gamebirds.

It is unlikely that a fox will present with clinical signs but, should one do so, diagnosis and treatment are as for domestic dogs and other wildlife (see Chapter 2). A dead but apparently uninjured fox should always be considered a suspect poisoning case.

Viral diseases

Rabies

Rabies is still widespread throughout the world, found on all continents except Australia and Antarctica. The disease is caused by the entry of a lyssavirus into a wound, usually inflicted by a bite from a rabid animal (though spread by aerosol can occur). The virus, which causes a fatal encephalomyelitis, may then replicate locally, prior to infection of the nervous system. The

incubation period varies but is usually about 3 months. Once the central nervous system is infected there is centrifugal viral dissemination, allowing spread of the virus particularly via saliva. Urine, faeces and other glandular secretions are not considered infectious.

Symptoms: The early signs of a rabid fox are subtle and non-specific, including a high temperature, malaise and inappetence. There may be paraesthesia at the site of entry of the virus. Two types of rabies may then occur: either the 'dumb' or the 'furious' form. Death occurs from either respiratory or cardiac failure.

Control: At present the British Isles are free from rabies and it has been the policy of successive governments to maintain this status. In the event of an outbreak of wildlife rabies, an eradication campaign would be mounted, involving either the poisoning or oral vaccination of foxes (Meldrum, 1988). Modelling has indicated that, for either of these methods of rabies control to work, in excess of 80% of foxes would need to find and consume the bait. This would work well in rural areas, but in urban areas it has been shown that only about one-third of foxes take the bait (Trewlella, 1991). Improved techniques are still being researched.

If a suspected case of rabies is presented, both DEFRA and the local police should be informed immediately. Those who routinely handle and work with foxes should consider having themselves vaccinated against rabies.

Canine distemper

The agent is a morbillivirus that causes an important disease in domestic dogs, mink and certain other species. Its significance in foxes is poorly understood, though they are susceptible to the canine distemper virus (Little *et al.*, 1998). Transmission of the virus is primarily by aerosol or contact with body excretions.

Presenting signs vary, depending on the viral strain and on the fox's age and immune status. Juveniles are most susceptible. The classic signs are of depression with mucopurulent oculonasal discharge and a dry or moist cough. Fever, anorexia, vomiting and diarrhoea frequently occur and central nervous system signs may also develop. Euthanasia is advocated. Differential diagnosis includes rabies, infectious canine hepatitis, poisoning and other causes of CNS signs.

Infectious canine hepatitis

Infectious canine hepatitis (fox distemper, enzootic fox encephalitis), caused by canine adenovirus I (CAV I), was first described in a silver fox in 1925 (Cabasso, 1981). Serological evidence of infection has been described all over the world but never apparently proved in the British Isles. Spread between foxes occurs via urine, nasal and conjunctival secretions, as well as in faeces.

Clinical presentation shows an anorectic fox, with a rhinitis. There may be a mucoid or haemorrhagic diarrhoea and hyperexcitability. In extremis, seizures, paralysis, coma and death occur (Cabasso, 1981). Euthanasia is recommended. On post-mortem examination, gross lesions are not as distinct as they are in dogs and are typically non-specific, involving generalized congestion with an enlarged liver, spleen and adrenal glands. Primary vascular damage is the basis for the pathology seen in foxes that die of CAV I infections. Rabies and canine distemper should be considered as differential diagnoses.

Bacterial infections

Historically, the wild fox population has shown little evidence of intrinsic bacterial disease. The most common lethal bacterial infection is caused by β-haemolytic streptococci (Blackmore, 1964). In this study it was also found that 61% of adult foxes were affected with an interstitial nephritis, probably of leptospiral origin.

Streptococci

Foxes are commonly presented with bacterial infections from bite wounds. These can be treated like any comparable infection in a dog. Abscesses can develop from either gunshot injuries or bite wounds. After anaesthetization, the abscess should be lanced and flushed clean. Intravenous fluids should be given to provide renal and hepatic support against toxic damage. In untreated cases streptococcal bacteraemia can occur, causing secondary lesions in the lungs or pericardial sac. Underlying disease should always be suspected.

Other bacteria

Epidemics of pasteurellosis have been reported in the silver fox (Lyubashenko and Dukur, 1983). An 8-week-old cub died from *Yersinia pseudotuberculosis* infection after apparently being caught by its right limb in a trap (Blackmore, 1964). *Salmonella* has been isolated on a number of occasions from foxes (Nielson *et al.*, 1981; Euden, 1990).

Beard *et al.* (1999) demonstrated *Mycobacterium avium* subsp. *paratuberculosis* in 89% of foxes examined. It may be that foxes act as a reservoir host in a more complicated epidemiology of Johne's disease than was previously thought.

Proteus infections have been recorded. An 8-week-old cub was found on post-mortem examination to be infected with *Proteus vulgaris* (Blackmore, 1964); the carcass was jaundiced, with degenerate areas in the liver, and heptachlor epoxide and dieldrin were detected in the muscles.

Fungal infections

Foxes can develop ringworm. Natural infection is by direct or indirect contact with a carrier or infected animal. Young foxes tend to be more susceptible than adults, and thus asymptomatic adults may act as the source. Severe infection may mean that there is an underlying systemic disease. The author has seen a case of ringworm (causal agent *Trichophyton equi*): the lesions were on the dorsal lumbar region, with a severe local exudation lesion, and there was sparse, patchy hair loss, with hyperkeratosis and erythema. The problem was resolved using weekly baths of enilconazole 10%, and systemic oral griseofulvin at 20 mg/kg daily for 6 weeks.

Ectoparasites

Sarcoptic mange

Two forms of mange caused by the parasite *Sarcoptes scabiei* can be seen in the fox: acute and chronic. Transmission between foxes may occur by direct or indirect contact. Miniature epizootics occur, having drastic effects on local fox populations.

The acute form is characterized by intense pruritus, erythematous eruptions, papule formation and seborrhoea but generalized alopecia is often absent. These signs are often not seen from a distance, as the fur may cover any lesions. However, the severely pruritic nature of the condition affects the ability of the fox to hunt. As the condition progresses, the animal becomes emaciated and debilitated; death comes from starvation and dehydration. This type of mange is rarely presented to the surgery.

A more generalized chronic form can develop (Figure 15.9). This appears especially along the dorsal body wall. There is often secondary bacterial infection, causing the sweet 'mangy' odour. Hair loss occurs in patches. The lesions often start near or on the base of the tail, progressing cranially along the back, but can also start on elbows and hocks. The fox may become listless and weak, and may die if untreated.

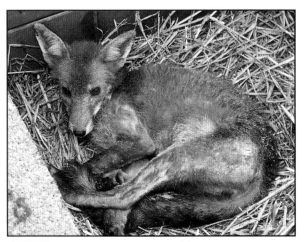

15.9 Fox with chronic mange (*Sarcoptes scabiei* infection). (Photograph: Secret World.)

Foxes may also develop a localized chronic mange, without systemic involvement. These foxes may be carriers of the parasite. The chronic form appears to be a more urban condition. This may be due to artificially high population densities with small territories, maintained due to good food availability. As these territories overlap, so there is a large amount of territorial dispute and incursions by itinerants. Stress will therefore be high, with concurrent higher levels of cortisol, increasing predisposition to mange (A. Routh, personal communication).

Diagnosis: A diagnosis of mange can be made from the characteristic skin lesions, as well as the presence of the mite in deep skin scrapings examined using microscopy. Biopsies can also prove helpful (see Chapter 4).

Treatment: Treatment should always include a full clinical examination to determine any underlying disease; for example, in one post-mortem study three foxes with sarcoptic mange were also infected with *Angiostrongylus vasorum* (Simpson, 1996). If there is no underlying problem, repeated treatments with amitraz at the recommended dose rates for dogs will effect a cure. Injections of ivermectin have also been used at dog dose rates given three times at 10-day intervals. Treatment with selamectin prior to release will provide longer-term cover.

Other mites: Other mites have also been observed in foxes – notably the harvest mite (*Neotrombicula autumnalis*), especially around the ears and eyelids of foxes in September and October. *Otodectes cynotis* has been identified in a fox and demodex mites (unidentified) have been found in fox faeces (Beresford-Jones, 1961) but not apparently as a causal agent of mange in a fox.

Fleas

Several species of flea have been found on foxes, most commonly *Ctenocephalides canis*, but there is no evidence that the fox has a flea exclusive to itself. All other fleas found are stragglers, normally found on other species. Treatment is with any proprietary dog flea treatment.

Ticks

Several different species of tick have been found on foxes but there is no specific fox tick. *Ixodes ricinus* (sheep tick) and *Ixodes hexagonus* are the most prevalent. Ticks are of importance in all wildlife, because of their potential to carry zoonotic diseases – notably Lyme disease (causal agent *Borrelia burgdorferi*), carried by the tick *Ixodes dammini*.

Lice

Various lice have been found on foxes, notably *Trichodectes melis* (normally found on badgers) and *Trichodectes vulpis*.

Endoparasites

Nematodes

Foxes can carry a heavy worm burden without showing any ill effects. Most commonly found are *Uncinaria stenocephala*, *Toxocara canis* and *Toxascaris leonina*.

Toxocara canis: Heavy burdens of *T. canis* can be found in cubs and may be harmful. These patients are normally in poor condition, with a swollen abdomen; however, the high number of parasites may be as a result of other factors creating suitable conditions for *Toxocara*. Once it has been confirmed that there is no underlying disease, treatment is with fenbendazole.

Angiostrongylus vasorum: *A. vasorum* (the heartworm) has been found at post-mortem examination in foxes in an area of mid-west Cornwall (Simpson, 1996). Clinical signs in an early case would include dyspnoea, cough and anorexia but most cases are likely to be seen after death. Adult worms and thrombi can be seen in the right heart and pulmonary circulation. Treatment is with 7.5% levamisole solution.

The presence of *A. vasorum* in foxes is significant, because of the part it may play in acting as a reservoir of the parasite in wildlife – particularly as the parasite increases its range in dogs. The disease is seen in dogs predominantly in south-west England and south Wales, where the climate favours the intermediate hosts. It has also been recorded in a captive fox outside the known range of the disease (A. Routh, personal communication) and the speculation was that it had been imported to the area by a dog that had infected local intermediate hosts (e.g. snails).

Hookworms: Many other canid nematodes have been noted in foxes, including hookworms such as *Trichinella spiralis*. Hookworms are common in foxes and *Uncinaria* spp. are probably commoner in foxes than in domestic dogs; *Ancylostoma* spp. have also been described in foxes in Britain (Beresford-Jones, 1961; Williams, 1976). Treatment is with fenbendazole.

Trematodes

A number of trematodes have been recorded in wild foxes in two surveys (Nicoll, 1923; Cook, 1965) but they are of no known clinical significance.

Cestodes

Tapeworms occur in a high proportion of foxes. The fox, being a carnivore and feeding on a wide range of prey species, has been exploited evolutionarily by a large number of endoparasites. Of particular importance are the genera *Taenia* and *Echinococcus*. *T. serialis* is the most common cestode found, although *T. pisiformis*, *T. taeniaeformis*, *T. ovis* and *T. hydatigena* have also been recorded. None of these tapeworms appears to cause any significant problem to the fox. Infection with the cyclophyllidean tapeworm *Mesocestoides* has also been recorded (Thompson, 1976).

Echinococcus granulosus has been repeatedly found in small numbers (average three per fox), with prevalence rates as high as 22% being reported (Cook, 1965). The significance of *E. granulosus* is particularly its zoonotic potential, as it can cause hydatid disease. Treatment is the same as for dogs, using praziquantel.

The fox is the definitive host for *Echinococcus multilocularis*, with intermediate hosts being the microtine rodents. The fox ingests the infected rodent, the larva evaginates and the cestode matures after the scolex attaches to the intestinal wall. This parasite, though apparently absent from Britain, is particularly significant because of its presence in mainland Europe and its zoonotic potential to cause a fatal alveolar echinococcosis in humans. Treatment would theoretically be the same as for *E. granulosus* but euthanasia should be considered in view of the serious zoonotic potential.

Protozoal diseases

Several species of *Eimeria* and *Isospora* have been found in foxes. *Cryptosporidium parvum* was isolated from the faeces of 9% of foxes (Sturdee *et al.*, 1999) and may be a source of cryptosporidia for humans. There have been no reported cases of protozoans causing a significant disease in a fox.

Hydrocephalus

Hydrocephalus seems to be a common finding amongst orphaned cubs, occurring once or twice in around every 50 cub admissions (A. Routh, personal communication). This apparently high incidence may reflect the likelihood that the cubs had been deliberately abandoned, found and then rescued. Clinical signs can range from the obvious to quite subtle (Figure 15.10). Most commonly seen is a relatively stunted appearance with abnormal behaviour, an inability to feed and fine tremors. The eyes may appear to deviate laterally and in time the domed forehead appears. Seizures manifest themselves as the condition deteriorates and these cases never recover. Euthanasia is recommended.

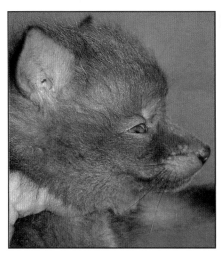

15.10

Fox cub with hydrocephalus. (© A Routh.)

Therapeutics

The ideal site for injection of drugs used subcutaneously is the scruff. Where intramuscular injections need to be given the muscle mass anterior to the femur (quadriceps) is the site of choice. Doses for drugs commonly used in foxes are given in Figure 15.11.

Drug	Dosage
Anti-infectives	
Amoxicillin + clavulanic acid	8.75 mg/kg s.c. sid for 3–5 days
Enrofloxacin	5 mg/kg s.c. bid for 7 days
Lincomycin	22 mg/kg s.c. sid
Amoxicillin trihydrate	15 mg/kg s.c. sid
Clindamycin	11 mg/kg orally on food sid
Antiparasitic	
Fenbendazole	Adults: 100 mg/kg once orally Cubs: 50 mg/kg orally sid for 3 days
Ivermectin	200 µg/kg s.c.
Levamisole	10 mg/kg s.c. sid for 3 days
Praziquantel	5 mg/kg orally
Selamectin	30 mg/2.6–5 kg 60 mg/5.1–10.0 kg

15.11 Drugs commonly used to treat foxes.

Management in captivity

The short-term housing and feeding of foxes in captivity has been described earlier (see 'First aid').

Housing

Longer-term accommodation requires specialized outdoor runs, with at least chain-link fencing at a minimum of 2 m high, plus an overhang – and foxes can even climb over this. There should be a raised sleeping platform, with screening to provide privacy and security. Newspaper or shavings can act as bedding. Large fir-tree branches make excellent foliage cover.

It is important to consider the minimizing of handling and stress, especially when cleaning the fox's quarters. Ideally any accommodation should allow discrete observation, without the fox being aware of the observer.

Foxes can be highly destructive. Wire mesh, on which they may damage their teeth whilst attempting to escape, should not be used and it is essential to avoid anything that they can chew, such as cables for heating, lighting or video equipment. Foxes are obsessively destructive.

Feeding

Although adult foxes can be fed on canned or dry dog food for a short while, this is not suitable on its own for longer periods. Other food such as rats, mice, day-old chicks and pieces of rabbit (e.g. road kills) should be added to the diet. Foxes are very adaptable and a group of foxes with a liver infection happily ate Hill's l/d diet until they recovered (personal observation). Requirements vary depending on the time of year but approximately 350–550 g of food per day is sufficient. Fresh water should be available at all times.

Rearing of cubs

Housing

The housing of cubs depends on their age at presentation. For the first 10 days the cubs should be held in isolation, with barrier nursing to prevent disease transmission. Younger cubs are unable to thermoregulate and so may need to be in an incubator, or have warmth provided. Later, older cubs can be housed in groups of up to six similarly aged conspecifics – preferably two dogs and four vixens (an ideal release group), though a mix of sexes in any ratio is often all that can be achieved.

Feeding

It is advisable to weigh orphans daily, to ensure satisfactory daily weight gain (which should be approximately 50 g/day between the ages of 4 and 10 weeks). Once cubs are weaned, the frequency of weighing should be reduced to avoid imprinting.

Very young cubs should be fed every 3 hours throughout the day and night. Any canine milk replacement can be used at standard dilutions, using a puppy feeder. It is necessary to stimulate urination and defecation by cleaning the perianal area.

At 4 weeks of age, cubs will begin to take solid food. Babyfood, scrambled egg, minced puppy food or minced meat, all with added vitamins and minerals, should be offered in small meals. Raw jointed pheasant, chicken and rabbit can also be fed. The size of meals should be gradually increased and more solid foods offered. Until this point, supplementary milk feeding should continue but can be reduced to every 4 hours and can be stopped when the cub is 6 weeks old.

At 5–6 weeks of age the cubs should gradually be moved on to larger food such as day-old chicks and 'pinky' mice. Vitamins and minerals should continue to be supplemented. Fresh water must be made available at all times.

Juvenile cubs being reared by hand should always be treated for endoparasites with fenbendazole at normal dog doses every 3 weeks for at least two treatments after weaning.

Release

Adults

Where possible, adult foxes should be released back to the area in which they were found. Suitable accommodation will be needed for transportation to the site (Figure 15.12).

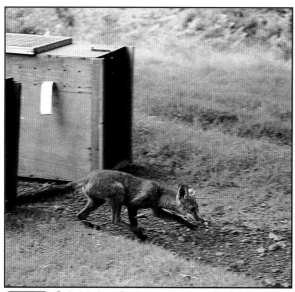

15.12 Suitable box for transportation of adult fox to release site. (Photograph: Secret World.)

Cubs

Close contact with humans can lead to habituation and even imprinting, especially when the foxes are young; therefore contact should be kept to a minimum, especially as habituated foxes are difficult to release and imprinted foxes impossible. Mixing with other cubs reduces this risk and allows social skills to develop. As cubs develop, they should be moved into more extensive and ultimately more naturalistic accommodation. The group should remain a closed unit, up to and including soft release (see Chapter 3) from a suitable and secure site.

Legal aspects

Legal considerations for foxes are given in Chapter 5.

Specialist information source

Website: www.abdn.ac.uk/mammal/redfox.htm

References and further reading

Beard PM, Henderson D, Daniels MJ, Pirie A, Buxton D, Greig A, Hutchings MR, Mckendrick I, Rhind S, Stevenson K and Sharp JM (1999) Evidence of paratuberculosis in fox (*Vulpes vulpes*) and stoat (*Mustela erminea*). *Veterinary Record* **145**, 612–613

Beresford-Jones WP (1961) Observations on the helminths of British wild red foxes. *Veterinary Record* **73**, 882–883.

Blackmore DK (1964) A survey of disease in British wild foxes (*Vulpes vulpes*). *Veterinary Record* **76**, 527–532

Boever WJ, Holden J and Kane KK (1977) Use of Telazol (C1-744) for chemical restraint and anaesthesia in wild and exotic carnivores. *Veterinary Medicine/Small Animal Clinician* 1722–1725

Buxton D, Maley SW, Pastoret PP, Brochier B and Innes EA (1997) Examination of red foxes (*Vulpes vulpes*) from Belgium for antibody to *Neospora caninum* and *Toxoplasma gondii*. *Veterinary Record* **141**, 308–309

Cabasso VJ (1981) Infectious canine hepatitis. In: *Infectious Disease of Wild Animals, 2nd edn*, ed. JW Davis, pp. 191–195. Iowa State University Press, Ames, Iowa

Chirkova AF (1955) *The Dynamics of Fox Numbers in Voarnesh Province and Forecasting of Fox Harvests*. Voprosy Biologii Pushmykh Zverery, Moscow, pp. 13–20

Cook BR (1965) *Incidence and epidemiology of* Echinococcus granulosus *in Great Britain*. PhD thesis, University of Liverpool

Doncaster CP and Macdonald DW (1991a) Ecology and ranging behaviour of red foxes in the city of Oxford. *Hystrix (NS)*, 11–20

Doncaster CP and Macdonald DW (1991b) Drifting territoriality in the red fox (*Vulpes vulpes*). *Journal of Animal Ecology* **60**, 423–439

Euden PR (1990) Salmonella isolates from wild animals in Cornwall. *British Veterinary Journal* **146**, 228–232

Farstad W (1998) Reproduction in foxes: current research and future challenges. *Animal Reproduction Science* **53**, 35–42

Harris S (1977) Spinal arthritis (spondylosis deformans) in the red fox. *Journal of Archaeological Science* **4**, 183–195

Harris S and Rayner JMV (1986) Urban fox population estimates and habitat requirements in several British cities. *Journal of Animal Ecology* **55**, 575–591

Jalanka HH (1990) Medetomidine and M/K induced immobilisation in blue foxes and its reversal by atipamezole. *Acta Veterinaria Scandinavica* **31**, 63–71

Kaplan C *et al.* (1977) *Rabies – the Facts*. Oxford University Press, Oxford

Little TWA, Swan C, Thompson HV and Wilesmith JW (1982) Bovine tuberculosis in domestic and wild mammals in an area of Dorset – the prevalence of tuberculosis in mammals other than badgers and cattle. *Journal of Hygiene* **89**, 225–234

Little SE, Davidson WR, Howerth EW, Rakich PM and Nettles VF (1998) Disease diagnosed in red foxes from the South Eastern Unites States. *Journal of Wildlife Diseases* **30**, 95–98

Lloyd HG (1980) *The Red Fox*. Batsford, London

Lyubashenko SY and Dukir II (1983) Pasteurellosis. In: *Diseases of Fur-bearing Animals*, ed. SY Lyubashenko, pp. 133–138. Amerind, New Delhi

Macdonald D (1995) *European Mammals – Evolution and Behaviour*. Collins, London

MAFF (1991) *Rabies Prevention and Control*. MAFF publication PB 0573, Ministry of Agriculture, Fisheries and Food, London

Meldrum KC (1988) Rabies contingency plans in the United Kingdom. *Parasitologia* **30**, 97–103

Nicoll W (1923) A reference list of the trematode parasites of British mammals. *Parasitology* **15**, 236–252

Nielsen BB, Clausen B and Elvestad K (1981) The incidence of salmonella bacteria in wild living animals from Denmark and in imported animals. *Nordisk Veterinarmedicin* **33**, 427–433

Osterholm H (1964) The significance of distance receptors in the feeding behaviour of the fox *Vulpes vulpes* L. *Acta Zoologica Fennica* **106**, 1–31

Simpson VR (1996) *Angiostrongylus vasorum* infection in foxes (*Vulpes vulpes*) in Cornwall. *Veterinary Record* **139**, 443–445

Sturdee AP, Chalmers RM and Bull SA (1999) Detection of *Cryptosporidium* oocysts in wild mammals of mainland Britain. *Veterinary Parasitology* **80**, 273–280

Swire PW (1978) Laboratory observations on the fox (*Vulpes vulpes crucigera*) in Dyfed during the winters of 1974/75 and 1975/76. *British Veterinary Journal* **134**, 398–404

Talbot JS (1906) *Foxes at Home*. Horace Cox, London

Thompson RCA (1976) The occurrence of *Mesocestoides* sp. in British wild foxes (*Vulpes vulpes crucigera*). *Journal of Helminthology* **50**, 91–94

Trewlella WJ (1991) A field trial evaluating bait uptake by an urban fox population. *Journal of Applied Ecology* **28**, 454–466

Williams BM (1976) The intestinal parasites of the red fox in south west Wales. *British Veterinary Journal* **132**(3), 309–312

Williams ES and Barker IK (eds) (2001) *Infectious Diseases of Wild Mammals*, 3rd edn. Manson Press, London

Acknowledgements

The author would like to thank A. Routh, Professor Trees, C. Brash and E. Mullineaux for all their comments and assistance in writing this chapter.

16

Deer

Peter Green

Introduction

Six species of wild deer may be encountered in the British Isles. For purposes of identification they can be divided into large deer (red, fallow, sika) and small deer (roe, Chinese water deer, muntjac). With the exception of the Chinese water deer, all are characterized by the growth of deciduous antlers on the frontal bones of the males, which are shed annually and regrown.

The identification of adult deer should not be difficult (Figures 16.1 and 16.2), though Chinese water deer may be confused with roe, and sika with red. Neonates and juveniles are often presented as casualties and these may prove more of a challenge to identify correctly.

Common name (species)	Size	Coat	Tail	Antlers	Distribution	Terms (male; female; neonate)	Other characteristics
Red deer (*Cervus elaphus*)	Largest in Britain: M up to 250 kg; F smaller	Coarse reddish to dark brown, no spots in adults M rough mane and thick neck autumn	Short	Several spikes or tines from beam; tines and beam round or oval cross-section	Widespread but not suburban Typical large deer of Scottish Highlands and West country, also East Anglia and Lake District; small groups elsewhere	Stag; hind; calf	Travel considerable distances
Sika deer (*Cervus nippon*)	Up to 60 kg	Similar to red but often retain juvenile spots More prominent lighter patch over rump perineum and caudal thighs	Short	Similar to red but tines shorter, more upright	S and W England, Scotland, Lake District, Ireland; isolated populations E Midlands	Stag; hind; calf	Closely related to red and will hybridize
Fallow deer (*Dama dama*)	Large: M up to 100 kg	Smooth sleek; colour varieties include menil (two-tone sandy, distinct spots, white belly), melanistic (dark brown to black), albino or cremello (nearly white) Many with black stripes down caudal thighs M thick neck but no mane autumn, usually elongated tuft of hair on prepuce F shorter coat, neck appears longer than other large deer	Much longer than other large deer	Mature M distinctive flattened (palmate)	Much of lowland Britain, not open moorland or mountain In some areas herds up to 50 on arable land	Buck; doe; fawn	Most likely of large deer to be close to urban areas
Roe deer (*Capreolus capreolus*)	Small, dainty; M and F up to 25 kg	Foxy red summer, greyer winter; always black muzzle, white chin, prominent white or cream caudal patch	None discernible; F may have prominent anal tuft of hair	Simple straight upright spikes, usually one forward-pointing tine and one rear-pointing on each antler	Almost all of Britain, wide range of habitats	Buck; doe; kid	May be nuisance in large gardens (especially roses)
Chinese water deer (*Hydropotes inermis*)	Long-legged; up to 18 kg	Rough greyish or sandy; large upright ears woolly	Short	None, but M grossly enlarged canines in upper jaw (up to 7 cm long)	Becoming more widespread E England in wetlands, open arable, small coppices	Buck; doe; kid	Small low-set eyes, square chin; face not unlike kangaroo or wallaby Gives birth to litter; often 3–4 neonates survive to weaning

16.1 Wild deer species in the British Isles (M, male; F, female). (continues) ▶

Common name (species)	Size	Coat	Tail	Antlers	Distribution	Terms (male; female; neonate)	Other characteristics
Reeves muntjac (*Muntiacus reevesi*)	Smallest, heavily muscled, with short very thin legs; up to 20kg	Foxy red summer, darker winter	Characteristic long; white ventral surface (signals danger)	Simple short curved spikes with or without tiny brow tine near base M prominent frontal ridge from eyes to pedicle and antlers, large curved canine teeth (up to 2 cm)	Common in many urban and suburban areas England; woodlands, parks, gardens, roadside verges, arable land, forest	Buck; doe; kid	Hunched back, almost pig-like appearance Tushes often broken off in fights with rivals

16.1 (continued) Wild deer species in the British Isles (M, male; F, female).

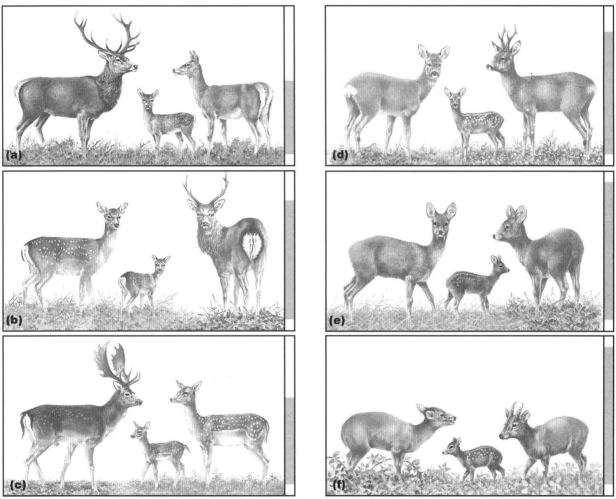

16.2 The six species of deer living wild in Britain. (a) Red deer; (b) sika deer; (c) fallow deer; (d) roe deer; (e) Chinese water deer; (f) muntjac. (© Crown copyright. Reproduced with permission from the Forest Commission.). Shaded bar = 1 metre.

Ecology

Social structure

All three of the large deer species (red, sika, fallow) are strongly socially bonded into small groups of between three and seven animals, which in turn become loosely associated into herds. The males form bachelor groups for most of the year and separate in the rut to hold groups of females (harems) for mating. This tendency to strong social bonding raises significant questions about the welfare of large deer kept in isolation for purposes of treatment, nursing or convalescence.

The three species of smaller deer (roe, Chinese water deer, muntjac) are less socially bonded, though maternal family groups are formed amongst some roe populations, and Chinese water deer appear to retain social bonding between dams and littermates for long periods. Muntjac are the most socially independent of the British deer, with the bucks often existing as isolated individuals, except for briefly courting females in oestrus, and the does keeping only the company of the most recent offspring.

Habitat and feeding
Deer are woodland animals, preferring mixed deciduous forest and scrubland. They are 'animals of the edge', dividing their time between open glades or pastures and dense areas of cover, where they lie up to ruminate. All deer tend to be browsers rather than grazers but the development and specialization of the rumenal system in certain deer approaches that of cattle, so that fallow, for instance, spend long periods grazing. All the small deer of Britain have primitive rumenal development; they are therefore true browsers, requiring frequent intake of small amounts of relatively low-fibre food, and depend upon considerable intake of succulent foods (Jackson, 1980). Red and sika deer are somewhere in between, eating a mixture of grazed pasture and browsed succulents.

Anatomy and physiology

Deer have typical ruminant anatomy, except that they do not possess a gall bladder. Skeletal anatomy is fundamentally goat-like, but the deciduous nature of antler growth is a significant difference and many deer possess distinct infraorbital structures, including a large infraorbital foramen and an infraorbital fossa, which in muntjac is as large as the orbit.

Breeding season and antler growth
Most deer are seasonal breeders, with both genders coming into fertile activity for a breeding period known as the rut, and antler growth and shedding are locked into this annual reproductive pattern. In muntjac, however, although the bucks grow new antlers through the British summer, both bucks and does are fertile all year round and parturition can occur at any time, with a rapid return to post-partum oestrus for the does. Roe deer are unusual in shedding their antlers much later than the other species and growing new ones through the winter months.

Osteogenesis
Antlers are composed of bone, which is laid down extremely rapidly as the new antlers grow within a covering of fragile, highly vascular skin known as velvet. Deer have the physiological ability to mobilize and precipitate very large quantities of bone minerals in a very short time, so that the entire circulating blood calcium and phosphate reserve is turned over and replenished within days. When the antlers are fully developed the vascular supply to the velvet becomes occluded and the velvet first becomes devitalized and is then shredded as the stag or buck 'cleans' the new antlers. At the end of the annual antler cycle a rapid invasion of osteoclasts into the base of the antlers occurs, so that the hard antlers are shed within a few days. Regrowth of the new set begins immediately. The impressive osteogenic capability of deer is reflected in very rapid bone healing in cases of fracture and in exaggerated disorganized bone deposition in cases of inflammatory or septic bone disease.

Dentition
In common with the domestic bovids, deer have no incisors in the upper jaw. The lower canine teeth are modified into an extra pair of incisiform teeth in the lower jaw and so deer appear to have four pairs of lower incisors. Unlike sheep and goats, it is unusual for wild deer to lose incisors in middle age and the appearance of a broken mouth, with incisors missing and very well worn, indicates extreme old age.

Ageing
In the wild, individual deer often live into their early teens and some for considerably longer. Ageing based upon teeth is a very unreliable science in deer and there is considerable variation between the species in the ages at which deciduous and permanent premolars and molars erupt. Added to this is the great difficulty of properly examining the molar arcades in living deer. Ageing should be based upon the size and appearance of the animal, the complexity of the antlers in males and the presence of permanent molars (i.e. more than four grinding teeth in each arcade). As a general rule, males develop larger antlers with each succeeding season and, in particular, the coronet at the base of the antler becomes more developed and prominent with age. It should be possible to classify a deer as juvenile, subadult, young adult, adult and old.

Seasonal metabolism
Most species of deer show a distinct seasonal variation in metabolic rate and appetite. During the winter they eat much less than in the summer and it is normal for them to lose up to 10% bodyweight over the winter, despite the availability of good food. Red deer stags and fallow bucks eat almost nothing during the autumn rut, when they are most active, and so they may suffer from exhaustion and debility to the point of collapse.

Senses
All deer have extremely well developed senses of hearing, smell and sight, enabling them to detect and avoid human contact if at all possible. Scent marking of territories is accomplished by secretions from interdigital, tarsal and sub-orbital glands and by urine marking. Male animals, especially in the larger species, become pungently smelly during the rut, principally from urine spraying and wallowing.

Capture, handling and transport

Dangers to handlers
The adults of all deer encountered in Britain are potentially dangerous to inexperienced or untrained handlers. Red, sika and fallow are large, strong animals with suicidal instincts to avoid contact with and handling by humans. Antlers and hooves are formidable weapons and the strength of these large deer far exceeds the strength of most healthy adult men. The smaller deer

are also violently fearful of human contact and will struggle, kick, plunge, rear and strike out in attempts to avoid being examined or restrained. The teeth and hooves of muntjac are notorious for inflicting deep wounds. Ill-advised or improperly planned attempts to corner or catch active, mobile deer are likely to result in injury to people or animals and must be avoided.

If the veterinary surgeon or staff are called to attend to a deer casualty, it is essential that a full range of appropriate equipment is available (Figure 16.3) and that complete evaluation of the animal *at a distance* is undertaken before making any initial approach.

Equipment

- Thick, dark towels, drapes or sacks for covering the head
- Thick blankets
- Soft ropes
- Soft cargo or freight netting
- Suitable crate for muntjac and Chinese water deer
- For large deer (red, sika, fallow): dart gun or pole-syringe
- Equipment and materials for euthanasia

Drugs

- Suitable alpha-2 adrenergic agonist sedative (xylazine, detomidine, medetomidine)
- Atipamezole
- Ketamine
- Diazepam
- Etorphine/diprenorphine (if experienced in use of this product)

16.3 Handling equipment for dealing with wild deer in the field.

Initial assessment of casualties by inspection

Casualties in the field

The most common circumstances under which large or adult deer are presented for veterinary examination are at the scene of a road traffic accident, or caught in fences, trapped in enclosures, tangled in netting, snared by fox-wires and poacher's traps or found recumbent in the field. It is important to realize that if an adult deer is not physically restrained in some way it will not tolerate the approach of a human. Juvenile deer, on the other hand, tend to crouch and cower rather than attempt to escape.

Adult deer that do not retreat from human contact are almost invariably injured or diseased to a terminal and irrecoverable extent.

Road accidents: At the scene of a road accident, if an injured deer remains recumbent despite the presence of police, bystanders, vehicles and general commotion, the veterinary surgeon arriving at the scene should assume that the animal has suffered severe orthopaedic and neurological trauma. Deer with multiple fractures of a single limb, soft tissue injuries and even internal organ rupture will not remain at the roadside but will make an escape into open countryside or woodland. Most will survive, though some will

succumb to their injuries later, far away from the scrutiny of people. The veterinary surgeon should therefore inspect the injured deer at a distance before approaching it. A strong torch is essential at night, a pair of binoculars useful by day.

To try to determine the reason why the deer has not moved away, it is necessary to look carefully for signs of haemorrhage, abnormally positioned and therefore possibly fractured limbs, and apparent alertness and responsiveness about the head. Dying deer will maintain sternal recumbency but have a floppy, waving or swaying head motion. Deer in lateral recumbency carry a hopeless prognosis.

The purpose of inspection without handling is to determine whether the animal should be euthanased, or approached and manually handled, or sedated from a distance with either a dart or pole-syringe.

Collapsed deer: Collapsed deer with no evidence of trauma are also likely to be terminally ill. In the winter significant numbers of young deer die because of winter inanition and environmental stress. Again, if called to such an animal, the veterinary surgeon must inspect it from a distance before deciding whether it should be approached.

Large deer are sometimes encountered suffering from severe myopathy; this is presumed to be the effect of prolonged chasing by hounds or dogs, though the association is not firmly established. These animals present as recumbent, hyperventilating and sometimes hyperthermic individuals with apparent hindquarter paralysis. By the time they collapse they have irreversible metabolic changes and kidney pathology and very rarely survive (see 'Specific conditions').

Welfare considerations: If an injured deer is active and mobile, consideration should be given to whether the stress and trauma of capture would present more of a welfare problem than the apparent injury. In the wild, deer frequently suffer wounds from fighting, superficial infestation with parasites, damage to the growing antlers in velvet and fractured limbs. There is considerable evidence that such injuries usually resolve without veterinary intervention.

The author therefore questions the need to catch and treat deer with injuries that are not grossly disabling to the animal. Deer manage very well on three legs and the author has encountered many wild deer with a distal limb missing – presumably as the result of fractures or injuries giving rise to ischaemic necrosis and shedding of the limb (see 'Limb fractures', below). The stress of captivity, handling, confinement and treatment may, in the author's opinion, make the long-term hospitalization of adult wild deer inhumane (Harris and Jeffries, 1991).

Injured deer that remain mobile and able to feed should not be captured for welfare reasons, even though their injuries may seem severe to veterinary surgeons used to dealing with domestic pets and farm stock. Exceptions to this rule include mobile deer entangled in foreign material, deer with mandibular or facial injuries that prevent them eating, and deer with more than one limb fracture.

If the deer can easily be captured, or is already restrained, and severe injury to a single limb is discovered, the ethics of releasing the animal without treatment may be reasonably questioned. Under such circumstances, amputation with swift post-operative release may be the best course of action.

Entrapment: Large deer entrapped in fencing or netting are candidates for remote sedation by darting or pole-syringe injection before any attempt is made to release them. Small deer may more safely be covered and restrained, but care must be taken not to convert a trapped limb into a fracture in the struggle. Sedation may be appropriate before untangling is undertaken.

Small deer may appear to be 'trapped' in gardens and enclosures; as a general rule, they are best left alone, since they will find the same way out as the way they entered. The presence of people will panic them and they may appear disoriented, but the optimum treatment is to leave them alone and withdraw all human observation.

Neonates: Neonatal deer of all species are left for long periods by the dams, usually concealed in undergrowth. If well-meaning people find or 'rescue' such an animal, they must be encouraged to take it back to the place it was discovered and to leave it alone. There is no point in watching for the return of the dam, since she will not approach whilst people are in the vicinity. Neonates can be successfully returned to the same spot up to 24 hours after being removed. It is a myth to say that human handling of the neonate will prevent the return and maternal attention of the dam.

Handling, restraint and sedation in the field

Should the decision be taken to handle or restrain a deer casualty, proper equipment (see Figure 16.3) must be available. Recumbent deer should be approached with caution, since they are likely to spring up and attempt to escape, even when seriously injured.

In the unusual circumstance where a number of healthy, conscious deer need to be moved (for instance, from a deer park or enclosed collection), inexperienced veterinary surgeons should seek the advice of specialist deer transporters. Individual deer should never be transported loose, without restraint. In the case of animals selected for treatment, a combination of sedation and physical restraint should be used (Jones, 1984). Large deer are best wrapped up in cargo nets with only the blindfolded head poking out and with the feet hobbled (Figure 16.4). A stout New Zealand-type horse rug will serve as well, though lots of rope must be used. Small deer can be wrapped in blankets. The trussed-up deer can then be transported in a vehicle or trailer.

Manual restraint of small deer: In the case of small deer or juveniles, manual restraint is more successful. The deer should be approached from behind, if it is recumbent, and smothered (i.e. covered and simultaneously restrained) with a blanket, net or coat (Figure 16.5). Roe deer and juvenile red, fallow and sika should then be masked, either with a conical hood

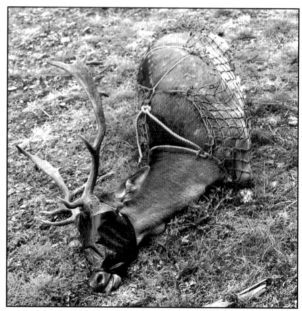

16.4 Larger deer such as this fallow buck are best restrained by masking, hobbling and then wrapping in a piece of cargo net. Fallow, roe and red deer restrained in this way will remain settled provided that the surroundings are quiet and talking is kept to a minimum. This buck, however, is becoming distressed: he shows evidence of mouth breathing, with his tongue protruding.

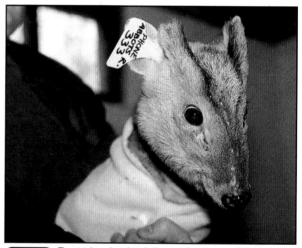

16.5 Restrained subadult muntjac buck. Small deer may be restrained by smothering in a blanket. This buck has since survived for 13 years after release and is regularly observed by the author.

made for the purpose or with a dark drape. Soft dark cohesive bandage may also be used in halter-like pattern to cover the eyes. Once masked, these deer will lie quietly if they are undisturbed by noise and if their four legs are tied together at the level of the metacarpi and metatarsi (cannons) using soft rope (hard or coarse ropes are not suitable). Hobbling in this way must be very carefully undertaken, so that the soft ropes are not too tight, and hobbling alone is insufficient restraint for more than a few minutes. To prevent further struggling, the deer should then be trussed up in a blanket or cargo net secured with further ropes (see Figure 16.4).

Vocalization: Some deer are very vocal when caught, injured or handled. The young of all species may whistle or bleat. Muntjac of all ages will scream loudly in an alarming and prolonged manner; some roe will also scream, although not so volubly and persistently.

The application of a blindfold will immediately calm species such as roe, but muntjac react with panic if they are unable to see and will thrash about in a frenzy.

Crating of muntjac and Chinese water deer: Muntjac and Chinese water deer continue to struggle even if masked, hobbled and trussed up. They must be either securely wrapped in a large blanket, with only the head exposed for breathing, or, preferably, placed in a strong wooden crate (Figure 16.6) (Chapman *et al.*, 1987). The crate size is important, since too large a box will result in panic and injury as the deer crashes around inside. There should be little room for manoeuvre. Veterinary practices dealing regularly with muntjac casualties are well advised to have a suitable crate constructed. Sliding doors at both ends are useful, since some muntjac will sulk in the box and need to be pushed out from behind when the time comes to release them.

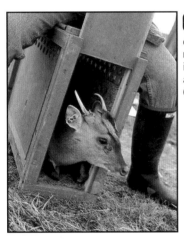

16.6 Transport and holding crate suitable for muntjac. Optimum internal dimensions are 25 cm x 80 cm x 60 cm high.

Zoonoses

All personnel should be warned that wild deer are regularly encountered with bovine tuberculosis (*Mycobacterium bovis*) and that they may carry ticks harbouring *Borrelia* (Lyme disease). There is therefore a small risk of zoonosis.

Examination and assessment for rehabilitation

If deer are brought to the clinic and they are presented without considerable difficulty and without being thoroughly wrapped up, tied up or crated, it is safe to assume that they are either critically injured or juvenile.

- Large adult deer brought to the clinic in the boot or on the back seat of a vehicle should be candidates for euthanasia unless the reason for their compliance to such transportation is obvious and easily reparable. The vast majority of such unfortunate creatures will have spinal or multiple limb fractures, or will be terminally ill with systemic disease
- Lively and alert deer, either restrained or in crates, should be inspected carefully before deciding on the best course of action
- Juvenile deer and neonates in good condition should be returned to the place of discovery immediately.

Sedation for examination

For complete and thorough examination of small deer casualties, it will probably be necessary to sedate the animal. This may be performed in the field, though it may be better to transport the animal back to the clinic. For routes and drugs of choice, see 'Sedation, anaesthesia and analgesia', below. Diazepam is a useful sedative for calming fractious deer for transportation but does not provide sufficient depth of sedation for relaxed examination.

Clinical examination

Full clinical examination is difficult in conscious deer and normal physiological parameters are almost worthless, as they are grossly moderated by the stress of handling or by the sedation. Because of their extreme distress at handling, heart and respiratory rates will be very high in conscious deer and are of little benefit to the clinical examination. Elevated temperatures (above 40°C) will be generated by struggling and stress; they are not reliable indicators of infection. Subnormal temperatures (below 37°C) may indicate metabolic shutdown or terminal collapse. Deer in great distress will adopt a panting, open-mouth mode of breathing (see Figure 16.4), regardless of exercise, exhaustion or respiratory compromise. Clinical examination of deer is therefore usually undertaken by observation, or when the deer is sedated.

Trauma

Inspection should include careful assessment of each limb for signs of fracture, trauma or joint swelling and the action of the deer must be evaluated for evidence of lameness or disability. (Clicking is often apparent and normal as deer walk, particularly in some larger species.) If the deer is handled and sedated, careful palpation of the limbs and spine may reveal the site of bone trauma. Palpation of the soft tissues will detect muscle injuries and body wall ruptures, which are common after road traffic accidents.

Recumbency

Recumbent deer must be subject to full passive orthopaedic examination, including cranial, spinal and pelvic radiography, as fractures of the spine and pelvis are common. If such fractures are discovered, the deer should be humanely destroyed.

Deer normally do not feed whilst in sternal recumbency, though they may ruminate whilst recumbent. Thus a recumbent deer that eats voraciously should be suspected of suffering from spinal injury, even though it may remain bright around the head. If no obvious bony trauma is discovered, blood samples should be taken to look for evidence of dehydration, bacterial infection or elevation of muscle enzymes. If the recumbent deer appears to be in good bodily condition, the differential diagnosis is virtually limited to trauma or myopathy. Both conditions will result in gross elevations of creatine kinase.

Reference values

The haematological and biochemical parameters of deer are remarkably consistent across the species but great variation occurs in response to stress, handling and trauma, presumably as a result of splenic contraction. Sedation and anaesthesia also affect the results. Blood biochemistry varies with the seasons, especially during winter metabolic shutdown. Laboratory blood sample analysis in wild deer may therefore be unrewarding. The data in Figure 16.7 are a guide and may be applied to all the British species.

Parameter	Reference range
PCV (l/l)	0.4–0.6
RBC (10^{12}/l)	9–12
Haemoglobin (g/l)	140–180
MCH (pg)	14–19
MCV (fl)	40–50
MCHC (g/l)	330–360
WBC (10^9/l)	3.5–6.0
Neutrophils (10^9/l)	1.9–2.5
Lymphocytes (10^9/l)	1.1–2.5
Platelets (10^9/l)	270–380
Total protein (g/l)	50–8
Albumen (g/l)	28–40
Globulin (g/l)	30–50
Fibrinogen (g/l)	< 6
Urea N (mmol/l)	6–10
Glucose (mmol/l)	2–10
Lactate (mmol/l)	< 15
AP (IU/l)	< 500
AST (IU/l)	< 200
Creatine kinase (IU/l)	< 2000
Gamma GT (IU/l)	< 300

16.7 Haematological and biochemical parameters for deer. (Sources: Kay, 1994; Jones, 1994; Knox *et al.*, 1988.)

Imaging

In small deer, ultrasonographic imaging of the abdomen with a 3.5 or 5 MHz probe has proved useful in the diagnosis of internal organ damage and haemorrhage into the peritoneal cavity. An abdominocentesis will confirm bowel rupture, peritonitis or haemorrhage.

Radiography is also valuable in the assessment of joint pathology. Deer are commonly encountered with severe proliferative septic arthropathy of several joints.

The affected joints are grossly swollen with a limited range of movement and radiography reveals massive periarticular exostosis. There is no treatment and humane destruction is indicated.

Cases of obvious respiratory disease should be assessed with the benefit of thoracic radiographs, since pulmonary tuberculosis gives rise to a typical miliary pattern within the lung tissue. Parasitic lung disease is relatively common in wild deer, especially roe, and may give rise to pneumonia-like signs. Further confusion is added by the frequent presence of nasal bots that may cause a snoring respiration.

Euthanasia

Criteria for euthanasia

The author strongly advocates that major surgery or prolonged convalescence should not be contemplated for wild deer. None of the British deer species is endangered, either in this country or worldwide. The salvaging of badly injured individual deer with no realistic prospect of release into the wild presents significant long-term welfare problems, since 'pet' deer are likely to be permanently confined to unnatural surroundings and isolated from their own species. Male deer of all species almost invariably become aggressive in captivity, especially if they have become habituated to human contact. For these reasons the author has grave reservations about the prolonged 'rescue and rehabilitation' of injured wild deer and, in his own practice, insists that any casualty treatment of wild deer is governed by the principle of *rapid rescue, repair and release*.

If the prospective period of treatment is likely to exceed 2 weeks and if repeated handling is likely to be necessary, the veterinary surgeon called to the scene of a wild deer casualty should consider only two options:

- Immediate treatment and release
- Euthanasia.

In the author's experience, deer showing the following clinical signs should be humanely destroyed without recourse to further investigation, examination or treatment:

- Deer that remain recumbent for more than an hour after obvious trauma (e.g. a road traffic accident)
- Deer with more than one fractured limb
- Deer with open abdominal or thoracic wounds
- Deer with fractured or severely traumatized mandibles or facial structures
- Deer that are recumbent with firearm wounds
- Deer that are severely lame with multiple joint disease.

Animals that might be suitable candidates for *rapid rescue, repair and release* may be those showing the following clinical signs:

- Neonatal deer that may be released immediately
- Deer with wounds that may be treated or sutured with one surgical intervention only
- Male deer with damaged antlers

- Deer with single leg fractures
- Female deer with dystocia
- Collapsed or recumbent deer with no evidence of trauma
- Deer entangled in fences or netting.

Techniques for euthanasia

For small deer that are restrained or anaesthetized, standard solutions of pentobarbital or secobarbital (quinalbarbitone) plus cinchocaine may be given intravenously.

The euthanasia of larger deer or mobile and active smaller deer presents something of a problem, especially at the scene of a road traffic accident or in the public view. There is no doubt that the most humane and instantaneous method of euthanasia is by the correct use of a firearm, though public scrutiny may dictate that the deer is deeply sedated and removed from the scene to be killed elsewhere. If the deer cannot be approached safely (for instance, in cases of pelvic or bilateral hindlimb fracture in which the deer may be dragging the hindquarters), the only sensible alternatives are darting or pole-syringe injecting, or shooting with a rifle. If firearms are not available the deer must be sedated, as described earlier, and then injected intravenously when the sedative has taken effect.

Shooting: To comply with the law in England and Wales, the rifle must have a calibre of no less than .240 inch (in Scotland the legislation is framed with reference to muzzle velocity and energy). Standard deerstalking rifles, such as the .243, .270, .308 and 30.06 calibres, are all high-velocity weapons and few veterinary surgeons will be equipped with such guns. Under these circumstances the services of a local Forest Authority ranger, experienced deerstalker, huntsman, reliable local gamekeeper or RSPCA inspector may be the best solution. In the experience of the author, police firearms officers are rarely well trained in the dispatch of deer or other large animals.

To achieve effective instantaneous dispatch the deer must be shot in the head, aiming to obliterate the brainstem at the base of the skull. For this reason the deer should not be shot from the front through the face but from the side, aiming at the base of the ear. Shots into the chest will not instantly kill the deer and may allow sufficient time for a panicking animal to cause further injury to itself or bystanders. Normal precautions of firearm safety must be observed throughout.

If the deer can be restrained, a pistol may be used. The standard .32 inch free-bullet horse-slaughtering pistol is suitable, as is the normal .22 captive-bolt weapon firing blue-labelled 2 grain cartridges. Under these circumstances the deer should be restrained securely and the pistol placed at the back of the skull, low down between the ears and pointed through the cranium towards the nose. This shot placement guarantees instant insensibility and avoids the thickened frontal bones of large stags and bucks. Only veterinary surgeons employed in large animal or equine practice are likely to be equipped with pistols, though huntsmen and RSPCA inspectors usually carry such weapons.

If the deer has been properly shot, with either a rifle or a pistol, there should be only brief reflex movement

and then complete cessation of breathing, as the respiratory centre of the brainstem will have been eliminated. Organized heart beating may be detected for up to 10 minutes; the animal will be instantly 'brain dead' and the remainder of the bodily tissues will succumb to anoxia. From the point of view of welfare, there is no need to pith or bleed deer shot in this way, but huntsmen and deerstalkers will have been trained to bleed the carcass because of carcass quality.

Carcass disposal: The disposal of deer carcasses may be difficult if chemical euthanasia has been employed and expensive arrangements for cremation or burial may be necessary. Animals that have been shot may be removed by the local hunt kennels.

First aid procedures

If at all possible, the veterinary surgeon should consider treating the deer and releasing it immediately. In the case of entanglement or entrapment and with some road traffic accident injuries, this may be accomplished in the field. After sedation or restraint the animal should be released from entanglement, removed to a quiet place away from road traffic and examined fully.

Fluid therapy

Recumbency of deer in poor condition extends the differential diagnosis, since the terminal effects of winter stress, bacterial infection, severe parasitism, tuberculosis and starvation will all result in emaciation and collapse. The best course of action in the case of a recumbent deer with no obvious trauma is to classify the deer as 'sick' rather than injured, to maintain the animal on intravenous lactated Ringer's fluids (Hartmann's) and supportive nursing for 24–48 hours and to monitor for improvement. An injection of soluble dexamethasone will be gluconeogenic and broad-spectrum antibiotic cover should be given, since clinical signs of sepsis are very variable. If capture myopathy (see 'Specific conditions') is suspected or diagnosed, the doses of dexamethasone will need to be higher and glucose should be added to the infusion.

It is possible to keep deer quiet for intravenous fluid administration by incorporating diazepam in the Hartmann's solution at a rate that does not exceed 1 mg/kg every 6 hours. Fluid lines should be of the extensible 'curly' equine variety, which allow some movement or attempts to rise without risk of spoiling the line; catheters should be sutured into the jugular vein.

Wounds

Superficial or granulating wounds are best treated with broad-spectrum antibiotic ointments such as chlortetracycline, sodium fucidate or neomycin/nitrofurazone.

Fresh deeper wounds may be lavaged according to normal principles and sutured using synthetic absorbable suture material (such as polyglactin or polydioxanone). It is worth noting that the skin of the neck and shoulders of mature male deer is extremely tough and the calibre of cutting needles suitable for cattle skin will be required. The wounds should be dusted with broad-spectrum antibiotic powder (e.g. chlortetracycline).

In the summer, some consideration of fly strike should be made: proprietary fly-repellent sprays may be applied. If no further injuries are discovered, the deer can be given intramuscular injections of a broad-spectrum antibiotic, e.g. long-acting tetracycline at 20 mg/kg (Wilson, 1983) and short-acting soluble dexamethasone (0.8 mg/kg), before being revived and released. In the author's experience, the gluconeogenic effects of the steroid, combined with the anti-inflammatory and anti-shock properties of this class of drug make it a better choice than non-steroidal anti-inflammatories.

Fractures

Some deer with obvious fractures of a limb may be released immediately, even if the fracture is compound and comminuted. Most deer with only a single limb fracture will remain mobile and will escape if possible. These deer should not be driven into nets or darted, since the best therapy is to leave them well alone. The author has followed the progress of several such cases and all have recovered very quickly. The criterion is the level of the fracture: all fractures above the carpus and tarsus can be left to heal without support and within a month the majority of these animals will be weight-bearing on the affected leg.

Fractures of the distal limb below the carpus and tarsus are more problematic, since they may succumb to ischaemia and slough. Although wild deer with such foreshortened limbs appear to manage adequately, there is a tendency for the stump to become abraded and ulcerated. For this reason it may be more humane to amputate the limb higher and then to release the deer soon afterwards. This will require removal to the veterinary clinic.

Veterinary surgeons are encouraged only to treat deer that have an excellent prognosis for rapid return to the wild; therefore long-term fracture immobilization with internal or external fixation is not recommended. Either no treatment or fracture amputation usually offers the most rapid return to the wild.

Dystocia

Rare cases of dystocia are suitable for laparotomy and caesarean section, followed by immediate release.

Short-term hospitalization

When the deer arrives at the clinic it must be taken either straight to the treatment room or to suitable accommodation.

It is not humane to kennel deer (even small and juvenile individuals) in the clinic kennel or cattery. They must be kept in isolated, quiet surroundings well away from disturbance by the barking of dogs or the general noise of people and pets.

As a short-term measure, larger deer can be kept in a stable or outhouse on a deep bed of straw. Small deer may be confined to an isolation kennel, which must be completely separate from other animals and people. If a recumbent deer is placed in a stable or shed and then recovers sufficiently to stand, further examination and treatment may be difficult. Such animals may leap blindly towards the light, either at a window or when the door is opened, and great care must be exercised.

Feeding

For short-term management, succulent food must be offered – cabbages, carrot tops, root vegetables and leafy branches of native deciduous trees (e.g. hazel, hawthorn, willow). In the first 24 hours the deer may eat nothing and will almost certainly not drink. Some succulent food should have been eaten by the end of 48 hours. Hay and proprietary dry foods or pellets will be ignored in the short term.

Sedation, anaesthesia and analgesia

Sedative and anaesthetic drugs for deer are summarized in Figure 16.8.

Drug	Dosage	Indications
Diazepam	0.5–1 mg/kg i.v., i.m.	Transportation, stress
Etorphine	0.5–0.75 ml/100 kg (1.125–2.2 mg/100 kg) i.m.	Field anaesthesia of red and sika deer
Etorphine + xylazine	As above + 1 mg xylazine/kg i.m.	Field anaesthesia of fallow deer
Xylazine	2 mg/kg i.m., i.v.	With ketamine for deep sedation and induction. Use 50% more for fallow deer
Detomidine/medetomidine	50–100 µg/kg i.m., i.v.	With ketamine for deep sedation. Use upper dose limit for fallow deer
Ketamine	2–3 mg/kg i.m., i.v.	For deep sedation with xylazine or detomidine/medetomidine and induction following xylazine
Glyceryl guacolate + thiopental	3% guacolate + 5% thiopental, to effect, slow i.v.	Induction of anaesthesia
Methohexital	10 mg/kg	Induction/field anaesthesia
Propofol	0.6–1.5 mg/kg i.v.	Prolongation/maintenance of anaesthesia
Pentobarbital	150 mg/kg	Euthanasia
Secobarbital (quinalbarbitone) + cinchocaine	100 mg/kg + 6 mg/kg	Euthanasia

16.8 Sedative and anaesthetic drugs for deer.

Sedation

Small deer

It is almost impossible to find the jugular vein in conscious muntjac and Chinese water deer without first sedating the animal by intramuscular injection to allow full extension of the head. Intravenous jugular injection is more simple in roe deer, in which the neck is longer and the vein more easily palpable.

For muntjac and Chinese water deer, the superficial aural veins on the caudal surface of the ear provide a convenient site for intravenous injection. The advantage of using an ear vein is that only the head of the deer (or even only the ear) needs to be withdrawn from the wrap-up blanket or net that has been used to restrain the animal during capture.

A 25 gauge butterfly cannula is preferable to a needle or over-the-needle catheter, as it may be left in place for top-up doses. The cephalic or saphenous veins may also be used if the deer is strapped to a stretcher.

Large deer

As deer are ruminants, it is important to prevent both bloat and inhalation of regurgitated rumen contents during deep sedation. This is more problematic in the large deer, with relatively larger rumen capacities. Sternal recumbency should be maintained if possible and patients should be monitored at all times for patency of the airway. If lateral recumbency is necessary, the deer should be laid on its right side. Profuse salivation is common, partly because of the parasympathomimetic action of the sedative combinations and partly because the swallowing reflex is easily abolished.

Etorphine: For the sedation of lively or mobile red or sika deer the drug of choice is etorphine, given from a dart or pole-syringe (Fletcher, 1994). As there are considerable human risks attached to the use of this drug, it is best reserved for open field situations where there are few bystanders. Etorphine alone is less satisfactory in fallow deer, which may suffer both respiratory and cardiac failure. The addition of an alpha-2 agonist such as xylazine to the etorphine will reduce this risk.

Xylazine and ketamine: A safer combination for intramuscular chemical restraint in large deer species is a combination of an alpha-2 adrenergic agonist and ketamine. Xylazine at a dose of 2 mg/kg combined with ketamine at 3 mg/kg will induce deep sedation in red and sika deer. Doses for fallow deer need to be increased by 50% since they appear to be more excitable and more intractable to such sedation. The so-called Hellabrun mixture of ketamine and xylazine is made by dissolving 500 mg xylazine powder (e.g. Rompun Dry Substance) in 4 ml of 10% (100 mg/ml) ketamine. Red deer can be sedated with 1–2 ml of this mixture; adult fallow deer will need up to 3 ml.

Medetomidine: A better alternative is the use of medetomidine or detomidine at 50–100 μg/kg in combination with ketamine at 2–3 mg/kg. Fallow deer should be dosed at the upper end of the dose range and other large deer given less (Jalanka, 1993). The use of alpha-2 adrenergic agonist sedation alone is not recommended, since the effect in wild deer is variable and the behaviour of the sedated animals is unpredictable. Animals given the combination of an alpha-2 sedative and ketamine will become amenable to handling within 10 minutes and the effect will last for up to 3 hours. Top-up doses of half the combined induction doses may be given intravenously if the sedation is insufficient or if the animal starts to recover from the initial dose. When the examination is concluded, or if the deer is to be released, an intravenous injection of atipamezole at five times the dose by weight of the detomidine or medetomidine will reverse the sedation, but this should not be administered for at least 30 minutes after the ketamine.

Anaesthesia

General anaesthesia may be induced with a bolus of ketamine at 3 mg/kg after premedication with xylazine at 2 mg/kg. The addition of diazepam to the induction bolus of ketamine at a dose of 0.5 mg/kg will aid intubation. Foal endotracheal tubes (14 mm and 16 mm) will be suitable for adult large deer; small animal tubes will be required for small deer and juveniles.

The use of atropine does not limit excessive salivation and so the head of the deer should be kept in a dependent position during surgery to allow drainage of saliva by gravity, or suction should be employed.

Anaesthesia may be maintained by inhalation of either halothane or isoflurane. Monitoring the depth of anaesthesia is not straightforward, since the palpebral and corneal reflexes are abolished in relatively light planes. The relaxation of the jaw and respiratory rate are better indicators.

Combinations of glyceryl guacolate (guaphenesin) in a 3% solution together with 5% thiopental may be given intravenously to effect as an alternative induction protocol and after premedication with xylazine (2 mg/kg). The effect is less predictable than with ketamine. Methohexital (methohexitone) sodium has been successfully used in the general anaesthesia of wild muntjac captured in nets in field situations; induction is smooth but recovery may be violent (Cooper *et al.*, 1986).

Where inhalation anaesthesia is not available for maintenance, an effective surgical plane of anaesthesia may be prolonged with a bolus of propofol (Jalanka, 1993). This extends the anaesthesia by up to 20 minutes and can be repeated without adverse effects upon recovery. The author has no experience of propofol as an induction agent in deer.

Specific conditions

Trauma

Limb fractures

Proximal fractures: As outlined earlier (see 'First aid'), proximal limb fractures are best left untreated, with the deer released immediately or confined to a large quiet convalescence pen for monitoring. The fractures usually become weight-bearing in 4 weeks and the author believes that they heal more quickly in the wild than if deer are confined for observation. On the occasions when the author has undertaken internal fixation of proximal limb fractures, the results have been disappointing because of the trade-off between the need for close confinement and rest post-operatively and the desire to rehabilitate the animal rapidly. Rapid release after surgery risks implant failure or wound breakdown; prolonged close confinement is stressful and inhumane.

Distal fractures:

Amputation: Distal limb fractures, especially compound and comminuted metatarsal and metacarpal fractures, are best managed by amputation and rapid release. Forelimbs should be removed at the level of the humerus and hindlimbs at the femur. General anaesthesia with intubation and maintenance by inhalation is essential. Bones should be sawn rather than cut with bone cutters, as longitudinal shattering is a problem. Post-operative pain relief with flunixin appears effective. Carprofen may also be used but has a very long half-life in ruminants and should be given only every 48 hours. Ketoprofen is very rapidly eliminated and must be given twice daily; for this reason it is not recommended in deer. Broad-spectrum antibiotic cover may be given with enrofloxacin in adult deer (growth plate dysplasia has been reported in juvenile animals of other species, though the drug is widely used in calves and piglets with no apparent ill effect), potentiated sulphonamides (trimethoprim–sulphonamide), or a single injection of long-acting oxytetracycline. Oral antibiotics should not be given to deer.

Self-healing: In the author's experience, closed simple distal limb fractures may be left untreated and will very rapidly form a large fibrous and then osseous callus. This process is not accelerated by the application of casts; deer will simply allow the uncast limb to hang and will avoid disturbing the fracture. Healing is remarkably swift.

Antler hypertrophy: A bizarre and unexplained phenomenon often occurs after limb trauma in male deer, in which one of the antlers subsequently fails to develop properly, so that the stag or buck grows a grossly asymmetrical pair of antlers (Antony-Davis, 1983). The hypertrophic antler is usually, but not invariably, on the contralateral side to the injured limb. This potential feature should be pointed out if male deer are consigned to captive collections after treatment of limb injury.

Pelvic fractures

Lame deer with pelvic fractures should be released, provided that they are mobile on the contralateral limb. The risk of dystocia should be considered in females. Bilateral lameness associated with pelvic fracture carries a poor prognosis, since neurological damage is usually present and both bladder and rectal control are usually lost. Such cases should be euthanased.

Spinal fractures are easily missed on radiography and the clinician must rely upon neurological examination. Evidence of hemiplegia after trauma is sufficient grounds for euthanasia.

Antler damage

As the antler is growing each year it is covered with highly vascular, soft and sensitive velvet (see 'Anatomy and physiology'). The developing bone is spongy and prone to trauma. Once the velvet is shed and the antlers are bare, hard and polished, they consist of dense bone continuous with the pedicular extensions of the frontal bones.

Damaged antlers may be amputated. In velvet, amputation will require local or general anaesthesia, and haemostasis must be achieved by the use of a tourniquet of rubber tubing around the base of the antlers. Nerves to be desensitized must include the infratrochlear nerve and the zygomaticotemporal nerve, both branches of the ophthalmic division of the trigeminal nerve (Adams, 1979). The sites for injection are well established in red deer, since velvet harvesting is a routine farming practice in some parts of the world (but illegal in the UK). Slight variation between species means that a ring block around the base of the antler may be more reliable in other deer. In hard antler, no haemostasis is necessary. Amputation must be undertaken at a level 2–3 cm *above* the coronet, which is the junction of the pedicle and the antler. If the pedicle is damaged in any way, future antler growth will be disrupted.

Dog-bite wounds

Young deer are often mauled by dogs and may be presented with multiple bite wounds on the hindquarters and neck. These animals warrant nursing for several days after routine wound cleaning, since deep soft tissue infections may take several days to become fulminant. Wounds must not be sutured. Daily enrofloxacin in adults appears to offer better antibiotic cover than other broad-spectrum drugs. If there is concern about the use of fluoroquinolones in juveniles, trimethoprim–sulphonamide can be given. Only a 3-day course is necessary and the animal should be released on the fourth day if the wounds are dry. Evidence of stress or myopathy as a result of chasing by dogs should be treated as outlined below.

Gunshot wounds

These should be treated as for dog-bite wounds. Surgery to retrieve bullets or pellets is completely unnecessary. Deer with shotgun wounds should be carefully assessed for evidence of blindness, as they are often shot when they are facing the gunman. Blind deer must be humanely destroyed.

Fox-snare and fence-wire wounds

These commonly affect the metacarpi or metatarsi and must be meticulously assessed to determine whether the vascular supply distal to the wound has been compromised. Deer that manage to escape from being caught in fences by degloving the distal limb invariably suffer sloughing of the limb distal to the site of the injury. If the vascular supply to the tissues below the wound has been lost, with cold soggy tissues and no bleeding to scalpel incision, the limb should be amputated and the deer released.

Foot-and-mouth disease

In the light of the 2001 outbreak of foot-and-mouth disease (FMD), it is worth noting that all British deer species are susceptible to FMD and that during the 2001 outbreak deer affected by oral and buccal lesions were encountered. It is also notable, however, that no positive laboratory confirmations of FMD in deer during the 2001 outbreak were reported, despite submission of samples from animals with typical signs.

In experimental infections lesions include typical oral, buccal, labial and lingual ulcers together with coronary band lesions. It is recognized that the smaller deer, particularly roe and muntjac, suffer severe morbidity with FMD and a large percentage of infected animals die. Those that recover do not become carriers. The larger deer (red, sika and fallow) suffer less severe disease but may carry the virus in the pharynx for at least 60 days.

Bacterial diseases

Enteritis

Deer may be presented with diarrhoea, for which several aetiologies are recognized. Systemic infection with *Yersinia* spp. is common in farmed deer and occasionally encountered in wild animals. Clinical signs include sudden death and peracute haemorrhagic diarrhoea, with concomitant dehydration and collapse. Severe intestinal parasitism is a problem where wild deer are grossly overstocked, for instance in some collections and within some 'deer refuges' provided to offer deer a sanctuary from hunting. Affected deer are usually thin, with a pasty, soft faecal consistency that results in soiling of the perineum (Dunn, 1983).

Much less common causes of diarrhoea include enterotoxaemia with *Clostridium perfringens* (which the author has encountered in wild roe), salmonellosis, Johne's disease (*Mycobacterium paratuberculosis*) and, in neonates, coliform enterocolitis (Fletcher, 1987).

Treatment: If a wild deer is presented with diarrhoea, it should receive appropriate rehydration by intravenous fluid administration and injections of oxytetracycline, since yersiniosis is the most likely bacterial cause of the enteritis. In addition, an injection of ivermectin should be given to eliminate parasites. Further therapy will depend upon response and laboratory investigation of the cause of the enteritis.

Tuberculosis

Acid-fast mycobacterial organisms are regularly recovered from wild deer tissues. Unlike domestic cattle and sheep, deer may succumb to severe disease because of infection with *Mycobacterium avium* as well as with *M. bovis*. Specific legislation covers tuberculosis in deer (the TB Deer Order), which makes the notification of suspicious infection mandatory.

Wild deer with TB are usually debilitated and may be found in an emaciated or collapsed condition. The author has also encountered muntjac with avian TB in good condition but recumbent and easy to catch. There are no specific external clinical signs but usually widespread internal abscessation is discovered.

Diagnosis:

Because TB in deer may form large abscesses with copious liquid pus, any internal abscess in a wild deer should give rise to suspicion of TB and samples should be forwarded to the Veterinary Laboratory Agency of DEFRA for examination.

More than 50% of *M. bovis* and *M. avium* infections in deer fail to stain by the Ziehl–Nielson technique. Negative ZN staining of tissues or pus is therefore not a reliable indicator that the abscess was not tubercular. Laboratory pathologists unfamiliar with deer are often not aware of this staining anomaly and the veterinary surgeon should insist upon culture of the tissues or pus, even if staining gives rise to a 'negative' TB report (Haigh and Hudson, 1993; Clifton-Hadley and Wilesmith, 1991).

The potential risk of TB in deer should alert the veterinary surgeon to adopt full precautions when performing post-mortem examinations of deer carcasses. The diagnosis is unlikely to be made in living deer, unless miliary lung lesions are revealed by radiography.

Johne's disease

Deer are also very sensitive to Johne's disease (*M. avium* subsp. *paratuberculosis*), which has a much swifter course than in cattle (McKelvey, 1987).

Septic arthritis

A common finding in casualty deer is evidence of severe arthritis, with massive periarticular exostosis and partial ankylosis of the affected joint (Figure 16.9). The author has isolated *Yersinia pseudotuberculosis* from a number of such joints and believes that the syndrome represents a non-pyogenic septic arthritis subsequent to haematogenous spread. Several joints are usually affected and the disease seems most common in muntjac, though it has also been encountered in fallow, roe and Chinese water deer. Swollen joints should be radiographed; severe cases of this condition have a radiological appearance that may suggest the disorganized repair of a fracture or dislocation. Some cases suffer collapse of affected joints, with consequent angular limb deformities.

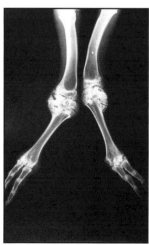

16.9 Dorsopalmar radiograph of forelimbs of a muntjac buck with severe carpal and metacarpophalangeal valgus secondary to septic arthropathy. Note the extensive proliferative carpal arthropathy, with destruction of the joint structure and production of new bone. *Yersinia* sp. was cultured from these joints. Enlarged or deformed joints in all deer species are more likely to be the result of this disease than of trauma. Affected animals should be euthanased.

There is no treatment and affected deer should be destroyed. The high percentage of road traffic casualties with this condition suggests that the debility of the arthropathy slows the animal down significantly.

Lyme disease
The association between deer, ticks and Lyme disease (borreliosis) has been noted. Clinical Lyme disease is most unlikely to be encountered in wild deer in Britain, though they may carry the organism.

Leptospirosis
Leptospirosis appears to be common among wild deer, based upon serological surveys, but clinical disease in wild animals is very rare (Fairley et al., 1984).

Ectoparasites
Most deer carry large numbers of external parasites, including ticks (*Ixodes* spp., *Dermacentor* spp., *Haemaphysalis* spp.), keds (*Lipoptena cervi*) and lice (*Bovicola* (*Damalinia*) spp., *Trichodectes* spp., *Solenoptotes* spp.). Muntjac have brought with them from China a host-specific louse, *Tricholipeurus indicus*, which is not found on any other British animal.

A routine injection of ivermectin will deal with these passengers. It may be considered that treatment of a low level of infestation is unnecessary.

Other conditions

Capture myopathy
Capture shock or exhaustion, also known as capture myopathy (CM), occurs in many wild artiodactyls and is always a risk when wild deer are chased, herded, netted or manually restrained (McAllum, 1985). The pathogenesis is not clear but CM manifests as a range of conditions from acute fatal shock through to a very severe analogue of the exercise-induced myopathy (rhabdomyolysis) encountered in horses, and even muscle rupture. The condition is so common that it has been suggested that it is a natural, inherent mechanism to hasten death and reduce the pain of prey species after chase and capture by a predator (Spraker, 1993).

Symptoms: The three factors that appear to contribute most to the development of the condition are fear, overheating and excessive muscular activity (Spraker, 1984; Nielsen, 1999). Acutely affected animals may die rapidly before signs of muscle necrosis appear, within 6–8 hours of capture or restraint. These animals show signs of depression, tachypnoea, tachycardia, hyperthermia and then death. Postmortem examination reveals widespread focal necrosis of the skeletal muscles, heart, brain, kidneys, liver and endocrine organs. Grossly, there is congestion of the lungs, small bowel and liver. There may be bloody bowel contents. Other deer may become affected with ataxic myoglobinuria several hours or several days after the stressor event. Affected deer are ataxic or recumbent, often hyperthermic and hyperventilating, and may show evidence of seizure or disorientation. There may be torticollis.

Serum creatine kinase and aspartate aminotransferase will be massively elevated, though care must be exercised in interpretation, because severe soft tissue trauma may have the same effect. A useful indicator of CM is a concomitant elevation of blood urea nitrogen (BUN). Myoglobinuria is common. Postmortem findings are similar to those for acute shock syndrome, with the addition of massive severe muscle necrosis and degeneration.

Deer in such an advanced state of myopathy that they cannot move have a hopeless prognosis, as secondary renal failure will be inevitable. Mild cases, with clinical signs of stiffness but an ability to rise and move about, may survive but there is a difficult cost/benefit balance to be assessed in the consideration of treatment, since further handling of the deer may stress the animal and worsen the condition to a fatal degree.

The final manifestation of the CM syndrome is rupture of the gastrocnemius/semimembranosus muscles on the caudal aspect of the thighs. This gives rise to a hunched and crouching posture with hock hyperflexion and may manifest several days after capture or manual handling. Most of these deer die a lingering death or, if they survive, are permanently crippled. Euthanasia should be considered early.

Prevention: Prevention of CM must be carefully considered when wild deer are to be caught. Chasing should be kept to a minimum, capture on hot days should be avoided and stress kept to a minimum by rapid blindfolding, quiet human activity and keeping the deer cool with water sprays if necessary. Deer casualties may have signs of CM in addition to their primary presenting condition. Unfortunately, there is some evidence that sedation (particularly alpha-2 adrenergic agonists and opioids) increases the incidence of CM, because of interference with thermostasis and hypotension.

Treatment: Once CM is apparent, treatment consists of large doses of glucocorticoid (e.g. dexamethasone 5 mg/kg, soluble methylprednisolone 20 mg/kg) dissolved in 5% glucose + 0.9% sodium chloride in water and given intravenously at a rate of 25 ml/kg bodyweight for the first 30 minutes, then at a reduced flow rate of 10 ml/kg/h. The addition of multivitamins, sodium bicarbonate, dimethylsulfoxide, non-steroidal anti-inflammatories and other systemic drugs appears to have little effect upon the outcome. In the author's experience, established CM is an unrewarding condition to treat.

Liver tumours
Scottish roe deer regularly suffer dramatic liver tumours, which may or may not affect their condition. The author has encountered these on routine postmortem examination more frequently than in living deer (Munro, 1991).

Therapeutics

Figure 16.10 gives details of some therapeutic drugs used for deer.

Drug	Dosage	Indications
Antibiotics		
Oxytetracycline LA	20 mg/kg i.m., once only	Wounds
Oxytetracycline 5%	10 mg/kg i.m., 5-day course	Enteritis
Enrofloxacin	5 mg/kg s.c. sid for 3 days	Dog bites and gunshot wounds
Trimethoprim sulfa	20 mg/kg i.m.	Soft tissue sepsis
Anti-inflammatories		
Soluble dexamethasone	0.8 mg/kg i.m., i.v.	Gluconeogenic and anti-inflammatory
Soluble dexamethasone	5 mg/kg i.v.	Capture myopathy with i.v. fluids and glucose
Soluble methylprednisolone	20 mg/kg i.v.	Capture myopathy with i.v. fluids and glucose
Anthelmintic		
Ivermectin	400 µg/kg s.c.	Internal and external parasites
Analgesics/NSAIDs		
Carprofen	1 mg/kg i.v. every 48 hours	Analgesia for trauma
Flunixin	2 mg/kg i.v. sid	Analgesia for trauma

16.10 Therapeutics for deer.

Management in captivity

Under the terms of the Deer Act 1991, special consideration must be given to certain aspects of the removal of deer from a site and their subsequent release. These are discussed below under 'Legal aspects'.

Housing of adults

The optimum accommodation for deer is a small low shed with straw or hay on the floor. For small deer, and juveniles of the large species, the maximum dimensions are 1.5 m x 1.8 m with a roof height of no more than 1.8 m. For large deer, a shed no bigger than 3 m x 2 m is suitable. There should be no windows, but good ventilation through slits at the top of the walls. Ideally, the door should comprise the whole of one wall, divided into a stable-door arrangement but with the top portion only 0.5 m high. The entire door should swing inwards so that it can be used as a swinging crush to restrain deer that are standing; the top portion can then be opened to allow access to the deer from above. Other traditional sheds may be dangerous, as deer will jump towards the light when the door is opened.

If an outdoor pen is provided, it should be sufficiently large to allow the deer to hide in undergrowth or within straw-bale shelters, otherwise the deer will crash about within the enclosure. The minimum for adult large deer is 20 m x 20 m, and for small deer 10 m x 10 m. The fence should be at least 3 m high for larger species or 2 m for small deer and should be constructed of tensile deer-fence mesh, which allows deer to bounce off if they panic and rush at the fence. The author has used several enclosures constructed in woodland within a few miles of the clinic for the convalescence of deer casualties, in areas where deer of the same species are known to exist. This greatly aids future release. With the cooperation of gamekeepers, pheasant release pens may be used out of season for muntjac, roe and Chinese water deer.

Feeding of adults

All deer prefer succulent food. Although fallow and red deer will eat grass and hay, the provision of grazing, cut grass or hay will not be sufficient for a confined or convalescing wild deer. The large species should be provided with hay and bulk succulent foods such as cabbages, fodderbeet, turnips or feed potatoes. In addition, small deer will need regular supplies of foliage, twigs and shoots. Favourites include ivy (*Hedera* spp., which is not poisonous to deer) and brambles (*Rubus fruticosus* agg., though there are more than 2000 closely related microspecies of bramble with complicated taxonomy and some are much more palatable than others). Leaves of hawthorn (*Crataegus monogyna*), blackthorn (*Prunus spinosa*), hazel (*Corylus avellana*), willow (*Salix* spp.) and wild cherry (*Prunus avium*) are readily consumed. Seasonal fruits such as crab apples (*Malus sylvestris*), horse chestnut conkers (*Aesculus hippocastanum*) and beechmast (*Fagus sylvatica*) are also eaten. Most deer can be weaned on to a proprietary coarse mix for goats, but some succulent food must always be available.

As a guide to optimum intake, an adult red deer needs 2–3 kg dry matter intake per day, which is equivalent to perhaps 12 kg of succulent food and hay. Small deer such as muntjac need less than 10% of this.

Rearing of orphans

Neonates that cannot be returned to the wild pose a real dilemma for the veterinary surgeon. Before embarking upon the intensive labour of orphan-rearing, it is advisable to make enquiries of local wildlife parks or private zoological collections to see whether a long-term home for the deer can be arranged. Male deer in particular do not make suitable pets or even semi-domesticated farm animals, since they often become unpredictably violent and dangerous. Castration should be considered if it is

179

decided that a hand-reared deer must be preserved and it is absolutely essential that this is undertaken before any antler growth occurs (i.e. before puberty), otherwise bizarre persistent pathological antler growth may occur (Wislocki *et al.*, 1947). In the author's opinion, castration and captivity present a more inhumane alternative to euthanasia for male deer.

Feeding orphans

Deer milk is considerably higher in protein and fat than cow's milk but has lower lactose content. A suitable deer milk replacer can be made up by adding one whole egg, 5 ml cod liver oil and 20 g glucose to 1 litre of full-cream cow's milk. For very young deer this must be fed every 3–4 hours at 37°C.

An orphan neonatal deer should be fed from a lamb bottle (in the case of the larger species) or a human-baby bottle (for the smaller species). A cross-slit in the teat is best. At each feed the anal region should be massaged with a wet warm tissue to stimulate defecation. If the young deer is obstinate, dehydrated or collapsed, intravenous fluids and milk substitute by stomach tube must be given, using a lamb tube, until the suck reflex returns.

Healthy young deer will nibble succulent foods from 1 week old but will not be fully weaned from the milk until they are at least 10 weeks old. Assessing the age of a baby deer is very difficult for the inexperienced veterinary surgeon and the procedure must be based rather on guesswork. Some orphan deer have been successfully persuaded to feed from a bowl or bucket, which enables the amount of human contact to be minimal and the prospect of release more realistic.

Release

Whenever possible, casualty deer should be released soon after treatment and at the place from which they were originally taken. It is, however, illegal to release muntjac into the wild, as they are subject to the restrictions of Schedule 9 of the Wildlife and Countryside Act (see Chapter 5); they may only be released under licence and then only within certain counties of England and within 1 km of where they were found. This adds to the difficulty of wild deer treatment and rehabilitation and adds weight to the principle of field treatment at the scene of the casualty and immediate release. Under such circumstances, the deer will not have been 'taken' from the wild and the veterinary surgeon is unlikely to fall foul of the law.

If adult deer are to be released after treatment they should be taken to an open woodland glade or ride, with thick cover nearby, and released either by opening the crate or by removing first the mask and then the wrapping and hobbles as one or two assistants restrain the animal by holding its head and draping themselves across its body. When all ties have been removed, the assistants should roll away to let the deer rise and run to cover.

Simply leaving the gate open and continuing to feed the animal less and less as it explores the surroundings may rehabilitate a deer confined to enclosures in woodland.

Legal aspects

The Deer Act (1991) consolidated earlier legislation and strictly controls the methods and seasons during which deer may be 'taken' from the wild in England, Wales and Northern Ireland. Similar laws exist in Scotland. Under these laws, it is an offence, without the consent of the owner or other lawful authority, intentionally to take, kill or injure deer, or to enter the land with the intention of taking, killing or injuring deer and to remove a deer carcass from the land. Even with the consent of the owner or lawful authority, it is an offence to take deer during the close seasons (basically spring through to autumn for both sexes of red, fallow and sika and for roe does; or from autumn through to spring for roe bucks). It is also an offence to kill deer in England and Wales with a rifle of calibre of less than .240 inch or muzzle energy of less than 2305 joules, or with an air weapon, crossbow arrow, spear or smooth-bore shotgun. In Scotland the prohibited firearms are defined entirely by reference to ballistics, not to calibre. In all parts of the UK it is an offence to 'take' wild deer by the use of 'poison, stupefying drug or muscle relaxant'. It is illegal to 'take' deer at night (between 1 hour after sunset and 1 hour before sunrise).

Fortunately, there are exemptions to this legislation that permit the veterinary surgeon engaged in wild deer work to treat casualties and for veterinary surgeons and deer farmers to pursue their normal duties. Close season and night-time 'taking' restrictions are waived if the purpose of taking the deer is to relieve suffering. In such circumstances a trap or net may be used. Strictly speaking, the use of 'poison' (which may be taken to include sedatives and tranquillizers) remains illegal under these circumstances. Any calibre or type of firearm may be used to destroy a deer to relieve suffering. If the deer is not suffering, it is illegal in England and Wales to 'take' a deer from one place and release it in another, without the issue of a licence granted by English Nature. Under section 14(1) of the Wildlife and Countryside Act it is an offence to release or to allow to escape into the wild any animal that is of a kind not ordinarily resident in, and not a regular visitor to, Great Britain in a wild state or to release or allow to escape any animal included in Part 1 of Schedule 9 of the Act (this includes sika and muntjac deer). See Harris and Jeffries (1991) and Chapter 5. Marking of deer, for example with ear-tags, requires a licence from English Nature.

Specialist organizations

British Deer Society
Burgate Manor, Fordingbridge, Hants SP6 1EF

Deer Commission for Scotland
Knowsley, 82 Fairfield, Inverness IV3 5LH

Northern Ireland Deer Society
Laurel Bank, Rugby Avenue, Newry Road, Banbridge, Co Down BT32 3NA

British Deer Farmers Association
Old Stoddagh, Penruddock, Penrith CA11 0RY

Veterinary Deer Society
7 Mansfield Street, London W1M 0AT

References and further reading

Adams JL (1979) Innervation and blood supply of the antler pedicle in red deer. *New Zealand Veterinary Journal* **27**, 200–201

Alexander TL and Buxton D (eds) (1994) *Management and Diseases of Deer*. Veterinary Deer Society, London

Antony-Davis T (1983) Antler asymmetry caused by limb amputation and geo-physical forces. In: *Antler Development in Cervidae*, ed. RD Brown, pp. 223–230. Caesar Kleberg Wildlife Research Institute

Chapman NG, Claydon K, Claydon M and Harris S (1987) Techniques for the humane capture of free living muntjac deer (*Muntiacus reevesi*). *British Veterinary Journal* **143**, 35–43

Clifton-Hadley RS and Wilesmith JW (1991) Tuberculosis in deer: a review. *Veterinary Record* **129**, 5–12

Cooper JE, Harris S, Forbes A, Chapman NG and Chapman DI (1986) A comparison of xylazine and methohexitone for the chemical immobilisation of Reeves muntjac (*Muntiacus reevesi*). *British Veterinary Journal* **142**, 350–357

Dunn AM (1983) Winter deaths in red deer: a preliminary report on abomasal parasites. *Publication of the Veterinary Deer Society* **1**(5), 17–23

Fairley RA, Schollum LM and Blackmore DK (1984) Leptospirosis associated with serovars hardjo and Pomona in red deer calves (*Cervus elaphus*). *New Zealand Veterinary Journal* **32**, 76–78

Fletcher J (1987) Veterinary aspects of deer management: disease. *In Practice*, May, 94–97

Fletcher J (1994) Sedation and immobilisation. In: *Management and Diseases of Deer*, eds TL Alexander and D Buxton, pp. 37–41. Veterinary Deer Society, London

Haigh JC and Hudson RJ (1993) *Farming Wapiti and Red Deer*. Mosby, St Louis, Missouri

Harris S and Jeffries DJ (1991) Working within the law: guidelines for veterinary surgeons and wildlife rehabilitators on the rehabilitation of wild mammals. *British Veterinary Journal* **147**, 1–17

Jackson JE (1980) The annual diet of the roe deer (*Capreolus capreolus*) in the New Forest, Hampshire, determined by rumen content analysis. *Journal of the Zoological Society of London* **192**, 71–83

Jalanka HH (1993) New alpha2adrenoceptor agonists and ant-agonists. In: *Zoo and Wild Animal Medicine: Current Therapy*, ed. ME Fowler, pp. 477–481. WB Saunders, Philadelphia

Jones DG (1994) Clinical biochemical reference ranges. In: *Management and Diseases of Deer*, eds TL Alexander and D Buxton, pp. 229-235. Veterinary Deer Society, London

Jones DM (1984) Physical and chemical methods of capturing deer. *Veterinary Record* **114**, 109–112

Kay RNB (1994) Blood composition. In: *Management and Diseases of Deer*, eds TL Alexander and D Buxton, pp. 229–235. Veterinary Deer Society, London

Knox DP, McKelveey WAC and Jones DG (1988) Blood biochemical reference values for farmed red deer. *Veterinary Record* **122**, 109–112

McAllum HJF (1985) Stress and post capture myopathy in red deer. In: *Biology of Deer Production*, eds PF Fennessy and KR Drew, pp. 65–72. Royal Society of New Zealand Bulletin **22**

McKelvey WAC (1987) Johne's disease in deer. *Publication of the Veterinary Deer Society* **2**(6), 24–28

Munro R (1991) Observations on ten liver cell tumours in Scottish roe deer. *Publication of the Veterinary Deer Society* **5**(1), 29–32

Nielsen L (1999) *Chemical Immobilisation of Wild and Exotic Animals*. Iowa State University Press, Ames, Iowa

Parkes C and Thornley J (2000) *Deer: Law and Liabilities*. Swan Hill Press, Shrewsbury

Putman R (1988) *The Natural History of Deer*. Christopher Helm, Bromley

Spraker TR (1984) An overview of the pathophysiology of capture myopathy and related conditions that occur at the time of capture in wild animals. In: *Chemical Immobilisation of North American Wildlife*, eds L Nielsen *et al.*, pp. 83–118. Wisconsin Humane Society, Milwaukee

Spraker TR (1993) Stress and capture myopathy in artiodactylids. In: *Zoo and Wild Animal Medicine: Current Therapy*, ed. ME Fowler, pp. 481–488. WB Saunders, Philadelphia

Stocker L (2000) *Practical Wildlife Care*. Blackwell, Oxford

Wilson PR (1983) Observations of a long acting formulation of oxytetracycline in red deer. *New Zealand Veterinary Journal* **31**, 75–77

Wislocki GB, Aub JC and Waldo CM (1947) The effects of gonadectomy and the administration of testosterone proprinate on the growth of antlers in male and female deer. *Endocrinology* **40**, 220–224

17

Marine mammals

James Barnett and Ian Robinson

Introduction

British marine mammals primarily belong to two groups: cetaceans and pinnipeds. Cetaceans, in particular, are rarely seen by most veterinary surgeons in general practice and specialist advice should be sought at an early stage of involvement with them.

The order Cetacea can be divided into two sub-orders: the Mysticeti (baleen whales) and the Odontoceti (toothed whales, dolphins and porpoises). The identification and distribution of those species found around British coasts is considered in Figure 17.1.

The group Pinnepedia is not strictly an order, as there is considerable evidence to warrant its inclusion in the order Carnivora. This group includes three families: the Phocidae (true seals), Otariidae (sealions and fur seals) and Odobenidae (walrus). The two resident species of seal found in British coastal waters are phocids: the grey seal (*Halichoerus grypus*) and common or harbour seal (*Phoca vitulina vitulina*). Occasionally Arctic ice-breeding phocids are found, including the ringed seal (*Phoca hispida*), harp seal (*Phoca groenlandica*) and hooded seal (*Cystophara cristata*). There are no sealions or fur seals in European waters.

Species	Group	Size	Appearance	Distribution	Behaviour
Harbour porpoise (*Phocoena phocoena*) (Figure 17.2)	Coastal odontocete	Up to 1.8 m (0.67–0.9 m at birth, 0.9–0.95 m at weaning)	Dark grey dorsally, paler on flanks; no 'beak'; small rounded pectoral flippers, small central triangular dorsal fin	Widely distributed and resident	Solitary or small pods
Bottlenose dolphin (*Tursiops truncatus*)	Coastal and pelagic odontocete	Up to 4.0 m (0.98–1.3 m at birth)	Dark grey or brown dorsally, light grey flanks, white ventrally; short 'beak'; centrally placed fairly tall usually sickle-shaped dorsal fin	Resident locally (Moray Firth, Cardigan Bay, SW England)	Usually small pods < 25
Common dolphin (*Delphinus delphis*)	Pelagic odontocete	Up to 2.6 m (0.8–0.85 m at birth)	Dark grey dorsally, 'hour glass' pattern of yellow/tan/grey on sides; long 'beak'; centrally placed sickle-shaped or erect dorsal fin	Seen off Atlantic and Irish Sea coasts	Forms large schools, sometimes hundreds of individuals
Striped dolphin (*Stenella coeruleoalba*) (see Figure 17.5)	Pelagic odontocete	Up to 2.4 m (1.0 m at birth)	Black dorsally, white ventrally, black lines from eye to anus and eye to pectoral fins, white blazes from eye to dorsal fin and eye to tail; mid-length 'beak'; centrally placed; sickle-shaped or erect dorsal fin	Seen off Atlantic and Irish Sea coasts	Forms large schools, sometimes hundreds of individuals
Atlantic white-sided dolphin (*Lagenorhynchus acutus*)	Pelagic odontocete	Up to 2.8 m (1.08–1.12 m at birth)	Black dorsally, elongated yellow-ochre band on flanks extending back from upper edge of long white oval blaze; short thick 'beak'; large often erect sickle-shaped centrally placed dorsal fin	Prefers colder northern waters: seen N. Scotland to Shetland and Atlantic coasts	
White-beaked dolphin (*Lagenorhynchus albirostris*)	Pelagic odontocete	Up to 2.7 m (1.2–1.6 m at birth)	Black dorsally around base of dorsal fin, pale grey/white areas on upper flanks cranial to fin and caudally over back and tail stock; short thick often white 'beak'; large often erect sickle-shaped centrally placed dorsal fin	Prefers colder northern waters, seen N Scotland to Shetland, central North Sea and Atlantic coasts	

17.1 Cetacean species found around British coasts (largely after Evans, 1995). (continues) ▶

Species	Group	Size	Appearance	Distribution	Behaviour
Risso's dolphin (*Grampus griseus*)	Pelagic odontocete	Up to 3.3 m (1.2–1.5 m at birth)	Dark grey dorsally and on flanks, lightening with age to light grey, particularly on head; multiple scratches and scars; no 'beak'; tall sickle-shaped centrally placed dorsal fin	Some resident inshore groups, e.g. Isle of Man	
Long-finned pilot whale (*Globicephala melas*)	Pelagic odontocete	Up to 5.9 m (1.75–1.78 m at birth, 2.5 m at weaning)	Grey-black dorsally, grey/white patch on chin; square, bulbous head, no 'beak'; low sickle/flag-shaped dorsal fin set well forward	Seen off Atlantic and northern coasts	Can form large schools
Orca (*Orcinus orca*)	Pelagic odontocete	Up to 9.75 m (2.06–2.5 m at birth, 4 m at weaning)	Black with white belly extending on to flanks, throat and chin, white patch behind eye, grey saddle caudal to dorsal fin; conical head, no 'beak'; tall triangular erect dorsal fin in adult males, smaller and curved in females and juveniles	Seen off Atlantic and northern coasts	Usually small pods < 25
Minke whale (*Balaenoptera acutorostrata*)	Pelagic mysticete	Up to 8.5 m (2.6 m at birth, 4.5 m at weaning)	Dark grey to black dorsally, pale grey/white ventrally, white band on dorsal surface of pectoral flippers; tall sickle-shaped dorsal fin set two-thirds along back	Commonest mysticete in British waters, resident inshore locally, e.g. Isle of Man, W. Scotland, Shetland	Solitary or small pods < 5

17.1 (continued) Cetacean species found around British coasts (largely after Evans, 1995).

Ecology and biology

Cetaceans

Cetaceans are usually considered to be coastal or pelagic (oceanic) in range (Figure 17.1). Mysticetes feed on plankton, krill or small fish; they take large quantities of water into their mouths, expelling it through the hairy plates of keratinous baleen that have replaced their teeth and retain any prey. Odontocetes hunt fish and squid, primarily using echolocation (see below).

Single births are normal and maternal care is highly developed. Lactation periods range from 4 months in the minke whale to 22 months in the pilot whale. The learning of life skills during prolonged lactation is considered critical for survival, throwing doubt on the wisdom of attempting to rehabilitate unweaned orphans. Harbour porpoises (Figure 17.2) strand more frequently as dependent calves than do other species: the calves are born mainly in June and July and suckle for 7–10 months.

Seals

The identification, distribution, behaviour and pup development of the two resident seal species are outlined in Figure 17.3. Both species moult annually. Pupping, mating and moulting take place in quick succession, with delayed implantation ensuring a 12-month pupping interval.

Grey seals travel long distances on feeding trips, often far out to sea, before returning to rest socially on traditional haul-out sites. Common seals (Figure 17.4) do not tend to disperse as widely but feed and haul out in the same area throughout the year.

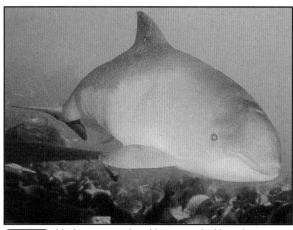

17.2 Harbour porpoise. Note rounded head, small rounded pectorals and triangular dorsal fin. (Courtesy of Florian Grana, International Fund for Animal Welfare.)

Grey seal pups are born with a long coat of creamy white hair ('lanugo'); they are able to swim but do not routinely take to the water. Breeding requires permanent land that is protected from disturbance, such as uninhabited islands and inaccessible coves, caves or beaches. The pups are abandoned by their mother at weaning and then undergo a period of starvation before taking to sea, by which time they have moulted completely. After weaning, they may lose more than 25% of their bodyweight while they learn to forage.

Common seals are adapted to life in the intertidal zone. The pups lose their white coat *in utero* and follow their mother into the water shortly after birth; thus they can be born below the high-tide line.

Species	Size	Appearance	Distribution	Feeding	Development of young
Grey seal (*Halichoerus grypus*) (see Figure 17.18)	Male up to 350 kg and 2.5 m Female up to 150 kg and 1.8 m	Coat colour generally darker in male Both sexes long muzzle (convex in adult male)	Exposed coasts and islands of Scotland, E and SW England, SW and N Wales	Range of fish (particularly sand eels), crustaceans and shellfish	Usually born July–January (earliest in SW England, latest in E England and Scotland) Birthweight 13–14 kg, length approx. 95 cm Born with 'lanugo' coat; start to moult after 10–21 days Weaned 16-21 days; typical weaning weight 45–55 kg (unlikely to survive first year if weaned at less than 35 kg male, 25 kg female)
Common or harbour seal (*Phoca vitulina vitulina*) (see Figure 17.4)	Males up to 120 kg, 1.8 m Females up to 100 kg, 1.5 m	Coats generally paler than grey seal but appear darker when wet Short muzzle and distinct stop in forehead	Sheltered coasts and estuaries of Scottish mainland and islands, Wash and E England coast, E coast of N Ireland	Diet similar to grey but also small flatfish and whelks	Birthweight 10–11 kg, length approx. 85 cm Lose white lanugo coat *in utero* Suckle 3–4 weeks; weaned abruptly at 20–30 kg

17.3 Resident pinniped species of the British Isles.

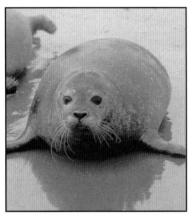

17.4 Common seal pup, in good body condition, being released into the Wash. (Courtesy of Anglian Newspapers Ltd.)

Anatomy and physiology

Cetaceans and seals have no intra-abdominal or intra-muscular fat. Instead, all fat is stored in a thick subcutaneous layer, the blubber. Blubber provides insulation and aids streamlining. Countercurrent heat-exchange systems in the flippers, flukes and fins control heat loss to the periphery.

Cetaceans achieve laminar flow over their smooth skin, lubricated by the continual shedding of epithelial cells and oil droplets. They propel themselves by vertical movement of the broad flat fibrous tail fluke. Seals flex the caudal spine and hind flippers laterally, spreading their webbed digits. Pectoral and fore flippers are used for steering and balance.

The nares ('blowholes') of cetaceans are on top of the head; they are single in odontocetes and paired in mysticetes. Cetaceans inhale before diving and exhale explosively on resurfacing, before immediately inhaling. Seals exhale on diving. In both, alveoli collapse at depth, the obliquely set diaphragm pushing air into non-absorbable air spaces. This prevents the occurrence of decompression sickness, where nitrogen absorbed into the circulation, under pressure at depth, comes out of solution as bubbles on surfacing. Marine mammals have a large oxygen storage capacity, with a relatively large blood volume, large red blood cells with a high haemoglobin content, and a high concentration of muscle myoglobin. During long dives, deoxygenated blood is pooled in large venous sinuses and there is pronounced bradycardia. Remaining oxygenated blood is diverted solely to nervous tissue and heart, while muscles respire anaerobically.

Marine mammals obtain water from food, as both free and metabolic water, and through the oxidation of fat in fasting animals. Water conservation and salt balance are ensured by production of concentrated urine and by restricted ingestion of sea water.

The eyes of marine mammals are adapted to low light intensities. The elastic lens of cetacean eyes allows effective focusing in water and air. The less elastic spherical lens of seals allows effective focusing underwater, but they suffer from astigmatism above water. Pupillary constriction corrects this in bright sunlight but vision is blurred in dim light. The cornea of marine mammals is heavily keratinized. A continually produced tear film also provides protection; it is particularly viscous in cetaceans. There are no functional nasolacrimal ducts and so tears continually overflow.

Marine mammals have well developed directional hearing underwater. Odontocetes also use 'echolocation': high-frequency clicks, emitted from the upper nasal passages, are focused by the 'melon' (fat pad in front of the skull) and, on being reflected, are received probably by the mandible and transmitted to the middle ear. Seals use sensitive vibrissae to detect vibrations and 'feel' their way along the seabed. They have a sigmoid flexure in the neck and can hunt in water of zero visibility by swimming with the neck flexed and suddenly extending it when vibration is detected.

Capture, handling and transportation

Health and safety aspects of handling

A wide range of potentially zoonotic bacteria may be carried by marine mammals, and even young seal pups are capable of delivering a nasty bite. Adult seals, particularly greys, have the potential to be very dangerous. Zoonotic infections include:

- *Brucella maris*: isolated from cetaceans and seals (Ross *et al.*, 1996) – may cause headaches, lassitude and severe sinusitis in humans (Brew *et al.*, 1999)
- Seal pox: isolated from seals – may cause skin nodules in humans (Hicks and Worthy, 1987)
- *Mycoplasma*: isolated from seals – may infect bite wounds in humans ('seal finger'); tetracyclines are the treatment of choice (Baker *et al.*, 1998)
- Opportunistic bacteria: isolated from cetaceans and seals – may infect humans via inhalation or contamination of wounds.

Capture and handling methods

Cetaceans

- To reduce lung compression, the animal should be supported in sternal recumbency
- Smaller animals, if necessary, can be moved in a tarpaulin, with the pectoral flippers folded ventrocaudally against the body
- Support on uncomfortable substrates can be provided with an air mattress or foam (Figure 17.5)
- Lifting by the dorsal fin, flippers or tail should be avoided
- Animals too large to move should be made comfortable, with shade and support, until the tide comes in; if available, a pontoon can be used for support (Figure 17.6).

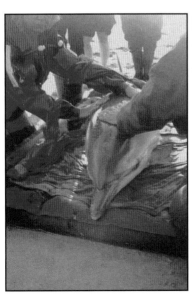

17.5 Striped dolphin supported on an air mattress. (Courtesy of British Divers Marine Life Rescue.)

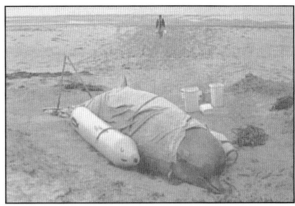

17.6 Northern bottlenose whale supported in a pontoon. (Courtesy of Gavin Gerard, Marine Mammal Rescue Team.)

Seals

- Seals weighing up to 50 kg (less if the handler is inexperienced) can be caught by covering their head with a towel and grasping the neck with both hands, just behind the head (seals can markedly extend their necks). The pup is then rolled on to its stomach and straddled
- Larger seals can be restricted against a solid barrier with a herding board for minor examination and sedation. Sedation is needed for more detailed procedures.

Transport requirements

Legal requirements should be borne in mind before transporting a marine mammal (see Chapter 5).

Cetaceans

- Transport is stressful and should only be carried out if absolutely necessary
- Journey times should be minimized and certainly should not exceed 2 hours
- The animal should be supported on an air mattress or foam
- Adequate temperature control (see 'First aid procedures') and ventilation are essential
- Poor transport can induce muscle damage and predispose to respiratory infections.

Seals

- Pups should be transported in cages, sky kennels, stretchers, or any suitable container with a secure cover
- Ventilation and temperature control are essential
- Older pups and adults in reasonable body condition are prone to overheating and should be sprayed regularly with water and bedded on damp towels
- Adult seals require purpose-built crates or cages, but loose transport in a horsebox is feasible.

Examination and assessment for rehabilitation

Cetaceans

Stranded cetaceans fall into one of three categories:

- **Candidates for reflotation** (i.e. release after a short period of treatment on the beach of origin or close by) include any weaned individual in good body condition (Figure 17.7), with no evidence of significant clinical disease or trauma, or with dehydration that is considered rapidly reversible. With prompt action, reflotation is a viable option primarily for pelagic species, which often strand in a healthy state through navigational error. It should be remembered that such animals might become severely compromised by the stranding event itself

- **Candidates for rehabilitation** may include any weaned individual in suboptimal bodily condition (but not emaciated) (Figure 17.7), or with evidence of disease or significant trauma that may respond to a limited period of care in captivity. Rehabilitation has been little used in the UK since 1995, as there is a lack of suitable facilities and successes have been few

- **Candidates for euthanasia** are those individuals that are emaciated (Figure 17.7) or showing evidence of severe disease or trauma carrying a poor prognosis, and dependent calves. As rehabilitation is not a viable option, candidates for euthanasia also include animals with any disease, trauma or condition loss likely to compromise their welfare and survival after reflotation.

Adoption of a two-option strategy in the UK does not appear to have hindered decision-making on the beach. A clinical triage to aid veterinary surgeons with this and the assessment of stranded cetaceans has been produced by veterinary surgeons of the Marine Animal Rescue Coalition (Baker *et al.*, 2000). The triage is reproduced, in part and modified, in Figure 17.8.

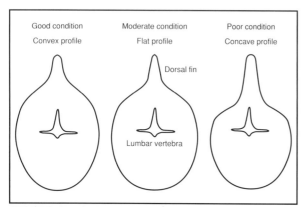

17.7 Lumbar muscle profile as an indicator of condition in cetaceans. (Courtesy of Mary-Ann Barnett; reproduced with kind permission of *In Practice*.)

1. Determine whether the animal is alive or dead.	
Small and medium sized cetaceans	Look for opening and closing of the blowhole
Big whales	May hold breath for up to 20 minutes, so (carefully) assess corneal and other reflexes (see below)
2. Determine whether any abnormal behaviour was observed before stranding.	
Abnormal behaviour	Twitching, muscle tremors, pronounced and sustained lateral or ventral flexion, listing, lack of responsiveness ± movement
May take several hours to correct. If it does not cease, the animal should be euthanased.	
3. Determine whether the animal was likely to be maternally dependent.	
Neonates	Umbilicus present; vibrissae may be present on maxilla
Older unweaned calves	With some species, dependent calves can be identified from length and season (see 'Ecology and biology'). May see lingual papillae
In the majority of cases, dependent calves will need to be euthanased, although, very occasionally, the mother may still be offshore.	
4. Assess the animal's body condition (see Figure 17.7).	
Poor condition	Lumbar muscles below dorsal fin concave. A visible neck may be present
Moderate condition	Lumbar muscles below dorsal fin flat
Good condition	Lumbar muscles below dorsal fin rounded
Animals in poor condition should not be refloated. Interpretation is complicated by a number of factors: blubber thickness is often season- and age-dependent and may be maintained despite atrophy of the underlying muscles. The shape of the animal may be distorted when beached, and animals in good body condition may, of course, be suffering from acute illness.	
5. Assess the extent of any injuries.	
Superficial trauma	Often occurs on stranding and is generally not clinically significant, despite often heavy bleeding
Significant injuries	Deeper wounds, penetrating the muscle layer, extensive abscesses or haematomas, fractures and dislocations
Animals with significant injury should not be refloated. Some significant injuries may be difficult to detect and the stress and trauma of stranding can cause significant muscle damage, which may not be clinically apparent.	

17.8 Clinical triage for stranded cetaceans (after Baker *et al.*, 2000). (continues) ▶

6. Assess degree of deterioration in skin condition due to being out of the water.

Signs of early skin deterioration	Wrinkling
Signs of more severe skin deterioration	Peeling, cracking and blistering

Animals with excessive skin loss should not be refloated, due to fluid loss and increased risk of secondary infection. Wind and high temperatures exacerbate deterioration.

7. Assess hydration.

Hydrated	Firm tone, no sponginess when hands placed against flanks
Dehydrated	Loss of tone, sponginess when hands placed against flanks

Dehydrated animals should not be refloated, unless easily corrected.

8. Assess muscle tone and reflexes.

Parameters to assess	Jaw and tongue tone, blowhole, flipper and palpebral reflexes
Poor reflexes and muscle tone	May be associated with shock and a decreased level of consciousness
Improvement in reflexes and muscle tone	May be seen with supportive treatment (oral fluids, intravenous steroids, etc.) and moving the animal into the water

If no reflexes or evidence of jaw and tongue tone are seen over the course of an hour, the animal should be euthanased.

9. Check for deep bleeding from anus, blowhole and mouth.

If these are seen, the animal should be euthanased.

10. Check for evidence of respiratory disease.

Signs of respiratory disease	Shallow respirations, strong-smelling exhalations, mucopurulent blowhole discharge, occasionally coughing and sneezing, adventitious lung sounds (only detectable in animals under 3 metres in length)

Animals with respiratory disease should not be refloated.

11. Determine the respiratory rate.

Small cetaceans e.g. harbour porpoise, common dolphin	2–5 breaths per minute: normal > 6 breaths per minute: mild stress or respiratory compromise > 10 breaths per minute: severe stress or respiratory compromise
Pilot whale	1 breath per minute: normal
Sperm whale	As low as 1 breath per 20 minutes: normal

If increased rate is due to stress, then removal of stressors should bring rate down in a few minutes. If due to hyperthermia, rate should come down quickly after extensive cooling. If no significant reduction is seen with time, the animal should not be refloated.

12. Determine gap between expiration and inspiration and assess capillary refill times.

Expiration–inspiration gap > 4 seconds	May be seen with respiratory disease, or with onset of shock
Capillary refill time > 2 seconds	May be seen with onset of shock
Improvement in expiration–inspiration gap and capillary refill times	May be seen with supportive treatment and moving the animal into the water

If no improvement is seen over the course of an hour, the animal should not be refloated.

13. If possible, take a rectal temperature.

36–37.5°C	Normal temperature
40–42°C	Critical. If no positive response to cooling, the animal should not be refloated
Above 42°C	Likely to be terminal: the animal should be euthanased

A standard digital thermometer can be used in animals under 50 kg. In larger animals, insert a thermistor probe at least 20 cm into the rectum, although a sealed digital thermometer securely attached to a length of stomach tubing may suffice. A positive response to cooling in hyperthermic animals is a good prognostic sign.

14. If possible, take a blood sample (see Figure 17.9).

Muscle enzymes	Check to see if significantly increased. Significant decrease in muscle enzymes may be seen with supportive treatment and moving the animal into the water – may take several hours to occur

If muscle enzymes remain significantly high despite supportive treatment and moving the animal into the water, the animal should not be refloated. Blood sampling site of choice: central tail veins, running near the midline of the ventral and dorsal surfaces of each tail fluke. Exceptions: can use caudal peduncle vein in very small animals (e.g. juvenile harbour porpoises) and, for safety in larger animals (pilot whales and upwards), the central arteriovenous complex in the midline of the dorsal fin (see Figure 17.9). N.B. Significant risk of necrosis distal to sampling sites. Needle sizes: see 'Therapeutics'. Reference ranges only available for the harbour porpoise (Koopman et al., 1995, 1999). Results (particularly from 'in practice' analysers) should be interpreted with caution. Serial bleeding during prolonged refloat may help indicate stability of condition. As speed of response is important, delaying refloat for results is not advisable.

17.8 (continued) Clinical triage for stranded cetaceans (after Baker *et al.*, 2000).

Mass strandings involve pelagic species with highly evolved social structures, such as long-finned pilot whales and Atlantic white-sided dolphins. Here, animals may strand with no evidence of significant infectious disease or trauma prior to the event (Mead *et al.*, 1980), or only one key animal is compromised (Rogan *et al.*, 1997). In other mass strandings, most animals involved have not been healthy at the time of intervention (Walsh *et al.*, 1990). Both reflotation and euthanasia may need to be carried out in any mass stranding event.

Clinical pathology

Blood collection is covered in the triage (see Figure 17.8) and collection sites illustrated in Figure 17.9. For other samples, blowhole swabs for culture are often of only retrospective use and bacteria that are cultured are not always representative (see Chapter 4). Blowhole swabs and discharges can also be examined for parasitic ova but false negatives may occur.

Methods of euthanasia

Large Animal Immobilon: Large Animal Immobilon (2.25 mg/ml etorphine and 10 mg/ml acepromazine; Novartis Animal Health) is injected intramuscularly at the following dose rates (RSPCA, 1997):

- Dolphins and porpoises: 0.5 ml per 1.5 m length
- Whales: 4.0 ml per 1.5 m length.

Ideally, injections should be given through the blubber into the lumbar muscles (see Figure 17.9). A 9 cm spinal needle (18 gauge) should be used in animals of over 2.5 m in length, but needles of up to 25 cm may be needed for large cetaceans. Injections with shorter needles should still prove effective, as the blubber layer is vascular. Blubber is fibrous and it is difficult to force in the liquid; care should be taken and the injection given over several different sites. In addition to considerations of public safety and disposal associated with its use, a marked excitatory phase may be seen prior to death, which can be distressing to onlookers. Prior administration of a sedative, e.g. diazepam, may help reduce the risk of this occurring.

Barbiturates: Barbiturates can be used intravenously (via blood sampling sites) or intraperitoneally in animals as large as pilot whales. Dose rates of 60–200 mg/kg are recommended (Greer and Rowles, 2000). Prior administration of a sedative, e.g. diazepam, is advisable before infusing large volumes in larger species.

Shooting: Animals under 3 m in length can be shot from close range through the blowhole, with a rifle of greater than .22 calibre, aiming towards a line midway between the pectoral flippers (RSPCA, 1997).

Large whales: As these are so difficult to euthanase, they may be best left to die naturally, which may be hastened by the animal's own bodyweight.

Seals

The majority of seals brought into care are pups, before or within a few months of weaning. As with other wildlife it is important to avoid unnecessary rescue of normal seal pups that are receiving maternal care. Similarly, recently weaned naïve pups may occasionally be brought into care unnecessarily. Seals breed seasonally in or close to colonies and so local knowledge is useful. If in doubt, the animal should be carefully observed *in situ* before the decision is made to rescue it.

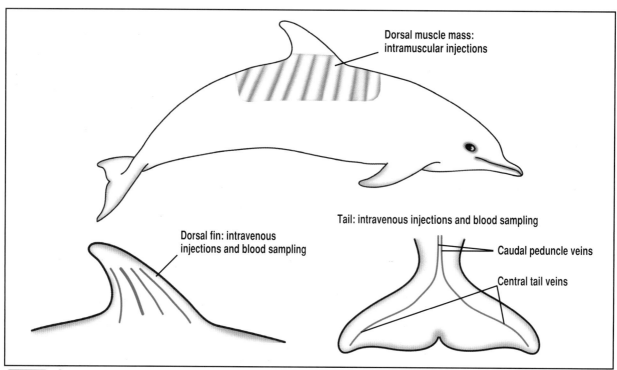

17.9 Cetacean injection and blood sampling sites. (Adapted from a drawing by Mary-Ann Barnett. Reproduced with kind permission of *In Practice*.)

Three options are available:

- Immediate release may be appropriate if the seal is weaned, healthy and well nourished, after allowing recovery from handling and transport.
- Malnourished, sick or injured seals should be transported to suitable rehabilitation facilities (see 'Specialist organizations').
- Animals in terminal condition should be euthanased.

Figure 17.10 contains a protocol for the clinical assessment of seal pups that are presented to the veterinary surgeon. Older seals can be assessed using the same guidelines but their nutritional state must be assessed without the help of specific guidelines for bodyweight. Seals that weigh over 50 kg may need sedation or anaesthesia to allow a full examination; adult male grey seals may weigh in excess of 200 kg.

1. Determine whether pup is dependent on mother.

Pups of less than 1 week old	Tend to have umbilicus (check this also for infection)
Older grey seal pups	Start to lose long white lanugo coat just before or around the time of weaning (16–21 days)
Older common seal pups	Usually lose lanugo coat *in utero*; time of weaning (3–4 weeks) difficult to determine

Dependent pups definitely require intervention (treatment in captivity prior to release).

2. If weaned, determine whether pup is at viable weight.

| Grey seals | Less than 35 kg (males) or 25 kg (females) at weaning – unlikely to survive to independence (Hall *et al.*, 2001) |
| Common seals | Minimum viable weaning weight probably around 18 kg for both sexes |

Seals weaned below these weights fail to thrive after weaning. Survivors weaned at adequate weight also undergo weight loss while learning to find food but eventually start to regain weight. Not really known how low pup's weight can drop during first year of life before becoming non-viable – decision cannot be based on weight alone, but requires physical and clinical assessment. Even emaciated pups will respond well to treatment and rehabilitation.

3. Assess condition.

Good condition	Visibly rounded, with no obvious bony protuberances
Emaciated	Distinct neck, pelvis and ribs, often with loose skin (NB pups below viable weight may not appear obviously thin)
Severely malnourished	May be hypoglycaemic, exhibiting muscle tremors and twitching

4. Assess alertness and demeanour.

Very young pups with fresh umbilicus	May seem thin, dull and unresponsive
Unweaned grey seal pups	Tend to be vocal
Unweaned common seal pups	Often quiet
Older pups, both species	Tend to be aggressive
Unresponsive pups	Withdrawal reflexes can be assessed; those that fail to respond to supportive therapy should be euthanased

5. Assess extent of any injuries (see 'Specific conditions').

| Minor abrasions and wounds | Clinically insignificant – heal readily; may not require intervention |
| Deeper infected wounds, abscesses and fractures | Will influence the option taken: pups with significant wounds should be treated and rehabilitated, unless likely to affect long-term viability or welfare in wild, in which case euthanasia is option |

6. Check skin for other lesions, particularly seal pox granulomas.

7. Check for evidence of respiratory disease.

Signs of respiratory disease	Mucoid or mucopurulent nasal, sometimes with ocular discharge, sneezing, coughing, dyspnoea and tachypnoea
Signs of pneumonia	As above plus dullness, pyrexia and audible lung sounds
Signs of parasitic pneumonia	Also often have wet productive cough, emphysema on auscultation, occasionally epistaxis and hypovolaemic shock

Lung auscultation complicated by forceful, irregular breathing pattern seen in healthy pups; normal rates 5–15 breaths/min. Pups with respiratory disease can be successfully treated and rehabilitated.

8. Assess cardiovascular function.

Murmurs	Associated with dehydration or, less frequently, congenital abnormalities, e.g. patent ductus arteriosus (may take up to 6 weeks to close physiologically; King, 1983)
Elevated heart rate	Sinus arrhythmia often found in healthy pups but heart rates consistently above 120 beats/min likely to be clinically significant
Pale mucous membranes	May be associated with hypovolaemic shock, peripheral vasoconstriction triggered by handling, or anaemia; assess in conjunction with capillary refill time

17.10 Clinical assessment protocol for seal pups. (continues) ▶

9. Carefully examine mouth and teeth, and manipulate mandible.	
Hyperaemia or ulceration of gums or hard palate	Relatively common finding; may not require intervention
Gingival regression and osteomyelitis	May be seen in severe cases; treatment and rehabilitation required
Teeth laxity, wear and fracture; symphyseal, and other fractures	Treatment and rehabilitation required
10. Examine eyes (see 'Specific conditions') and ears.	
Significant ocular lesions	Treatment and rehabilitation required
Aural discharge	Often persistent and unresponsive to antibiotic therapy; usually clears spontaneously with time
11. Assess hydration.	
Dehydrated pups	Dry mucous membranes and sunken eyes ('skin pinch' test unreliable, due to inherent skin elasticity); severely dehydrated pups should be treated
Hydrated pups	Tend to have 'tear stains' surrounding eyes due to absence of nasolacrimal ducts (King, 1983)
12. Check for diarrhoea.	
Parasitic causes	Heavy infestations of ascarids and acanthocephalans (may also see melaena); treatment and rehabilitation required
Bacterial causes	*Salmonella bovimorbifficans* (Robinson, 1995; see 'Specific conditions'); treatment and rehabilitation required
Stress-related causes	Handling and transport; intervention not necessary
13. Take rectal temperature.	
Normal temperature	36.0–37.2°C
Causes of hyperthermia	Include transport and handling, so not always a reason for intervention
Causes of hypothermia	Age (neonates), emaciation, critical illness; treatment and rehabilitation required

17.10 (continued) Clinical assessment protocol for seal pups.

Clinical pathology

Blood collection: Blood samples can be obtained from the extradural intravertebral vein, with the pup held in sternal recumbency. This vein is accessed via the L3/L4 intervertebral space, halfway between the last rib and the iliac crests (Figure 17.11). In pups under 25 kg, the space can be palpated and a 2.5–5 cm, 21 or 20 gauge needle can be used. In larger seals, the space is found by 'walking' a 6–9 cm, 20 to 18 gauge spinal needle over the vertebrae. Adults may need to be sedated for blood sampling if no suitable physical restraint (e.g. a crush cage) is available.

Blood samples clot rapidly and should be placed immediately in tubes containing standard anticoagulants (see Chapter 4). Samples can also be collected for retrospective serology. Hypoglycaemia in severely malnourished pups can be assessed quickly with blood glucose test strips or a glucometer. Haematology and biochemistry results can be compared with reference ranges (Figure 17.12).

Other samples: Nasal swabs are of limited use but laryngeal swabs may help to isolate underlying pathogens in bacterial pneumonia. Bacterial isolates from traumatic lesions may be clinically significant but faecal contaminants are a problem. Faeces can be screened for helminth ova (see also 'Lungworm') and subjected to bacterial culture.

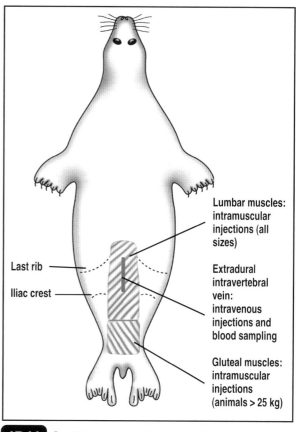

17.11 Seal injection and blood sampling sites.

Parameter	Common seal		Grey seal	
	Range	(No. samples)	Range	(No. samples)
Haemoglobin (g/dl)	15–26	(144)	17–24	(79)
Red blood cell count (10^{12}/l)	4–7	(134)	4–7	(78)
Packed cell volume (l/l)	0.45–0.70	(136)	0.45–0.70	(78)
Mean cell volume (fl)	90–125	(134)	90–130	(78)
Mean cell haemoglobin (pg)	30–45	(134)	30–50	(78)
Mean cell haemoglobin concentration (g/dl)	30–40	(136)	30–40	(78)
Reticulocytes (% RBC) [a]	0–8	(134)	0–4	(78)
Heinz bodies (% RBC) [a]	0–1	(130)	0–3	(79)
Total white blood cell count (10^9/l)	3–17	(142)	5–19	(79)
Neutrophil count (10^9/l)	2–11	(137)	2–12	(79)
Lymphocyte count (10^9/l)	0–5	(137)	0–6	(79)
Monocyte count (10^9/l) [a]	0–4	(137)	0–3	(79)
Eosinophil count (10^9/l) [a]	0–3	(139)	0–2	(79)
Basophil count (10^9/l) [a]	0–1	(139)	0–1	(79)
Platelet count (10^9/l)	80–740	(116)	180–780	(68)
Fibrinogen (g/l)	2–6	(109)	1–5	(66)
Total protein (g/dl)	50–90	(41)	50–90	(25)
Albumin (g/dl)	29–50	(41)	29–50	(25)
Urea (mmol/l)	7–23	(41)	7–22	(25)
Creatinine (μmol/l)	0–100	(41)	0–100	(25)
Alanine transaminase (IU/l)	0–200	(41)	0–100	(25)
Aspartate transaminase (IU/l)	0–500	(39)	0–200	(24)
Alkaline phosphatase (IU/l)	0–200	(41)	0–600	(25)
Gamma glutamyl transferase (IU/l)	0–80	(39)	0–100	(25)
Bilirubin (μmol/l)	0–10	(39)	0–10	(25)
Cholesterol (mmol/l)	4–8	(40)	4–10	(25)
Phosphate (mmol/l)	0.7–3.0	(41)	1.3–2.7	(24)
Sodium (mmol/l)	145–160	(38)	145–155	(25)
Potassium (mmol/l)	3.5–5.5	(38)	3.5–5.5	(25)

17.12 Haematology (adapted from Bennett *et al.*, 1991) and biochemistry (adapted from RSPCA Norfolk Wildlife Hospital) reference ranges for common and grey seals, originally calculated as mean ± 2 S.D. [a] Observed range

Other diagnostic aids

Radiography is useful, particularly in the assessment of injuries involving bone. Sedation or anaesthesia will be required. Ultrasound has been used to assess suspected cardiac problems.

Methods of euthanasia

Seals can be euthanased with intravenous (see 'Blood collection' and Figure 17.11) or intraperitoneal barbiturates. Canine dose rates are applicable and needles of up to 9 cm may be required.

Large seals *in extremis* on the beach can be shot from point-blank range with a free-bullet humane killer. If the seal cannot be shot from point-blank range, the provisions of the Conservation of Seals Act 1970 apply and a soft-nosed bullet of over 45 grains (i.e. 2.9 g) with a kinetic energy of at least 600 ft lb (i.e. 813 J) is needed. Under these circumstances, competent marksmen must be used.

First aid procedures

Cetaceans

In addition to the handling procedures already described, trenches can be dug under the pectoral fins to reduce cramping and overheating. Hyperthermia can be corrected by applying cool water; the tail stock appears to be an important site of heat dumping. Very cold water or ice on the flukes and fins, however, may cause peripheral vasoconstriction (T. Williams, personal communication). The skin can be kept moist with damp sheets, and obstetrical jelly or zinc oxide cream. Hypothermic individuals should be sheltered from the wind and covered with sheets soaked in mineral oil. Noise and disturbance should be minimized, though individual human contact and quiet talking may help to calm nervous animals.

Dehydration, a common finding in stranded animals, can be corrected with oral fluids. Proprietary oral rehydration solutions, Ringer's, Hartmann's and glucose–saline solutions have been used. Many small cetaceans open their mouths when a lubricated equine stomach tube is introduced, but towels can also be used to pull the jaws apart gently. After negotiating the central dorsally pointing larynx, the tube is passed to a point between the pectoral and dorsal fins to enter the stomach. Before fluids are passed, the animal is allowed to take a breath to ensure that the larynx has not been dislodged.

Due to the small size of the cetacean forestomach, fluids should be given at a maximum of 1% v/w, up to 1 litre for small cetaceans and, to minimize stress, no more frequently than every 6 hours. Oral rehydration of animals over 4 m in length is unlikely to be practicable. Intraperitoneal fluids have also been used (Sweeney, 1989).

Refloating

At the earliest opportunity, small cetaceans suitable for refloating should be carried into waist-deep water; larger animals can be refloated on the tide in a pontoon. The animal is supported with its blowhole above water, until control of breathing is regained, and rocked gently to alleviate any muscle stiffness or circulatory impairment and to help to restore equilibrium. Careful attention should be paid to the animal's behaviour and response to being in the water (see Step 2 of the triage in Figure 17.8). Handlers supporting cetaceans in the water are at risk from hypothermia and should keep clear of thrashing tails.

When the animal appears to be able to support itself and is making an effort to swim, it should be moved into deeper water to see whether it can swim unaided. If it can, it should be guided quietly seawards. Boats (and pontoons) can be used to take an animal further out to sea before final release. A successful refloat may take several hours to complete.

In mass strandings, ensuring adequate assessment and care for all individuals requires a high level of organization. Early detection and euthanasia of those unsuitable for refloating is required. Refloating involves amassing suitable candidates in sheltered shallow water and releasing them together when tidal and weather conditions are suitable (Needham, 1993).

Seals

Seal pups, particularly if malnourished, are usually dehydrated, and fluid therapy is given as a routine. With the pup restrained in sternal recumbency, proprietary oral rehydration solutions are given via a lubricated stomach tube (approximately 1 cm external diameter) at volumes of 100–200 ml for common seal pups and

150–250 ml for grey seal pups. Additional glucose can be given where hypoglycaemia is suspected, and tubing should be carried out every 3–4 hours. Severely debilitated pups can be given intravenous fluids (using blood sampling sites; see 'Blood collection' (above) and Figure 17.11). The tight application of the skin to the blubber layer makes it difficult to give adequate volumes subcutaneously but it can still be a useful technique. The intraperitoneal route is possible but sterility is always in question as the skin of the abdomen is in constant contact with contaminated surfaces. Hyperthermia and hypothermia should be corrected.

Oral rehydration of adult seals will be possible only in weaker animals. More lively adults can be encouraged to drink from a freshwater pool or hose, or fed fish injected with fluids. Intravenous fluids can be given to moribund individuals, or to animals sedated for examination.

Short-term hospitalization of seal pups

Housing

It is advisable to move all seals to appropriate rehabilitation facilities as soon as initial assessment and treatment have been completed. If this is not possible, seal pups at least can be housed for short periods. They should be isolated initially, to minimize stress and reduce the potential for disease spread. They can be kept without continuous access to swimming water, especially in the early stages of rehabilitation, but will benefit from daily exercise in water from an early stage. Small emaciated seals cannot maintain core body temperature in water and so must be given short 'floats' only and their body temperature carefully monitored. Supplementary heat and some floor insulation (e.g. rubber matting, towels) may be necessary. Access to water can be increased with clinical and physical progress. Larger seal pups that are thriving well may suffer from hyperthermia without access to water to cool down, though this can be provided in the short term by cold-hosing.

Feeding

After initial assessment and treatment, seal pups are given rehydration fluids at intervals of 3–4 hours throughout the first 24 hours. After 24 hours a liquid diet is gradually mixed with the rehydration fluid, in increasing proportions until the pup is on full-strength diet (see 'Rearing of seal pups'). The speed of transfer to liquid diet depends on the progress of the individual but on average takes 3–4 days. Volumes of feeds are initially small (see above) and build up to a maximum of 350 ml for common seals and 500 ml for grey seals over a period of 3–5 days.

Anaesthesia and analgesia

Cetaceans

Non-steroidal anti-inflammatory drugs (NSAIDs) at canine doses may help with analgesia and inflammation (see Figure 17.13). If these are used, the animal should not be refloated until any masking of clinical signs has worn off.

Intramuscular diazepam (see Figure 17.13) has been used to sedate cetaceans before transport to rehabilitation facilities but its use prior to refloating is not advisable. Most sedatives are contraindicated, due to their effects on respiration and thermoregulation (Sweeney and Ridgway, 1975).

Anaesthesia is not an option in the management of stranded cetaceans.

Seals

Figure 17.13 gives analgesics, sedatives and anaesthetic drugs that have been used in seals.

When anaesthetizing seals, premedication with atropine sulphate 20 μg/kg i.m. is advisable. Anaesthetized animals should be intubated immediately and given oxygen. Apnoea and bradycardia (as low as 2–3 beats per minute) may occur during anaesthesia, associated with physiological adaptations to diving. Even during light sedation of a seal, the operator should always be prepared to intubate and use intermittent positive pressure ventilation (IPPV) should apnoea and associated bradycardia occur. Thermoregulation may also be affected and rectal temperatures should be monitored. Anaesthesia can be prolonged with halothane or, preferably, isoflurane.

Drug	Dose rate; route in seals	Indications, side effects and comments	Use in cetaceans[a]
Analgesics/anti-inflammatories			
Carprofen	4 mg/kg i.m. sid; 2 mg/kg orally bid initially, reducing to sid after 7 days	Musculoskeletal disorders	2–4 mg/kg orally sid during rehabilitation
Meloxicam	0.2 mg/kg orally sid on day one, 0.1 mg/kg sid thereafter	Musculoskeletal disorders	
Ketoprofen	2 mg/kg i.m. sid (max. 3 days); 1 mg/kg orally sid (max. 5 days)	Musculoskeletal disorders, pneumonias Maximum 3–5 days' use, as risk of gastric ulceration	
Flunixin	1 mg/kg i.m. sid (max. 3 days)	Musculoskeletal disorders and pneumonias Maximum 3 days' use, as risk of gastric ulceration	1 mg/kg i.v. sid (max. 3 days) during reflotation and rehabilitation
Sedatives			
Medetomidine	50–100 μg/kg; i.m.	Light to heavy sedation in grey seal pups, lasting up to 1 hour; reverse with atipamezole (5 x medetomidine dose rate in mg; i.m.)	
Medetomidine and butorphanol	M: 20 μg/kg; i.m. B: 80 μg/kg; i.m.	Sedation of grey seal pups for radiography and ocular examination; reverse medetomidine with atipamezole (5 x medetomidine dose rate in mg; i.m.)	
Midazolam	0.5 mg/kg; i.v., i.m.	Light to moderate, 10–15 min sedation of adult seals and pups for minor procedures; premedication before induction of general anaesthesia with propofol or isoflurane	
Diazepam	0.1 mg/kg; i.v. (*not* i.m.)	Light to moderate sedation of adult seals and pups for minor procedures; premedication	0.15–0.2 mg/kg; i.m.; for transporting to rehabilitation facilities
Anaesthetics			
Medetomidine and ketamine	M: 60 μg/kg; i.m. K: 2.0 mg/kg; i.m.	Grey seal pups; up to 1 hour of anaesthesia	
Medetomidine, butorphanol and ketamine	M: 25 μg/kg; i.m. B: 100 μg/kg; i.m. K: 2.0–2.5 mg/kg; i.m., 15 min after M+B	Grey seal pups; up to 1 hour of anaesthesia	
Ketamine and midazolam	K: 6 mg/kg; i.m. M: 0.15 mg/kg; i.m.	Common and grey seals; induction agent or short periods of anaesthesia	
Tiletamine and zolazepam	Up to 1 mg/kg combined dose; i.m.	Field use primarily; sedation and light anaesthesia; not licensed for use in UK and not easily available to UK practitioners	
Propofol	5–6 mg/kg; i.v.	Induction agent; short periods of anaesthesia	
Isoflurane	To effect; masking down	Use with or without initial sedation in seals of any size, but handling can be problem for larger animals	

17.13 Analgesics, sedatives and anaesthetics: seals (sources: unpublished data; Baker *et al.*, 1990; Robinson, 1995; Barnett, 1998; Paul Riley and Richard Lucas, personal communications). [a]Sources for use in cetaceans: unpublished data; Sweeney (1989); Kastelein *et al.* (1997); RSPCA (1997); Barnett (1998).

Specific conditions

Cetaceans

As cetacean rehabilitation is generally not an option in the UK at present, prognosis is made on the basis of clinical signs in the stranded animal, rather than the diagnosis of specific conditions. Discussion of specific conditions will therefore be limited to seals.

Seals

Trauma

Seal pups may be bitten by other seals or dogs, pecked by gulls, or injured in rough seas and when caught in nets. Bites on the hindflippers often involve bones and joints; nets often cause deep wounds primarily cranial to the shoulders or pelvis (Figure 17.14). The latter may worsen initially, as the skin breaks down due to pressure necrosis. Pups with deep infected wounds, abscesses and fractures should be taken into rehabilitation facilities for treatment, or euthanased if their long-term viability or welfare will be compromised.

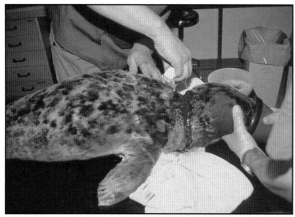

17.14 Encircling neck wound caused by monofilament netting in a grey seal pup. (Courtesy of Alison Charles, RSPCA Norfolk Wildlife Hospital.)

Soft tissue trauma and infection usually respond to regular topical flushing and debriding and to antibiotic therapy, which may need to be protracted if osteomyelitis is present in underlying bone. Suturing is usually contraindicated, but infected, exposed or fractured phalanges can be removed and digits amputated, using tension-relieving sutures through salvaged healthy tissue, to minimize the risk of dehiscence. Suturing may also be useful with deep net wounds, reducing the area that has to heal by secondary intention. Dressings readily become contaminated; animals have to be kept dry and changes are stressful. Liquid plastic dressings (e.g. Germolene Nu Skin) may be a useful alternative (Lucas *et al.*, 1999).

Seals with amputated digits appear able to swim and dive normally. A pup released in Holland after removal of an entire hindflipper was spotted in good condition several months later (SRRC Pieterburen, 1999).

Viral diseases

Morbillivirus: A morbillivirus caused thousands of deaths in predominantly common seals in Northern Europe in 1998 and again in 2002, largely through acute pneumonia. Signs include respiratory disease, subcutaneous emphysema of the head and neck and, less commonly, nervous signs. Diagnosis in live animals is by serology and virus isolation. Treatment involves supportive care, and trials with a modified live vaccine are ongoing in 2002. Survival rates, however, are poor.

Herpesvirus: Phocine herpesvirus can cause peracute viraemia, encephalitis, pneumonia, adrenocortical necrosis and hepatitis in seals admitted to rehabilitation units, associated with high morbidity and, in some cases, mortality, particularly in the very young. Signs of severe infections include nasal discharge, oral mucosal inflammation, vomiting, diarrhoea and pyrexia, coughing, anorexia and lethargy. Herpesvirus appears to be enzootic in the wild but is not commonly associated with serious disease. Diagnosis in live animals is by serology and treatment is supportive (Borst *et al.*, 1986; Robinson, 1995; Gulland *et al.*, 1997, Harder *et al.*, 1997).

Poxvirus: Seal pox is seen commonly in seal rehabilitation facilities: it infects both species but common seals appear to be less susceptible than greys. Lesions appear as raised circular granulomas, which may ulcerate, and pups may be incubating this highly infectious disease on arrival. Infection is confirmed with electron microscopy. Both orthopox and parapox virions are found and mixed infections do occur. Lesions regress typically within 8 weeks. Affected animals may suffer from pruritus and secondary bacterial infection; here, antibiosis may be justified. Rarely, pups develop a severe widespread infection. Seal pox has zoonotic potential, occasionally causing nodules on the fingers of handlers (Hicks and Worthy, 1987).

Bacterial diseases

Septicaemia: A number of bacteria associated with traumatic injuries and pneumonia may cause septicaemia, such as *Pseudomonas aeruginosa* and *Pasteurella haemolytica* (Barnett, 1998). With *Pseudomonas aeruginosa* in particular, a poor response to antibiosis may occur, due to antibiotic resistance; *P. aeruginosa* contamination and secondary infection of wounds and eye lesions in rehabilitation facilities are significant problems and can only be eliminated with strict hygiene and isolation procedures.

Diarrhoea: Diarrhoea commonly occurs with handling and transport in seals. *Salmonella bovimorbifficans* can also cause severe febrile diarrhoea, which generally responds to antibiosis (e.g. enrofloxacin) and symptomatic and supportive treatment. Diagnosis is by faecal culture.

Parasites

Lungworm: Two species of lungworm, *Parafilaroides gymnurus* and *Otostrongylus circumlitis*, infest seals. Both have intermediate hosts and therefore only weaned pups and adults tend to be infested. *P. gymnurus* infests the lung parenchyma and alveoli, causing oedema, inflammation, excessive mucus production and, occasionally, pulmonary and pleural haemorrhage; *O. circumlitis* infests the bronchial tree, causing obstruction. Larvae can be found in the sputum and faeces, and adult worms may be coughed up.

Treatment with anthelmintics may cause anaphylaxis and physical obstruction; pups should first be stabilized and then monitored carefully. Mucolytics, bronchodilators, anti-inflammatories and oral fluids are given to help to reduce side effects, and also antibiotics as bacterial pneumonia is often present. Ivermectin is the anthelmintic used most frequently but fatal side effects have been seen following its use in heavily parasitized common seal pups. Fenbendazole is a relatively safe alternative but treatments often need to be repeated.

Coccidiosis: *Eimeria phocae* can cause fatal dysentery in seal pups that are undergoing rehabilitation.

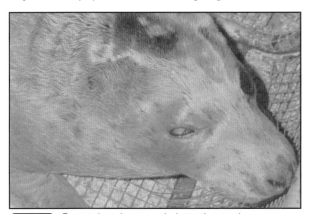

17.15 Corneal oedema and ulceration and blepharospasm in a grey seal pup. (Courtesy of Paul Riley, Head and Head Veterinary Surgeons.)

Diagnosis is confirmed by observing coccidial oocysts in the faeces of clinically affected animals. Prompt treatment with potentiated sulphonamides and supportive therapy, including rehydration, is essential. Outbreaks can be controlled by pen cleaning and water changes at least every 48 hours, i.e. under the likely sporulation time of the parasite (Munro and Synge, 1991).

Ocular conditions

Ocular conditions (Figure 17.15) include: corneal oedema; corneal ulceration (including melting ulcers with *Pseudomonas aeruginosa* infection); anterior uveitis; hypopyon; conjunctivitis; conjunctival or bulbar abscesses; and bilateral persistent pupillary membranes.

Treatment is usually topical and pups often have to be kept dry for long periods, which can be stressful. Subconjunctival injections of antibiotics, administered under sedation, can be used in intractable pups and adults. Non-responsive corneal ulcers have been managed with conjunctival pedicle grafts, protected by third-eyelid flaps. Severely traumatized and infected eyes, or those where glaucoma has developed, can be enucleated.

Loss of sight in one eye does not rule out release, as many such seals have been observed surviving well in the wild. This is also true of some totally blind adult seals but the release of a naïve blind pup into an unfamiliar environment would not be recommended.

Therapeutics

Cetaceans

Drugs used in the treatment of stranded cetaceans are listed in Figure 17.16. Many drugs used in animals taken into rehabilitation facilities are of limited use or, in some cases, contraindicated for animals to be refloated (e.g. anthelmintics). Due to considerable variation in the weight of animals encountered, allometric scaling of doses may be appropriate for larger animals (Kirkwood, 1983). Some weight-related doses are given in the literature (e.g. Sweeney, 1989).

| Drug | Cetaceans | | Seals | |
	Dose rate; route	Indications and comments	Dose rate; route	Indications and comments
Antibiotics				
Amoxicillin	15 mg/kg i.m. depot preparation as single injection	RF, RH	7 mg/kg i.m. sid	First choice broad-spectrum
	5–10 mg/kg orally bid, depending on size	RH	10 mg/kg orally bid	
Potentiated amoxicillin	12.5 mg/kg orally bid (double dose in refractory cases)	RH	12.5 mg/kg orally bid (double dose in refractory cases)	First choice broad-spectrum
	8.75 mg/kg i.m. sid		8.75 mg/kg i.m. sid	

17.16 Drugs used in treatment of cetaceans and seals. Sources: Unpublished data; Sweeney (1989); Stoskopf (1990); Robinson (1995); Kastelein *et al.* (1997); RSPCA (1997); Barnett (1998); Andrew Greenwood and Paul Riley (personal communications). RF: Refloated animals. RH: Animals taken into rehabilitation. SR: Used based on sensitivity results. (continues) ▶

| Drug | Cetaceans | | | Seals | |
	Dose rate; route	Indications and comments	Dose rate; route	Indications and comments
Antibiotics continued				
Clindamycin	8 mg/kg orally bid	RH	11 mg/kg orally bid	Abscesses, osteomyelitis, gum disease
Enrofloxacin	2.5–5 mg/kg orally sid 2.5–5 mg/kg i.m. sid	RH; may cause anorexia in some animals	5 mg/kg orally sid 5 mg/kg i.m. sid	Septicaemias
Gentamicin	2–3 mg/kg i.m. tid	RH	5 mg/kg i.m. bid on first day, sid thereafter	*Pseudomonas* infections
Cefalexin	20 mg/kg (wt < 500 kg) orally bid 15 mg/kg (wt > 500 kg) orally bid	RH RH	10–15 mg/kg orally bid	SR
Amikacin	4 mg/kg i.m. tid	RH		
Baquiloprim/ sulfadimethoxine			30 mg/kg orally every other day	SR; also effective against *Eimeria phocae*
Trimethoprim/sulfadiazine			30 mg/kg orally, i.m. sid	SR
Oxytetracycline	20 mg/kg i.m. (depot preparation)	RF	initially 50 mg/kg then 25 mg/kg thereafter orally bid 10 mg/kg i.m. sid	SR
Anti-inflammatories				
Shock treatment				
Methylprednisolone	30 mg/kg i.v.	Primarily RH		
Dexamethasone	5 mg/kg i.v.	Primarily RH		
Mucolytics				
Bromhexine	1 mg/kg orally bid	RH	2 mg/kg orally bid 0.5 mg/kg i.m. sid	Respiratory disease
Dembrexine			300 µg/kg orally bid	Respiratory disease
Carbocisteine			75–125 mg orally qid	Respiratory disease
Bronchodilators				
Clenbuterol			0.8–5 µg/kg orally, i.m., i.v. bid	Respiratory disease
Anthelminthics				
Fenbendazole			10 mg/kg sid for 3 days	Respiratory and GIT nematodes
Ivermectin	200 µg/kg i.m.	RH	200–300 µg/kg; i.m.	Respiratory and GIT nematodes
Praziquantel	10 mg/kg orally	RH		
Drugs acting on gastrointestinal tract				
Butylscopalamine and metamizole			0.4 mg/kg B and 50 mg/kg M i.m., i.v.	Gut sedation
Cimetidine	6 mg/kg orally tid	RH	5–10 mg/kg orally, i.m. qid	Gastric ulceration
Ranitidine	2–3 mg/kg orally bid initially, then sid	RH	2–3 mg/kg bid orally initially, then sid	Gastric ulceration
Kaolin and pectin	1 ml/kg/day orally in divided doses	RH	1 ml/kg/day orally in divided doses	Diarrhoea

17.16 (continued) Drugs used in treatment of cetaceans and seals. Sources: Unpublished data; Sweeney (1989); Stoskopf (1990); Robinson (1995); Kastelein *et al.* (1997); RSPCA (1997); Barnett (1998); Andrew Greenwood and Paul Riley (personal communications). RF: Refloated animals. RH: Animals taken into rehabilitation. SR: Used based on sensitivity results. (continues)

Drug	Cetaceans			Seals		
	Dose rate; route	Indications and comments		Dose rate; route	Indications and comments	
Drugs acting on gastrointestinal tract continued						
Bismuth, kaolin and charcoal	6–18 g orally bid–tid	RH		6–18 g orally bid–tid	Diarrhoea	
Liquid paraffin	1 ml/kg/day orally in divided doses	RH		1 ml/kg/day orally in divided doses	Constipation	
Ispaghula husk	5–15 ml orally sid	RH		5–15 ml orally sid	Constipation	
Attapulgite and bone charcoal				2.5–5 g/feed orally	Diarrhoea	
Sucralfate	25 mg/kg orally bid	RH		0.25–1 g orally tid	Gastric ulceration	
Topical eye treatments						
Chloramphenicol	As required	RF, RH		2 drops 3–6 times daily	SR	
Gentamicin	As required	RF, RH		1–2 drops 4–6 times daily	SR; treatment of choice for melting corneal ulcers caused by *P. aeruginosa*; improved response often seen if enriched with injectable gentamicin	
Fusidic acid				1–2 drops 3–6 times daily	SR	
Cloxacillin				Applied 3–6 times daily	SR	
Ofloxacin				1–2 drops 4–6 times daily	SR; also used for melting corneal ulcers caused by *P. aeruginosa*	
Ciprofloxacin				2–3 drops 4–6 times daily	SR; often treatment of choice for persistent corneal ulcers	
Dexamethasone, hypromellose, neomycin, polymyxin B				3–4 drops 3–6 times daily	To reduce scarring	
Ocular lubricant	As required	RF and RH				
Vitamin supplementation						
Injectable multivitamin/vitamin B complexes	2–30 ml i.m. depending on product and size	RF, RH		2–10 ml i.m. depending on product and size	May be given when pup is first admitted	
Oral multivitamin preparations for fish-eaters (Aquavits, International Zoo Veterinary Group) (Alternatively use human oral multivitamin preparations at twice recommended dose rate, ensuring 50 mg thiamine per kg feed and 100 mg vitamin E per kg feed)	1 tablet bid; oral	RH		1 tablet bid; oral		
Iron supplementation						
Ferrous sulphate				200 mg orally bid	Dose can be increased in non-regenerative anaemias	

17.16 (continued) Drugs used in treatment of cetaceans and seals. Sources: Unpublished data; Sweeney (1989); Stoskopf (1990); Robinson (1995); Kastelein *et al.* (1997); RSPCA (1997); Barnett (1998); Andrew Greenwood and Paul Riley (personal communications). RF: Refloated animals. RH: Animals taken into rehabilitation. SR: Used based on sensitivity results.

Intravenous injections can be given into vessels used for blood sampling and the same risks of ischaemic necrosis apply. Needles of 2.5–9 cm, 18–21 gauge, will be required, depending on patient size. Intramuscular injections are administered into the lumbar muscles (see Figure 17.9).

Eye and wound care

The eyes of stranded cetaceans can be flushed with saline and ocular lubricants. Topical antibiotics may also be beneficial. Superficial wounds can be cleaned and flushed but topical preparations usually wash off on immersion, except possibly Orabase (Bristol Myers). Suturing of wounds is not advisable, as dehiscence is likely.

Seals

Drugs used in the treatment of seals are included in Figure 17.16. Canine dose rates are generally applicable, though allometric principles should be borne in mind with large adult seals (up to 300 kg).

Intravenous injections are given via the extradural intravertebral vein. Intramuscular injections are into the lumbar muscles, or the gluteals in larger animals (see Figure 17.11). Needles of up to 9 cm, 18 gauge, may be required. Oral drugs may not be appropriate during stabilization, due to poor gastrointestinal absorption, but later in rehabilitation these can be added to tube feeds or inserted in fish.

Management in captivity

Cetaceans

Possible candidates for rehabilitation are given under 'Examination and assessment'. For reasons already discussed, this option is not widely used at present and should not be undertaken lightly. Facilities required include: an oval or round pool (minimum diameter 9 m) with padded sides; an isolated and fully treated supply of salt water; a controlled environment; and specialist support and handling facilities for the animal (Mayer, 1996). Rehabilitation in suboptimal facilities cannot be condoned.

Adult seals

Adult seals, particularly greys, are potentially very dangerous and require specialist accommodation, which is unlikely to be available in the ordinary veterinary practice. Immediately after initial assessment and treatment, these animals should be moved to a facility that is able to house them appropriately.

Rearing of seal pups

Although initial management of seal pups in captivity can be carried out in a veterinary practice isolation facility, it is advisable to move seals at an early stage to an appropriate rehabilitation centre. The full rehabilitation process cannot be attempted without access to adequate facilities, including suitable pools (Figure 17.17).

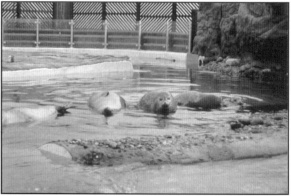

17.17 If large numbers of seals are to be catered for, large outdoor pools, such as this one at Scarborough Seal and Marine Life Sanctuary, need to be provided.

Feeding: Several liquid diets can be used successfully to rear seal pups but it is difficult to emulate the high fat content (about 40–50%) of natural seal milk. Seals are intolerant of lactose, and diets containing cream must be treated with the enzyme lactase before being administered; thus they are best avoided unless in experienced hands. Suitable diets easily available include the following:

- **Fish soup**. Ingredients: 500 ml rehydration fluid, three (500 g) medium-sized mackerel or herring (heads and tails removed, but not gutted), vitamin/mineral supplement (see Figure 17.16). Liquidize until of a consistency that will pass down a stomach tube. The fat content of the final mix is low and is variable, as the fat content of the fish will vary with the season in which they are caught. However, it is simple and readily available. It is the first choice for older pups that have been weaned for some time and will rapidly progress to a diet of whole fish
- **Lactose-free milk replacer**. Zoologic 30/55 (Pet Ag, Hampshire, Illinois), mixed at maximum recommended concentration with water (1:1 by weight). This provides a good milk substitute, especially for unweaned pups, but the fat content of the reconstituted milk is only about 15%
- **Oil-enriched mixtures**. By adding fish oil to the milk replacer, a higher fat content can be achieved. Up to one third salmon oil by volume can be added. Lethicin, easily available from health food shops, can be added as an emulsifier. A vitamin/mineral supplement is also added. The fat content of the final diet is about 40%.

All diets should be freshly made up each day and kept refrigerated.

Pups continue to be fed by tube every 4 hours for 1–3 weeks, though some older stronger animals (particularly greys) may be able to go without middle-of-the-night feeds sooner than this. As they start to progress, the night feeds are eliminated until feeding is at 4-hour intervals through a 12-hour day.

When pups start to thrive and gain weight, they begin to show swallowing movements as the tube is passed. At this stage they are gradually weaned on to whole fish and in older stronger animals (particularly greys) this may occur sooner than 1 week after arrival. Tube and fish feeds can be mixed during the transition. Herring or mackerel is used as fish feeds for the high oil content. The fish are 'force-fed' by restraining the pup in sternal recumbency, introducing a fish into the corner of its mouth and then gently pushing the fish over its tongue until swallowing is stimulated. The use of gags or heavy gloves to force open the mouth is discouraged, as it tends to increase aggressive resistance, cause discomfort and increase the time until self-feeding is established.

From this time on a fish is always left with the seal. Usually seals will start to self-feed, or will first progress from 'force-feeding' to 'hand-feeding', in which the pup does not need to be restrained but still requires the fish to be pushed over its tongue to stimulate swallowing. Each seal progresses at its own pace and this process depends on the skill and experience of the operator.

Once self-feeding is established, feed quantity is increased according to appetite to a maximum of 4.5 kg/day in three feeds. Seals should be weighed at least weekly to assess progress.

Seals are able to obtain water from the fish on which they feed and it is not necessary to provide drinking water. Even where water is provided (in a bowl), not all seals will take it.

Release

Cetaceans

Survival rates

Nearly half the animals involved in mass strandings between 1992 and 1995 were assumed to have survived but the number from single strandings that survived was less than a quarter. Refloating appears to have been more successful than rehabilitation. All harbour porpoises that stranded failed to survive, indicating the poor prognosis with this species (Mayer, 1996). In view of this, only one rehabilitation attempt has been made since 1995, but there has been continued apparent success with refloating (Barnett *et al.*, 2001).

At present, no animals in the UK have been monitored in the long term following release and the success of refloating can only be assumed. Therefore, there is a danger that unsuitable animals are being refloated, only to die later. To monitor success requires satellite telemetry but there are legal (see Chapter 5) and welfare concerns associated with its use, including attachment of tags to the dorsal fin with bolts, and effects on hydrodynamics, health and behaviour.

Seals

Seals are released when they are clinically and behaviourally normal and in good body condition. Naïve pups may take some time to learn to feed adequately in the wild and undergo weight loss similar to naturally occurring post-weaning weight loss. Therefore, as a guideline, pups should be released at average expected weight at weaning, though they will be considerably older. The authors recommend release weights of 40–45 kg for grey seals and 30–35 kg for common seals.

On average the rehabilitation process can take from 3 to 6 months. A short-term rehabilitation option has been investigated for very young common seal pups (Wilson, 1999) and is under further investigation.

Survival rates

Survival rates of over 80% (grey seal pups) and 70% (common seal pups) can be expected during rehabilitation. Hind flipper rototags, commonly used on released animals, have yielded little information on survival rates after release but greater returns have been achieved with head tags. Satellite Relay Data Loggers (Figure 17.18) have yielded information on diving behaviour (Vincent *et al.*, in press). The effects of these on health and behaviour require further evaluation.

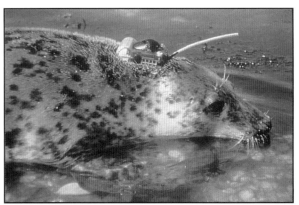

17.18 Satellite tag on a grey seal pup. (Courtesy of Cecile Vincent, University of La Rochelle.)

Legal aspects

Aspects of the law relating to wildlife rehabilitation that is pertinent also to marine mammals are covered in Chapter 5.

Legislation specific to cetaceans includes the Statute Prerogative Regis, 17 Edward II (AD 1324), which states that cetaceans are classified as 'Royal Fish' and belong to the Crown. The exceptions to this are animals that strand within the limits of a Manor, where title passes to the Lord of the Manor. In Scotland, pilot whales, northern bottlenose whales and cetaceans less than 7.5 m in length are not classed as 'Royal Fish' (RSPCA, 1992).

In practical terms, this law requires that stranded cetaceans be reported to the Receiver of Wrecks, via the local coastguard. Alternatively, the stranding can be reported to the Strandings Co-ordinators for England and Wales and for Scotland, appointed by the Department of the Environment, Food and Rural Affairs. In both cases, the report will be passed on to the Natural History Museum, which has been recording strandings since 1911 (RSPCA, 1992).

Legislation specific to seals includes the Conservation of Seals Act 1970, which restricts the category of firearms that can be used in the euthanasia of seals (see 'Methods of euthanasia'). The Act also makes it an offence to capture healthy seals, which well-meaning members of the public may inadvertently contravene.

Specialist organizations

Veterinary advice

Cetaceans and seals

James Barnett
Vetlab Services and British Divers Marine Life Rescue
Tel.: (day) 01403 730176, mobile 07703 855399

Ian Robinson
RSPCA Norfolk Wildlife Hospital
Tel.: 01553 842336

Cetaceans

Paul Jepson
Institute of Zoology, London Zoo
Tel.: (day) 020 7449 6691, mobile: 07768 498622

Tony Patterson
SAC Veterinary Services, Inverness
Tel.: (day) 01463 243030

Seal rehabilitation facilities

(This list is not exhaustive.)

Orkney Seal Rescue
Tel.: 01856 831463

Isle of Skye Environmental Trust
Tel.: 01471 822487

National Seal and Marine Life Sanctuary
Oban, Argyll
Tel.: 01631 720386

SSPCA Animal Centre
Dunfermline, Fife
Tel.: 01383 412520

Scarborough Seal and Marine Life Sanctuary
North Yorkshire
Tel.: 01723 376125

Animal and Bird Gardens
Mablethorpe, Lincolnshire
Tel.: 01507 473346

Natureland Marine Zoo
Skegness, Lincolnshire
Tel.: 01754 764345

Welsh Mountain Zoo
Colwyn Bay, Conwy
Tel.: 01492 532938

RSPCA Wildlife Hospital
Stapeley Grange, Nantwich, Cheshire
Tel.: 0870 442 7102

Hunstanton Seal and Marine Life Sanctuary
Norfolk
Tel.: 01485 533576

RSPCA Norfolk Wildlife Hospital
King's Lynn, Norfolk
Tel.: 01553 842336

RSPCA Wildlife Hospital
West Hatch, Taunton, Somerset
Tel.: 01823 480156

National Seal Sanctuary
Cornwall
Tel.: 01326 221790/221361

References and further reading

Baker AS, Ruoff KL and Madoff S (1998) Isolation of *Mycoplasma* species from a patient with seal finger. *Clinical Infectious Diseases* **27**, 1168–1170

Baker JR, Fedak MA, Anderson SS, Arnbo T and Baker R (1990) Use of a tiletamine-zolazepam mixture to immobilise wild grey seals and elephant seals. *Veterinary Record* **126**, 75–77

Baker J, Barnett J, Cooke M, Jepson P, Patterson T, Robinson I and Simmonds M (2000) Assessment of stranded cetaceans. *Veterinary Record* **147**, 340

Barnett J (1998) Treatment of sick and injured marine mammals. *In Practice* **20**, 200–211

Barnett JEF, Woodley AJ, Hill TJ and Turner L (2000) Conditions in grey seal pups (*Halichoerus grypus*) presented for rehabilitation. *Veterinary Record* **147**, 98–104

Barnett J, Knight A and Stevens M (2001) *Marine Mammal Medic Handbook*. British Divers Marine Life Rescue, Gillingham

Bennett PM, Gascoyne SC, Hart MG, Kirkland JK and Hawkey CM (1991) Development of Lynx: a computer application for disease diagnosis and health monitoring in wild mammals, birds and reptiles. *Veterinary Record* **128**, 496–499

Borst GHA, Walvoort HC, Reijnders PJH, van der Kamp JS and Osterhaus ADME (1986) An outbreak of a herpesvirus infection in harbor seals (*Phoca vitulina*). *Journal of Wildlife Diseases* **22**, 1–6

Brew SD, Perrett LL, Stack JA, MacMillan AP and Staunton NJ (1999) Human exposure to *Brucella* recovered from a sea mammal. *Veterinary Record* **144**, 483

Dierauf LA and Gulland FMD (eds) (2001) *CRC Handbook of Marine Mammal Medicine: Health, Disease and Rehabilitation, 2nd edn*. CRC Press, Boca Raton, Florida

Evans PGH (1995) *Guide to the Identification of Whales, Dolphins and Porpoises in European Seas*. Sea Watch Foundation, Oxford

Geraci JR and Lounsbury VJ (1993) *Marine Mammals Ashore. A Field Guide for Strandings*. Texas A&M Sea Grant, Galveston, Texas

Greer L and Rowles T (2000) Humane euthanasia of stranded marine mammals. *Proceedings AAZV and IAAAM conference, New Orleans*, pp. 374–375

Gulland FMD, Lowenstine LJ, Lapointe JM, Spraker T and King DP (1997) Herpesvirus infection in stranded Pacific harbour seals of coastal California. *Journal of Wildlife Diseases* **33**, 450–458

Hall AJ, McConnell BJ and Barker RJ (2001) Factors affecting first year survival in grey seals and their implications for life history strategy. *Journal of Animal Ecology* **70**, 138–149

Harder TC, Vos H, de Swart RL and Osterhaus ADME (1997) Age-related disease in recurrent outbreaks of phocid herpesvirus type-1 infections in a seal rehabilitation centre: evaluation of diagnostic methods. *Veterinary Record* **140**, 500–503

Hicks BD and Worthy GAJ (1987) Sealpox in captive grey seals (*Halichoerus grypus*) and their handlers. *Journal of Wildlife Diseases* **23**, 1–6

Kastelein RA, Bakker MJ and Staal C (1997) The rehabilitation and release of stranded harbour porpoises (*Phocoena phocoena*). In: *The Biology of the Harbour Porpoise*, eds AJ Read *et al.*, pp. 9–61. De Spil Publishers, Woerden, The Netherlands

King JE (1983) *Seals of the World*. Oxford University Press, Oxford

Kirkwood JK (1983) Influence of body size on animals in health and disease. *Veterinary Record* **113**, 287–290

Koopman HN, Westgate AJ, Read AJ and Gaskin DE (1995) Blood chemistry of wild harbour porpoises *Phocoena phocoena* (L.). *Marine Mammal Science* **11**, 123–135

Koopman HN, Westgate AJ and Read AJ (1999) Haematology values of wild harbour porpoises (*Phocoena phocoena*) from the Bay of Fundy, Canada. *Marine Mammal Science* **15**, 52–64

Lucas RJ, Barnett J and Riley P (1999) Treatment of lesions of osteomyelitis in the hind flippers of six grey seals (*Halichoerus grypus*). *Veterinary Record* **145**, 547–550

Mayer SJ (1996) *The Veterinary Care of Stranded Cetaceans*. Report for the Whale and Dolphin Conservation Society, Bath

Mead JG, Odell DK, Wells RS and Scott MD (1980) Observations on a mass stranding of spinner dolphin, *Stenella longirostris*, from the west coast of Florida. *Fishery Bulletin* **78**, 353–360

Munro R and Synge B (1991) Coccidiosis in seals. *Veterinary Record* **129**, 179–180

Needham DJ (1993) Cetacean strandings. In: *Zoo and Wild Animal Medicine. Current Therapy 3*, ed. ME Fowler, pp. 415–425. WB Saunders, Philadelphia

Robinson I (1995) The rehabilitation of seals at the RSPCA Norfolk Wildlife Hospital. *Journal of the British Veterinary Zoological Society* **1**, 13–17

Rogan E, Baker JR, Jepson PD, Berrow S and Kiely O (1997) A mass stranding of white-sided dolphins (*Lagenorhynchus acutus*) in Ireland: biological and pathological studies. *Journal of the Zoological Society of London* **242**, 217–227

Ross HM, Jahans KL, MacMillan AP, Reid RJ, Thompson PM and Foster G (1996) *Brucella* species infection in North Sea seal and cetacean populations. *Veterinary Record* **138**, 647–648

RSPCA (1992) *Stranded Whales, Dolphins and Porpoises. A First Aid Guide*. Royal Society for the Prevention of Cruelty to Animals, Horsham

RSPCA (1997) *Stranded Cetaceans: Guidelines for Veterinary Surgeons*. Royal Society for the Prevention of Cruelty to Animals, Horsham

SRRC (1999) *Annual Report 1998/1999*. Seal Rehabilitation and Research Centre, Pieterburen, The Netherlands

Stoskopf MK (1990) Marine mammal pharmacology. In: *CRC Handbook of Marine Mammal Medicine: Health, Disease and Rehabilitation*, ed. LA Dierauf, pp. 139–161. CRC Press, Boca Raton, Florida

Sweeney JC (1989) What practitioners should know about whale strandings. In: *Small Animal Practice, 10th edn*, ed. R Kirk, pp. 721–727. WB Saunders, Philadelphia

Sweeney JC and Ridgway SH (1975) Procedures for the clinical management of small cetaceans. *Journal of the American Veterinary Medical Association* **167**, 540–545

Vincent C, Ridoux V, Fedak M and Hassani S (in press) Mark-recapture and satellite tracking of rehabilitated juvenile grey seals (*Halichoerus grypus*): dispersal and potential effect on wild populations. *Aquatic Mammals*

Walsh MT, Odell DK, Young G, Asper ED and Bossart G (1990) Mass strandings of cetaceans. In: *CRC Handbook of Marine Mammal Medicine: Health, Disease and Rehabilitation*, ed. LA Dierauf, pp. 673–683. CRC Press, Boca Raton, Florida

Wilson S (1999) Radiotelemetry study of two rehabilitated harbour seal pups released close to the natural time of weaning in the wild. *Journal of Wildlife Rehabilitation* **22**, 5–11

Acknowledgements

The authors would like to thank: Andrew Greenwood, Paul Jepson, Richard Lucas, Paul Riley and Terrie Williams for their technical input into this chapter; the Zoological Society of London for use of data from the Lynx programme; and *In Practice* for the use of illustrations previously published in an article by James Barnett in 1998. They would also like to thank the staff of the RSPCA Norfolk Wildlife Hospital and the National Seal Sanctuary, the directors of British Divers Marine Life Rescue and their wives for their support and patience over the years.

18

Seabirds: gulls, auks, gannets, petrels

Emma Keeble

Introduction

Seabirds belong to three main orders: Procellariiformes ('tube-noses' such as albatrosses, fulmars, shearwaters, petrels and storm petrels); Pelecaniformes (gannets, pelicans, cormorants and shags); and Charadriiformes (waders, skuas, gulls, and auks such as razorbills, guillemots and puffins). This chapter will consider only the common species of seabirds that may be presented to the veterinary surgeon in practice. For wading birds, see Chapter 19.

Species found in the British Isles

The coastline of Britain and Ireland provides the most important breeding sites for seabirds in the north-east Atlantic Ocean and 24 species breed here regularly. There are great variations in adaptive anatomical features and in nutritional and captivity requirements for the different species; therefore species identification is of great importance. Biological parameters for commonly encountered species are given in Figure 18.1.

Anatomy and physiology

There are several anatomical and physiological adaptations of seabirds in general to their aquatic lifestyle. (Plumage is discussed later under 'Oiling'.)

Posture

The feet are placed far back on the body, which is more effective for propulsion and agility. The posture is upright and weight is borne on the caudal lower limb, which means that severe leg and foot problems are common in captivity.

Adaptations to diving

Diving birds are adapted anatomically to resist pressure and physiologically to withstand shortage of oxygen (see 'Anaesthesia and analgesics'). The muscles are deep red due to large amounts of myoglobin for storing oxygen, used during diving. Deep-diving birds have the ability to close the external ear canal. The eyes of most diving birds (except terns) are specially adapted to amphibious vision.

Order and family	Commonly encountered species	Bodyweight [a]	Natural diet
Procellariiformes			
Procellariidae	Fulmar (*Fulmarus glacialis*)	1 kg	Zooplankton, live fish
	Manx shearwater (*Puffinus puffinus*)	350–545 g	Pilchards, herrings, sprats
Hydrobatidae	British storm petrel (*Hydrobates pelagicus*)		
Pelecaniformes			
Sulidae	Northern gannet (*Sula bassana*)	2.1–3 kg	Herring, mackerel, sprats, whiting
Phalacrocoracidae	Cormorant (*Phalacrocorax carbo*)	2.1–3.6 kg	Trout, eels, flat fish, perch
	Shag (*Phalacrocorax aristotelis*)	1.8–2.2 kg	Trout, eels, flat fish, perch
Charadriiformes			
Laridae	Herring gull (*Larus argentatus*)	Weights variable, depending on species	Omnivorous
	Black-headed gull (*Larus ridibundas*)		
	Lesser black-backed gull (*Larus fuscus*)		
	Kittiwake (*Rissa tridactyla*)		
Sternidae	Sandwich tern (*Sterna sandvicensis*)	120 g	Whiting, herring, squid, sand eels, crustaceans
	Common tern (*Sterna hirundo*)		
	Arctic tern (*Sterna paradisaea*)		
Alcidae	Razorbill (*Alca torda*)	372–645 g	Sand eels, small sprats, crustaceans, molluscs
	Guillemot (*Uria aalga*)	618–870 g	Sand eels, sprats, annelids, crustaceans, molluscs
	Puffin (*Fratercula artica*)	490 g	Sprats, whiting, sand eels

18.1 Biological parameters for seabirds. [a] Average bodyweights vary according to time of year, breeding season, age and sex of bird.

Gastrointestinal tract

Seabirds have simple stomachs, with an elongated glandular proventriculus leading into a small ventriculus. Bills are adapted to the type of food eaten, which is primarily fish.

Body temperature

The body temperature ranges from 39 to 41°C. The arteriovenous countercurrent flow mechanism in the tarsi conserves heat.

Salt glands

Seabirds excrete large amounts of salt, ingested with food and water. Excess salt is eliminated not through the kidneys but through salt glands, which open into the nasal fossa. Paired glands are situated at the anterior angles of the orbit. Secretions run along the beak, or into the mouth, in those species with internal nares (e.g. gannet). These glands excrete chlorine, sodium, potassium and water. They function intermittently, depending on the blood salt concentration; hence birds are able to adapt from a freshwater environment to a marine one. Uptake of electrolytes across the intestinal mucosa triggers secretion from the nasal glands; thus hindrance of intestinal absorption will affect the bird's ability to survive in a saltwater environment. Failure to provide salt in captivity may, in theory, result in atrophy of these glands, leading to dehydration when the bird drinks salt water on release.

Order-specific adaptations

Procellariiformes

- Nares: covered dorsally by a keratinized tubular flap, the operculum
- Stomach oils: produced from complex species-specific mixtures of monoester waxes, oils, triglycerides and other organic substances and stored in large amounts (100–200 ml) in the proventriculus. Regurgitation of stomach oils is a means of defence.

Pelecaniformes

- Nares: closed by opercula as an adaptation to diving from a great height. Breathing is through the corners of the mouth, via normal extensions of the keratinaceous plates of the upper bill (Figure 18.2). The horny lid closes during diving
- Airsac diverticula (gannets): track subcutaneously, along fascial planes, between skeletal muscles, over neck and sternum. They act as pneumatic shock absorbers when diving and may inflate when stressed.

Charadriiformes: auks

- Diving: aided by heavier skeletal structure and reduced air sacs
- Body temperature: layer of fat acts as heat insulator against cooling of water (see 'Anaesthesia and analgesia')
- Seasonal moult: flightless period associated with decreased appetite and disease.

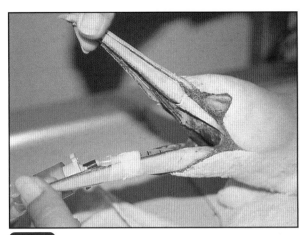

18.2   Gannet bill.

Capture, handling and transportation

Seabirds often vocalize loudly on capture but their main defensive weapon is the beak, though the claws may cause scratches. Extreme care should be taken when handling these birds and they should never be held close to the face. Goggles or safety glasses are recommended. In species with internal nares (gannets), care must be taken that the beak is not held closed.

Capture

1. Always stand between the water and the bird, since it will try to return to water.
2. Approach slowly from the side. Throw a net, towel or coat over the bird.
3. Once it is covered, locate the bird's head and grasp its neck firmly, just behind the head.
4. Keeping hold, remove the covering but keep the bird's head covered at all times, to reduce stress.
5. Wrap a towel lightly around the wings, to prevent flapping. In large species, restrain the wings and body between the knees. Take care not to contaminate or disrupt feathers (this would affect waterproofing).
6. Control the beak with a rubber band or tape. In species with internal nares, place a small gag such as rubber tubing, toothbrush or syringe plunger between the two halves of the beak before applying tape, to ensure that the bird can breathe.

Handling

- Use subdued lighting; cover the head; minimize time
- Do not use leather gloves or gauntlets – they are cumbersome and make gripping difficult
- Do not handle dyspnoeic birds; place in oxygen first
- Goggles or masks should be worn when handling cormorants or gannets
- Grasp the neck firmly just behind the head and restrain the wings (Figure 18.3).

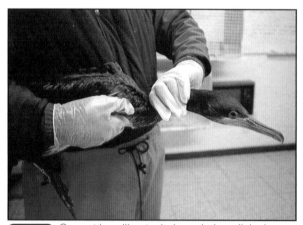

18.3 Correct handling technique during clinical examination of a cormorant.

Transportation

Any ventilated container may be used, as long as it is large enough for the bird to sit in without damage to its tail feathers. There should be a non-slip base, such as a towel, blanket, cloth or mat. Cases of splay leg and bilateral partial paresis occur in auks following transportation in cardboard boxes with no lining. The beak restraint should be removed before transportation, as seabirds commonly regurgitate under stress, and asphyxiation may occur.

Dangers

Gannets, cormorants and auks are the most dangerous seabirds to handle, their powerful beaks being used for defence. The gannet's beak has sharp serrated edges, which can cause severe lacerations to a bare arm.

Zoonoses

Seabirds, particularly gulls, may transmit zoonoses, though this is extremely rare. Good hygienic practice (washing hands, use of disinfectants) should prevent transmission.

Examination and assessment for rehabilitation

General principles as detailed in Chapter 2 apply to the examination and assessment of seabird casualties. The following points are important in seabirds:

- Assessment of the oral cavity (for mucous membrane colour, presence of fishing hooks or lines)
- Thoracic auscultation (aspergillosis is common in captivity)
- Assessment of body condition by pectoral muscle mass palpation (a good indicator of health status in these species). Birds that are underweight may have a reduced post-release survival rate; they often have systemic disease or heavy endoparasite burdens. Seabirds are more likely to be underweight at certain times of the year (e.g. the moulting season in auks)
- Assessment of plumage condition (ectoparasites are common in debilitated birds; also seabirds are commonly presented with oil contamination of the feathers)
- Palpation of wings and legs for fractures (common findings in debilitated seabirds).

Clinical techniques

Basic diagnostic tests, which can be carried out with minimal stress to the bird, include radiography and blood sampling. Faecal parasitology and bacterial culture are also commonly used.

Radiography

Fractures may not be detected on clinical examination, and radiographs help to assess the severity and prognosis. The author has commonly seen airgun and shotgun pellet injuries in seabirds. Ingested fishing hooks (common in cormorants and gulls) are easily detected on radiography.

Blood sampling techniques and clinical values

The maximum safe volume of blood that can be collected from a healthy bird is 1% of bodyweight. The following points should be noted:

- For blood sampling and administration of intravenous fluids, the medial tarsal vein is best. The ulnar and jugular veins are also useful
- Red blood cells are larger in seabirds than in other birds (an adaptation to diving)
- Leucocytosis is commonly seen, associated with bacterial, fungal or protozoal infections, with an absolute heterophilia in the former two cases.

Normal haematological and biochemical values are given in Figures 18.4 and 18.5.

Parameter	Gannet	Cormorant	Herring gull	Guillemot[c]
RBC (10^{12}/l)	2.64	3.02 1.6–2.3[a]	2.92 1.8–2.4[b]	2.43–3.94
PCV (%)	41	45 27–41[a]	43 40–42[b]	33–58
HB (g/l)	140	140.5 80.4–130.1[a]	150.9 110.14–140.86[b]	100.2–160.8

18.4 Haematological values in certain species of seabird. (Source: Balasch *et al.*, 1974, except as indicated.) [a] Bennett *et al.* (1991). [b] Averbeck (1992). [c] Newman and Zinkl (1996) (continues) ▶

Parameter	Gannet	Cormorant	Herring gull	Guillemot[c]
WBC (10⁹/l)	–	6.1–15.5[a]	12.4–18.6	2.0–9.5
Heterophils (10⁹/l)	–	5.37–13.2[a]	2.6–8.2[b]	1.26–4.86
Lymphocytes (10⁹/l)	–	0.4–2.17[a]	6.4–12.4[b]	0.08–1.68
Monocytes (10⁹/l)	–	0–0.12[a]	0–1.4[b]	0
Eosinophils (10⁹/l	–	0[a]	0–1.6[b]	0.48–4.46
Basophils (10⁹/l)	–	0–0.49[a]	0.5–1.4[b]	0–0.24
Thrombocytes (10⁹/l)	–	25–50[a]	–	–
Fibrinogen (g/l)	–	2.06–3.86[a]	–	–
Total protein (g/l)	40.5	30.3	30.7	–

18.4 (continued) Haematological values in certain species of seabird. (Source: Balasch *et al.*, 1974, except as indicated.) [a] Bennett *et al.* (1991). [b] Averbeck (1992). [c] Newman and Zinkl (1996)

Parameter	Reference range
Creatinine (µmol/l)	35.4–70.2
Uric acid (µmol/l)	267–1118
Inorganic phosphate (mmol/l)	1.41–2.94
Calcium (mmol/l)	2.08–2.77
Total protein (g/l)	39–48
Albumin (g/l)	11–14
Globulin (g/l)	26–34
Total bilirubin (µmol/l)	0–5.13
Conjugated bilirubin (µmol/l)	0–1.71
Cholesterol (mmol/l)	8.22–10.95
Glucose (mmol/l)	12.26–17.19
Alkaline phosphatase (IU/l)	22–149
Alanine transaminase (IU/l)	53–216
Gamma glutamyl transferase (IU/l)	0–10
Aspartate transaminase (IU/l)	117–1491
Creatinine kinase (IU/l)	537–3801
Bicarbonate (mmol/l)	17–33
Chloride (mmol/l)	103–121
Sodium (mmol/l)	152–163
Potassium (mmol/l)	3.3–10

18.5 Biochemical values in the guillemot. (Source: Newman and Zinkl, 1996)

Assessment

Poor prognostic signs include emaciation, a heavy ectoparasite burden and wing or leg fractures, especially if open or adjacent to a joint. Euthanasia should be considered in these cases. It is essential that seabirds, once released to the wild, are able to fly, swim and dive in order to catch food and survive. Fracture repair would need to be 100% effective to ensure that this was the case. These birds do not take well to prolonged periods in captivity.

Euthanasia

The preferred method of euthanasia is intravenous barbiturate injection using the medial tarsal vein. Intrahepatic injection of barbiturate can be used when the peripheral circulation is compromised.

First aid procedures

Basic principles of wildlife first aid and treatment are discussed in Chapter 2.

Urate deposition leading to visceral gout is a common post-mortem finding in seabirds and is thought to be associated with dehydration. Immediate fluid therapy is therefore paramount in a dehydrated bird.

Initial therapy

The bird should be placed in a quiet environment and housed on soft substrates such as rubber or foam matting, to avoid keel and foot injuries. A warm environment may predispose to overheating in these species, but in a shocked or oiled bird a thermally neutral environment should initially be provided, such as ambient room temperature (15–20°C). At first, access to open water should be denied since ill or oiled seabirds will rapidly become waterlogged and hypothermic. The bird should be encouraged to feed on its own and should be weighed daily.

Fluid therapy

If necessary, fluids should be administered and nutritional support by gavage should be started. The medial tarsal vein is preferred for intravenous catheter placement and this is well tolerated by seabirds. Intraosseous fluids may be given as for other avian species (see Chapter 2).

Continued supportive care with oral fluid may be necessary if dehydration persists, despite feeding. Gavage is as described for other bird species (see Chapter 2). Initially electrolyte solutions such as Lectade Plus (Pfizer) should be used. After 24 hours, two tins of Hill's a/d diet (Hills Pet Nutrition), 10 ml Ensure Plus (a human liquid nutrition product, Abbot Laboratories), half an Aquavits tablet (International Zoological Veterinary Group) and 1 x 200 mg ferrous sulphate tablet (Robinson, 2000) should be added to 50 ml Lectade Plus. The estimated capacity of the proventriculus of seabirds is 50 ml/kg bodyweight and this volume should be tolerated for each feed (Stoskopf and Kennedy-Stoskopf, 1986).

Anaesthesia and analgesia

General principles of avian anaesthesia apply to seabirds but the diving ability of many of these species may lead to breath-holding on induction and predispose to metabolic acidosis. Seabirds are adapted anatomically to resist pressure and physiologically to withstand shortage of oxygen, which is a problem when gaseous induction techniques are used. Drugs and doses for analgesia are given in the Avian Formulary. Specific considerations for anaesthesia are as follows.

Pre-operative period
Overnight fasting is required, since regurgitation on handling and induction is common. Prolonged fasting is not recommended as it leads to hypoglycaemia and dehydration, due to the high metabolic rate.

General anaesthesia
- Interdigital webbing pinch and corneal reflexes should be used for monitoring levels of anaesthesia
- Hyperthermia is common, particularly in anaesthetized auks: a layer of fat acts as a heat insulator against the cooling action of water as an adaptation for diving in a cold environment for prolonged periods
- Hypothermia may also occur and should be prevented as in other avian species (see Chapter 2). Cloacal temperature should be recorded throughout anaesthesia and on recovery.

Inhalation anaesthesia
Induction using isoflurane gaseous anaesthesia with an open facemask is preferred. It should be remembered that breath-holding is common.

For birds with long beaks (e.g. gannet), a latex glove may be attached to the facemask and the bird's beak introduced through a hole cut in the fingers (Figure 18.6).

Nitrous oxide should not be used in diving birds with subcutaneous air pockets, such as the gannet. This may lead to subcutaneous emphysema, since the gas rapidly diffuses into closed gas spaces.

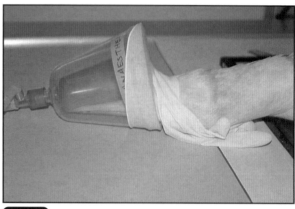

18.6 Facemask adapted for a gannet.

Injectable anaesthesia
General principles apply (see Chapter 2). For drugs and doses, see the avian formulary in Appendix 1.

Specific conditions

Trauma
Traumatic injuries secondary to entanglement in fishing line or nets, ingestion of fishing hooks and lines, and shotgun or air rifle pellets are common in seabirds. Cormorants, shags and gulls more commonly encounter humans than do other species and are particularly prone to traumatic injuries. The author has also seen gannets with humeral and femoral fractures caused by shotgun pellets. Lead toxicity secondary to ingestion of lead weights or shot is theoretically possible but seems to be rare (see Chapter 20). Fishing-hook and line injuries should be treated as in other avian species (see Chapter 20).

When surgically preparing the operation site, care should be taken not to pluck too many feathers as this will prevent the bird returning to the water immediately following surgery. Care should also be taken with surgical skin preparations, since these may affect feather waterproofing.

Wing or leg fractures in seabirds carry a poor prognosis. It is essential that the bird is totally fit before being released back to the wild following repair. This is difficult to achieve in a gannet, for example, which hits the water from a height of 35 m when diving. Avian bone healing on average takes 3 weeks, during which time the bird will be vulnerable to captivity-associated problems (see 'Management in captivity'). Gulls are an exception: they tolerate fracture repair exceedingly well.

Toxins and natural poisons
Seabirds are positioned near the top of the food chain, making them susceptible to accumulation of toxic compounds. Substances such as heavy metals (zinc and lead) and pesticides (e.g. DDT) accumulate in heavily contaminated areas in fish, on which seabirds feed. DDT may affect the salt gland, inhibiting secretions and also osmoregulation. Clinical signs include muscle tremors, which do not respond to atropine. Deaths occur, often in large numbers.

Polychlorinated biphenyls (PCBs) are industrial byproducts that have been implicated in reproductive failure, increased susceptibility to infection and chronic debilitation. Natural toxins also occur; for example, the 'red tide' organism (*Gonyaulax tamarensis*), which causes paralytic shellfish poisoning in humans, may affect seabirds.

In general, toxic poisoning (or infectious causes) should be suspected if different species of seabird are presented from the same area with similar clinical signs.

Botulism

Botulism is a common problem, occurring particularly during the summer in gulls. It is caused by the ingestion of the neuroparalytic toxin of the anaerobic bacterium *Clostridium botulinum*, the most common toxin type affecting birds being Type C, although Type A has been reported in gulls in Britain (Ortiz and Smith, 1994) (see Chapter 20). Intoxication is rare in seabirds other than gulls since *C. botulinum* does not survive well in sea water. Occasional deaths do occur and these may be associated with shallow water during the summer months. Dead animals and maggots feeding on them provide the medium for bacterial growth and toxin production. These in turn may be eaten by fish or birds and outbreaks commonly occur concentrated in one area. Gulls scavenging from rubbish tips are also at risk of ingesting the toxin.

Oiling

Large oil spills have inevitable knock-on effects on marine life, particularly surface-swimming and diving seabirds. Fortunately these incidences are relatively rare and protocols are in place in the UK to deal with oiled seabirds should such a disaster occur. What is more likely is that the veterinary surgeon in practice may encounter individual birds that have become oiled through minor spills, illegal dumping and background pollution. Oiled birds can be presented at any time of the year and in varying states of body condition (Figure 18.7).

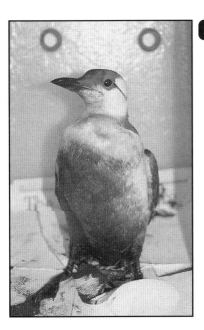

18.7 Oiled guillemot.

Oil pollution has two main effects on seabirds:

- It coats the feathers, affecting buoyancy and waterproofing and leading to hypothermia
- It causes direct toxicity, particularly affecting the gastrointestinal tract.

Environmental effects

Large oil spills may result in catastrophic environmental effects, such as contamination of food sources and nesting habitats, reduction in fertility and egg hatchability, and reduction in production of future food sources. The severity will depend on the type of oil spilt, the size of the spill, environmental conditions and the proximity of susceptible marine life and their habitat.

External effects

Waterproofing: Intact feathers have interlocking barbs and barbules, which act to provide the basis of waterproofing and insulation. A lattice structure is formed, with air pockets inbetween. The feather repels water due to the air/water interface that is formed. The extent of the waterproofing depends on the anatomy of the contour feathers, with cormorants having a less efficient structure that requires them to dry out on land after a period in water. It should be noted that oils from the uropygial or preen gland play no part in waterproofing the feathers.

Preening: The act of preening has two primary functions in birds. First, it spreads the oils from the uropygial gland on to the feathers. The gland secretes an oily substance, which is primarily comprised of fatty acids. This acts to maintain the strength and suppleness of the feathers, increasing their lifespan and preventing them from becoming dry and brittle. Secondly, preening rearranges feathers that are misaligned, reuniting barbs and barbules to maintain a waterproof layer.

When a bird becomes oiled the interlocking structure is destroyed, leading to a loss in waterproofing and insulation. The bird may be unable to fly, cannot feed and may drown. Metabolic rates are increased to maintain body temperature and the bird loses weight. Hypothermia is life-threatening and ensues rapidly once the feathers are disrupted and cold water contacts the skin. Seabirds in this condition will seek land, coming ashore on beaches (Miller and Welte, 1999).

Burns and lesions: Other common external effects include chemical burns, with skin irritation and blistering, and ocular lesions such as corneal ulceration and conjunctivitis.

Internal effects

Many systemic toxic effects of oil have been documented in seabirds and the severity of these will depend on the oil type encountered. The most toxic are refined lighter oils, which have had the tar fraction removed (Robinson, 2000). Toxins affect the respiratory tract, gastrointestinal tract, pancreas, liver, kidney and haematopoietic system. Hypothermia, dehydration and stress combine to worsen the clinical picture.

Preening, a normal behavioural response to oiling, increases ingestion of toxin. Toxin ingestion and stress result in mucosal ulceration and haemorrhage throughout the gastrointestinal tract. This disrupts electrolyte balance and prevents nutrient absorption, leading to dehydration, diarrhoea, bloody faeces, anaemia and reduced plasma total protein levels.

Pneumonia is common, with pulmonary haemorrhage and oedema following inhalation of the lighter volatile fractions. This is usually fatal. Inhalation of oil or regurgitated fluid may also occur, leading to aspiration pneumonia.

Renal failure secondary to direct toxicity and dehydration is often encountered. Visceral gout is a common post-mortem finding in oiled seabirds.

Other less obvious toxic effects of oil include reduced growth rates, reduced fertility rates, reduced function of the salt gland, increased hepatic mixed-function oxidase activity and reduced endocrine gland function, such as adrenal activity. Problems associated with keeping seabirds in captivity, as discussed later, are extremely common in oiled birds.

Haemolytic anaemia following oil ingestion has been well documented, with birds becoming severely anaemic 4–6 days after intoxication (Yamato *et al.*, 1996). Packed cell volume (PCV) may initially be falsely elevated, due to dehydration effects.

Initial assessment and triage
This may take place at the site of capture or nearby. Birds should be transported only short distances prior to assessment and stabilization. Initial assessment should include the following steps:

1. Record bodyweight. Body condition may be assessed by palpation of the pectoral muscle mass. Normal bodyweights (see Figure 18.1) will vary according to the time of year, age and sex of the bird and so these should be used only as an approximate guide. Oiled guillemots have been found to weigh on average less (499–713 g) than those that have been found drowned in nets (851–1095 g) (V. Simpson, personal communication).
2. Record body temperature. Normal values in seabirds vary between 39 and 41°C. A temperature below 32.5°C carries a poor prognosis (Robinson, 2000).
3. Assess hydration status.
4. Carry out a brief clinical examination, with least stress to the bird. There should be a quick visual inspection of the eyes, periorbital area, nares, beak and oropharynx. The neck, abdomen, vent and feather condition should be assessed. Auscultation of the heart (over the sternum), lungs (over the dorsum) and caudal air sacs (over the ventral abdomen) should be carried out. Birds with underlying disease should be isolated or euthanased.
5. A single drop of blood should be taken to assess PCV and total protein. These are useful indicators of hydration status, anaemia and hypoproteinaemia. Normal values in seabirds are PCV 35–55%, total protein (TP) 35–55 g/l, glucose 8.33–13.88 mmol/l

(for values for certain species, see Figures 18.4 and 18.5). PCV values below 25% and TP values below 20 g/l may give rise to concern.

Birds with hypothermia, poor body condition and severe dehydration have little chance of survival and should be euthanased. Moribund birds, dyspnoeic birds or birds with severe traumatic injuries may also be candidates for euthanasia at this stage.

Initial treatment
Birds should be stabilized prior to washing. Treatment is aimed at correcting dehydration and hypothermia and preventing further preening and ingestion of oil.

Fluid therapy: In any oiled bird presented for treatment, 10% dehydration should be assumed. A bird that can lift its head should be given a warm electrolyte solution (e.g. Lectade, Pfizer) by crop tube. For calculation of fluid volumes, see 'First aid procedures'. Severely debilitated birds may be given intravenous fluid boluses but care should be taken to be as aseptic as possible, to avoid contamination with oil. For this reason, the routine use of indwelling catheters is not recommended in oiled birds.

Adsorbents and activated charcoal should be added routinely to the electrolyte solution to reduce further absorption of toxins.

Hypothermia: Prior to washing oiled birds, it is essential to provide warmth. Warming should be gradual until a core body temperature of 39–41°C is reached. Heated air or heat lamps should be used.

Ingestion of oil: Oil should be removed from inside and around the beak with paper towels. The use of 'ponchos' to cover the bird and prevent further preening is not recommended, since they cause further stress to the bird.

Prophylactic antifungal and antibiotic treatment: In high-risk cases prophylactic antifungal (oral itraconazole) and antibacterial (neomycin) treatment may be indicated.

Ocular lesions: Corneal ulceration and conjunctivitis are commonly encountered secondary to initial oil contamination and also following washing with a detergent. Clinical signs include blepharospasm, corneal oedema and epiphora. Ulcers may take up fluorescein dye. Topical eye preparations should be used and may be applied prophylactically prior to washing.

Chemical burns and skin irritation: Depending on the type of oil pollution, varying degrees of skin irritation and blister formation may be present. Oil should be removed from the legs and feet on arrival to minimize the topical effects. Topical treatment may be indicated. The feet and legs should be cleaned daily with dilute warm salt water, and a barrier ointment such as petroleum jelly applied to prevent drying and cracking of the skin. Once the bird has been washed, topical treatments should be avoided in case of feather contamination. Pressure sores related to time spent in captivity are discussed later.

Traumatic injuries: Severe open wounds and open fractures are difficult to treat in an oiled bird since oil contamination follows rapidly. These cases should be assessed individually but a decision to euthanase the bird may need to be made. Beak fractures, wing-tip fractures, carpal luxations, keel wounds and traumatic leg injuries are common. Treatment, if possible, is as for similar injuries in other birds.

Continual assessment

After stabilization, daily continual assessment is essential. Individual birds should be identified and a record card of treatment, weight, feeding, blood test results and washes should be updated daily. Birds should be monitored carefully for clinical signs of chronic effects of oil pollution, such as regurgitation, melaena, haemorrhagic faeces, biliverdinuria, dyspnoea, pressure sores and mucous membrane pallor.

Washing techniques

Once a bird is feeding on its own, appears bright and shows no evidence of ill health, it may be considered for washing. The washing process itself is highly stressful and is poorly tolerated by debilitated birds.

Hand washing: Traditionally, washing by hand with an appropriate detergent has been the method of choice for cleaning oiled birds. The detergent of current choice in the UK is Fairy Liquid (Procter & Gamble). The process is highly specialized and should be attempted only if suitable facilities and trained staff are available.

A sink is required with a continuous supply of hot (42°C) water through a high-pressure (minimum 5.5 bar) hand-held shower head. Two operators are required for the cleaning process, one to hold the bird, the other to clean the feathers (Figure 18.8). To prevent operator injuries, the bird's beak may be taped using a rubber band or rubber nozzle. Extreme care should be taken not to cover the nares. In species with internal nares, a pencil or toothbrush should be used inside the beak prior to taping (see 'Capture') so that the bird may still breathe.

The bird is immersed in a solution of detergent at 42°C and the person washing moves the feathers between finger and thumb from base to tip to clean the oil from them. A standard procedure should be followed, working cranially to caudally. The inside of the

beak is cleaned using a toothbrush. Cleaning progresses along the neck, back and tail feathers, then the bird is rotated on to each side to wash the wing and flank area. Finally the ventral neck, sternum, abdomen and ventral tail feathers are cleaned.

Several cleaning cycles may be necessary, either in one session or on separate occasions, if the bird appears distressed. Once the bird is clean, all traces of detergent are removed from the surfaces, sink and operators prior to rinsing the bird. Rinsing follows the same order as cleaning, making sure that detergent runs away from areas already rinsed and directing the shower jet against the lie of the feathers. Beading of water indicates successful cleaning of feathers. Areas where water runs into the feathers will need to be cleaned again.

Other cleansing agents have been tried with some success, such as iron powder (Orbell *et al.*, 1999).

Machine washing: A relatively new automated machine-washing method has been described (Westerhof *et al.*, 1997). This may be useful after large oil spills if washing facilities are not available within a reasonable distance. Washing times are reduced to 10 minutes (compared with 20–40 minutes for hand washing). The bird is placed in a cage with wings held in extension and the head protruding from the top away from the cleaning area. Rotating nozzles spray detergent and then rinse with water. The head is cleaned by hand.

Husbandry after washing

Once washed, birds should be dried in a separate room with a warm air current supplied by heated fans; for individual birds a hairdryer may be used. Birds are left overnight and are placed on outside pools the following morning to assess waterproofing. Failures at this stage do occur and may be secondary to incomplete removal of oil or detergent during the washing process, inadequate skimming of the pool or contamination of the water with fish oils, oily faeces or detergent. Birds that are too weak to preen will also be poorly waterproofed.

Birds may take 4–5 days on pools to preen and regain waterproofing prior to release. They should be monitored carefully during this time for chronic effects of oil toxicity.

Release

Appropriate sites and weather conditions are essential for release. Oiled birds should not be released where they are in danger of recontamination. Depending on the species and time of year, they may be released on beaches or cliffs or from boats. They should be released into wind in calm conditions, preferably in groups, at a site where food sources are readily available.

Survival rates of oiled birds vary according to many different factors, such as the species affected, type of oil spilt, weather conditions and facilities available. Survival to release may be as high as 60% (Robinson, 2000) but post-release survival rates in auks have been disappointingly low (Sharp, 1996; Wernham *et al.*, 1997). Mute swans and jackass penguins have higher post-release survival rates and the reasons behind this are still unknown. Suggestions have been

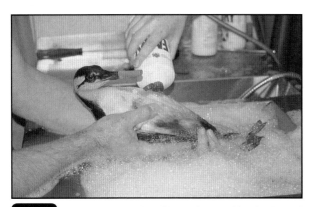

18.8 Holding an oiled guillemot for washing by hand.

made that inadequate food sources and persistent immunosuppression are factors involved in low post-release survival rates. Further work needs to be done to address this welfare problem and the rehabilitation of oiled birds may need to be questioned if high post-survival rates are not achieved in the future.

Viral diseases

'Puffinosis'
The most documented viral disease in seabirds is 'puffinosis', which is endemic in Europe. The virus has yet to be classified. Clinical signs include conjunctivitis, blistering of the foot webbing and spastic paralysis of the legs. Mortality is high in the Manx shearwater but low in other species, with the exception of the chicks of lesser black-backed and herring gulls. The virus has been described in oystercatchers, shags, herring gulls, lesser and greater black-backed gulls and fulmars, where it causes only foot lesions with or without conjunctivitis. It is thought that the virus persists in trombiculid mites overwintering in nesting burrows. It has been suggested that doxycycline may reduce mortality in affected Manx shearwater chicks (Brooke, 1990).

Newcastle disease
Paramyxovirus Type 1 (Newcastle disease) has been identified in seabirds, which may act as a reservoir of infection. Reported cases have occurred in guillemots, puffins, cormorants and gannets, with clinical signs only in gannets (Stoskopf and Kennedy-Stoskopf, 1986). Clinical signs, diagnosis and post-mortem changes are as for other avian species.

Other viruses
Several virus types have been isolated in birds following oiling or stress but these are not thought to be a significant cause of disease. Examples include adenovirus in guillemots and herring gulls, and influenza viruses.

Bacterial diseases
Bacterial infections are common in seabirds and numerous types have been reported, usually at post-mortem examination. Most infections are enteric, resulting in lethargy, urate soiling of the vent and anorexia. Diagnosis is based on cloacal swab culture. Treatment with fluid therapy and antibiotics may be indicated. These infections may be more common in captivity, associated with stress. Typically encountered bacteria include *Escherichia coli*, *Klebsiella* spp., *Salmonella typhimurium*, *Campylobacter* spp. and *Listeria* spp.

The latter three have often been found in gulls and these birds have been implicated as potential health hazards to humans via zoonotic spread (Quessy and Messier, 1992). *Chlamydophila psittaci*, another zoonotic organism, has also been reported in gulls (Franson and Pearson, 1995). Where there is a serious zoonotic risk, the decision to euthanase the bird may be necessary. The risk is high only where large numbers of gulls are in contact with humans, e.g. at seaside resorts.

Mycobacterium avium is common in gulls, associated with lameness secondary to bone infections. Diagnosis is based on clinical signs, radiography and post-mortem examination. Prolonged culture is necessary for this organism but special stains (Ziehl–Neelson) may demonstrate the presence of acid-fast bacteria. Other bacterial causes of lameness, resulting in septic arthritis in the author's experience, include *Staphylococcus aureus* and *Salmonella typhimurium* joint infections. Treatment with systemic antibiotics and joint lavage is rarely successful.

Fungal diseases
Aspergillus fumigatus is frequently found in seabirds in captivity and is often fatal. *Aspergillus flavus* is more rarely encountered. Other fungal infections seen include *Mucor* spp., *Geotrichum candidum* and blastomycosis.

Aspergillosis
Aspergillosis (see Chapter 20) has been reported in puffins, cormorants, guillemots, razorbills and gannets. Seabirds are thought to be predisposed to infection by stress and lack of previous exposure to the fungus. They should never be housed on straw or hay, which are sources of fungal spores.

Clinical signs include open-mouthed breathing, inappetence and increased respiratory effort. Diagnosis is primarily based on clinical signs but radiography may also be useful in advanced cases. Treatment is rarely successful once the infection is established. Prophylactic treatment with itraconazole is recommended.

Parasites

Endoparasites
Heavy endoparasite burdens are often encountered in seabirds, in particular in moribund or emaciated individuals. It is thought that endoparasite infections in healthy birds rarely cause problems, but they lower resistance to other stressors such as oil pollution or bad weather (Jauniaux *et al.*, 1998). Cestodes, trematodes, nematodes and protozoans have all been regularly reported in seabirds (Stoskopf and Kennedy-Stoskopf, 1986). Cestodes have been commonly reported in petrels (Jones, 1988), as have trematodes (Robinson, 2000).

The most common endoparasites encountered in seabirds are *Contracaecum* spp., nematodes that inhabit the proventriculus. Infection occurs secondary to ingestion of fish containing encapsulated larvae. Treatment with an anthelmintic, such as fenbendazole, is effective.

Gapeworm (*Syngamus trachea*) has been seen in gulls; earthworms are the intermediate host (Robinson, 2000). Diagnosis is based on clinical signs (open-mouthed breathing, increased respiratory noise) and faecal microscopy for ova. Treatment with fenbendazole is successful.

Ectoparasites
Feather lice are common in rescued seabirds. Although they do not cause primary disease, they are an indication that the bird is debilitated. Many different species of

lice and mites have been described; they do not directly affect the bird but they can be an irritation to the handler. Care should be taken with topical treatments, since these can affect the waterproofing of the feathers. Ivermectin is successful when applied topically.

Nutritional disease

Beak and skeletal deformities associated with vitamin D deficiency have been recorded in cormorants in captivity. This should be borne in mind when rearing juvenile seabirds (see 'Supplements', below). Abnormal rotation of the carpal joint ('slipped wing' or 'angel wing') has also been seen in well fed, rapidly growing wild juvenile cormorants (Kuiken et al., 1999). This condition is common in waterfowl, where it is thought to be related to excessive intake of protein and deficiencies in calcium, magnesium and vitamin D.

Starvation and emaciation

Seabirds are extremely vulnerable to climatic changes when at sea. Juvenile birds in particular are at risk. Stormy weather, high winds, lack of food sites and heavy parasitism may lead to emaciation and weakness. Many birds may die while out at sea but some are found on the shore or even inland. Supportive care with fluid therapy, anthelmintics and feeding of high quality fish is indicated. Euthanasia is indicated in severely emaciated and weak birds.

Occasional mass seabird 'die-offs' occur and these are often the first indication of a problem within the marine environment. Pollution with oil or PCBs is most commonly implicated (Pokras, 1996).

During winter months, it is common to find seabirds that have 'crash-landed' inland. Fulmars, gannets and Manx shearwaters seem particularly predisposed. These individuals are normally in good body condition with no obvious abnormalities and should be released as soon as possible at a suitable site.

Therapeutics

Routes of administration of drugs in seabirds are as for other avian species. Oral medications may be administered inside fish, if the bird is eating. Doses are given in the avian formulary in Appendix 1.

Management in captivity

Housing

There are common problems associated with keeping seabirds in captivity for prolonged periods. To avoid these, high standards of hygiene and husbandry, along with good housing and ventilation, are essential.

Seabirds are gregarious in nature and should be housed as groups. Initially they may be housed separately to monitor food intake. Larger species such as gannets and cormorants may be easier to handle if kept singly. They are extremely sensitive to disturbance by sudden noise, which should be avoided.

The nature of the substrate is of utmost importance. Decubitus ulcers are common in seabirds in captivity, involving the sternum, hock and tarsometatarsal area.

Secondary infection with bacteria is common, necessitating euthanasia in severe cases. Substrates should be easy to clean and soft, such as Astroturf, rubber matting, deep layers of blankets or wood shavings. Straw or hay must be avoided. Netting and waterbed substrates have been used successfully to prevent these lesions from developing. Cormorants will climb on to structures such as wooden boxes or overturned buckets and this will keep the feet and tail feathers free from faecal soiling. Auks will climb on to rocks if provided.

Build-up of ammonia from droppings is common and could predispose to respiratory disease. Ventilation should be adequate to cope with this, and 12 air changes per hour are recommended (Robinson, 2000). A room temperature below 15°C is recommended for auks (Stoskopf and Kennedy-Stoskopf, 1986).

Access to open water should be provided for all but debilitated or oiled seabirds. Diving birds prefer water deep enough for their feet not to touch the bottom. A padded ramp and platform should be provided for access out of the water if needed. The pool edges should be cleaned regularly to prevent accumulation of faeces; they should be free draining and roughened to avoid pressure sores developing by constant weight-bearing on one part of the lower limb and foot. Water should be constantly skimmed with drains at the level of the water surface to prevent build-up of fish oils, which impair the waterproofing of the plumage and cause thermoregulatory problems.

Feeding

For fish-eating birds, the provision of good quality fish is essential. Seasonal variations in fish quality occur. A balanced diet may be achieved by providing a variety of fish species. Strict hygiene is essential to prevent bacterial contamination of fish and ensuing gastrointestinal infections. Seabirds may be encouraged to eat by moving the fish through the water or injecting fish with air so that they float.

Debilitated birds should be fed by tube, which stimulates intestinal peristalsis and appetite. As a general rule debilitated birds will initially take smaller fish. Petrels may be fed using defrosted krill, available from aquarist suppliers. Gulls are omnivorous and adults may be fed diets described for juveniles (see 'Rearing of orphans'). Assisted feeding may also be necessary (Figure 18.9) and may commence with small sprats for most species or small mackerel for gannets. The bird's mouth is opened and the fish is placed head first in the oropharynx. The beak is then closed and the bird should swallow the fish.

Weight of bird (kg)	Whole fish (g)	Frequency of feeds (per day)
< 0.5	10–35	6–7
0.5–1.5	25–100	5–6
1.5–3	60–180	4–5
3–5	180–369	4

18.9 Recommended amounts for assisted feeding of seabirds (Stoskopf and Kennedy-Stoskopf, 1986).

Supplements

Deficiencies in fat-soluble vitamins are common in fish-eating birds in captivity. Oily fish, such as mackerel and tuna, are low in vitamin E and feeding such fish to birds may lead to steatitis. Vitamin E should be added to the diet at 100 IU/kg of fish fed. Water-soluble vitamins leach out of frozen fish thawed at room temperature; the fish should therefore be defrosted slowly in a closed container in a refrigerator for 24–48 hours and then used immediately.

Marine fish contain high levels of thiaminases, which destroy thiamine, leading to ataxia, abnormal posture, respiratory effort, coma and death. Thiaminase levels are highest in clams, herring and smelt. Thiamine should be added to the diet at 25–30 mg/kg of fish fed. Commercial vitamin supplements are available (e.g. Aquavits, International Zoo Veterinary Group; Fish Eater tablets, Mazuri Zoo Foods).

Problems associated with captivity

Salt gland atrophy

Salt glands will atrophy rapidly in seabirds given fresh water in captivity. In species living in fresh or brackish water, such as cormorants and gulls, salt supplementation may not be necessary. Salt glands should be reactivated by gradually increasing the salt content of the diet. Salt tablets are available but sea salt is just as good.

Decubitus ulcers

These are common in captivity. Application of petroleum jelly may prevent drying of the feet and webbing. Care should be taken not to contaminate the plumage, which would necessitate washing of the bird.

Cloacal impaction

This is common in some diving species. Feathers around the cloaca become rapidly soiled with urates and faeces, leading to impaction. Diagnosis is based on clinical signs and confirmed radiographically. Chronic impaction may lead to stretching of the cloaca and atony, predisposing to further impactions.

Respiratory disease

Aspergillosis is frequently encountered in seabirds in captivity and is often fatal (see 'Fungal diseases'). Seabirds should never be housed on straw or hay, which are sources of fungal spores.

Rearing of orphans

With the exception of the gull family, it is rare to encounter orphaned seabirds. This is because juvenile seabirds fledge and migrate out to sea for the first few years of their lives.

Rehabilitation centres may become overrun with 'orphaned' gull chicks during the breeding season each year. They are rarely true orphans and have either fallen from inappropriate nest sites, been picked up by other birds and dropped, or been picked up by well meaning members of the public. They rapidly become imprinted on people unless housed in social groups. Release sites are often a problem since herring gulls are present in large numbers in southern England, where they may be seen as a nuisance and public health concern.

Orphaned gulls should be housed in social groups on padded mats or towels to prevent foot lesions. The accommodation should be cleaned out twice daily to prevent build-up of ammonia in the environment. The birds may be fed a variety of food items, such as mashed fish-flavoured cat food, finely chopped whitebait, herring, mackerel or day-old chicks. Appropriate vitamin and mineral supplements should be added (see above).

Release

The release of adult seabirds is usually by a 'hard release' technique (see Chapter 3) in a suitable marine environment, at a time when conspecifics are present and in good weather conditions. Following oiling incidents, release sites away from oil contamination will need to be found.

Legal aspects

Leach's petrels may occasionally be encountered. This species is covered by Schedule 4 of the Wildlife and Countryside Act and as such requires to be registered if in captivity.

Specialist organizations

Advice on oil spill incidents and care of oiled seabirds can be sought from the following organizations, which will provide details of local contacts.

RSPCA West Hatch Wildlife Hospital
West Hatch, Taunton, Somerset TA3 5RT
Tel.: 01823 480156

RSPCA Norfolk Wildlife Hospital
Station Road, East Winch, Kings Lynn, Norfolk PE32 1NR
Tel.: 01553 840045

RSPCA Stapeley Grange Wildlife Hospital
London Road, Stapeley, Nantwich, Cheshire CW5 7JW
Tel.: 01270 610347

RSPCA Headquarters
Wilberforce Way, Southwater, Horsham, West Sussex RH13 9RS
Tel.: 08700 101181

SSPCA Middlebank Wildlife Centre
Masterton Road, Dunfermline, Fife KY11 8QN
Tel.: 01383 412520

SSPCA Oiled Bird Cleaning Centre
Tirlandie, Gott, Shetland
Tel.: 01595 840321

References and further reading

Averbeck C (1992) Haematology and blood biochemistry of healthy and clinically abnormal great black-backed gulls (*Larus marinus*) and herring gulls (*Larus argentatus*). *Avian Pathology* **21**, 215–223

Balasch J, Palomeque J, Palacios L, Musquera S and Jiminez M (1974) Haematological values of some great flying and aquatic diving birds. *Comparative Biochemistry and Physiology* **49**, 137

Bennett PM, Gascoyne SC, Hart MG *et al.* (1991) *The Lynx Database*. Department of Veterinary Science, Zoological Society of London

Brooke M (1990) *The Manx Shearwater*. T and AD Poyser,

Cramp S, Bourne W and Saunders D (1974) *The Seabirds of Britain and Ireland*. Collins, London

Croxall JP (ed.) (1987) *Seabirds: Feeding, Ecology and Role in Marine Ecosystems*. Cambridge University Press, Cambridge

Flammer K (1999) Zooonoses acquired from birds. In: *Zoo and Wild Animal Medicine, Current Therapy 4*, eds ME Fowler and RE Miller, pp. 151–156. WB Saunders, Philadelphia

Franson JC and Pearson JE (1995) Probable epizootic chlamydiosis in wild Californian (*Larus californicus*) and ring-billed (*Larus delawarensis*) gulls in North Dakota. *Journal of Wildlife Diseases* **31**, 424–427

Furness R and Monaghan P (1987) *Seabird Ecology*. Blackie and Son, Glasgow

Jauniaux T, Brosens L, Meire P, Offringa H and Boignoul F (1998) Pathological investigations on guillemots (*Uria aalge*) stranded on the Belgian coast during the winter of 1993–94. *Veterinary Record* **143**, 387–390

Jones HI (1988) Notes on parasites in penguins (Spheniscidae) and petrels (Procellariidae) in the Antarctic and Sub-antarctic. *Journal of Wildlife Diseases* **24**(1), 166–167

King AS and McLelland J (1984) *Birds: Their Structure and Function*. Baillière Tindall, London

Kuiken T, Leighton FA, Wobeser G and Wagner B (1999) Causes of morbidity and mortality and their effect on reproductive success in double-crested cormorants from Saskatchewan. *Journal of Wildlife Diseases* **35**, 331–346

Miller EA and Welte SC (1999) Caring for oiled birds. In: *Zoo and Wild Animal Medicine, Current Therapy 4*, eds ME Fowler and RE Miller, pp. 300–309. WB Saunders, Philadelphia

Newman S and Zinkl J (1996) Establishment of haematological, serum biochemical and electrophoretogram reference intervals for species of marine birds likely to be impacted by oil spill incidents in the state of California. Baseline Marine Bird Project for the Californian Department of Fish and Game, Office of Oil Spill Prevention Response

Orbell JD, Tan EK, Coutts M, Bigger S and Ngeh L (1999) Cleansing oiled feathers – magnetically. *Marine Pollution Bulletin* **38**, 219–221

Ortiz NE and Smith GR (1994) *Clostridium botulinum* type A in the gut contents of a British gull. *Veterinary Record* **135**, 68

Pokras MA (1996) Clinical management and biomedicine of sea birds. In: *Diseases of Cage and Aviary Birds, 3rd edn*, eds W Rosskopf and R Woerpel, pp. 987–988. Lea and Febiger, Philadelphia

Quessy S and Messier S (1992) Prevalence of *Salmonella* sp., *Campylobacter* sp. and *Listeria* sp. in ring-billed gulls (*Larus delawarensis*). *Journal of Wildlife Diseases* **28**(4), 526–531

Robinson I (2000) Seabirds. In: *Avian Medicine*, eds TN Tully *et al.*, pp. 339–363. Butterworth Heinemann, Oxford

Sharp B (1996) Post-release survival of oiled, cleaned seabirds in North America. *IBIS* **138**, 222–228

Stoskopf M and Kennedy-Stoskopf S (1986) Aquatic birds (Sphenisciformes, Gaviiformes, Podicipediformes, Procellariiformes, Pelecaniformes and Charadriiformes). In: *Zoo and Wild Animal Medicine, 2nd edn*, ed. ME Fowler, pp. 293–313. WB Saunders, Philadelphia

Wernham CV, Peach WJ and Browne S (1997) Survival rates of rehabilitation. Unpublished report prepared for Sea Empress Environmental Evaluation Committee (SEEEC)

Westerhof I, Berrevoets M and Kaemingk JG (1997) A washing machine for birds. *Proceedings, 4th Conference of the European Association of Avian Veterinarians*, pp. 171–174

Yamato O, Goto I and Maede Y (1996) Haemolytic anaemia in wild seaducks caused by marine oil pollution. *Journal of Wildlife Diseases* **32**, 281–284

Acknowledgements

Acknowledgements are due to Vic Simpson and Ian Robinson for their help with references.

19

Wading birds, including herons

Dick Best and Becki Lawson

Introduction

This chapter will consider all long-legged wading birds, namely waders and herons, as one group. This may not be strictly correct in taxonomic terms but birds in these groups share similar morphology and natural history.

Wildlife casualties from this grouping are not presented in large numbers to veterinary practices or rehabilitation units. In a recent survey from a number of British wildlife rehabilitation units, recorded over a 7-year period, wading birds represented less than 1% of all avian casualties (BWRC, 1999 and unpublished data). Although not common, wading-bird casualties in rehabilitation units do require special care, due to their highly specialized habitat and feeding requirements.

Species found in the British Isles

Figure 19.1 gives details of the classification of the families containing species that commonly occur in the British Isles.

Family/ Subfamily	Common name	Diet	Feeding strategy	Resident/migrant	Typical habitat: breeding	Typical habitat: winter
Order Charadriiformes Waders (also includes gulls, skuas, terns and auks)						
Haematopodidae	Oystercatchers	Bivalve molluscs Also earthworms on grassland	Deep probing	Resident	Seashore and coastal grassland	Seashore and coastal grassland
Charadriinae	Plovers	Small invertebrates, especially insects	Surface feeding on wet ground	Resident and winter migrant	Moorland, coastal grassland, inland wetlands	Estuaries
Vanellinae	Lapwing	Invertebrates	Surface feeding on wet ground or grassland	Resident and winter migrant	Moorland and coastal grassland	Coastal and inland wetlands
Calidridinae	Sandpipers	Invertebrates	Mainly intertidal shores, surface feeding or probing soft mud	Mostly winter visitor; some breed on UK moorland	Moorland or tundra	Flocking on estuaries
Gallinagininae	Snipe	Invertebrates	Probing deeply into soft mud, wet grasslands	Resident and winter visitor	Wetland, both coastal and inland	Wetland, both coastal and inland
Scolopacinae	Woodcock	Invertebrates	Surface or probing wet ground	Resident and winter visitor	Open, damp woodland	Marsh and wet woodland
Tringinae	Curlew, 'shanks', godwits	Invertebrates	Probing soft ground	Resident and winter visitor	Grassland, moorland, tundra	Grassland, estuaries, beaches
Phalaropodinae	Phalaropes	Invertebrates	Surface feeding on wet ground or whilst swimming	Passage migrant, some breed Northern Isles	Tundra	Mostly at sea
Order Ciconiiformes Herons, egrets and bitterns						
Ardeidae	Herons, egrets, bitterns	Fish, amphibians, also small mammals, birds and invertebrates	Stalking in shallow water	Resident and winter visitor	Wetlands and reed beds Herons and egrets nest in trees	Wetlands

19.1 Classification and natural history of British wading birds.

Waders

Identification of casualty waders 'in the hand' can be difficult, especially with juvenile birds in the autumn and with adults in non-breeding plumage in the winter. Accurate identification might not be essential for the initial stages of rehabilitation but is required for the successful release of a casualty. Reference can be made to one of the many excellent field guides to British and European birds but may still require the assistance of an experienced naturalist.

Herons

The grey heron (*Ardea cinerea*) is a common species that occurs mainly in wetland areas but will fly into urban areas to feed, sometimes causing problems in fish farms and garden ponds.

Ecology and biology

Waders

The majority of wader species acquire distinct breeding and non-breeding plumages. They nest on the ground, laying small clutches (usually up to four eggs); the chicks are generally precocial, nidifugous and self-feeding and are usually independent soon after fledging. Mortality in first-year waders is high, ranging from 65% to 80%, or higher in some years with adverse weather conditions. Adult annual mortality is 30–40% in most species.

In a breeding territory, many of the small waders will perform a distraction display to entice predators away from their nest or offspring. The display usually involves a distress-type call, with the bird feigning injury by drooping one or both wings. This display might lead the unwary to assume a bird to be a casualty.

Waders have developed highly specialized feeding techniques. Those with shorter bills forage for small invertebrates on the surface of mud and wet sand, while those with longer bills probe for larger prey deep into mud.

Herons

Herons are gregarious during the breeding season, nesting in traditional sites high in trees overlooking wetland areas. Breeding occurs early in the year, starting in February in the British Isles. The young are altricial and nidicolous, fledging at approximately 50 days; they remain at or around the heronry for a further 10–20 days, after which they are independent.

Herons feed by stalking a wide variety of prey, mainly in shallow water on the edge of lakes or rivers. They develop feeding territories, which they will defend against other herons. This behaviour causes problems in finding a suitable site for the release of a rehabilitated casualty.

The mortality of first-year grey herons in Britain is almost 70%, whereas the annual loss of older birds is approximately 30%.

Anatomy and physiology

Waders

Those waders that specialize in feeding by probing in mud have long, thin, often curved bills. These are very delicate structures, with a fine bony architecture and elastic zones along the length of the bone that allow movement of the rostral section of the beak (rhynchokinetic). This is particularly well developed in snipe (*Gallinago* spp.; Figure 19.2), where just the tip of the bill moves to catch food whilst probing. In these probing waders the bill is covered not with a hard keratinized sheath (rhamphotheca), as in most birds, but with a soft leathery epidermis that contains many specialized mechanoreceptors (Herbst corpuscles) at its tip (King and McLelland, 1984). Damage to the bill seriously compromises the bird's ability to detect and capture prey items. Waders that do not probe with their bills but feed from the surface of the ground, notably the plovers (Charadriinae), do not have a sensitive bill tip with Herbst corpuscles.

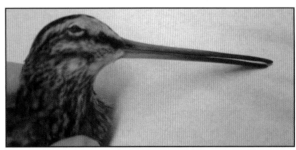

19.2 Common snipe. The long bill is very delicate and easily damaged by rough handling while in captivity. (Courtesy of G Cousquer.)

Most waders are swift runners and are able to swim. They have long thin legs with simple feet (anisodactyl), which are partially webbed in only a few species. As part of their thermoregulation, some waders possess a countercurrent tibiotarsal rete on the leg distal to the stifle. Many species, especially those living in coastal environments, possess nasal salt glands. Most species do not possess a crop.

Herons

Herons possess a long and very powerful bill with a horny rhamphotheca (see Figure 19.3). Their feet are very large, to assist in walking over very soft ground and perching in trees.

Handling and transportation

The methods of handling and transporting wading birds follow the basic techniques for birds as described in Chapter 2.

Handling waders

The smaller waders are delicate birds and great care must be taken not to cause damage, especially to the sensitive beak-tip in those species with long bills. They must not be restrained for any period with their legs in forced flexion, as the circulation will be compromised and this may result in paralysis.

Handling herons

Great caution is required when capturing and handling casualties of the heron family. These species are all capable of making sudden stabbing movements at a handler's face, particularly the eyes. The wearing of industrial eye-protectors would be a wise precaution when handling such species, especially during capture.

When handling any member of the heron family it is essential first to restrain the head by grasping the uppermost part of the neck carefully yet firmly, and then to restrain the body, wings and feet within a suitable towel, blanket or coat. A short length of rubber tubing can be placed for short periods on the tip of a heron's beak during handling and clinical examination but the bird should never be left unattended, due to the potential risk of regurgitation and choking. As with long-legged waders, it is essential that herons are not retained with their legs in flexion for any length of time.

Transportation

Waders can be transported safely in a suitably sized box that must be sufficiently tall to allow the bird to stand. Containers should be darkened and well ventilated and the floor should be covered with a towel or carpeting to provide a non-slip surface that allows the bird to grip and steady itself. Where suitable boxes are not available for larger species, the casualty can be safely transported (for a short time) wrapped in a suitable cloth, towel or blanket, with the head restrained and the legs placed in extension behind the bird. Long journeys should be avoided whenever possible.

Examination and assessment for rehabilitation

The examination of a wading bird casualty follows the basic techniques and criteria outlined in Chapter 2.

Careful examination and assessment of the functioning of the limbs and bill must be made before attempting to treat a wader casualty. To prevent damage to the delicate maxilla and mandibles, the bill of a wader should be held at its base when being opened. The strong beak of a heron may need the use of an improvised gag, such as a disposable syringe barrel wrapped in adhesive tape, to hold it open for examination of the mouth or for passage of a gavage tube.

Assessment of body condition should be made by palpation of the pectoral musculature, as with other groups of birds. Experience may be required for condition scoring of herons in particular, since their keels are especially prominent.

The commissures of the mouth and frenulum of the tongue should be checked carefully for evidence of nylon fishing line. The leading edge of the wing (propatagium) should be checked for evidence of abrasions caused by entanglement in netting.

First aid procedures

First aid for a wading bird casualty follows the basic techniques of wound and fracture management, fluid and energy replacement and warmth outlined in Chapter 2.

Fluid replacement therapy

The smaller waders are similar in weight to small passerines and the approach to re-establishing their fluid and energy levels is similar (see Chapter 25). In the larger waders (>100 g bodyweight) and in the heron, the medial tarsal vein is readily accessible for administering a bolus of fluid or for placing an intravenous catheter. When administering fluids by gavage, it is important to hold the beak of a long-billed wader as close to its base as possible, to prevent iatrogenic damage, and to use a gag with herons to prevent damage to the handler's fingers (see 'Examination and assessment').

Short-term housing

Satisfactory short-term housing for waders requires a quiet, secure, dark and warm enclosure. This could be provided by a cardboard box, or a cage with the bars covered with cloth or towelling. Non-slip flooring should be provided. Further details are given in Chapter 2.

Herons require short-term housing of sufficient height to allow the bird to stand upright. A large kennel, away from the sight and sound of dogs and cats, would be satisfactory.

Feeding

It can be particularly difficult to encourage wader casualties to feed in captivity. If birds are unable or unwilling to feed for themselves on admission, nutritional support can be given by feeding by gavage tube with liquid feeding formulae (e.g. Hill's a/d, Hill's Pet Nutrition; Reanimyl, Virbac; Critical Care Formula, Vetark Animal Health). Anorexic herons can be fed by gavage tube with liquidized fish or fed by hand with small fish (Figure 19.3) or day-old chicks.

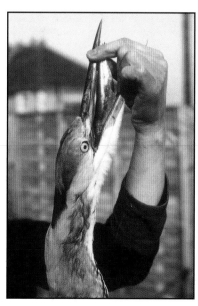

19.3 Hand feeding an anorexic grey heron, with its head in gentle extension.

Care should be taken to minimize the frequency of feeds to that considered to be essential, since the repeated stress of capture and handling may lead to regurgitation and discourage the bird from starting to self-feed. A delicate compromise must be reached in these cases and every effort made to stimulate the bird to recognize the offered foodstuffs as its natural diet. For example, herons may be encouraged to feed by injecting air into some of the sprats being fed and presenting them in a shallow tray of water so that some of the fish float and others sink, giving the food a more 'natural' appearance.

Anaesthesia and analgesia

The details of avian anaesthesia and analgesia given in Chapter 2 apply to wading bird casualties.

Care must be taken when handling the delicate smaller waders and caution taken to protect handlers when dealing with members of the heron family (see 'Handling and transportation', above). During anaesthesia, long-legged birds should always have their legs in extension.

Inhalation anaesthesia using isoflurane is, whenever practicable, the method of choice. The length of the bill in some larger waders may complicate the use of masks for induction. This can be overcome by extending the length of a Hall's rubber mask by gluing to the open end a 'skirt' made from a rubber rebreathing bag or by fashioning a mask from a plastic bottle.

Larger birds, especially herons, can injure themselves during recovery. They should be restrained in lateral or ventral recumbency wrapped in towelling with their legs extended behind them until they are able to stand.

Specific conditions

Trauma
The majority of casualties of free-living wading birds are associated with trauma. For example, woodcock commonly feed in woodland and roadside ditches and, being crepuscular, are often involved in road traffic accidents. Herons, especially juvenile birds, commonly collide with overhead cables and sustain wing fractures, which are usually open and comminuted and rarely operable. Due to their feeding habits, herons may become entangled in discarded fishing line or enmeshed in netting over ornamental garden ponds.

Natural poisoning
Poisoning could occur in waders that are feeding on molluscs that have accumulated, by filtration, toxins produced by certain types of phytoplankton (dinoflagellates) in a marine algal bloom – the so-called 'red tides'. Such incidents would involve deaths of wading and other birds, especially marine waterfowl.

Oil pollution
Waders may be involved in incidents of marine oil pollution when the oil, especially if fresh, contaminates beaches. Details of treatment of oil pollution are given in Chapter 18.

Nutritional problems
In hard winters, herons – especially immature birds – are frequently found suffering from emaciation caused by starvation. If supportive treatment (including treatment with anthelminthics, if indicated) results in a rapid increase in weight, the casualty may be a suitable case for release to the wild when local conditions are favourable. If no increase in weight occurs, it is likely that the bird is suffering from a chronic infectious disease or organ failure and as such would not be suitable for release.

Therapeutics

Allometric scaling and methods of administering medication as detailed in Chapter 2 apply to wading birds.

For very small waders (< 50 g) an intramuscular injection is a painful and stressful procedure and should be avoided whenever possible. Oral dosage by gavage, using medications suitable for that route, may be preferable, taking care not to damage the delicate beak. Intramuscular injections using the pectoral muscles are less of a problem in larger species but are associated with the potential problem of damage to the flight muscles. Indirect methods of medication, using food or water, are unreliable unless the medicated food can be given in measured amounts.

Doses for various agents are given in the avian formulary in Appendix 1.

Management in captivity

Accommodation for hospitalization during a period of medium- to long-term treatment should follow the details outlined in Chapter 2. In addition, wading birds benefit from access to drinking and bathing water placed in suitably sized shallow containers, which will need regular cleaning. Waders, especially the smaller and more sensitive species, should be placed in hospital cages that are protected from disturbance. A wet substrate should be used on the floor of the cage, such as moist sand or newspaper.

For a recuperation period, waders will settle in a grassed or gravel-floored aviary with access to a shallow pond and, for marshland species, some natural cover. Herons require a large secluded aviary with a pool and high perches (see Chapter 3).

Diet for waders
Following supportive treatment, waders should be introduced to an artificial diet that resembles their natural diet of invertebrates (insects, molluscs, annelids) or fish. An appropriate diet should be fed as a wet mash in a suitable shallow container and can be constructed from a selection of the following constituents, depending on the size and natural diet of the casualty species (Koivisto, 1977; Wildlife Information Network, 2002):

- Mealworms and starved ('clean') maggots
- Earthworms, lugworms (fisherman's bait)
- Finely chopped or minced fish, meat or hard-boiled egg
- Proprietary insectivorous diets (e.g. Sluis Insectivore Diet, Sluis; Prosecto, Haith's)
- Mashed tinned dogfood or catfood
- Chick, turkey or fish rearing crumbs or crushed pellets
- Small seeds in canary mixture
- Vitamin and mineral supplement.

Many waders, especially those feeding on seashores, have nasal salt glands (see Chapter 18) and addition of salt to their diet may help to prevent atrophy of these glands.

Diet for herons

Heron casualties, once feeding on their own, can be provided with a diet comprising the following:

- Small fish (sprats) or strips of fish
- Dead mice or day-old chicks
- Solid chunks of tinned dog food
- Vitamin and mineral supplement (supplementation with thiamine and vitamin E becomes essential when feeding white fish for a prolonged period).

Rearing orphans

Waders

Wader chicks rarely come into captivity. They are actively and noisily protected by the adults and should only be taken into care once the absence of parents has been established definitively.

The young of all species of wader are precocial, nidifugous and self-feeding. Following supportive treatment and the provision of heat, and in the absence of any underlying injuries or disease, they should feed without assistance on a diet based on similar, but finer, constituents to that suggested above for adult waders. The diet may be presented in a shallow container as a moist mash. A source of light placed over the feed container might encourage the chicks to find the food.

Imprinting in precocial species occurs within hours of hatching and so is not a problem with artificially reared wader chicks. Once fully fledged (at approximately 3 weeks of age for the smaller waders and up to 6 weeks for the larger species), the chicks are independent. This is the optimal time for release.

Herons

Heron nestlings and fledglings are occasionally dislodged from the nest or surrounding branches. Young nestlings need to be fed by hand but once fledged they should have learnt to self-feed, as at this stage in the wild they are presented with regurgitated food by the adults. A diet based on similar constituents to those in that suggested above for adult herons should be suitable. Careful attention should be paid to appropriate mineral supplementation of the rearing

diet to avoid the development of nutritional osteodystrophy. Young herons need regular exercise to prevent abnormal growth of the long bones of the leg (Humphries, 1988).

Release

Adults

The release of adult waders is usually by a 'hard' release technique (see Chapter 3) in a suitable wetland environment, at a time when conspecific individuals are known to be present and the weather conditions are appropriate.

Young herons

Returning a hand-reared fledgling to its heronry is rarely practicable. Heron chicks are fully fledged by 50 days of age and usually remain at the heronry for a further 10–20 days before becoming fully independent. At this age they can be released in a suitable location in the proximity of their natal heronry.

Legal aspects

Legal aspects of handling wildlife casualties are outlined in Chapter 5. Many species of wading birds that are rare breeding birds in the British Isles are included in Schedule 4 of the Wildlife and Countryside Act 1981 and must be registered with DEFRA if they are to be kept in captivity for treatment.

Specialist organizations

Population studies:
British Trust for Ornithology
The Nunnery, Thetford, Norfolk IP24 2PU

Conservation of wetland habitats:
Wildfowl and Wetlands Trust
Slimbridge, Gloucestershire GL2 7BT

Captive management of waders:
Federation of Zoological Gardens of Great Britain and Ireland
Zoological Gardens, Regent's Park, London NW1 4RY

References and further reading

BWRC (1999) Report on the Wildlife Casualties Recording Scheme 1993–1997. *Rehabilitator* **28**. British Wildlife Rehabilitation Council, c/o RSPCA Wildlife Department, Horsham
Cramp S (1977) *The Birds of the Western Palearctic, Vols I and III.* Oxford University Press, Oxford
Humphries PN (1988) Rearing orphan birds. *Companion Animal Practice* 2(4), 45–49
Jordan WJ and Hughes J (1982) *Care of the Wild.* Macdonald, London
King AS and McLelland J (1984) *Birds: Their Structure and Function.* Baillière Tindall, London
Koivisto I (1977) The breeding and maintenance of some northern European waders, Charadrii, at Helsinki Zoo. In: *International Zoo Yearbook, 17*, pp. 150–153. Zoological Society of London, London
Perrins C (1987) *Collins New Generation Guide to the Birds of Britain and Europe.* Collins, London
Stocker L (2000) *Practical Wildlife Care.* Blackwell Science, Oxford
Wildlife Information Network (Wildpro®, Royal Veterinary College, London) (April 2002) *UK Wildlife First Aid and Care,* www.wildlifeinformation.org

20

Waterfowl: swans, geese, ducks, grebes and divers

Stephen W. Cooke

Introduction

An indication of the species most commonly presented for veterinary care is given in Figure 20.1. Casualties presented for treatment also include a number of feral domesticated species (e.g. domestic duck and goose breeds), wild species that have been introduced into the country (e.g. mute swan, Canada goose) and some less common species such as escaped captive-bred black swans, oiled seabirds (e.g. great northern diver) or lead-poisoned migratory whooper swans.

Order Family	Genus and species	Diet	Feeding strategy	Resident or migrant	Typical habitat
Gaviiformes					
Gaviidae (divers)	*Gavia* Red-throated diver (*G. stellata*) Black-throated diver (*G. arctica*) Great northern diver (*G. immer*)	Fish	Diving	Summer migrants to Scotland Winter migrants elsewhere	Summer: inland lakes and pools Winter: mainly at sea
Podicipediformes					
Podicipedidae (grebes)	*Tachybaptus* Little grebe (*T. ruficollis*)	Aquatic invertebrates Small fish	Diving	Resident	Freshwater lakes, ponds and rivers
	Podiceps Great crested grebe (*P. cristatus*) Slavonian grebe (*P. auritus*) Black-necked grebe (*P. nigricollis*)	Fish	Diving	Resident	Summer: inland lakes Winter: freshwater and coastal
Anseriformes					
Anatidae (swans, geese and ducks)	*Cygnus* (swans) Mute swan (*C. olor*) Bewick's swan (*C. columbianus*) Whooper swan (*C. cygnus*)	Aquatic vegetation Grasses	Grazing and upending	Mute: resident Bewick's and whooper: winter migrants	Mostly open fresh water, marshes, wet pasture
	Anser (grey geese) Greylag (*A. anser*) Pink-footed goose (*A. brachyrhynchus*) White-fronted goose (*A. albifrons*)	Aquatic vegetation Grasses Vegetation, including grain and root crops	Grazing	Greylag: mainly resident Others: winter migrants	Marshes, wet grassland and winter arable crops
	Branta (black geese) Barnacle goose (*B. leucopsis*) Brent goose (*B. bernicla*) Canada goose (*B. canadensis*)	Grasses	Grazing	Canada and some barnacle geese: feral and resident Others: winter migrants	Fresh water, marsh and wetlands Brent and barnacle geese: winter coastal marshes
	Tadorna (shelduck) Shelduck (*T. tadorna*)	Invertebrates, mainly crustaceans/ molluscs	Filtering mud	Resident, adults migrate for post-breeding moult	Coastal
	Anas (dabbling ducks) Mallard (*A. platyrhynchos*) Teal (*A. crecca*) Wigeon (*A. penelope*) Shoveler (*A. clypeata*) Pintail (*A. acuta*)	Mainly aquatic vegetation, grasses Some aquatic invertebrates	Grazing and upending Shoveler: sieves vegetation and invertebrates from water surface	Resident and winter migrants	Freshwater lakes, rivers and marshes Spread to coastal marshes in winter

20.1 Classification and biology of commoner species of British waterfowl. (continues) ▶

Order Family	Genus and species	Diet	Feeding strategy	Resident or migrant	Typical habitat
Anseriformes *continued*					
	Aythya (diving ducks) Pochard (*A. ferina*) Tufted duck (*A. fuligula*) Scaup (*A. marila*)	Invertebrates, mainly small molluscs Aquatic vegetation	Diving	Resident and winter migrants	Mainly freshwater lakes Scaup: winter at sea
	Somateria (sea ducks: eiders) Eider (*S. mollissima*)	Mainly molluscs	Diving	Resident in north Winter migrants elsewhere	Coastal
	Mellanita (sea ducks: scoters) Common scoter (*M. nigra*)	Mainly molluscs	Diving	Summer migrant to Scotland Winter migrant: coasts	Summer: inland lakes Scotland Winter: coastal
	Buchephala (goldeneyes) Goldeneye (*B. clangula*)	Aquatic invertebrates	Diving	Mainly winter migrant	Freshwater lakes, coastal
	Mergus (sawbills) Goosander (*M. merganser*) Red-breasted merganser (*M. serrator*) Smew (*M. albellus*)	Fish	Diving	Goosander: breeds inland rivers and lakes Others: winter migrants	Merganser: coastal Others: inland lakes and rivers

20.1   (continued) Classification and biology of commoner species of British waterfowl.

Ecology and biology

By definition, waterfowl are birds that depend on or are associated with water to a greater or lesser degree. Most waterfowl float on water using a boat-like 'hull' of feathers that have waterproofing and insulating properties. Damage to the hull will compromise the bird's ability to survive and every effort must be taken to ensure that the waterproof characteristics and integrity of the feathering are not damaged by ill-considered intervention.

Some species have specialized feeding requirements (see Figure 20.1) but most are herbivorous and relatively tolerant of new diets and of the commonly used recovery feeds designed for companion species.

The young of some species are self-feeding (e.g. ducks and geese); others, such as the divers and grebes, produce young that are dependent on parental feeding for some time. Most of the young imprint very readily (see Chapter 3).

Anatomy and physiology

With few exceptions, waterfowl tend to be medium-sized to large birds with well developed fat deposits and a good resistance to stressors when healthy. Metabolic rates range from one (swans and large geese) to four (small ducks and grebes) times those of the dog.

Specialized organs include nasal glands that secrete concentrated salt solutions in marine species (see Chapter 18) and the copulatory organ of male ducks and geese.

Most waterfowl pass through an eclipse moult during the breeding season and take on an immature or female plumage colouring. Most have a synchronized moult of the flight feathers, leading to a temporary loss of flight.

Some species – most obviously divers and grebes – have adapted to swimming to the point where they cannot walk easily on land. Individuals of these species should be assessed on water for pelvic damage.

Capture, handling and transportation

Capture

Swans and some large geese tend to be easy to catch with appropriate equipment; most rescue centres have swan hooks and access to boats or canoes and people who can use them. In many cases the birds' willingness to accept food from humans allows close contact and easy capture. In other cases birds are often very difficult to catch and the assistance of experienced rescuers is required.

Handling

Most species are best restrained in some form of wrap that will prevent the wings from flapping. The most basic form is a tea towel with the ends wrapped diagonally across the body to form a parcel, with the head and neck exposed. The towel is secured with tape or open-weave bandage to prevent loosening. In a similar manner a large sheet or blanket may be wrapped around swans, geese or ducks recovering from anaesthesia. Specially made wraps have been described (Figure 20.2) and there are appropriate sizes for most waterfowl. Simple disposable restraints may be created from suitable bags (e.g. pillowcases, plastic feed-bags, hessian sacks) with one corner cut off to allow the bird's head and neck to protrude.

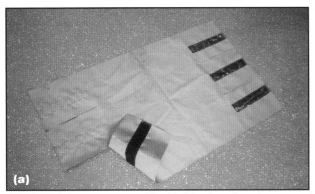
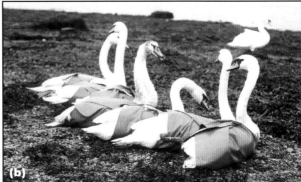

20.2 (a) A swan wrap. The bird is placed on the opened wrap, preferably with the legs extended, and held caudally. The flaps are folded over the back and secured (in this case with Velcro strips). (Courtesy of Dick Best.)
(b) Mute swans held in swan wraps prior to release. Such wraps are useful for restraining large waterfowl during clinical examinations, radiography, administration of medication and transportation. (Courtesy of Colin Seddon.)

In most cases (where anatomy or injury allows) it is advisable to use soft bandages, strips of linen or old neckties to secure the legs together over the tail. The 'shanks' are crossed and secured with a double-bow knot that can be loosened easily if the bird is distressed. This prevents the bird from pushing its way out of the restraint. Close confinement will cause a bird's body temperature to increase and may induce hyperthermia if prolonged.

Boxes may be used to carry the smaller species (up to goose size) but care needs to be taken when opening the box. It is best to place a large blanket over the top of the box first and then to push the top inwards and grasp the bird blind under the blanket.

Protective gloves may be worn at this stage but should be discarded as soon as adequate restraint has been established, as their use hinders accurate clinical examination. Sharp-billed species (e.g. grebes, mergansers) can inflict deep lacerating wounds by pecking and should have the head held by an assistant or the beak tied closed with easily removed dressing material.

Feather damage caused by improper handling and restraint must be avoided as it may prevent the bird from being returned promptly to the wild.

Examination and assessment for rehabilitation

The examination and assessment of a waterfowl casualty follow the basic techniques and criteria outlined in Chapter 2.

Members of the public often present debilitated birds and this fact alone usually implies that there is a good reason for their capture. In the absence of obvious physical causes (e.g. oiling, fishing tackle entanglement), the presence of severe injury or systemic disease must be inferred and carefully investigated.

In all instances it must be appreciated that the sequelae to some disabilities will prevent the individual from being returned to the wild. Some rescue groups are able to place disabled birds (especially swans) in 'protected' environments but places are limited and increasingly difficult to find.

Euthanasia

The intravenous administration of any one of the standard small animal euthanasia solutions at recommended dosages is an appropriate means of euthanasia in the larger species, where venous access is readily available via the medial tarsal, right jugular (the left is absent) or basilic vein. Details of appropriate techniques are given in Chapter 2. Smaller birds will resent a wing being lifted, preventing access to the basilic vein, and the jugular vein often is difficult to visualize in debilitated birds. In these cases consideration should be given to intraperitoneal, intracardiac or intracranial administration (see Chapter 2).

First aid procedures

First aid for a waterfowl casualty follows the basic techniques of wound and fracture management, fluid and energy replacement and warmth outlined in Chapter 2.

Feeding

Once the bird has been stabilized, appropriate preparations for gavage include Hills a/d (Hill's Pet Nutrition), Lectade (Pfizer), proprietary babyfoods and homemade diets tailored to individual species (e.g. sardines put through a blender for anorectic grebes or marine birds). As a guide, 120 ml three times a day may be given to mute swans, with proportionately less for geese and ducks.

Spontaneous regurgitation will occur in response to force-feeding and handling, especially with divers and grebes. The best method is to handle the bird carefully and retreat immediately, leaving it quiet for at least an hour.

Short-term hospitalization

For short-term (less than 5 days) hospitalization of most species, all that is required is an easily cleaned substrate or cage environment and provision of water in good-sized bowls. A 'small dog' kennel is appropriate for species up to goose size and a walk-in kennel would easily house a swan (Figure 20.3) or goose.

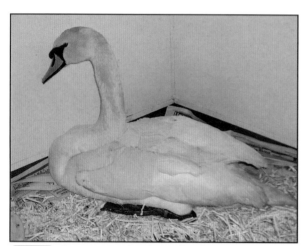

20.3 A mute swan in a heated walk-in pen, suitable for short-term hospitalization. This bird is showing a 'kinked' neck suggestive of lead toxicity.

Anaesthesia and analgesia

Details of avian anaesthesia and analgesia are given in Chapter 2.

Many minor procedures, such as removal of fishing tackle, may be carried out safely on conscious birds.

Small individuals are best induced with isoflurane, either by mask or by the use of an anaesthetic chamber. Struggling as an avoidance response to high induction concentrations of isoflurane may be prevented by gradually increasing the inhaled concentration from 0.5 to 4.5% over a period of 1 minute or so.

Care must be exercised when maintaining anaesthesia, as high concentrations of isoflurane (3–4%) are often necessary; prolonged anaesthesia or the use of circle absorber systems may reduce these values to 0.5–1.5% in some individuals.

Larger species are difficult to induce by inhalation and a suitable injectable induction is required. The author prefers alfaxalone/alfadolone given as an intravenous bolus at approximately 7 mg total steroids/kg bodyweight; however, this may lead to a brief period of apnoea – especially if the bird's head is allowed to drop below the level of its heart, as this will induce the positional apnoea reflex and compound that of the injection. If the blood's oxygenation is monitored by pulse oximetry (the tongue is the best place for sensor positioning), appropriate intermittent positive pressure ventilation (IPPV) may be used to maintain a good pO_2 and allow the bird to inhale the maintenance agent at the same time.

A ketamine/xylazine anaesthetic protocol has been described (Routh and Painter,1999) and is in widespread use (see avian formulary in Appendix 1).

Intubation

Intubation and the use of cuffed tubes is recommended for waterfowl in all except the shortest of procedures (the avian tracheal ring is complete and so overinflation of a cuff may rupture the trachea or cause pressure necrosis of the epithelium).

Specific conditions

Trauma

Wing injuries

A description of wing injuries and their treatment is given in Chapter 2. Techniques are further discussed in Chapter 22, in relation to birds of prey.

If the whole wing is drooping, a high limb site is involved and a radiographic examination of the shoulder area should be undertaken. The area is highly sensitive to irreversible damage, which usually results in inhibition of normal flight ability. Physical damage to the coracoid and associated tissues almost always causes loss of flight ability. One exception is nerve (brachial plexus) trauma without bony damage and a significant percentage of such cases will resolve if given sufficient time (weeks or a few months). If conservative treatment is justified in waterfowl, reducing the weight of the wing by clipping primary and secondary feathers prevents the limb from becoming waterlogged and drooping further or becoming traumatized.

If the carpus is drooping, damage to the humerus, elbow and radius or ulna is suggested. Most fractures of the humerus become open and contaminated and so high limb amputation is indicated, if inflicting such permanent deformity can be justified. The site for amputation is the proximal third of the humerus and routine surgical technique is appropriate. It is difficult to justify amputation at the radius and ulna, as most amputation wounds at this position become damaged and infected at some time. It should be noted that the humerus is pneumatized and so contamination of the air sac system may have already occurred. Appropriate antibiosis is usually sufficient but *Aspergillus* spp. may contaminate the wound and produce severe secondary lesions or even sudden death.

Pinioning: Pinioning – the elective removal of the metacarpal bones to prevent flight in captive birds or to treat aeroplane wing (angel wing, carpal rotation) – is an acceptable technique for many waterfowl where the loss of flight ability does not compromise their wild existence. The alula should be preserved. Haemostasis should be confined to a pressure bandage left in place for 48 hours.

Leg injuries

Femoral, tibiotarsal and tarsometatarsal bone injuries in waterfowl have to be considered life-threatening in all instances. Birds are bipedal and loss of use, loss of limb or immobilization after surgery will cause a number of sequelae (e.g. keel bone exposure; loss of waterproofing; inability to fly, mate or escape predation). All open fractures must be considered as untreatable: the loss of periosteum, infection, bone necrosis and consequent malunion of the fracture are virtually inevitable.

Most injuries to the foot (phalanges and web) may be successfully treated if they are not too extensive. Healing of fractures is usually rapid, though this may be seen as well organized pseudo-arthroses as a consequence of non-union. Even quite extensive loss of web tissue is well tolerated.

Neck and head injuries

Neck bone injuries are commonly found during routine radiographic examinations. The flexible nature of the extremity usually hides and compensates for apparently severe injury and, assuming no neurological damage is found, most bony damage will heal without interfering with the bird's survival ability.

The loss of an eye is commonly seen in waterfowl but many survive well despite the disability.

Fishing-hook injuries

Hooks retained in the beak are easy to detect and remove (Figure 20.4). Swelling usually signals those further down the oesophagus. Simple cases may be dealt with by removing the hook either with endoscope grasping forceps (the bird having been anaesthetized) or externally through a small incision directly through the skin to the hook tip, if it can be palpated and immobilized manually. Here the bird may remain conscious, if it will tolerate the handling (usually only geese and swans), and the lack of skin sensation obviates the need for local anaesthesia. There is a very good blood supply to the neck and care must be taken when cutting down in such a manner.

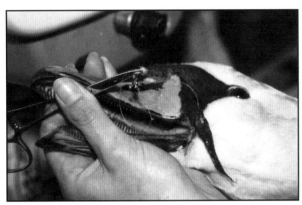

20.4 Discarded fishing line in a mute swan. Radiography is essential to identify the presence of an embedded hook in birds that have ingested fishing line.

Hooks with nylon attached may be removed by passing a thick-walled tube over the line down to the hook, which is then dislodged by being forced further down the oesophagus. Tension on the line brings the hook tip into contact with the end of the tube wall, allowing it to be withdrawn safely.

In cases where hooks have been under tension for some time, especially where a length of line is dangling from the bird's beak, there is a good chance that a linear laceration of the oesophageal wall will be present. This is usually signalled by a long fusiform abscess with crepitus and dysphagia. General anaesthesia is necessary to allow good wound preparation and a long incision over the full length of the laceration. Wound cleansing is often difficult but in most long-term cases a good abscess membrane will have formed; this will strip away under the influence of dry swab abrasion, leaving a granulating bed that will only require skin closure for excellent healing. The oesophageal lesion should be debrided and freshened before closure with absorbable monofilament material in a single layer (to avoid stricture). If the lesion is extensive, two or more repeat closures over a period of a few weeks may be required to repair the defect.

Hooks in the proventriculus should be removed endoscopically. Hooks in the gizzard may be left *in situ*, as they will be removed rapidly by normal gizzard action. The exception to this is in the case of very large (pike) hooks, which may have to be removed by ventriculotomy via an abdominal exploratory laparotomy approach.

Fishing-line injuries

Discarded fishing line is usually of nylon and resistant to ultraviolet degradation, especially when submerged. Thus it is a long-term environmental contaminant and may cause injury in a number of ways:

- The line may become wrapped around legs and wings causing tourniquet-type wounds
- Loops of line may pass over the tongue or lower or upper bill, acting as constricting foreign bodies; here the effect is more like that of cheese wire, with deep lacerations of the tongue frenulum or erosion into the mandibles or maxillae.

It may be very difficult to detect such foreign bodies and careful investigation of any deep fissures at these sites is essential. The cheese-wire effect is often compounded because the rest of the line passes into the gizzard as a mass that is continually moved as the gizzard works.

Line hanging from or attached to the beak has to be assessed for the presence of a hook, radiographically or by gentle traction. If a hook is present it may be visualized as movement of the oesophagus in the neck or as a pain response if it is in the proventriculus. If no hook is present, gentle continuous traction is applied on the line, with the bird restrained so that there is a straight line from the beak to the gizzard to avoid damage to the oesophagus. If there is a mass of line and food material in the gizzard, it may require prolonged tension before the gizzard muscles relax and allow the mass to be extracted.

Lead toxicity

A particularly pure, concentrated and widely used form of lead introduced into the environment is lead shot, in the form of shotgun pellets and angler's split-shot (sinkers), both of which are known to sink into soil at a very slow rate (approximately 2.5 cm every 10 years in undisturbed pasture) and thus remain available for ingestion over a very long period of time. All animal species are potentially at risk from these two sources of lead poisoning but swans (Figure 20.5) and Canada geese are the species most commonly presented for veterinary care in the UK.

The reasons for the vulnerability of waterfowl are related to feeding behaviour. Many bird species utilize grit as a grinding medium in their gizzards to break down food into a more readily digestible form. Small quantities of grit are ingested on a regular basis in order to 'top up' the grit in the gizzard as required, and the bird has the ability to select grit of the correct size for its own requirements. Thus small species will select small particles of grit, large species select large pieces; also herbivorous species use more grit than do carnivorous species.

Sinkers and shotgun pellets are produced in size ranges commonly sought out by swans and geese as grit and are also often concentrated in areas used by these birds. Recent legislation has banned the sale of lead sinkers in the size range 0.06–28.36 g (the sizes most commonly found in swans suffering from lead toxicity) and their place has been taken by 'non-toxic' material of various compositions.

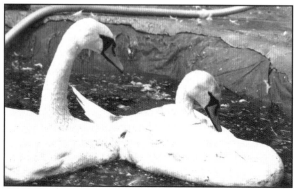

20.5 Mute swans showing the 'kinked' neck posture suggestive of lead toxicity.

Clinical signs

Clinical signs vary depending on the species, the amount of lead ingested, the rate at which it is absorbed by the bird and the period of time over which it is absorbed. The grinding action of grit in the gizzard produces fine particles of shot material, which, combined with the acid environment of the gizzard, allows significant amounts of lead to be absorbed into the bloodstream using the same pathway as calcium.

Lead competes with calcium in physiological processes as well as having a strong chemical affinity for many biochemically reactive compounds. It inactivates enzymes involved in major metabolic pathways and is a pansystemic toxin and so may be expected to have an adverse effect on all tissues in the body. Three clinical descriptions of lead poisoning are appropriate: peracute, acute and chronic.

Peracute: This is normally seen in cases where a large number of shotgun pellets have been ingested. The soft nature of this material allows it to be ground down rapidly in the gizzard, ensuring that large amounts of lead are absorbed quickly. Deaths are often so rapid as to be asymptomatic and the bird will be in good or very good body condition if this is the first episode.

Acute: This is the 'typical' presentation, where signs suggest a provisional diagnosis. It should be noted that there are no pathognomonic signs of lead toxicosis. Several signs are cited as being associated with this condition, seen in combination or singularly; they include: dysrexia; anorexia; a bright green watery diarrhoea (often staining the feathers around the cloaca and sometimes the buccal mucous membranes through

preening); progressive weight loss; a 'kinked' neck; anaemia; changes in behaviour (becoming more aggressive or self-isolation from the flock) or vocalization; muscle weakness (staggering gait and increased risk of flight accidents); reflux of water up the cervical oesophagus; ketotic breath; fluffy head feathers; 'olive-shaped' eye; dehydration; poor feathering; drooping wings; and an inability to eat or digest food normally.

Chronic: This is now the more common presentation since the ban on the sale of lead sinkers. It is mainly seen in cases where non-lethal amounts of lead have been ingested over a long period (many weeks to many months). Signs relate to chronic organ damage complicated by lead toxicosis. Many of the changes are similar to those seen in starvation and chronic malnutrition: muscle atrophy, loss of fat deposits, liver atrophy with an enlarged gall bladder, intestinal contraction, reflux of gizzard contents (especially grit) into the proventriculus, flaccid heart muscles with associated cardiac insufficiency, and severe anaemia. Impaction of the oesophagus and proventriculus due to flaccid paralysis of the gizzard is a common finding; it is usually seen in chronic poisoning in swans but may also be seen in acute poisoning in Canada geese, which may also show a cephalic oedema that is possibly unique to this species.

Diagnosis

Radiography: Adult swans are usually placed in sternal (ventral) recumbency, restrained within a body wrap. It is essential that gizzard radiography is performed. Whole-body radiographs of most species are easily undertaken without anaesthesia and should be considered an absolute minimum diagnostic work-up. Centring the beam just caudal to the ziphisternum in the midline or at the level of the elbow joints will always show the gizzard and proventriculus. The advent of non-toxic alternatives for fishing weights complicates the diagnosis of lead toxicity, as the alternatives are also strongly radio-dense and have the same morphology as those containing lead. Sometimes the overlying pelvic or wing bones will obliterate the gizzard and a lateral view may be necessary, the bird being restrained within a body wrap and suitably supported in lateral recumbency.

Blood samples: Blood lead levels are a useful adjunct to clinical signs and radiography for confirmation of a diagnosis. Diagnostic laboratories vary in their sample requirements; some prefer heparin as an anticoagulant but most accept EDTA, which has a longer sample life *in vitro*; the minimum volume is 1 ml but 2 ml is preferred.

Blood lead values greater than 20 µg/dl (0.2 ppm, 0.2 µg/ml or 0.97 µmol/l; conversion factor µg/dl x 0.0483 = µmol/l) should always be interpreted as a sign that lead has been ingested in sufficient quantities to produce some form of toxic effect. This fact, together with clinical signs or radiographic evidence of lead in the gizzard, would strongly suggest a diagnosis of lead toxicosis. Lead values greater than 60 µg/dl (0.6 µg/ml or 2.9 µmol/l) indicate clinical toxicosis; values above 100 µg/dl (1 µg/ml or 4.83 µmol/l) indicate acute lead toxicosis. In the mute swan, apparently healthy breeding individuals have been recorded with very high values (> 500 μg/dl) and some chronic cases respond to treatment even with only mildly elevated values. The final diagnosis must therefore be made with full consideration of all the elements of a good diagnostic work-up, including response to trial therapy with chelating agents.

Other diagnostic tests (e.g. blood biochemistry and haematology) have proved to be non-specific in the majority of cases. The author has carried out numerous 'blood profiles' on swans suffering from lead toxicosis and has found no single test or combination of tests to be of diagnostic or prognostic value in that species. The typical red blood cell morphological changes seen in humans do not exist in birds but poikilocytosis is reported and reflects the anaemia often associated with the condition.

Post-mortem examination: Post-mortem examination may provide a diagnosis, especially when elevated tissue lead values are found. Various histopathological findings have been documented, most of which are related to the effects of long-term tissue damage (especially red blood cell destruction and the sequelae). Lead is excreted as a metalloprotein complex deposited in the proximal convoluted tubules of the kidneys and is visible as eosinophilic inclusion bodies therein. Tissue values are often used to confirm the diagnosis. Normal liver lead values are considered to be < 2 μg/g wet weight, with elevated values indicating exposure to toxic quantities of the metal. Kidney values are usually in the region 50–100% of liver values.

The presence of characteristic metallic material in the gizzard also helps to ensure that it is lead rather than a non-toxic alternative before progressing with a diagnosis. Metallic lead is soft, has a shiny metallic cut surface and easily marks paper, whereas the alternatives are harder, have a granular gritty cut surface and are likely to tear paper.

Blood or tissue lead values above zero indicate that the bird has ingested the element in some form and that normal excretion pathways have failed to clear it from the system. Lead is a toxin and any positive value must imply a degree of toxicity.

Treatment

Chemical methods: Chelating agents are indicated whenever a definite or presumptive diagnosis has been made. Sometimes the response to therapy will aid in reaching a more certain diagnosis, especially when other factors are involved (such as concomitant disease where lead toxicity may be exaggerating the problem). Several agents have been used but only calcium disodium EDTA, available as sodium calcium edetate (strong) (Animalcare, York) has satisfied the needs for a routine drug of choice in wildlife. The author uses a standard dose of 62.5 mg/kg, which is administered once, twice or three times a day depending on the severity of signs and the amount of lead expected to be present in the bird's body (as determined by radiography or clinical assessment of the chronicity of exposure

to the element). The preparation has been used undiluted and subcutaneously (over the proximal tibial muscles) with adverse reactions limited to a small number of animals exhibiting skin thickening, pain reaction and hyperaemia only after long periods (> 3 weeks) of administration. This is recognized as being 'off datasheet recommendations' but does cause very much less tissue trauma than that produced by intramuscular injections and is easier for lay staff to perform than the intravenous route.

For other treatment regimens, see the avian formulary in Appendix 1. Other classes of drugs will have to be used during the treatment of a primary lead toxicosis in order to counteract the pansystemic tissue damage that often ensues. Antibiotics, antifungals, anthelmintics, anabolic steroids, multivitamins, vitamin K (clotting defects), nutritional support, cardiac stimulants and so on will all find their place in the supportive care of such cases and good clinical acumen is essential if there is to be a successful outcome.

Gizzard flushing: Physical removal is appropriate in cases where more than five pieces of shot of any size are present. Fewer than five pieces of less than 5 mm in diameter may usually be left *in situ* and chelation treatment continued for at least the 3 weeks necessary for this material to be ground down and lost naturally. Young birds have a faster throughput of material (including lead shot) through the gastrointestinal tract and so this period may be reduced to 2 weeks.

The following gizzard flushing technique was first described for use in swans by the author (Cooke, 1981):

1. The bird is anaesthetized and carefully intubated with a cuffed endotracheal tube.
2. The bird's core temperature is determined and preferably monitored by a rectal (entering the rectum, not just the cloaca) electronic thermometer in order to reduce the risk of hypo- or hyperthermia induced by the fluid introduced.
3. A suitable volume of the flushing fluid (water or physiological saline) is brought to body temperature. As large volumes of fluid (well in excess of 5 litres for swans) are often required, a source of water at a reliably controlled temperature (e.g. a shower unit or mixer tap) may be considered. Monitoring the water temperature before and during use is essential. The procedure produces large volumes of waste water and so the operation should be performed over a sink or surface drain.
4. An open-ended stomach tube 1.5–2 m in length, of maximum diameter 12 mm (swans) or 6 mm (ducks), with a reasonable wall thickness to prevent kinking and with an adapter to fit the supply of flushing fluid, is used.
5. With the bird in ventral recumbency and its neck held horizontally, the tube is passed through the oesophagus and proventriculus to the level of the gizzard where further advancement is impeded. At this point the bird is tilted to an angle of between 45 and 60 degrees with its head down (using either a tilting table or a purpose-built sloping surface) and the flushing supply is connected.

225

6. The flushing begins at a low flow rate and the tube is gently advanced, with slight pressure, in order to enter the gizzard sphincter (this will relax at regular intervals of approximately 15–35 seconds).

7. A change in character of the waste water issuing from the bird's beak will occur when the tube has entered the gizzard: the fluid will then contain grit, small pieces of plant material and, hopefully, the shot. At this point the fluid flow is increased to enhance the flushing action and the tube is moved gently backwards and forwards to flush material from both the anterior and posterior grit pockets of the gizzard.

8. The progress of the flushing may be monitored by counting the shot retrieved or by radiographing the bird. If the latter procedure is used, care must be taken to include the whole oesophagus to ensure that the shot has been completely removed.

9. Once the shot has been removed, the bird is allowed to recover and chelation therapy is continued for at least 7 days to reduce bone deposits of lead. Routine antibiosis would be indicated as the technique may cause surface damage to mucous membranes.

Ventriculotomy: Large foreign bodies (most commonly lead ledger weights) may be removed by a ventriculotomy technique:

1. The approach is through the cranial part of the linea alba. Wound preparation should be confined to a small area of feather plucking so that regrowth is rapid.

2. The gizzard is located by blunt dissection through the falciform fat and held in the abdominal wound by stay sutures placed in the lateral muscle walls. Packing with swabs will prevent contamination of the peritoneal cavity.

3. A 2–4 cm incision is made in the fibrous caudal gizzard wall between and parallel with the lateral (grinding) muscle masses. The area is muscular and vascular but with relatively thin walls, and this approach will allow direct access to the lumen of the gizzard, where the foreign bodies may be identified and removed with long forceps.

4. Closure of the wound is routine; the gizzard is closed using a sturdy absorbable monofilament material in three layers: simple interrupted in the mucosa, horizontal mattress in the muscularis, followed by an inverted Lembert pattern to cover the incision with serosa.

5. Chelation is continued as above and routine antibiosis instituted. Stainless-steel suture staples offer the most effective skin closure and should be considered the method of choice in birds.

Prognosis

As a general rule, if a wild bird casualty is recovering as indicated by a progressive improvement in clinical signs such as weight gain, reduction in severity of presenting signs, change in behaviour back to a 'wild' state and so on, it should be returned to the wild as soon as possible. However, in the case of lead toxicity, this may not be enough to guarantee a good prognosis for full recovery.

The possibility that a degree of 'maladaptation syndrome' (see below) will occur or already be present must be considered and borne in mind when considering release dates, sites and post-release monitoring. Practically, it is best to release clinically healthy birds whenever possible but to arrange for the individual to be identified (by ring or microchip) so that, if it is re-presented for treatment, its previous history will be available and 'maladaptation syndrome' included in the differential diagnosis if appropriate.

'Maladaptation syndrome'

A sequel to treatment, recovery in care and release back to the wild is termed 'maladaptation syndrome' (more accurately 'malreadaptation syndrome') by the author and is seen in individuals that have been systemically damaged by lead toxicosis. Liver, kidney, heart, gut and immune system are the commonest organs affected.

In the protected environment of a care centre the bird is able to 'cope' and even thrive, despite the irreversible damage that is present, and thus may be released when the criteria for health are present. In the wild state there are other stressors (e.g. temperature extremes, lack of high quality food, peer pressure, breeding) that were not encountered in care. If the organ damage is severe enough, there may be insufficient functional reserve to compensate for an extra drain on resources and organ failure will result.

If noticed in time, the bird may be re-admitted for care in a very poor state that requires careful assessment in order to identify the source of the malaise. Remobilization of lead from bone may complicate this assessment, as blood lead values may be high enough to produce a diagnosis of lead toxicity in a case of multisystem insufficiency. To date there is no diagnostic methodology that can aid in the assessment of birds for the presence of this syndrome (it being impractical to harvest multiple organ biopsies) and it is likely to remain an unavoidable sequel to the treatment of lead toxicosis for some time yet. Affected birds often live out a short life in care.

Other toxins

Botulism

Clostridium botulinum produces a number of powerful exotoxins, which produce a flaccid paralysis in mammals and birds. Type C and sometimes type E are responsible for disease in waterfowl in the UK. The toxin is produced by the organism whilst multiplying and is released into the immediate environment. The toxin is relatively stable and persists even when its source has disappeared or is dormant.

C. botulinum is an anaerobe and multiplies in putrefying animal and plant material, where the toxin concentrates and may be ingested by insect larvae, which are unaffected by it. (A common source is from contaminated maggots – the bacteria being present in putrefying offal upon which commercially produced maggots are fed – used as fishing bait; as few as two maggots may cause clinical signs in a duck.) The toxin may become accessible to birds when contaminated food is exposed as water levels drop; thus the disease is often associated with the summer months but it may also be seen at any time of the year, due to its persistence in the environment.

Clinical signs and diagnosis: When ingested by susceptible species that have either eaten contaminated plant foods or selectively ingested insect larvae and pupae, the toxin rapidly enters the bloodstream and passes to nerve presynaptic membranes, where it specifically blocks release of acetylcholine. This results in a flaccid paralysis affecting all muscles, the severity of which depends on the muscle type (cardiac is relatively resistant to the effects) and amount of toxin ingested. Diagnosis is based on the presence of typical signs of flaccid paralysis. Three grades of clinical sign have been described that are useful in predicting prognosis:

Grade 1: unable to fly but able to walk and swim
Grade 2: unable to fly or walk but able to swim and move by a flopping motion assisted by the wings; unable to lift head out of water or off the ground
Grade 3: almost totally paralysed.

Respiration is usually laboured, bradycardia and diarrhoea are pronounced, and a useful (almost pathognomonic) sign in swans is the production of excessive saliva, which mats the feathers between the wings when the bird rests its beak there. The neck may be held up, with the beak touching the ground, or the whole neck may be flaccid and lying on the ground, between the wings or alongside the body. Body temperature may be lowered.

Laboratory aids to diagnosis are no replacement for clinical acumen. The diagnosis is usually easy once a few cases have been seen in practice.

Death is often due to drowning (the terminal convulsions of drowning may be confused with acute cases of duck virus enteritis, see below) but respiratory failure, dehydration or opportunist predation are also commonly seen. Post-mortem examination will aid diagnosis only by excluding other differentials.

Treatment: Oral preparations such as activated charcoal may be given in an attempt to prevent further absorption of toxin from the intestinal tract. Rehydration with oral, intravenous or intraosseous fluids and the supply of nutrients such as glucose should be instigated immediately and continued until the bird is able to drink without risk of drowning. Antibiotic cover (not penicillins, aminoglycosides or tetracyclines, all of which may exaggerate clinical signs) should also be provided and it would be prudent to administer a parasiticide to reduce any endoparasite infestation. Air sac administration of oxygen via a large-bore catheter placed in the abdominal air sac often aids respiration and is a useful adjunct to other treatments.

A specific antitoxin is available in the USA. In the UK, where the preparation is not readily available and where birds are often presented for treatment many hours or a few days after showing signs, most birds will not benefit from such treatment unless it can be given promptly, since the toxin will have already bound irreversibly to nerve cells.

Prognosis: A significant percentage of birds assessed as exhibiting Grade 2 and 3 signs have a poor or hopeless prognosis for recovery but some will make dramatic and complete recoveries. No long-term effects have been recorded in recovered individuals and early release is usually appropriate.

It is often possible to identify geographical areas of high risk to birds and efforts may be made to reduce the microenvironmental conditions responsible for the growth of the causal organism. Local knowledge by carers is often of vital importance in such preventive measures.

Blue-green algae
Blue-green algal toxicity is recognized as a separate source of systemic toxicity but is very difficult to diagnose and in practical terms may only be implicated by conjecture – for example, the presence of 'typical' algae in a body of water where birds are dying, or other species (e.g. domestic animals) are also being affected. Supportive treatment is logically applied but neuro- and hepatotoxicity effects are often too extensive to be anything other than fatal in many cases.

Oil contamination
A detailed description of the treatment of oiled birds is given in Chapter 18. Oil contamination of feathers is more serious in waterbirds because they are in contact with the surface of the medium upon which the contaminant floats. As a consequence the head and neck are often uniformly coated when the bird dabbles for food under water. There is also contamination of the whole hull area, with spread by preening to the upper parts of the body, when the bird swims through the contamination. The main effect of most oil contamination is to damage the waterproofing and insulating properties of the feathers, with obvious consequences for the individual affected.

As well as notorious crude-oil spill disasters at sea, common contaminating substances include heating and diesel fuel oils (including those lost from boats), lubricating oils, frying fats and oils, and heavy industrial waste, tar or crude oils. Paints, including anti-barnacle paints, are also sometimes encountered as a feather contaminant. Some substances, notably diesel, cause chemical burns to the skin as well as being a systemic toxin when they are ingested by the bird preening itself. Used cooking oil leaves a waxy coating with a characteristic chipshop smell and is very difficult to remove. The author has noted contamination with Waxoil, a waterproof/anti-rust compound used in the motor trade; the compound was impossible to remove and the bird succumbed to renal failure.

The government-funded Environment Agency (see Appendix 2) should be contacted in all cases of pollution. The Agency should be able to act to prevent further contamination and remove that already present.

Viral diseases

Duck virus enteritis

Duck virus enteritis (DVE) is caused by a herpesvirus (duck enteritis herpesvirus, DEHV) specific to Anatidae, which results in acute (1–5 days after onset of illness) or peracute (< 24 hours) death. Many outbreaks are seen as multiple deaths over a short space of time in a flock or mixed population of waterfowl. As with other herpesviruses there is a carrier state, which may last for up to 4 years. Some carriers may show a transient ulcerated lesion at the opening of the sublingual salivary gland, especially when stressed. The carrier remains an asymptomatic source of infection and may in turn produce offspring that are also carriers.

Spread of the virus is usually via water, as all fomites can carry the infective particles. Entry to the host is via exposed mucous membranes. Incubation periods are 3–7 days in domestic ducks and 10–14 days in wild waterfowl. In the UK the disease shows seasonal peaks (April to June) and this may be related to breeding activity, mixing of populations or increased stressors in carrier birds. Cases have been recorded throughout the year and this probably indicates that carrier birds have mixed with other immuno-compromised birds.

Clinical signs: These are usually severe and varied but are typically pansystemic, ranging from photophobia through polydypsia and watery bloody diarrhoea to ataxia and convulsions. None is pathognomonic and so all cases of sudden death, haemorrhagic enteritis or severe illness should be treated as if DVE were responsible and appropriate barrier nursing should be instigated. Of especial note is the bloody diarrhoeic discharge left after affected birds have been moved for treatment or disposal.

Diagnosis: Diagnosis is usually made by post-mortem examination, where the typical lesions associated with severe peracute viral damage to the gastrointestinal tract (petechiation, haemorrhagic fluid contents, diphtheritic oesophageal lesions and haemorrhagic enteritis with annular ulcers in ducks or button ulcers in swans and geese, representing lymphoid tissue damage), abdominal organs (petechiation), liver (petechiation or focal necrosis), spleen (congestion) and lung (oedema) are found in most cases. Some young birds may show only limited signs. Fresh liver, spleen and kidney may be submitted for confirmation by viral isolation.

Prevention and treatment: DVE is a disease of flocks, collections and overcrowding. Wild mallard may be one of the most significant reservoirs of infection, and steps should be taken to try to prevent their ingress into care facilities where water movement is limited (in a river or lake, the dilution of excreted virus is great; in restricted ponds, little dilution occurs and the risk of infection is significantly higher). Recurrent episodes of mortalities in a swan rescue facility have been associated with surviving swans of one disease outbreak being retained and mixed with new admissions.

Appropriate advice regarding the fate of survivors from a DVE outbreak must be given, including euthanasia, as the risks to the wild population must be carefully considered if potential carriers are to be released. A vaccine (Nobilis Duck Plague, Intervet) is available and may be used if circumstances are clinically appropriate. It is useful in a flock outbreak as protection is provided rapidly (within 24 hours) but it will not prevent the carrier state being produced in some individuals.

Treatment is limited to supportive therapy but the ethics of treatment when the disease has been diagnosed must be carefully assessed.

Bacterial diseases

Hot cygnet syndrome

Hot cygnet syndrome (HCS), a common presentation for juvenile birds, is a 'pyrexia of unknown origin'.

Clinical signs: Dramatic temperature spikes occur and mortality is high unless aggressive antibiosis is administered promptly. Some birds are found dead, often apparently sleeping on a riverbank, whilst others present in a state of complete collapse that may be confused with botulism (the high temperature seen in HCS differentiates the two) or similar acute-onset diseases. Terminal convulsions are possible but seldom reported, due to their short duration. Affected individuals are usually in very good body condition, with no obvious wounds or concurrent pathology.

Diagnosis: The condition is seen as single, isolated cases in almost all instances and so differentiation from duck virus enteritis is usually straightforward. The organisms responsible have not been identified but it may be assumed that they could include *Escherichia coli*, *Pasteurella* spp., *Erysipelothrix* spp. and other similar pyrogenic bacteria.

Post-mortem investigation will reveal signs consistent with a generalized septicaemia and pansystemic organ damage. The bacteria responsible may be isolated from appropriate samples.

Treatment: Treatment is usually successful if initiated quickly. The use of broad-spectrum antibiotics such as the fluoroquinolones (adult birds), potentiated penicillins or macrolides (especially gentamicin, if renal perfusion can be maintained) is considered by the author to be essential.

Bumblefoot (pododermatitis)

This is a proliferative swelling of the plantar surface(s) of the feet and usually affects the 'heel' (tarsometatarsal-phalangeal joint) but also occurs over the other interphalangeal joints. The lesions are induced by pressure and physical damage and reflect the fact that most waterfowl in their preferred habitats do not spend much time on land. Where they do, as in hospital situations, bumblefoot is likely to develop.

Clinical signs: The tissue is mainly thickened hyperkeratotic epithelium with an underlying chronic active inflammatory and fibrous tissue response. Some lesions have necrotic areas; others are just large fibrous swellings. Contamination with *Staphylococcus aureus*, *Escherichia coli*, *Proteus* spp., *Candida albicans* and other microorganisms tends to complicate the tissue trauma, which continues because the area is swollen and so progressively more prone to damage. Because birds are bipedal, they cannot avoid using the affected limb.

Treatment: Surgery is indicated if bumblefoot is causing problems such as pain, interference with normal activities, or secondary infections. Surgical intervention is limited in most instances to debulking of the lesion in order to return the foot to a more normal anatomy or the removal of caseous material or foreign bodies. Few lesions in waterfowl show the deep involvement of tendons, as is commonly found in birds of prey, and surgery is usually uncomplicated (see Chapter 22).

The skin is highly vascular and a tourniquet may be used to reduce perioperative bleeding. It is undesirable to reduce bleeding by ligation: the final skin closure and an appropriate dressing are all that is necessary, without introducing more foreign material into the wound. Stainless-steel suture staples are excellent for closing such surgical defects, as they provide rapid and secure closure and haemostasis in a short time without introducing suture material deep into the subcutaneous tissue, where contamination is inevitable. Post-operative antibiosis is essential. Dressings are best removed after 48–72 hours and the bird may be released after suture removal at 10 days.

Mycoplasmas

These organisms are often associated with respiratory and reproductive disease in adult birds and with generalized and nervous symptoms in juveniles. Typically a tenosynovitis is reported as being caused by the serofibrinous cell-mediated inflammatory response initiated by this group of bacteria but this systemic effect is not localized in joints: it may also affect other serous membranes, such as the sinuses, lung, other parts of the respiratory system and any abdominal organ. Secondary opportunist bacterial invaders will complicate the clinical picture, treatment and prognosis. Specific diagnosis is often not possible and broad-spectrum antibiosis is often necessary, to provide a 'catch-all' treatment.

Avian tuberculosis

This is a chronic, insidious and debilitating disease caused by bacteria of the *Mycobacterium intracellulare/ M. avium* complex, of which *M. avium* is the organism most commonly associated with disease in birds. It is a ubiquitous soil contaminant that builds in concentration with time in any site where waterfowl are housed. Infection is initially introduced by wild birds and its portal of entry in healthy birds is the gastrointestinal tract.

Clinical signs: Weight loss, muscle mass depletion, weakness and bright green diarrhoea have all been reported as classical signs; they are commonly seen in most debilitated waterfowl and cannot be considered pathognomonic. Various post-mortem signs have been described that parallel those seen in other systemic granulomatous reactions. Amyloidosis is also frequently associated with the chronic nature of the disease and care should be taken not to discount concomitant disease, such as *M. avium* infection, when diagnosing amyloidosis at post-mortem examination.

Diagnosis: Diagnosis in the live bird is difficult, despite the availability of several laboratory tests. It may be prudent to consider laparoscopy of the abdominal contents (especially liver), while at the same time harvesting biopsy samples of any tissues (e.g. liver nodules) that appear to be abnormal for histopathological analysis.

Treatment: Treatment is theoretically possible but difficult to justify in most cases.

Fungal diseases

Aspergillosis

Some waterbird species are highly susceptible to infection with *Aspergillus* spp., especially when debilitated or otherwise immunocompromised (see Chapter 18). Exposure to infective spores is enhanced in care facilities, especially those using hay and straw as bedding (shredded paper is far better) or where hygiene standards are allowed to deteriorate. Thiamine deficiency, especially in piscivores, also predisposes to infection.

Clinical signs: Signs are often subtle and may be hidden or mimic other conditions such as chronic lead toxicity, tuberculosis and pseudotuberculosis, amyloidosis and other chronic systemic pathology. The disease must always be considered if progressive weight loss (with or without respiratory signs) occurs despite treatment for the more clinically obvious causes; however, a definite diagnosis is often difficult to establish. Antibodies are rarely present, as seroconversion is often slow or non-existent; an ELISA test is claimed to detect infection after 7 days and should be requested rather than the gel diffusion antibody test. Radiographic changes may be too subtle to detect. Respiratory distress may not always occur and haematological signs may be limited to a transient heterophilia followed by a vague anaemia, monocytosis and the presence of toxic heterophils. An acute presentation, which is often indicated by a number of sudden deaths at a care centre, may be attributed to the use of a heavily contaminated bale of straw or hay; in such cases the risk of human infection should also be considered.

Treatment: The use of antifungal drugs (see the avian formulary in Appendix 1) will be curative if given early enough in the course of the disease but treatment is usually ineffective, as the fungus is well established before its presence is diagnosed. Indeed, diagnosis is often made only at post-mortem examination.

Parasites

Cestodes, nematodes, acanthocephelans, trematodes, feather lice and leeches are all commonly found. Some are pathogenic, others a nuisance and some are commensals. It would be prudent to instigate parasiticidal treatment of all debilitated individuals presented for care.

Gizzard worm

Gizzard worm (*Amidostomum* spp.) causes extensive damage to the mucous membranes at the proventriculus/gizzard border and subsequent classic signs of chronic debilitating disease (listlessness, lack of thrift, dysrexia/anorexia, emaciation, weight loss, diarrhoea, anaemia). This and some other pathological species may be resistant to commonly used drugs and a 3–5-day course of fenbendazole is often necessary to treat such infestations.

Leeches

Leeches, which often inhabit the nasal sinuses, cloaca and palpebral conjunctiva, respond well to ivermectin as a single dose.

Heartworm

A heartworm, *Sarconema eurycera*, is well documented in some swan and geese populations but is not considered to be pathogenic in all affected individuals. The presence of microfilariae in circulating blood has been reported to be as high as 22% of some populations but care should be exercised when considering treatment, for the same reasons as those cited for canine heartworm cases.

Myiasis

Infestation of traumatic wounds by fly larvae is common and should be treated appropriately. Care must be taken when using insecticides as treatment for myiasis as most birds are very susceptible to the toxic side effects of organophosphates. Flushing with copious amounts of water and drying with a hairdryer are often the best techniques. Ivermectin may also be used systemically.

Other diseases

Amyloidosis

This is often seen in long-term patients, older birds and those suffering from chronic disease such as aspergillosis, avian tuberculosis or bumblefoot. Domestic breeds and collections of birds seem to be most commonly affected, with prevalences approaching 25% in one study. It is likely that the disease is under-reported at post-mortem examination and so may be much more common than the usually reported 2–5% of individuals examined.

Carpal rotation

In this condition, a lateral rotation of the carpal joint (angel wing, aeroplane wing) allows the primary feathers to point upwards and outwards from the body. It is thought to be caused by a number of environmental or genetic factors and many birds appear to survive well in the wild. Surgical removal of the carpus at the mid point of the fused phalangeal bones, retaining the alula, will remove the affected feathers.

Slipped tendon (perosis)

Lameness and rotation of the foot are seen clinically and this developmental abnormality occurs in young birds and is believed to be caused by the same factors as the equivalent condition in poultry. There seems to be no successful treatment and euthanasia must be considered appropriate in most cases.

Keel bone exposure

Debilitated waterbirds tend to allow their centre of gravity to move forward, so that the keel is scraped along the ground (especially when entering and exiting pools). This first damages the feathers, then the skin and finally the sternum (keel bone) itself. This process obviously destroys the waterproof hull structure and prevents the bird from floating and thus behaving normally. It is an irreversible and progressive event that may only be modified if the bird is returned to full health quickly, whilst only feather damage has been sustained. It is the author's opinion that there are no medical, management or surgical treatments that can be advocated with confidence, and euthanasia must be considered appropriate if the skin is breached.

The condition is often seen in juvenile birds and may be treated with appropriate antibiotic creams that have a waterproof base. Systemic antibiosis is also often required.

Management in captivity

Waterfowl are accustomed to feeding on or about water and so housing requires specialized facilities that are often best provided by appropriately equipped centres (Figure 20.6).

Specialized feedstuff is usually readily available, such as pelleted diets and grass for grazing birds, or frozen and fresh fish (sprats, whitebait, sardines) or even day-old chicks for piscivores.

Most ill individuals will have lost bodyweight and have a reduced body score. Release should be considered only if these parameters are improving, as well as the reason for attention in the first instance being corrected. Indications that a bird is suitable for release should include:

- An increase in bodyweight
- Normal feeding and faecal character
- Normal behaviour towards humans (usually avoidance) and other individuals of the same species (either aggression or mating display)
- Full recovery from the original injuries
- Full waterproofing with good feather condition.

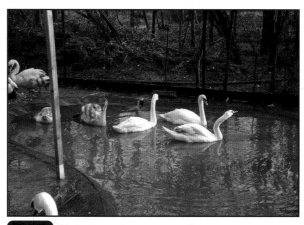

20.6 Mute swans in a recuperation pen

Rearing of young

Many juveniles are 'rescued' by members of the public but it requires a great deal of experience to provide the appropriate sets of social skills, food selection and survival traits for a juvenile wild bird to thrive. This is best provided by the bird's own parents, next best by surrogate parents of the same species and least best by humans. The assistance of specialized rescue and rehabilitation centres should be sought whenever possible.

The criteria for suitability for release are as follows.

Bodyweight

For most species of waterbird, juveniles will start the winter heavier than their parents and this should be a prerequisite when considering release. As they are growing, they also need to be heavier than when admitted.

Plumage

The plumage must be free from damage that could adversely influence waterproofing or insulation. The flight feathers are of little practical importance in species such as swans (if released appropriately) but are essential for others that rely on flight as a means of predator avoidance (e.g. ducks – especially teal, which panic and fly up vertically if challenged). The waterproof body plumage that makes up the hull of the bird when it is in water should be undamaged, as any breach will allow ingress of water and a sensation of sinking that drives most birds back on to land, where they may be more vulnerable to predation.

Imprinting

Imprinting of any kind must be avoided (see Chapter 3). The best environment in which to raise them is one in which they maintain contact with others of the same species.

Release

Where there is a limitation on return to full body function (usually as a result of wing amputation), the release environment should be chosen with care. It is common practice to release large waterfowl with such injuries to 'protected' environments but here the birds must be under good observation – ideally daily and for life – to ensure that the environment is suitable and the birds remain healthy.

Legal aspects

It should be noted that some species (e.g. Canada geese and other non-indigenous species) may have restrictions placed on their release after treatment. Schedule 4 birds, such as the divers and rarer grebes, scoters and long-tailed duck, require registration with DEFRA (see Chapter 5).

Reference

Routh A and Painter KS (1999) The use of intravenous ketamine and xylazine for induction of general anaesthesia in the mute swan (*Cygnus olor*): a review of 130 Cases. *Proceedings of the Autumn Meeting of the British Veterinary Zoological Society, November 20–21*, 17–20

Specialist organizations

National Swan Convention
Co-ordinator: Ellen Kershaw
Tel: 01633 895241
Mobile: 07801 472788
E-mail: ellswan@aol.com

21

Crakes and rails – coot and moorhen

Dick Best

Introduction

Coots and moorhens are common birds of British freshwater habitats and are frequently presented as casualties to rehabilitation units and veterinary practices, usually as abandoned chicks or victims of road traffic accidents.

Species found in the British Isles

Although having many of the characteristics of waterfowl, the crakes and rails (forming the family Rallidae) are classified in a separate order, the Gruiformes. Figure 21.1 gives details of the taxonomy and natural history of the commoner members of the Rallidae found in the British Isles. The coot (Figure 21.2) and the moorhen (Figure 21.3), both of which are usually found close to fresh water, are distributed throughout the country. Less common species – such as the water rail, a ubiquitous bird of marshes, and the corncrake, a highly endangered pastureland species – tend to be very skulking and difficult to observe.

Ecology and biology

Details of the feeding behaviour, natural diet and habitats of common British species are given in Figure 21.1.

The moorhen feeds mainly on invertebrates, whereas the coot has a diet predominantly of plant material. Both the coot and the moorhen nest in vegetation at the water's edge and their young are precocial and nidifugous. Hatching is usually synchronous, i.e. incubation starts with the last egg laid and all eggs hatch at the same time; however, with moorhens, the hatching of the second clutch in the year is often asynchronous and the young from the first brood frequently care for and feed the younger siblings. This behaviour would allow moorhen chicks to be safely replaced with their siblings, even if one or both of the adults are known to be absent.

Coot and moorhen chicks are self-feeding at 25–30 days of age, fledge at 50–60 days and become independent from about 50–70 days old. The mortality in the first year of life is approximately 70%.

Species	Diet	Feeding strategy	Resident/migrant	Typical habitat
Water rail (*Rallus aquaticus*)	Small aquatic invertebrates, some vegetation	Foraging on wet marshy land	Resident and winter migrant	Marshes, reedy fringes of fresh water
Corncrake (*Crex crex*)	Mainly invertebrates, some plant material	Foraging	Summer migrant	Pastureland
Moorhen (*Gallinula chlorpus*)	Wide range of plant and animal material	Surface feeding on water; foraging in wetlands	Resident	Fresh water, from rivers to ditches
Coot (*Fulica atra*)	Mainly aquatic vegetation	Surface feeding on open water and diving	Resident and winter migrant	Fresh water

21.1 Taxonomy and natural history of common British rails and crakes (Order Gruiformes, Family Rallidae).

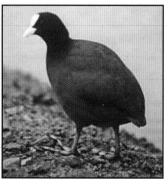

21.2 Adult coot (*Fulica atra*). The toes have lateral fringes of flattened lobes of skin. (Courtesy of C Seddon.)

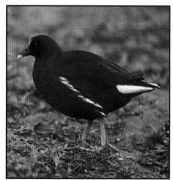

21.3 Adult moorhen (*Gallinula chlorpus*). (Courtesy of C Seddon.)

Anatomy and physiology

The coot is more aquatic in its behaviour than the moorhen, spending more time swimming and diving. This is reflected in the anatomy of its feet (see Figure 21.2). The moorhen and the coot both have a complete post-breeding moult and lose all wing flight feathers at the same time, becoming flightless for a period in late summer.

The young chicks of moorhens and coots look fairly similar. Coot chicks can be distinguished 'in the hand' by their emarginated toes.

Capture, handling and transportation

The catching, handling and transportation of these birds is similar to techniques described in Chapter 2.

Examination, assessment, first aid and anaesthesia

The basic principles of examination, assessment, first aid and anaesthesia are as described in Chapter 2. For short-term hospitalization, coots and moorhens may be housed in secure enclosed cages but will benefit from access to water in shallow trays.

Specific conditions

Moorhens appear to be prone to road traffic accidents, presumably as a result of their habit of foraging away from water. Male coots are very territorial and aggressive during the breeding season. Injured and exhausted males are frequently found and will usually respond to first aid and supportive treatment.

Therapeutics

The use of medications and techniques for administration in crakes and rails are similar to those described in Chapter 2. Doses are given in Appendix 1.

Management in captivity

Accommodation for medium- to long-term periods of hospitalization should follow the details outlined in Chapter 2. In addition, these species will benefit from access to drinking and bathing water placed in shallow containers of a suitable size. A wet substrate, such as moist newspaper, should be used on the floor of the cage.

Following supportive treatment, the birds should be introduced to an artificial diet that resembles their natural diet of invertebrates. An appropriate diet may be fed as a wet mash in a suitable shallow container and can be constructed from a selection of the following constituents (Wildlife Information Network, 2002):

- Mealworms and starved ('clean') maggots
- Finely chopped or minced fish, meat or hardboiled egg
- Proprietary insectivorous diets (e.g. Sluis Insectivore Diet, Sluis; Prosecto, Haith's)
- Mashed tinned dog food or cat food
- Chick, turkey or fish-rearing crumbs or crushed pellets
- Small seeds in canary mixture
- For coots: green food, especially aquatic vegetation
- Vitamin and mineral supplements.

For recuperation and assessment before release, the birds should be placed in suitable grass or gravel-floored aviaries, preferably with a pond large enough for swimming and, for moorhens and other secretive species, plenty of cover.

Rearing of young

As with many apparently 'abandoned' nidifugous chicks, it is possible that so-called orphans have been temporarily separated from the adults. If such chicks are uninjured and in good bodily condition, consideration should be given to returning them, whenever possible, to the site where they were found.

As coot and moorhen chicks will not start to self-feed naturally until 25–30 days of age, they will need to be fed by hand when very young. Food particles can be offered held in fine forceps and the chick stimulated to gape by presenting the food from above and gently moving the forceps up and down.

It has been shown experimentally that moorhen and coot chicks will peck at objects that are brightly coloured, especially red, yellow and (to some extent) white (Kear, 1966). Painting the tips of forceps bright red and yellow might encourage young chicks whilst being fed by hand.

A hand-rearing diet can be made using suitably sized particles of the foods used for mature birds (as outlined above). Additional heat must be provided and water in shallow containers should be placed in their accommodation to encourage them to swim. Food material can be sprinkled on the surface of the water to encourage self-feeding.

Once self-feeding and fully fledged, the young can be moved to aviaries as described above and, when assessed as being able to swim and retain their water-proofing, released in a suitable location (see Chapter 3).

Accurate identification of newly hatched coot and moorhen chicks (see 'Anatomy and physiology') is important if attempts are to be made to return them to wild broods. This might be worth considering with moorhen chicks, especially those of broods hatched later in the year (see 'Ecology and biology').

Release

Coot casualties caused by territorial aggression raise problems with their release: they can be returned to the location where found, where they possibly have a territory and a mate but where they have already shown themselves to be at risk, or they can be released on a lake that holds a flock of non-breeding birds. Such decisions are more easily made with the assistance of a knowledgeable local naturalist.

Legal aspects

The corncrake and the spotted crake are included in Schedule 4 of the Wildlife and Countryside Act (1981) and need to be registered with DEFRA when kept in captivity. Further details of legal aspects of handling casualties are given in Chapter 5.

References

Kear J (1966) The pecking response of young coots (*Fulica atra*) and moorhens (*Gallinula chloropis*). *Ibis* **108**, 118–122

Wildpro® (Wildlife Information Network) (April 2002) *UK Wildlife First Aid and Care*, Royal Veterinary College, London, www.wildlifeinformation.org

Birds of prey

Neil A. Forbes

Introduction

The term 'raptor' encompasses all birds of prey, whether diurnal (hawks, falcons, eagles) or nocturnal (owls).

Species found in the British Isles

This chapter will refer only to species indigenous to the British Isles. Figures 22.1 to 22.5 give taxonomic, biological, identification and ecological data for the six most common British raptors.

Order	Behaviour	Diet	Sexual dimorphism	Chicks	Beak and claws	Caeca and crop	Perching
Falconiformes and Accipitriformes (diurnal raptors – hawks, harriers and eagles)	Active searchers and hunters; generally catch prey by flying high and then stooping down at great speed; spend much of the time perching or in flight	Carnivorous	Reverse, often marked (i.e. female often 30% larger than male)	Altricial	Hooked beak and talons for holding and eating prey	Small caeca; significant sized crop	Anisodactyl: perch with three toes forward and one toe back
Strigiformes (owls)	Principally nocturnal; spend much of time perching or in flight	Carnivorous	Slight or absent	Altricial	Hooked beak and claws for holding and eating prey	Large caeca; no crop	Semi-zyodactyl: will perch with two toes forward and two back but also with three forward and one back

22.1 Orders of common British raptors.

Family	Species	Length	Wing span	Bodyweight	Eye colour	Identification	Behaviour
Falconidae	Kestrel (Common) (*Falco tinnunculus*)	31–39 cm	68–82 cm	Male 180–200 g Female 227–266 g	Dark	Medium-sized with long wings and tail Adult male blue-grey upper tail and head, brown upper back, black wing tips Adult female tail and upper back barred brown Juvenile similar to adult female but generally yellower	Frequently seen hovering
Accipitridae (hawks and eagles)	Sparrow hawk (Eurasian) (*Accipiter nisus*)	Male 29–34 cm Female 35–41 cm	Male 58–65 cm Female 67–80 cm	Male 110–196 g Female 185–342 g	Yellow iris	Small with broad blunt-tipped wings, long tail; tail always longer than width of wing, with 4–5 bars; small beak, slender body, very fine legs Adult male small, slate grey upper parts, rufous cheeks, barring on breast Adult female significantly bigger, slate grey upper parts, barring below is brown grey Juvenile dark brown upper parts Coarse barring of underparts, broken up and irregular	Flies at low level making surprise attack
	Common buzzard (*Buteo buteo*)	46–58 cm	113–128 cm	Male 525–1183 g Female 625–1364 g Both sexes heavier in winter, lose av. 20% bodyweight during breeding season	Juvenile eye colour slightly paler than in adult	Medium-sized, broad-winged, tail medium length (shorter than width of wing) Plumage very variable, from very dark to very light; buff breast with variable streaking, all show pale band across lower breast Adult blackish terminal tail band; chest obviously barred Juvenile chest streaks with tendency to vague bars; tail slighty longer than in adult	Often seen still-hunting whilst sat on fence/ telegraph post; also often seen soaring

22.2 Biology, taxonomy and identification of common British diurnal birds of prey (Order Falconiformes, Suborder Falcones).

Species	Distribution	Feeding	Nesting	Clutch	Incubation	Age at fledging	Sexual maturity	Lifespan
Kestrel (*Falco tinnunculus*)	Commonest 'falcon' in UK, well adapted to variety of terrains: wooded, farmland, rural, urban; seen in open countryside, often hovering above food	Voles (90%) and insects	In trees, often in old corvid nest, or hole or niche in building	3–6 eggs	27–31 days	27–35 days, fed by parents for further 2–4 weeks	1 year	Mortality in 1st year 50–70% Potential longevity 16 years
Sparrowhawk (*Accipiter nisus*)	Woodland (coniferous, deciduous) or open farmland; common even in urban areas	Small and medium-sized birds	In trees, often close to a clearing, 6–12 m up; rebuilds each year	3–6 eggs; up to 2 replace-ment clutches if eggs lost	32–34 days	26–30 days, fed by parents for further 3–4 weeks	1–3 years	Rarely live over 7 years
Common buzzard (*Buteo buteo*)	Common; variable habitat but must include woodland for nesting and roosting; feeds in areas that are more open in winter	Adaptable food intake according to availability; mainly voles, rabbits, reptiles, insects, earthworms, carrion	In large trees close to edge of wood; bulky platform of twigs, lined with greenery; usually alternate nests year by year	2–4 eggs	33–38 days	50–60 days, fed by parents for further 6–8 weeks	3 years	Oldest recorded 25 years Pre-breeding territorial disputes often lead to severe potentially fatal talon puncture wounds

22.3 Ecology of common British diurnal birds of prey.

Family	Species	Length	Wing span	Bodyweight	Eye colour	Identification	Behaviour
Tytonidae	Barn owl (*Tyto alba*)	33–39 cm	80–95 cm	Male 231–381 g Female 295–395 g	Dark	Medium sized, slim body, long wings and legs. Face (white) pale with distinctive heart shape. Plumage typically pale (male lighter in colour); upper parts grey. Juvenile similar to adult but more heavily spotted	Sedentary and nocturnal, daytime hunting witnessed occasionally Silent in flight
Strigidae	Tawny owl (*Strix aluco*)	37–43 cm	81–104 cm	Male 304–465 g Female 385–716 g	Black	Medium sized, with wings broad and rounded. Brown (usually rufous but varies from very pale to greyish-brown) with large round face, cinnamon facial disc, thin whitish extra eyebrows; whole plumage mottled, finely streaked, noticeably shaggy and loose. Tarsus and most toes feathered. Bill pale brown to pale yellow. Juvenile plumage paler	
	Little owl (*Athena noctua*)	23–27.5 cm	54–58 cm	Male 139–230 g Female 137–260 g	Yellow	Small (far smaller than any other UK owl), compact, plump, with large broadly rounded head, long legs, short tail. Brown upper parts, buff-whitish underparts clearly streaked brown. Juvenile plumage pattern duller and less well defined. No white spots on crown	Hunt predominantly dusk to midnight and again at dawn Partially diurnal; often seen perching on posts in daylight

22.4 Biology, taxonomy and identification of common British owls (Order Strigiformes).

Species	Distribution	Feeding	Nesting	Clutch	Incubation	Age at fledging	Sexual maturity	Lifespan
Barn owl (*Tyto alba*)	Now rare in UK but locally distributed; farmland Sedentary but will also disperse if under pressure for food or nest sites	Predominantly voles (absolutely dependent on permanent pasture for voles), also frogs and insects Use hearing extensively during hunting	In holes in trees or within farm buildings, 2–20 m from ground	4–7 eggs (clutch replace-ment occurs) May have 2–3 broods if food plentiful	29–34 days	7–10 weeks, dependent on parents for further 3–5 weeks, then disperse within 2–8 weeks; disperse within 20 km	< 1 year	Monogamous but polygamy recorded Licence required (from DEFRA) to release captive or rehabilitated wild barn owls in UK

22.5 Ecology of common British owls. (continues) ▶

Species	Distribution	Feeding	Nesting	Clutch	Incubation	Age at fledging	Sexual maturity	Lifespan
Tawny owl (*Strix aluco*)	Most common British owl; breeds in woodland, wooded farmland, large gardens, urban parkland Sedentary and nocturnal	Mainly voles (56%), also birds, amphibians, reptiles, earthworms and insects, caught on ground by still-hunting	In holes in trees or buildings, cliff, second-hand squirrel or magpie nest	Usually 3–5 eggs	28–30 days, brooded until 15 days	32–37 days Fratricide if food shortage	25–30 days as 'branchers', dependent on parents until 3 months after fledging Leave nest when young, before able to fly (often presented as orphans) Disperse within few km of natal nest in autumn	1 year Mortality in 1st year 71%; potential lifespan 19 years Monogamous, pair for life
Little owl (*Athena noctua*)	Breeds in open mixed countryside or built-up areas Sedentary; partially diurnal	Insects (70%), birds, small amphibians, snakes	In cavity of tree, wall etc.	3–6 eggs	28–33 days	30–35 days, dependent on parents for further month	Mortality in 1st year 70%, annual adult mortality 35%	Monogamous Introduced into UK in 19th century

22.5 (continued) Ecology of common British owls.

Anatomy and physiology

The most significant anatomical features are listed in Figures 22.1 and 21.3. All raptors eat whole carcasses, thereby consuming meat (flesh), bones (required to satisfy the Ca:P:vitamin D_3 balance) and also indigestible material (such as fur or feather), which is regurgitated as a pellet or 'casting'. Whilst most birds have a distinct proventriculus (enzyme and acid-secreting area of the stomach) and ventriculus (or gizzard – the muscular grinding part of the gut), in birds of prey both parts are confluent, with only minor ventricular function present. The digestible part of the meal is acted upon in the proventriculus and then passes to the small intestine, leaving behind the indigestible fibrous material. The bird will 'cast' a pellet some 12–18 hours after eating. It is important not to feed a raptor again before it has cast. Although many falconers and rehabilitators have a fixation about the fact that raptors require casting, this is not strictly true.

Capture, handling and transportation

Handlers should beware the talons of raptors. Although the bird may bite with its beak, this will not cause any significant damage (except, possibly, with eagles). Even when dealing with birds with sharp pointed talons, a clean towel should be used rather than gloves (see Figure 2.5c) to catch and restrain any injured wild bird. A long-handled fisherman's landing net or similar may be useful.

In handling and transportation, it is crucial that the full integrity and condition of the flight (tail and wing) feathers are maintained. The bird must never be placed in a wire cat basket (see 'Short-term housing'). Any travelling box should be readily disinfectable or disposable and should be ventilated but dark. Clean carpet or similar should be placed on the floor of the box to allow traction with the talons. If the container is of sufficient size a perch may be placed within it, such that a perching bird will keep its wing feathers off the floor of the container. With any wild raptor being boxed or hospitalized, a tail guard must be applied to prevent damage to tail feathers (see later).

Zoonoses

Zoonotic infections that might be contracted from wild raptors include *Chlamydophila psittaci* (very rare), salmonellosis (common), campylobacteriosis (common and probably under-diagnosed) and Newcastle disease (rare and usually rapidly fatal in avian hosts). The greatest risk is salmonellosis, primarily as so much poultry-derived food (which may be infected) is fed to raptors, so that keepers or clinicians may become infected when either feeding or handling the birds.

Examination and assessment for rehabilitation

As with all wildlife casualties, the patient may initially be suffering from extreme cardiovascular shock. The bird must only be handled in a minimal manner until the shock has been reversed. Doing too much too soon is very detrimental and may lead to the bird's premature demise. Therapy for shock involves the administration by gavage tube of warm electrolyte solution at 10 ml/kg bodyweight, repeated after 2 hours, and maintenance in a dark, warm and quiet environment. The use of intravenous, intraosseous or subcutaneous fluid therapy may have a preferable response in addressing hypovolaemia. In each case the improved benefit should be assessed against any potential increase in stress in undertaking the procedure.

Figure 22.6 summarizes the steps to be taken for common causes of admission of wild raptors. There is also a useful schematic approach to the assessment and nursing of traumatic raptor wildlife casualties in Redig (1996).

Orphan

Options in order of preference
1. Return to nest for parental care.
2. Return to another wild nest of same species under DEFRA licence.
3. Rear in captivity under foster parents of same species.
4. Crèche rear in captivity.
5. Rear in captivity under foster parents of similar species.
6. Hand rear by puppet feeding.

Starved/exhausted

Action list by order
1. Control shock.
2. Gavage feed, small amounts and often.
3. Full physical, radiological, clinical pathology and ophthalmic examination to find reason for starvation. Check and treat as required for endo- and ectoparasites.
4. If considered to be long-term releasable, feed up, increase fitness and prepare for assessment for release.
5. If not long-term releasable, euthanase.

Trauma

Action list by order
1. Treat shock and stabilize.
2. Triage for long-term release.
3. Full investigation of trauma and other disease or infestation. Check and treat as required for endo- and ectoparasites.
4. Administer further nursing, medical or surgical therapy as indicated.
5. Reassess with respect to potential release.
6. Euthanase or increase fitness and prepare for final assessment for release.

Poisoned

Action list by order
1. Remove any crop contents and store.
2. Administer fluid therapy i.v., charcoal by mouth, nursing, any specific antidote and support therapy
3. Notify police or DEFRA Wildlife Incident Officer.
4. Testing of toxic agent.

Infected/infested

Action list by order
1. Often present as starved or exhausted.
2. Control shock and give support care.
3. Full clinical pathological investigation. Medical therapy as indicated. Check and treat as required for endo- and ectoparasites.
4. Recheck to assess for resolution.
5. Increase fitness and prepare for final assessment for release.

22.6 Common causes of admission of wildlife raptors and actions required.

Clinical examination

Once shock has been controlled, the bird should be examined thoroughly and systematically. For a raptor to be released back to the wild, it must be able to fly well enough, see well enough and hunt well enough to be able to catch, despatch and consume quarry in sufficient volumes to maintain its bodyweight and at the same time be able to interact normally with members of its own species and not present an undue risk to human safety.

Factors that would prevent the release of an injured wild raptor include:

- Impaired eyesight or loss of eye
- Loss of function of, or any part of, any limb
- Loss of beak or ability to ingest wild-caught diet
- Loss of first or second toe, permanent loss of talon or loss of foot holding ability
- Inability to catch suitable wild-caught food
- Inability to relate safely to birds of its own kind
- Inability to survive in the wild without being a danger to humans.

The last two points would include, for example, young wild birds admitted into care that have become 'imprinted' on humans. Imprinting must be avoided if release is to be successful (see 'Rearing and release of young birds').

Ocular examination

One of the commonest causes for a raptor to be presented in an emaciated condition, as well as a common sequel to traumatic incidents, is damage to ocular function. It has been shown that 30% of raptor trauma cases have eye damage; in 70% of these cases the damage affects only the posterior segment of the eye and hence is not visible to a rehabilitator or a veterinary surgeon without use of an ophthalmoscope. It is important that all incoming raptor trauma cases receive an ophthalmoscopic examination. The retina and pecten should be examined in all cases, which with experience is often possible in conscious birds. The high incidence of posterior segment damage is linked to contrecoup effect following head trauma, especially to the attachment of the pecten, which floats in the vitreous humour, providing nutrition to the avascular retina.

The cornea, presence of tears (Schirmer tear test: 10–15 mm in 1 minute is normal), anterior pressure (reference values using Tonopen XL, 9–22 mmHg; owls typically 9–11 mmHg, kestrels 13 mmHg, buzzards 17 mmHg) and anterior and posterior segment should all be examined. Iris light reflex should be tested; a positive response is indicative of retinal function but absence of response may be due to a degree of voluntary iris control, since birds, in contrast to mammals, have striated musculature in the iris.

Mammalian mydriatics are ineffective. The fundus in raptors reflects red (in nocturnal species) or grey (in diurnal species), the colour emanating from the sclera, as there is no tapetum behind the retina. In some clinical cases, the posterior segment can be adequately examined without mydriasis. Topical vecuronium may on rare occasions be effective; alternatively systemic (intravenous) vecuronium at 0.2 mg/kg may be administered (latent time 26 seconds, duration 25 minutes, paralysis of body musculature 7 minutes) to achieve mydriasis. A 3% solution of D-tubocurarine (0.01–0.03 ml) may be injected (using a 27–30 gauge needle) into the anterior chamber: this technique will facilitate extensive examination of the posterior segment, but iris damage, transmission of corneal flora into the anterior chamber, increase of the intraocular pressure or systemic side effects can occur. Alternatively, air sac perfusion anaesthesia (Chapter 2) will induce mydriasis.

Whether examined with or without mydriasis, the pecten and retina must be visualized. In many trauma cases haemorrhage will have occurred from the attachment of the pecten, with a concurrent uveitis. Any significant haemorrhage is likely to affect long-term eyesight. Topical ocular steroid preparations should not be used in birds.

First aid

The general principles of first aid as detailed in Chapter 2 apply to raptor casualties. Details are also to be found in Figures 22.6 and 22.7.

Short-term housing

When dealing with short-term casualties, it is imperative that appropriate food, fluids, warmth and seclusion are provided, whilst at the same time preventing undue stress and self-trauma (in particular to flight feathers,

cere and wings). Hygiene and prevention of the transmission of infections must be considered. Either disposable containers (e.g. cardboard cat carriers) or readily cleanable cages should be used.

Birds should never be placed in cat carriers or cages with mesh sides or doors, as feathers are severely damaged when forced through these. Tail guards and perches should be used to prevent feather damage (see 'Capture, handling and transportation').

Newly admitted casualty birds should be maintained at 26.7–32.2°C. Birds are best kept at a height off the floor and should have sufficient light to feed but otherwise be kept in the dark. They should be kept away from excessive noise (e.g. barking dogs).

Short-term feeding

After initial shock therapy (see 'Examination and assessment'), nutrition is most easily provided by gavage feeding (Hill's a/d diet, Hill's Pet Nutrition: little owl 2 ml every 6 hours; kestrel, sparrowhawk, tawny owl and

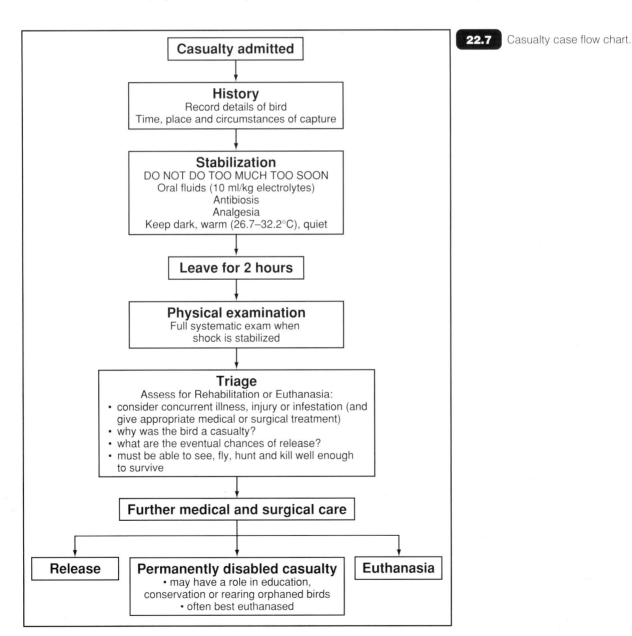

22.7 Casualty case flow chart.

Casualty admitted

History
Record details of bird
Time, place and circumstances of capture

Stabilization
DO NOT DO TOO MUCH TOO SOON
Oral fluids (10 ml/kg electrolytes)
Antibiosis
Analgesia
Keep dark, warm (26.7–32.2°C), quiet

Leave for 2 hours

Physical examination
Full systematic exam when
shock is stabilized

Triage
Assess for Rehabilitation or Euthanasia:
• consider concurrent illness, injury or infestation (and give appropriate medical or surgical treatment)
• why was the bird a casualty?
• what are the eventual chances of release?
• must be able to see, fly, hunt and kill well enough to survive

Further medical and surgical care

Release

Permanently disabled casualty
• may have a role in education, conservation or rearing orphaned birds
• often best euthanased

Euthanasia

barn owl 4–5 ml every 6 hours; buzzard 15 ml every 8 hours). This technique is far quicker and less stressful to birds than force feeding with meat. Birds should be weighed daily to ensure that they are maintaining or gaining bodyweight.

Once the casualty has overcome its initial trauma, day-old chicks or mice can be offered, as long as they have first been skinned. It is important to offer small regular meals (half a cropful of food, repeated as soon as the crop is empty) and this can be achieved only if no casting material is present in the meal.

Analgesia and short-term therapy

The value of analgesia cannot be overemphasized, not only from a welfare standpoint but also as a method of reducing unnecessary stress and as an aid to voluntary food consumption (birds in pain will typically not eat). NSAIDs are preferred: carprofen, ketoprofen and butorphenol have proved safe and effective in the hands of many clinicians.

Birds are very susceptible to the deleterious side effects of glucocorticoids. The use of ultra short-acting steroids such as hydrocortisone sodium succinate or prednisolone sodium succinate minimizes these risks. Where glucocorticoid therapy is essential, its duration should never exceed 48 hours, and doses should be kept to a minimum (see the avian formulary in Appendix 1 for dose rates).

Anaesthesia

The general principles of anaesthesia in birds as detailed in Chapter 2 apply to raptor casualties. It must always be remembered that, for wildlife casualties, proximity to humans is an intensely terrifying and stressful event. The time spent being handled and examined must be minimized, in particular when first admitted. If any significant procedures are required – even a full physical examination – this is generally best performed under isoflurane anaesthesia.

For all birds receiving an anaesthetic of more than 10 minutes in duration, the author favours an open intravenous port (intravenous jelco catheter sutured into the superficial basilic vein) for administering intravenous fluid therapy.

Birds should preferably have an empty crop prior to anaesthesia. Where this is not possible, entubation and maintaining the head above the level of the crop is even more important.

Where oxygen, gaseous anaesthesia or support staff experienced at monitoring avian anaesthesia are not available, parenteral anaesthetics may be employed (see Appendix 1). Further details of avian anaesthesia may be found in Forbes (1999).

Specific conditions

Raptor casualties can be broadly divided into the groups specified in Figure 22.2 and should be treated accordingly. For orphans, see also 'Rearing young birds', below.

Trauma

In a major review of wildlife raptor admissions, Howard and Redig (1993) demonstrated that 33% are likely to have suffered a fracture incident; of these, 40% are likely to be euthanased on account of that fracture, 10% are likely to be euthanased for other reasons and 15% to die spontaneously. The percentage of wild raptor fracture cases that are eventually released is 36% for closed fractures but only 15% for open fractures.

Assessment for orthopaedic surgery

The two factors that have the greatest influence on the successful release of orthopaedic cases are whether a fracture is compound and how close it is to a joint. Normal joint function is unlikely to be regained if the fracture is closer to the joint than 150% of the affected bone's diameter. Wing fractures account for 86% of wild raptor fracture cases. If a bird has suffered severe enough trauma for a bone to be fractured, consideration must be given to what else might have been damaged.

The aims of orthopaedic surgery in raptors are as follows:

* To treat contaminated or infected wounds
* To preserve soft tissues, if necessary by applying splints or other dressings. In view of the extreme fragility of avian skin and the small volume of soft tissue, special care is required in many cases to prevent desiccation of muscle and tendon tissues
* To realign fractures or replace luxations
* To stabilize the fracture site rigidly, preventing any movement or rotation. This may require a combination of surgical techniques, together with a full understanding of the husbandry of the bird, such that it may be properly controlled during its convalescent period
* To maintain full early function of all joints and tendons. No bird should have a wing strapped up (so as to prevent normal joint function) for more than 48 hours following surgery
* To return the limb to full, normal function, without adversely affecting the healing process and as quickly as possible.

An important point to remember is that wing-amputee male birds are highly unlikely ever to copulate successfully. Leg-amputee birds over 150 g almost inevitably develop bumblefoot or arthritis in their remaining foot sooner or later.

It is the author's experience that all orthopaedic cases should have surgery delayed by 24 hours. In the interim, desiccation and further trauma should be prevented. The bird should be stabilized with fluid therapy, analgesia, antibiosis, parasiticides (if necessary) and nutritional support.

Timing and method should always be considered on an individual case basis. Decisions will vary depending on the nature and lifestyle of the bird, as well as the nature of the fracture and the state of the proximate tissues.

Surgical techniques

Surgical approaches to avian fracture repair have been discussed by Orosz *et al.* (1992), Harcourt-Brown (1994) and others. Orthopaedic techniques are very varied, depending on the bone, fracture type and the size and species involved. For surgical techniques the following references should be consulted: Hess (1994), Howard and Redig (1994), Coles (1996) and Harcourt-Brown (1996).

Current recommendations are in line with newer procedures in humans and domestic mammals. Surgical intervention, and in particular bone fragment manipulation at the fracture site, should be minimized or, better still, avoided. The aim should be to stabilize the fracture in correct alignment and length, permitting full joint movements. This is often best achieved by the use of a hybrid or tie-in fixator, which involves the combination of a half-pin external fixator joined to a single intramedullary pin.

Thoracic limb fractures

Coracoid: These fractures are relatively common and are most often seen in sparrowhawks following collision, especially with windows. Good quality radiographs are required in order to delineate exactly the coracoid, furculum and scapula. Smaller species (< 300 g) generally respond well to immobilization of the affected wing and rest. Sparrowhawks in particular are very susceptible to stress, and the placement of bandages around the thorax can be deleterious. Larger species, especially those in which there is significant displacement, may benefit from fracture reduction and internal fixation. The cranial portion of the pectoral musculature is elevated to expose the fractured coracoid; a pin is passed retrogradely and after reduction of the fracture a blunt end is passed into the proximal fragment, great care being taken not to advance the pin normograde too far in view of the position of the heart in relation to the surgical field.

Proximal humerus: Humerus fractures are the most frequent type of fracture in wild raptors, especially in the goshawk and sparrowhawk, and commonly occur following similar injuries to those described above. The humerus is pneumatized, being joined to the clavicular air sac. Flushing of the proximal bone segment is dangerous in view of the possibility of encouraging infection to pass from the humerus into the air sac. The fractures may be repaired by single intramedullary pinning or stack pinning but a pin and tension band connected to a hybrid fixator is generally preferable. The natural curve of the humerus lends itself to pins being exited either proximally near the shoulder or distally near the elbow, without interference with the joints.

Mid-shaft humerus: These fractures frequently become grossly displaced and often (59%: Redig *et al.*, 1993) result in compound fractures, with exposed necrotic bone. For closed, simple fractures of the mid-shaft, any of the techniques mentioned above may be employed. During surgery, great care must be taken

not to traumatize the radial nerve, which is located just beneath the skin on the dorsal aspect. Care must be taken to ensure the correct alignment of the humerus – malrotations can easily occur. As with many other long bones in avians, there is a great propensity for longitudinal cracking; such cracks should be evident on good quality radiographs. In cases of comminuted mid-shaft fractures, where the radial nerve is functional, a half-pin external fixator on the dorsal or lateral aspect of the wing may be used, but the result is significantly improved when combined with an intramedullary device, creating a hybrid fixator.

Distal humerus: The same devices as above may be used or, if the fracture is very close to the joint, a cross-pin technique joined to an external fixator or a transarticular external fixator may be used, in which case at least five pins are required: two in the proximal humerus, one in the distal humerus and two in the proximal ulna.

Dislocation of the elbow: This injury carries a poor prognosis for return to normal flight. The author has used a half-pin transarticulation technique, applied for 7 days only, as described by Martin *et al.* (1993), and has achieved a success rate similar to the 50% release rate reported in injured wild birds in that review.

Ulna and radius: In a series of orthopaedic cases in wild raptors, 30% of fractures to the forearm involved only the ulna, 60% involved the ulna and radius and 10% involved only the radius (Redig *et al.*, 1993). These bones have little soft tissue support, the soft tissue being prone to desiccation.

In birds with a fracture of only the ulna, where there is no significant displacement, cage rest alone is generally sufficient. In such cases the bird should be maintained in a 'night quarter' (e.g. tea chest), so that it can move its wings but not extend or flap them fully, for a period of 2–3 weeks.

If the radius is fractured, this generally needs to be stabilized by internal fixation with a single fine intramuscular pin, on occasions reinforced by incorporation into a hybrid fixator. When repairing the radius, the pin may be placed retrograde or normograde, as it can be passed out through the carpus without undue trauma to the joint. If the ulna requires repair, a single pin is generally inserted in the proximal ulna just beyond the point of attachment of the triceps tendon, i.e. gaining entry from the level of the second or third last secondary feather, on the dorsocaudal aspect of the wing. Cerclage wires may also be necessary. In larger birds, especially if there is contamination of the wound, an external fixator may be used.

During healing of fractures where the ulna and radius are involved, a synostosis bridging callus between the radius and ulna may develop. Careful surgery with an air drill to remove this, and the placement of a fat pad (readily harvested, in most species, from the subcutaneous site in the ventral abdominal midline) between the bones, will often be effective in preventing recurrence.

Hybrid fixator (external fixator/intramedullary pin tie-in)

This is the newest and most widely recommended technique for many avian fracture cases. Any device inserted should promote load sharing. As healing progresses, parts of the fixator may be removed – a process referred to as dynamic destabilization (Redig, 2000).

The technique has been present in various forms for a number of years. It was refined and further developed (Redig, 2000) as an answer to provide longitudinal and rotational stability to humeral fractures, without having to resort to total wing fixation. With good fixation and good overall vascular condition at the fracture site, healing will often be achieved in $2^1/_2$–$3^1/_2$ weeks. Loosening of pins should not occur and can be prevented by the use of threaded pins.

In simplistic terms, a single intramedullary pin is placed along the full length of the bone but avoiding any damage to or interference with full functioning of the joints. External fixator pins are then placed in safe sites (to avoid major blood vessels and nerves or contusion of tissues in subsequent limb movements), with at least two either side of the fracture, spread out as far as possible along the length of the bone. The free end of the intramedullary pin is bent through 90 degrees and attached to a bar, which in turn joins with all the external fixator pins, thereby linking the intramedullary pin and the external fixators.

Pesticide toxicity

Birds of prey have been persecuted (often unjustifiably) for centuries by farmers and gamekeepers, often by means of deliberate poisoning. This has led to the extinction of various species, including the red kite (*Milvus milvus*) and the northern goshawk (*Accipiter gentilis*), in the UK in recent times.

In the 1950s and 1960s many global raptor populations were severely decreased by the accidental ingestion of organochlorine and organophosphate pesticides. These substances sometimes caused acute deaths; in other cases birds presented with central nervous system signs, in particular hypersensitivity and fits, whilst in others there was general debility, reduced hunting ability leading to inanition, or eggshell thinning leading to infertility. Since that time most of the chemicals involved in accidental poisonings have been banned in the developed world, though many are still sold to and used freely in the Third World.

At present, organophosphates are the commonest cause of poisoning and are often found in agricultural areas. The UK has an international obligation for the conservation of indigenous birds of prey, with 11 of its 16 raptor species being recognized as birds of high conservation concern. However, despite their legal protection, the level of intentional and malicious poisoning of raptors in the UK increases year on year. In 2000 there were 186 reported incidents of illegal destruction of birds of prey, with 109 cases involving the reported use of poisons. In 64 cases poisons were considered to have been responsible and were proved to be so in 56 cases but the true national figure must greatly exceed this.

Alphachloralose, mevinphos (an organophosphate insecticide) and strychnine (in that order of frequency) account for some 95% of all wildlife poisoning incidents. Target species are typically poisoned using baited eggs or meat. Carrion- and egg-eating species are at greatest risk. Birds are commonly found dead, often close to the source of the bait. Baiting is indiscriminate; hence the carcasses of other predatory species may be in the vicinity. If poisoning is suspected, crop and stomach contents should be retained and the police wildlife liaison officer or DEFRA wildlife incident officer should be notified immediately.

Cholinesterase inhibitory (ChEI) poisons (organophosphate and carbamate chemicals) act by inhibiting acetyl cholinesterase activity (AChE). Clinical signs are explained by the persistent action of acetyl choline at the nerve endings, where it normally stays only momentarily. Carbamates are rapid in onset but described as reversible ChEIs, whilst organophosphates are slower in onset but irreversible. Clinical signs include flaccid paralysis of the limbs, whilst the head is upright and alert. There is a marked bradycardia, ataxia, diarrhoea, tremors, dyspnoea and death. Treatment within 24 hours of ingestion with pralidoxine (10–20 mg/kg i.m.), repeated after 8 hours, can be highly efficacious but it should not be administered more than 24 hours after ingestion, as it can cause toxicity in its own right. Atropine can be administered (0.2–0.5 mg/kg i.m.) at any stage following poisoning and should be repeated every 3–4 hours.

Clinical signs caused by alphachloralose are lethargy, incoordination or stupor. If birds are kept warm, they will typically make a full recovery in 24–36 hours.

Birds poisoned with strychnine are very rarely found alive. Poisoning is peracute, with marked opisthotonos, rigor and severe muscle contracture. Typically several carcasses are found immediately adjacent to the poisoned bait.

Although birds are more resistant to anticoagulant rodenticides compared with mammals, accidental poisoning of wild raptors does occur on occasion. The commonest signs are oral, subcutaneous haemorrhage or acute death (Shawyer, 1985).

A thorough review of poisoning in raptors is given by Cooper (2001).

Infectious diseases

Bacterial and fungal diseases

Even if a primary reason for presentation is traumatic, there will often be secondary bacterial or fungal infections.

Bacterial infections should generally be treated subsequent to microbial culture and sensitivity testing. However, in the first instance, the author favours the use of amoxicillin long-acting preparations, clavulanic acid-potentiated amoxicillin or marbofloxacin.

Primary fungal systemic infections in wild raptors are extremely rare. Once diagnosed, treatment is not justified – taking into account response rates, survival in the wild and welfare implications.

Parasites

It is estimated that 65% of wild raptors carry a parasitic infestation. Whilst host and parasite will normally live harmoniously, once the host bird suffers an injury and is taken into captivity (suffering unprecedented levels of stress) the parasite will often gain the upper hand over the host. Parasite infestations should be checked on admission and treated if there is indication of significant burdens. Ectoparasites, endoparasites and blood parasites should all be considered.

- Ectoparasites are treated with fipronil
- The commonest nematode infestation is caused by *Capillaria* spp. It is worth noting that this worm on occasions demonstrates multiple drug resistance. It may be treated with benzimidazoles (e.g. fenbendazole) or avermectins (e.g. ivermectin). In such cases repeat faecal analysis should always be performed to assess efficacy of therapy
- Tapeworm infestations may be treated with praziquantel
- Blood parasites, including *Haemoproteus* spp. and *Leucocytozoon* spp., are most commonly treated with chloroquine or mefloquine.

Starvation or exhaustion

This occurs most commonly after any period of extreme weather (cold, storms or drought), on return from migration or during dispersal at the end of the breeding season (when young birds leave the rearing location in search of their own territories). These are acceptable reasons for exhaustion and such cases will respond well to support and nutritional care (see 'Short-term feeding', above). However, other cases may be suffering as a result of an inability to see or fly well enough to catch sufficient food to maintain normal body condition. Such cases should be carefully assessed for eyesight and flight ability and it is vital that ocular function is assessed prior to release (see 'Ocular examination').

Once the bird has gained condition, it must be carefully assessed to ensure that it can fly, hunt and kill well enough to survive in the wild.

Therapeutics

Medication may be given by gavage or buried in a food morsel for voluntary ingestion, prior to a full meal. Standard intramuscular, intravenous or subcutaneous injections are readily administered (see Chapter 2; see also the avian formulary in Appendix 1).

Management in captivity

Housing

After initial attention to its injuries, a casualty should be housed in an aviary (see Chapter 3). Mixed-species aviaries are contraindicated. Groups of the same species can usually be mixed in one aviary, with the exception of more aggressive species, such as goshawks. Any aviary used must be safe for the bird (to prevent trauma or stress from any other bird, mammal or human), whilst at the same time also preventing it

from damaging itself (including feathers, feet or beak) in such a manner that the release might have to be delayed. For example, many traditional aviaries have chainlink fencing, which is unsuitable for many species and should have vertical battens or electrician's conduit piping erected inside the mesh at intervals of 3.5–5 cm (depending on the species), to prevent birds from damaging themselves on the wire.

An aviary should be a safe and hygienic staging post and must not in any way present a danger to the bird in respect of any build-up of parasites or pathogens. Compost heaps and, in particular, hay must never be kept in the proximity of raptors, in view of the inherent risk of aspergillosis. Birds of unknown disease status will pass through this aviary and the possibility of contamination (e.g. by mycobacteria), which might pose a threat to future inhabitants of the aviary, should be considered. The base of the floor should comprise concrete or a builder's vapour membrane, so that it is possible to clean down to an impervious layer prior to refilling with fresh soil, sand or pea gravel. Sharp gravel should never be used.

Birds should have some form of refuge within the aviary, in which to hide from aviary mates or perceived predators (including humans). An evergreen shrub planted in a tub is ideal, as it can be removed when the aviary is cleaned.

Perches

Perch design and fabrication are critical, especially when dealing with falcons. No single perch material is perfect for all birds. Astroturf (resembling tough artificial grass and sold in hardware stores as doormats) is the most frequently used material; its multiple plastic spikes spread the bird's weight across the plantar aspect of the foot, preventing pressure necrosis, which is the underlying predisposing factor in the majority of bumblefoot cases. However, research has shown that pathogens persist for extended periods and so ease of cleaning and disinfection is important.

Generally block perches (Figure 22.8) are used for falcons and bow perches (Figure 22.9) for hawks, but a clean hessian sack or towel tied around a block of stone

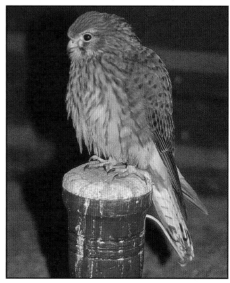

22.8

Kestrel on a block perch.

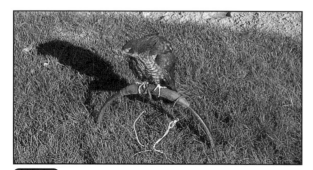

22.9 Sparrowhawk on a bow perch.

or wood will suffice. The purpose of the perch is simply to raise a bird's tail off the ground in order to prevent it from becoming damaged. Within the aviary, perches should be situated as high as possible, as this gives the bird a good vantage point; birds in an elevated position feel more secure and are probably less stressed.

Observation
Observation of birds by eye is difficult, as those that know they are being watched often appear to behave normally. If observations are recorded with a video or CCTV camera, the natural behaviour will be apparent and this will give an improved indication as to the suitability for release. Factors that preclude release have been listed above (see 'Examination and assessment for release').

Tail guards and imping
All incoming raptors should have a tail guard applied to the distal portion of their tail, in order to prevent soiling or damage. Tail guards can be made from spent X-ray film and attached to the tail with a single strip of adhesive tape.

No bird should be released with any broken or damaged tail or wing flight feathers. Should feather damage be present, it may be repaired by 'imping'. This is a traditional falconry technique, whereby a previously discarded but perfect feather (from exactly the same position and the same sex, age and species of bird) is glued into the stump of the damaged or missing feather. The central shaft (calamus) of the broken feather is trimmed 1 cm above the skin border. The replacement feather is cut to exactly the correct length. A small length (3–4 cm) of bamboo, fibreglass or carbon fibre peg is trimmed to fit snugly within the shaft of both the replacement feather and the existing stump. The peg is then glued into the shaft, prior to gluing into the stump. Care is taken is ensure that the feather is set at the correct angle before the glue hardens.

Records
Detailed records must be maintained of all casualty raptors admitted: by whom found, from where and in what circumstances. There must be a record of the aviaries in which a bird has resided whilst in care, in case a future health condition implies that an area may be contaminated. Birds should be marked (e.g. BTO ringed) prior to release, such that some long-term data may be collected on survival rates (see Chapter 3 for details on telemetry).

Rearing young birds

It should be noted that displaced juvenile tawny owls are commonly found in woodland and should not be taken into care unless they are injured. They are able to climb trees and regain safety but will benefit by being placed as high and as close as possible to the site where they were found.

Young raptors that are still of an age where they would be dependent on their parents (the age varies according to species) will become imprinted on their keeper, their nest site and their food, all of which can have detrimental consequences on their subsequent release. Birds that are imprinted on humans have no fear of them and may occasionally even attack them. Also, on reaching sexual maturity such birds may attempt to seek a suitable human with which to breed and this can lead to perceived attacks on children, for example. For these reasons, and because they are unable to associate normally with their own species, imprinted birds cannot be released to the wild.

Young 'imprintable' birds should never be reared on their own in captivity (see Figure 22.6). If the keeper does not have further young of that species, contact should be made with other rehabilitators until a group of birds of a suitable age can be found for the orphan to join. Even if reared in captivity, 'orphans' that are kept in a group of their own species will not be psychologically crippled.

Young birds should be fed on a food type resembling that which they will find in the wild. If only white mice or day-old chicks (hatchery waste) are available, then these should first be skinned.

Release

Assessment
The activity of a bird in an aviary can give a reasonable impression as to its flight ability but the most reliable method of release is the training and flying of a bird using traditional falconry techniques. In this way it can be ascertained that the bird can fly, see, hunt, kill and eat well enough to survive in the wild.

Habitat selection
The area that is chosen for release must be natural terrain for that species. It is also advisable to consider other avian species that may already inhabit the area – especially rooks, carrion crows and magpies, and also woodpeckers, tits and some other songbirds. Such species tend to mob the released bird persistently and it will be kept constantly on the move, allowing little time to rest or hunt and in the meanwhile burning up precious energy by staying on the wing for extended periods.

Timing of release
The longer a bird is kept in captivity, the more problematic the release may become. If an adult bird is fit for release within 14 days of the initial injury, it should go back to its original territory. If release has

been delayed, the bird is usually better released in another area.

Winter is not an easy time of year to release birds, as their metabolic rates will be higher (because of the cold weather) and hence food requirements greater. During winter, the prey base tends to be lower, with few insects, small mammals and reptiles available. The summer months are ideal for release; the days are long, the breeding season is over and food is more plentiful.

For non-migratory species the autumn can also be good, as ground cover is diminishing, making hunting easier, whilst prey is still relatively plentiful. Diurnal birds should be released early in the day; owls should be released shortly before sunset.

Methods of release

Each method has its own inherent advantages and disadvantages; each has its place and different ones will be most suitable on different occasions.

Release subjects can be divided into the following categories:

- Adult bird, experienced hunter; hospitalized for 4–6 weeks; good condition
- Adult bird, experienced hunter; more than 8 weeks in captivity; fair condition
- Young bird, inexperienced at flying and hunting; less than 6 weeks in captivity; good condition.

As birds regain fitness, intra-abdominal fat is utilized and muscle tone throughout the body is developed and strengthened. Manoeuvrability and stamina will increase daily, as long as the bird is given the opportunity to fly. Variations of the traditional 'hack' (see below) and falconry techniques are often appropriate and adequate. Birds can be flown to the fist or the lure to achieve this fitness.

Fitness training

Adults, and juveniles that have not hunted for themselves, can be trained and flown at wild prey. Once the bird is killing proficiently it can be released, preferably leaving it with its last kill after having all of its hardware (i.e. jesses and bells) removed. Where possible, this fitness training should be carried out in the area into which the bird is to be released. The advantage of this technique is that of continual assessment of the bird's suitability for release and its increased fitness. The bird is only released when it reaches its optimum condition.

Lure training

Alternatively, raptors can be trained to be flown to the lure (falcons) or to the fist (hawks) to feed. Once habituated to this feeding method, the bird can be released without its jesses and bells and the falconer or rehabilitator goes daily to call the released bird down to be fed. This technique enables the released bird slowly to gain independence and regain its hunting skills; the only disadvantage is the continual reinforcement of the rehabilitator being a food source.

Hacking

The falconer's definition of 'hack' is a period of liberty offered to a young inexperienced bird to enable it to develop naturally the skills required in flying and hunting. In the casualty situation, 'young inexperienced bird' is replaced by 'convalescent bird'. Several techniques are used, two of which are discussed briefly below. Figures 22.10 and 22.11 show a hack box and tower.

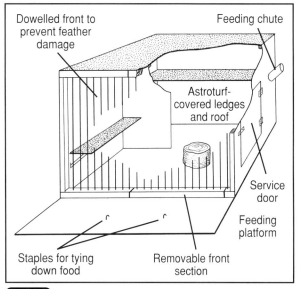

22.10 Hack box.

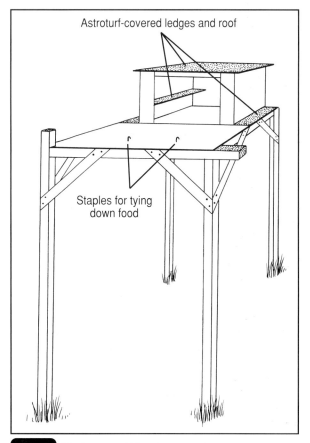

22.11 Hack tower. (After Fox, 1995.)

Feeding board or hack board:

1. A platform is placed in a tree or other secure site that offers the bird a good view of the surrounding countryside. Food is secured to the hack board.
2. The bird, unhooded, is carried on the fist to the hack board so that it becomes familiar with its new surroundings. It is then tethered to the board and allowed to feed.
3. Initially the bird is left on the board for only 10 minutes after feeding. This is repeated daily until it attempts to fly to the board as it approaches in order to reach its food. Throughout this process the bird is offered food only on the board.

The day a decision is made to release the bird, it should be given only half the normal food. As it is still hungry, it is more likely to remain near the hack board. The rehabilitator now has to cut off the bird's jesses and this negative stimulus will help to break the rehabilitator/patient bond. From then on, food is continually placed out on the board and tied to it, at a regular time each day. Food should continue to be left out for a considerable period after the bird is last seen.

Hack flight

The principle involved here is similar to the hack board system, except that it involves far less human contact. The technique makes use of a simple aviary, rather than a platform, built along similar lines to a recuperation aviary (see Chapter 3). The aviary is best kept simple and preferably collapsible and transportable, so that different hack sites may be used. Food is tied to a platform inside the flight. When the bird is feeding well, the flight is opened to allow it to venture out and investigate the surrounding countryside. Again, the bird must be kept hungry in order to discourage it from departing before it is fully fit and ready.

Birds released in this way do not acquire the same degree of territoriality about the feed station as those hacked using a platform. For this reason, they must not be frightened or disturbed during the delicate procedure.

Legal aspects

Any member of the public is permitted to take an injured raptor into care, as long as they provide suitable care and support, prevent anything occurring that would prevent the bird's later release, and release it as soon as it is fit into suitable environmental conditions. Species listed in Schedule 4 of the Wildlife and Countryside Act (golden eagle, red kite, goshawk, osprey, all harriers, peregrine, hobby and merlin) need to be registered with DEFRA (see Chapter 5).

Assessment for release

Veterinary surgeons may sometimes be asked to certify a raptor as temporarily or permanently unsuitable for release. This task should be undertaken only by those who are certain that they are suitably experienced to make such an assessment. The decision is particularly difficult in cases of imprinting, which may not be clear-cut. It is a sad truth that a member of the public wishing to 'launder' an ex-wild injured bird so that it can be kept permanently in captivity will not seek such an opinion from an experienced avian veterinary surgeon. A suitable certification form may be found at www.lansdown-vets.co.uk

Specialist organizations

Hawk and Owl Trust
c/o Zoological Society of London, Regent's Park, London NW1 4RY

Raptor Rescue
8 Carlisle Grove, Buxton, Derbyshire SK17 6XP
Helpline: 0870 2410609
Website: www.raptorrescue.org.uk

References and further reading

Beynon PH, Forbes NA and Harcourt-Brown NH (eds) (1996) *Manual of Raptors, Pigeons and Waterfowl*. BSAVA, Cheltenham

Coles BH (1996) Diseases of the wing. In: *Manual of Psittacine Birds*, eds NA Forbes *et al.*, pp. 134–146. BSAVA, Cheltenham

Cooper JE (2001) *Birds of Prey: Health & Disease, 3rd edn*. Blackwell Science. Oxford

Cooper JE and Greenwood AG (eds) (1981) *Recent Advances in Raptor Diseases*. Chiron Publications, Keighley

Del Hoyo J, Elliott A and Sargatal J (eds) (1994) *Handbook of the Birds of the World, Vol. 2*. Lynx Edicions, Barcelona

Del Hoyo J, Elliott A and Sargatal J (eds) (1999) *Handbook of the Birds of the World, Vol. 5*. Lynx Edicions, Barcelona

Forbes NA (1999) Avian anaesthesia. In: *Manual of Small Animal Anaesthesia and Analgesia*, eds C Seymour and R Gleed, pp. 283–294. BSAVA, Cheltenham

Harcourt-Brown NH (1994) *Diseases of the pelvic limb of birds of prey*. FRCVS Thesis, RCVS Library

Harcourt-Brown NH (1996) Foot and leg problems. In: *Manual of Raptors, Pigeons and Waterfowl*, eds NA Forbes *et al.*, pp. 147–169. BSAVA, Cheltenham

Heidenreich M (1997) *Birds of Prey Medicine and Management*. Blackwell Science, Oxford

Hess RE (1994) Management of orthopedic problems of the avian pelvic limb. *Seminars in Avian and Exotic Pet Medicine* 3, 63–72. WB Saunders, Orlando, Florida

Howard DJ and Redig PT (1993) Analysis of avian fracture repair: implications for captive and wild birds. In: *Proceedings of the Association of Avian Veterinarians Annual Conference, Lake Worth, Florida*, pp. 78–83

Howard DJ and Redig PT (1994) Orthopedics of the wing. *Seminars in Avian and Exotic Pet Medicine* 3, 51–62. WB Saunders, Orlando, Florida

Lumeij JT, Remple D, Redig PT, Lierz M and Cooper JE (eds) (2000) *Raptor Biomedicine III*. Zoological Education Network, Lake Worth, Florida

Martin HD, Brueker KA, Herrick DD and Scherpelz J (1993) Elbow luxations in raptors: a review of eight cases. In: *Raptor Biomedicine*, eds PT Redig *et al.*, pp. 199–206. University of Minnesota Press, Minneapolis

Mullarney K, Svensson L, Zetterstrom D and Grant PJ (1999) *Bird Guide*. Harper Collins, London

Orosz SE, Ensley PK and Haynes CJ (1992) *Avian Surgical Anatomy: Thoracic and Pelvic Limbs*. WB Saunders, Philadelphia

Redig PT (1996) Avian emergencies. In: *Manual of Raptors, Pigeons and Waterfowl*, eds PH Beynon *et al.*, pp. 30–42. BSAVA, Cheltenham

Redig PT (2000) Trauma related medical conditions. In: *Avian Medicine*, ed. J Samour, pp. 131–165. Mosby, London

Redig PT, Cooper JE, Remple D and Hunter DB (eds) (1993) *Raptor Biomedicine*. University of Minnesota Press, Minneapolis

Shawyer C (1985) *Rodenticides: a Review and Assessment of their Potential Hazard to Non-target Wildlife with Special Reference to the Barn Owl (Tyto alba)*. The Hawk Trust, Zoological Society of London

23

Gamebirds

John R. Chitty

Introduction

Gamebirds are those that are hunted for the table or for sport. While this description may include wild duck and certain waders, such as snipe (*Gallinago gallinago*) and woodcock (*Scolopax rusticola*), this chapter will concentrate on galliform birds to avoid duplicating information that can be found in Chapters 19 and 20.

Species found in the British Isles

The Galliformes are related to poultry. Some of these species are not indigenous to the British Isles but have become established over several centuries. Many are farmed semi-intensively prior to release (typically the pheasant and both partridge species); therefore many of those birds presented to rehabilitators will not be truly 'wild' and may be harbouring or exhibiting clinical signs of diseases that are more typical of intensive-rearing situations. For this reason a brief description of rearing practices will be included here. Game species can only be hunted in legally defined seasons and naturally it is sensible to avoid these periods when releasing rehabilitated birds. Figure 23.1 describes the characteristics and ecology of British gamebirds.

Species	Description	Weight	UK distribution	Habitat	Diet
Common pheasant (*Phasianus colchicus*)	Male red-brown with bright head/back colours; long tail lost after breeding Female dull brown with shorter tail	Male approx. 1500 g Female approx. 1000 g	All except N Scotland	Generally edges of woodland/ hedgerows	Seeds, insects
Red-legged (French) partridge (*Alectoris rufa*)	Red tail, white face with dark eye-stripe, barring on flanks, red bill and legs	450–600 g	England as far north as Yorkshire moors; not Wales	Open countryside, heaths, downland, etc	Seeds, insects
Chukar partridge (*Alectoris chukar*)	Closely related to red-legged; chukar and hybrids with red-legged extensively released 1980s to improve 'quality'; release of pure-breds and hybrids illegal since 1992 but still sometimes practised Distinguished by bolder eye-stripe and flank barring, and single stripe on neck	450–600 g		Open countryside, heaths, downland, etc.	Seeds, insects
Grey (English) partridge (*Perdix perdix*)	Grey-brown; orange-red face, red-brown tail Male brown horseshoe mark on breast; duller in female	320–400 g	All except N Scotland and mountainous areas	Open countryside, some cover	Seeds, insects
Common quail (*Coturnix coturnix*)	Resembles very small partridge Male black-and-white stripes on throat and neck (absent in female)	150–180 g	Summer visitor S England, some parts Scotland and Ireland	Open countryside	Seeds
Red grouse (*Lagopus lagopus*)	Male dark red-brown plumage, red eye wattles, white legs Female smaller and paler	400–700 g	Scotland, N England, Wales, Ireland	Moorland	Heather shoots

23.1 Characteristics and ecology of gamebirds. (continues) ▶

Species	Description	Weight	UK distribution	Habitat	Diet
Ptarmigan (*Lagopus mutus*)	Summer: male dark brown upper parts, white wings and belly, red eye wattles; female paler with smaller wattles Winter: white with black tail; male has black face patch (lacking in female)	250–600 g	N Scotland	Mountain top	Heather shoots, ground berries, leaves
Black grouse (*Lyrurus tetrix*)	Male (blackcock) black with red head wattles, black-and-white lyre-shaped tail Female (greyhen) smaller; similar to red grouse but greyer and forked tail	Male: 1000–1750 g Female: 750–1100 g	Scotland, N England and Wales	Moorland	Heather shoots
Capercaillie (*Tetrao urogallus*)	Male huge; dark plumage, bushy throat feathers, rounded tail Female similar to greyhen but larger and with chestnut breast	Male: 3700–4800 g Female: 1600–2500 g	Scottish Highlands	Pine forest	Pine shoots

23.1 (continued) Characteristics and ecology of gamebirds.

Ecology and behaviour

Gamebirds are ground-nesters that generally form territories, usually set up and defended by the males. These may be centred around good food sources (e.g. for pheasants) or at ritual breeding grounds where many males come together (black grouse).

The chicks are precocial and have pale down with dark mottles or stripes.

Game farming

Pheasants (Figure 23.2) and both species of partridge are reared for release. Reared birds will make up the vast majority of the casualties that may be presented to rehabilitators.

Traditionally, at the end of the shooting season, adult males and females are caught up and placed into breeding pens. However, this results in selection of

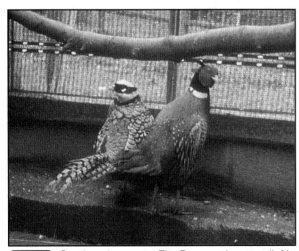

23.2 Captive pheasants. The Reeves pheasant (left) is a non-native species and may not be released. (Courtesy of Wiltshire Wildlife Hospital.)

birds with an innate tendency to run rather than fly when alarmed. As this tendency is inherited by the offspring, the 'quality' of the shoot declines. Therefore, new breeding strategies have developed alongside the traditional methods.

One system is to maintain a permanent captive breeding stock; this is the basis of game farms, which supply chicks to the rearing fields in June each year. The other system is to encourage breeding in the wild and this (it is supposed) produces a wilder, more strongly flying bird.

Many shoots continue to feed 'wild' birds through spring and early summer by means of strategically placed hoppers. These enable male birds to form a territory around a feeder and attract females. This approach has many advantages for the environment: gamebirds will not do well without insects in the diet and therefore breeding areas are not sprayed, and small copses and mature hedgerows are left intact to encourage the formation of territories.

Where birds are captive-bred, chicks are initially reared in houses and then moved to covered runs, before being moved to a large release pen – typically in late July. The release pen is intended to act as a 'home base' and the birds are fully released after a few weeks. Fox-proof re-entry funnels enable the birds to return to feed if they are unable to fly back into the release pen.

Anatomy and physiology

The anatomy is essentially chicken-like. There is a short straight beak for prehending food items from the ground. Gut adaptations to the natural diet consist of a large crop, powerful grinding gizzard and well developed paired caeca to enable hindgut fermentation.

Capture, handling and transportation

Capture

Capture of injured birds is not always easy. They are all good runners, even with damaged legs, and tend to head towards thick undergrowth. Catching birds in the wild is best done with several people 'flushing' the bird into an open area where a net can be used. It is important to note that male capercaillie are extremely aggressive; they should be approached with caution.

Gamebirds are very nervous and will cause themselves a great deal of damage in evading capture. In the clinic or rehabilitation centre, where the bird is more confined, it is best to dim the lighting before attempting handling as this might help to calm the bird. It can then be caught using a net or by being enveloped in a large towel.

Handling

A strong grip is necessary and large hands are useful. Gamebirds are strong and will struggle violently, which can result in injury to the bird. They are also extremely loose-feathered and the loss of large amounts of body feathering will delay release, as the feathers play an important role in the bird's thermo-regulatory system.

Males often possess large spurs just proximal to the foot (Figure 23.3). These can inflict deep wounds on a handler and so the legs of male gamebirds must be held firmly.

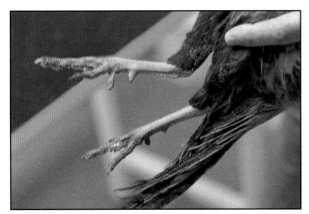

23.3 The feet of a male pheasant, showing the prominent spurs.

Wrapping the bird in a towel to restrain the wings and feet will help greatly when it is being moved. It is important that the legs are not crushed together, as this may result in bruising of the lower limb and injuries to the opposite leg from the spur and claws. Part of the towel can be used to cover the head, which should calm the bird.

The wrap may need to be removed during examination. The hands should be placed on either side of the bird's body, with the thumbs between its shoulder joints. The index and middle fingers are held around the wings while the ring and little fingers hold the upper legs (Figure 23.4). Smaller gamebirds (quail and young partridge) may be held in one hand in much the same manner as for passerines.

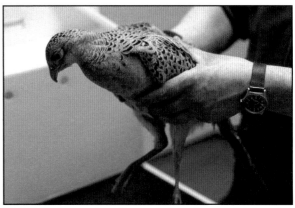

23.4 Correct handling technique for an adult female pheasant.

Transportation

These are nervous birds and so a dark box (or covered cage) is essential. It should be sturdy and should open from the top. Extricating a flapping pheasant from a cat box with a small door is very difficult. Cardboard boxes or BSAVA-standard cat carriers are ideal.

Zoonotic risks

The main risk is salmonellosis. It is important to maintain strict hygiene and to wash and disinfect hands, surfaces and handling equipment after use.

Chlamydophilosis is unusual but should be suspected in birds showing upper respiratory signs. In these cases, facemasks and goggles should be worn by handlers.

Examination and assessment for rehabilitation

The general principles of examination and assessment, as detailed in Chapter 2, apply to gamebird casualties.

Body condition can be assessed by feeling the pectoral muscles. It is important to note that chicks and poults should feel thinner than full adults, as the pectoral muscles will be less developed.

Birds should also be weighed, as this enables correct calculation of drug dosages and, where a pheasant or partridge is in good body condition, will enable some degree of ageing of young birds. Tables of bodyweights may be found in Beer (1988).

Droppings should be examined. Farmed game are very prone to a range of parasitic infections (see below) and so gross evaluation and faecal flotation may be useful. Microscopic examination of a wet preparation of fresh faeces is useful for the diagnosis of protozoal enteritis (e.g. trichomoniasis, hexamitiasis). A soiled vent and tail feathers may indicate problems.

Anaesthesia may be useful to facilitate examination in the following circumstances:

- Very nervous birds, where detailed examination may cause more stress
- Dyspnoeic birds (allows supply of oxygen as well as reducing stress)

- Examination of the upper legs. These are very well muscled and held tightly against the body, so that full extension and examination of the femurs, hips and stifles may be difficult in the conscious bird
- Examination of the posterior segment of the eye. Anaesthesia is necessary to dilate the (small) pupil. This examination should be performed whenever head trauma is suspected.

Criteria for euthanasia

Birds should be returned to the wild only if they can meet the following criteria:

- Full use of both legs. Inability to use both legs fully will reduce the capacity of these heavy birds to escape predators. A unilateral lameness will inevitably result in bumblefoot (pressure sores) in the 'good' foot
- Ability to fly. These are not 'performance fliers' in the manner of raptors and they do not rely on their wings to get food, nor are they migratory (except quail). Indeed there is some argument that poor fliers are more likely to survive the shooting season. However, some flight is necessary to avoid predators and so those unable to fly should not be released
- Vision in both eyes. The need for binocular vision is less important than in a raptor but lack of vision makes birds more prone to predation. The side-facing position of the eyes gives these birds a large field of vision (typical in prey species). Defects in one or both eyes will be a hindrance
- Free from infectious disease. A bird that is suspected of carrying or that is suffering from infectious disease should not be released. A bird that does not gain weight or body condition even though it is eating well may well fall into this category.

Euthanasia *at first examination* is recommended in the following cases:

- Open, complicated fractures
- Fractures involving joints
- Extensive soft tissue injuries (especially where there is penetration of the coelomic cavity or where there are large tissue deficits of the leg muscles or tendons)
- Obvious loss of an eye (e.g. rupture, hypopyon).

Euthanasia techniques

Ideally euthanasia should be performed using intravenous pentobarbital into the ulnar or tibial veins. The jugular vein is difficult to find in gamebirds.

This may be difficult or impossible in the field, where it may be deemed inhumane to transport a bird to a veterinary clinic. In these cases, euthanasia by rapid cervical dislocation is acceptable (see Chapter 2).

First aid

This subject is covered in Chapter 2.

In the non-collapsed bird, oral fluids (e.g. Critical Care Formula, Vetark; Lectade, Pfizer) may be given by crop tube at a rate of 12 ml/kg and repeated as necessary.

In the collapsed bird, bolus intravenous fluids can be given into the ulnar vein at 5–10 ml/kg (Hartmann's is ideal). Intravenous and intraosseous drips do not appear to be well tolerated.

Repeated intravenous injections may require extensive handling and where this is not desirable the subcutaneous route may be used. Injection of Hartmann's at 20 ml/kg into the precrural fold is simple and not traumatic to the bird. Fluid appears to be absorbed completely within 20–30 minutes.

It is advisable to give a broad-spectrum antibiotic, such as amoxicillin.

Fracture stabilization

The general principles set out in Chapter 2 apply to gamebirds. Injuries following road traffic accidents are the most frequent reasons for gamebirds being presented and fractures are therefore commonly seen. In these cases, analgesia should always be provided at first presentation. The author uses carprofen at 5 mg/kg by intramuscular injection initially; this may be repeated once daily as required.

Leg fractures

A ball bandage may be applied to immobilize broken toes, and aluminium finger splints may be used to support fractures of the tarsometatarus. It is not advisable to apply support to fractures higher than the intertarsal joint: the legs are short, muscular and held close to the body, which makes it impossible to immobilize the joints above and below a fracture as well as making it likely that the dressing will slip. In these cases, it is better to confine the bird in a small dark box until it can tolerate surgery and internal fixation can be performed.

Wing fractures

The short rounded wing is very difficult to stabilize with a figure-of-eight bandage. It is usually best to confine the bird in a small dark box until surgery can be tolerated. Where support is essential (e.g. where the wing is trailing and being stepped on), the wing can be held against the body using conforming bandage.

Short-term hospitalization

Gamebirds have few specific needs. The enclosure must be secluded and there should be no potential predators (e.g. dogs, cats, raptors) in view.

In the short term a conventional dog or cat kennel is acceptable. It should be large enough for the bird to move freely without damaging wing or tail feathers, but not so large that catching becomes difficult. Perching is not required.

Anaesthesia and analgesia

The general principles of anaesthesia and analgesia, as detailed in Chapter 2, apply to gamebird casualties.

Anaesthesia

Isoflurane can be administered by open mask and is the anaesthetic agent of choice. The bird can then be maintained on mask, or intubated for longer procedures.

Where gaseous anaesthetic agents are not available, medetomidine/ketamine combinations may be used. Medetomidine can be reversed by an equal volume of atipamezole but it should be noted that this combination carries more risks than isoflurane.

Gamebirds are extremely nervous and may be prone to catecholamine-induced dysrhythmias and death while anaesthetized. If the capture of the bird before induction has been difficult (e.g. it has escaped and been chased), it is generally better to replace the bird in its box or hospitalization unit and leave it quietly in the dark to calm down before proceeding.

On recovery, birds should be wrapped to prevent flapping and injury or feather loss.

Analgesia
Carprofen and meloxicam are particularly useful and appear to be safe in these species (see the avian formulary in Appendix 1).

Specific conditions

For full reviews see Curtis (1987), Beer (1988) and Coles (2000). It should be noted that, commercially, diagnoses are generally reached following necropsy and most textbooks reflect this. It is important that any gamebird that dies or is euthanased while being cared for is submitted for post-mortem examination; this will enable detection of infectious disease agents and so reduce risks for other birds.

Trauma

Eye haemorrhage
Trauma will often result in damage to the pecten and haemorrhage into the eye. Where haemorrhage is visible, therapy using topical ophthalmic corticosteroid preparations should be started promptly (see Appendix 1) and the eye re-examined before release.

Orthopaedic problems
Gamebirds tend to have relatively large bones with thin fragile cortices, which shatter easily, and it is unusual to see simple fractures. In addition, many fractures will be open and infected, giving a poor prognosis for return to the wild in most cases. The nature of the bones reduces the options for repair and the vast majority of cases are unsuitable for surgery.

General principles for avian fracture repair are discussed in Chapter 2. Some details specific for gamebirds are as follows.

Coracoid: Fractures of this bone may be seen as a result of in-flight collisions. Surgical repair is rarely indicated. Confinement to a cage or aviary for 4–6 weeks is sufficient.

Humerus and femur: These bones are pneumatized. They have a large internal diameter and very thin cortices. Simple intramedullary pinning requires a very large pin such that the sheer weight of the pin will cause problems. This technique also gives no rotational stability. The methods of choice in these birds are stack pinning or hybridization techniques (see Chapter 22).

Fractures distal to the carpus: It is difficult to apply and maintain external support in this area due to the shape of the wing. The primary feathers should be trimmed and heavy tape or Vet-lite (Runlite SA, Micheroux, Belgium) should be applied to the feather bases to align the bones and maintain their length. The bird needs to be maintained in captivity until the primaries have regrown.

Tibiotarsus: Heavy muscling around this bone makes the use of external fixators less desirable. Stack pinning techniques give a good success rate.

Tarsometatarsus: Surgical intervention is likely to damage surrounding tendons. Most cases will do well with external support using an aluminium finger splint or Vet-lite. The support should immobilize the intertarsal joint and the tarsometatarsophalangeal joint (with a 'stirrup' beneath the foot). Care should be taken to maintain normal standing joint angles so that the bird is able to move and stand comfortably.

Toe fractures: These do well in a ball bandage, which should be removed after 5 days and the bird confined for a further fortnight.

Infectious diseases
Infectious diseases of gamebirds are outlined in Figure 23.5. It is important that equipment is not shared between birds and that it is disinfected thoroughly after use.

Disease	Causal agent	Clinical signs	Diagnosis	Therapy
Viral diseases				
Newcastle disease	Paramyxovirus-1 (PMV-1)	Neurological, including incoordination and staggering Diarrhoea Polydipsia Respiratory signs less common than in poultry	**Notifiable disease**: local Divisional Veterinary Manager should be notified *on suspicion* Diagnosis (based on serology and post-mortem signs) carried out by Veterinary Laboratories Agency	No specific therapy
Pheasant ataxia	Unknown	An 'emerging' disease Leg paresis/paralysis, which must be differentiated from spinal/ pelvic injuries	Suspicion aroused if several birds present from same site or if examination/necropsy reveals no sign of injury Definitive diagnosis by histopathology of central nervous system tissue	None

23.5 Infectious diseases of gamebirds. (continues) ▶

Disease	Causal agent	Clinical signs	Diagnosis	Therapy
Viral diseases continued				
Marble spleen disease	Adenovirus	Pheasants 'fall out of the sky' Unusual to see in rehabilitation set-up but important differential for sudden death in adult birds	Enlarged mottled ('marbled') spleen seen on post-mortem examination	None
Pheasant coronavirus	Coronavirus	Wasting Polyuria/polydipsia in adult birds	Enlarged pale kidneys on post-mortem examination	None
Pox	Poxvirus	Multiple masses around head, limbs and sometimes upper alimentary tract	Histopathology or cytology of needle aspirates	Symptomatic care until lesions resolve Bird's welfare must be considered during treatment Some lesions may result in permanent scarring in sensitive positions (e.g. eyelids) Highly contagious – birds under treatment should be barrier nursed until completely resolved
Bacterial diseases				
Colibacillosis	*Escherichia coli*	Chicks and poults Fluffed birds, wasting Death due to septicaemia Often secondary to other diseases (e.g. coccidiosis) or in unhygienic conditions	Typical signs Culture/sensitivity of faeces (or heart blood, liver, or bone marrow on post-mortem examination)	Antibiosis, ideally based on culture/sensitivity Correction/treatment of underlying factors/disease
Salmonellosis	*Salmonella* spp.	Haemorrhagic enteritis typically but signs may appear similar to colibacillosis	Signs Culture/sensitivity (as for colibacillosis) Hard white caecal cores may be seen on post-mortem examination; wet preparation of these should always be examined to differentiate from other causes of caecal cores, especially coccidiosis and *Heterakis* (roundworm) infestations	Antibiosis, ideally based on culture/sensitivity
Avian tuberculosis	*Mycobacterium avium*	Wasting in adult birds	Ante-mortem diagnosis difficult but clinical signs may be suggestive Acid-fast stains of faeces, haematological signs (high white blood cell count with heterophilia and monocytosis) and intracoelomic endoscopy probably methods of choice White nodules found in liver, spleen and intestines on post-mortem examination	Anti-mycobacterial therapies available but treatment not recommended as success rate so poor Massive numbers of bacteria shed in faeces, emphasizing need for good hygiene and strict isolation of ill/thin birds
Mycoplasmosis	*Mycoplasma* spp.	Sinusitis and/or tenosynovitis (typically lame birds with swelling above intertarsal joint) Highly infectious to other birds	Clinical signs Cytology of fluid aspirates Mycoplasmal culture/serology	Antibiosis, especially tetracyclines or fluoroquinolones Advanced cases develop large cores of inspissated pus in sinuses; need to be removed surgically
Fungal diseases				
Aspergillosis	*Aspergillus* spp.	Dyspnoea and death due to formation of fungal colonies in lungs and airsacs following inhalation of spores from rotting organic matter (e.g. bark chip, mouldy hay)	Typical signs in young birds Radiography and coelomic endoscopy of greatest value with cytology and culture/sensitivity of colonies	Itraconazole or terbinafine systemically with nebulization of F10 Unlikely to be successful Prevention best by removing organic matter from rearing/hospitalization areas

23.5 (continued) Infectious diseases of gamebirds. (continues) ▶

Disease	Causal agent	Clinical signs	Diagnosis	Therapy
Parasitic diseases				
Coccidiosis	*Eimeria* spp.	Usually affects young birds Wasting Sometimes scour May predispose to colibacillosis	Finding coccidial oocysts in faecal smears/flotation	Toltrazuril ideal but available only in 1-litre bottles Amprolium/sulphadimethoxine licensed in pigeons and available in much smaller quantities
Protozoal dysentery	*Hexamita* spp. or *Trichomonas* spp.	Frothy yellow scour, wasting and death	Finding motile flagellates in fresh (< 30 min old) faecal samples Note that these organisms may be present in low numbers as gut commensals in healthy birds (stress of illness/captivity may trigger overt disease)	Dimetridazole (preferably) or metronidazole
Histomoniasis	*Histomonas meleagridis*	Especially seen in red-legged partridge Young birds may die suddenly; older birds may scour and become emaciated	Organisms may be found in fresh wet preparations of faeces	Dimetridazole
Gapes	*Syngamus trachea*	'Gapes' (open-mouthed breathing) and dyspnoea	Typical signs Tracheal endoscopy reveals adult worms Microscopy of sputum and faecal samples to reveal ova	Flubendazole, ivermectin or fenbendazole
Strongylosis	Various species	Wasting *Trichostrongylus tenuis* is major cause of mortality in red grouse and partridge; in the former is one of the major causes of large population fluctuations in wild	Finding ova by faecal flotation	Flubendazole, ivermectin or fenbendazole
Ectoparasitic infestations	Feather lice, mites, hippoboscid flies	Rarely cause of clinical disease but may be sign of debilitated bird		Permethrins, fipronil

23.5 (continued) Infectious diseases of gamebirds.

Therapeutics

The general principles in Chapter 2 apply to gamebirds. It should be noted that intramuscular injections should be given into the pectoral muscle masses, not the leg muscle, to avoid an injection reaction or abscess in these important muscles.

It is important to note that gamebirds are officially classed as food-producing animals and therefore drug withholding periods must be observed. Birds should not be released within 28 days of the end of treatment and, more sensibly, not during the shooting season or for a month before its start (Figure 23.6).

Management in captivity

Housing

Small flights or aviaries are ideal. It is also possible to keep gamebirds on the floor of an aviary used for passerines. Some perching should be provided to allow the birds to roost at night if they wish.

Ideally flooring should be cleanable and not soil-based, to reduce build-up of parasites and enable disinfection between batches. Concrete answers these

Species	Season
Pheasant	1 October to 1 February
Partridge	1 September to 1 February
Quail	Protected at all times
Red grouse	12 August to 10 December
Black grouse	20 August to 10 December
Ptarmigan	Protected at all times, except Scotland (12 August to 10 December)
Capercaillie	1 October to 31 January

23.6 Hunting seasons in the UK.

criteria but may result in foot lesions in long-term patients. Gravel may therefore be more acceptable.

To reduce the risk of spreading infectious disease, birds from different areas should not be housed together.

Feeding

Diet is simple, as these birds will readily take poultry pellets or mash, or chick crumb. For debilitated birds these can be liquidized and fed by crop tube. Corn or commercial diets for mynah birds may be added to increase palatability for reluctant feeders. Drinking water should be provided in a shallow dish.

Rearing young

Orphaned birds are not commonly presented. When they are, they should be reared in groups. Gamebird chicks are precocial and social imprinting is not an issue. They will readily take chick crumb, and feeding by hand should not be necessary.

Release

Birds may be released after recovery from the presenting illness or injury. Their fitness for release can be determined by:

- Demeanour and vision
- Ability to prehend food
- Body condition
- Ability to walk or run
- Ability to fly.

These criteria should be assessed thoroughly before release. This can be done in much the same way as for other birds (see Chapter 3) but it may be difficult to assess the last criterion, as gamebirds are often reluctant fliers. Where there are doubts about any of the criteria, the bird should be either euthanased or kept and reassessed at a later date if it is felt that the problem will resolve.

Ideally, birds should be released where they were found. This should be done just after the shooting season (see Figure 23.3). It is sensible to discuss release activities with local landowners and gamekeepers: access to land requires their permission (see Chapter 5) and they may be willing to help with post-release monitoring and feeding. Brightly coloured leg tags are available to aid post-release monitoring.

Two forms of release may be employed: hard or soft (see Chapter 3).

Hard release

Many of these species are amenable to hard release. Birds may simply be released, as long as there is suitable habitat. The presence of other birds of the same species should be an indicator of the suitability of that area.

Soft release

Soft release is the preferred option and is particularly suitable for pheasants. As discussed earlier, male pheasants can be induced to form a territory around a feeding station in a hedgerow or on the edge of woodland. If access to land is possible, a feeding hopper containing game or poultry feed should be placed in a suitable position. A male pheasant can then be released (or one will soon arrive) and released females will generally join his harem. Feeding can be gradually tapered off at the end of the breeding season.

This technique involves close cooperation with the local gamekeeper. As 'wild' breeding is now very important, opposition is unlikely (outside the shooting season) unless the released birds are placed too close to existing release pens.

Legal aspects

The legal aspects pertaining to holding and re-release of injured birds (see Chapter 5) also apply to gamebirds. It is important to have knowledge of the legal hunting seasons so that birds are not released during or immediately prior to these (see Figure 23.6).

References and further reading

Beer JV (1988) *Diseases of Gamebirds and Wildfowl*. Game Conservancy, Fordingbridge
Coles BH (2000) Galliformes. In: *Avian medicine*, eds TN Tully *et al.*, pp. 266–295. Butterworth-Heinemann, Oxford
Curtis P (1987) *A Handbook of Poultry and Gamebird Diseases*. Liverpool University Press, Liverpool

24

Pigeons and doves

John R. Chitty

Introduction

With the exception of the turtle dove (a summer visitor to southern England and the Midlands) and the rock dove (confined to Ireland and Scotland), pigeons and doves can be found year-round throughout the British Isles, except in the Scottish mountains. They are the most common avian species presented to rehabilitators, either as injured birds or as orphaned young. British Wildlife Rehabilitation Council (BWRC) wildlife casualty recording scheme figures for 1993–1997 show that 14% of all bird casualties were feral and racing pigeons and 9% were wood pigeons.

Species found in the British Isles

The characteristics and ecology of the different species are summarized in Figure 24.1.

Ecology and behaviour

The sexes are essentially alike in all species. Breeding occurs almost year-round; nests are made off the ground and the young are altricial. Young birds are covered in coarse tufts of yellow down; they have fleshy beaks, often with a tiny hook on the upper part, and are therefore often presented as 'raptors'. Very young birds (up to 4 weeks of age, still covered in down) are referred to as squabs; slightly older birds (until fledging) are squeakers (Figure 24.3).

Anatomy and physiology

All species are granivorous. The crop is large, for food storage, and is also adapted (in both sexes) to produce

Species	Characteristics	Weight	UK distribution	Habitat	Diet
Rock dove (*Columba livia*)	Ancestor of ubiquitous 'feral pigeon' (latter essentially grey but wide range of markings due to intermixing with racing and show pigeons)	250–500 g	Pure in N Scotland, Scottish isles and Ireland	Rocky coastal areas Feral pigeon mainly urban areas	Seeds, leaves
Stock dove (*Columba oenas*)	Same size as rock dove Lacks white rump of rock dove and has shorter wings, less obvious dark bars on wings	250–450 g	Throughout, except N Scotland	Widespread, especially farmland, woodland edges	Seeds, leaves
Wood pigeon (*Columba palumbas*)	Larger Distinctive white patches on wings and dorsal neck (Figure 24.2)	450–700 g	Throughout	Widespread, especially farmland, woodland edges	Seeds, leaves
Collared dove (*Streptopelia decaocto*)	Smaller Pale grey with distinct black 'collar' on dorsal neck	150–200 g	Throughout	Mainly suburban	Seeds, leaves
Turtle dove (*Streptopelia turtur*)	Chestnut upper parts, pink breast, black-and-white neck patch	150–180 g	Summer migrant to S and E England, less common now	Woodland edges, thick hedges	Seeds, leaves

24.1 Characteristics and ecology of pigeons and doves.

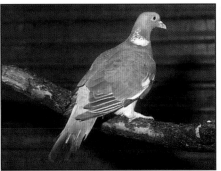

24.2 Adult wood pigeon (*Columba palumbas*). (Courtesy of C Seddon.)

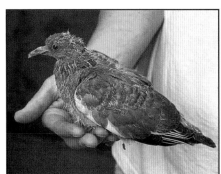

24.3 A 'squeaker'.

'crop milk' for feeding squabs, when the lining will hypertrophy. The gizzard is large and well developed. In mature male rock doves the cere may show extensive hypertrophy to give white 'crusty' growths.

Capture, handling and transportation

Capture is most easily accomplished by using a net. If no net is available, birds may be cornered and enveloped with a towel or simply picked up.

Pigeons and doves pose no physical risk to handlers. The smaller species may be held easily in one hand, with the keel in the palm and the head facing the handler's wrist. The bird's feet, tail and wing tips are held between the little, ring and middle fingers, respectively (see Figure 2.5b). Wood pigeons may flap vigorously and are loose-feathered; they should be towel-wrapped or held in two hands.

Any pet carrier or cardboard box will suffice for transportation but should be darkened in order to calm the bird. Specialist cardboard carriers are also available.

Zoonotic risks

Pigeons and doves can pose a considerable health risk. The main dangers are salmonellosis and chlamydophilosis. Many healthy birds are asymptomatic carriers and will excrete these organisms; the stress of illness and captivity may increase this excretion rate. Campylobacteriosis may also be a risk.

Certainly any bird with loose droppings or swollen joints must be regarded as a high risk for salmonellosis. Clinical chlamydophilosis must be suspected in birds that are fluffed or have loose droppings or any upper respiratory signs, in which case the risk to handlers is so high that it may be advisable to euthanase such birds.

Strict personal hygiene should be followed after handling pigeons. When working with these birds, in particular when cleaning out, handlers should wear disposable waterproof gloves, facemask and goggles, as chlamydophilosis may be contracted via the conjunctivae.

Examination and assessment for rehabilitation

The general principles of examination and assessment are as detailed in Chapter 2. Particular attention should be paid to the droppings, vent and body condition. Neurological disorders are common and the bird's demeanour, head position and reflexes should be carefully observed.

The mouth and pharynx should be thoroughly examined for the characteristic white plaques typical of trichomoniasis ('canker') (Figure 24.4). It is important to 'smell the breath': crop infections are common, especially in young birds, and a foul smell may be an early sign. The crop itself should be observed for excessive size, thickening (though this may be normal in parent birds), inability to empty and wounds.

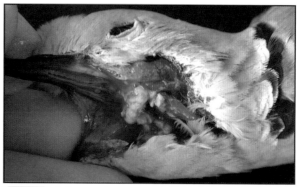

24.4 Advanced caseous lesions of trichomoniasis (canker) in the exposed pharynx of a collared dove. (Courtesy of G. Cousquer.)

Euthanasia

Pigeons are strong fliers, with a reliance on flight to escape and to reach nesting and roosting sites; they should not be released if flight is impaired. Repair of open or complicated wing fractures is unlikely to be fully successful and so euthanasia should be considered. Birds will also frequently present with septic arthritis (often caused by *Salmonella* spp.); this may resolve with antibiosis but treatment may be inadvisable as some arthritis and loss of joint mobility will remain (as well as the zoonotic implications).

Infectious disease is a major consideration. Signs of the major zoonotic diseases should preclude admission and treatment. There are also several diseases (especially paramyxovirus and poxvirus) that may be highly infectious to other birds. Signs suggestive of these infections should be a reason for euthanasia. Although mild canker is simple to treat, advanced cases with extensive crop lesions should be euthanased as therapy is less successful and the organism is highly contagious.

Euthanasia technique is as for gamebirds (see Chapter 23). The jugular vein is hard to locate, as there are no suitable aptera (featherless tracts) and the skin is very thick.

First aid

The general principles of first aid, as detailed in Chapter 2, apply to pigeon and dove casualties. It is important to emphasize the role of fluids, analgesia and the early use of broad-spectrum antibiosis. Amoxycillin is often appropriate but many birds will be presented following cat attacks. These wounds quickly become septicaemic, and antibiotics with a good spectrum of activity against anaerobes and Gram-negative organisms should be given as soon as possible (e.g. amoxicillin/clavulanate, piperacillin).

Short-term hospitalization

For short-term hospitalization a cat kennel is adequate. The kennel should be placed as high as possible (to increase the bird's feeling of security) in a quiet place away from cats, dogs, raptors and people. Strict biosecurity should be maintained and initially the casualty should not be kept in the same airspace as other birds.

Anaesthesia and analgesia

The general principles of anaesthesia and analgesia, as detailed in Chapter 2, apply to pigeon and dove casualties. Endotracheal tubes should be used with caution, as very narrow gauges (< 2.5 mm) are required. These may easily become blocked with mucus.

Specific conditions

For a full discussion of pigeon disease see Beynon *et al.* (1996).

Trauma

Fracture repair

The general principles of fracture repair, as detailed in Chapter 2, apply to pigeon and dove casualties (Figure

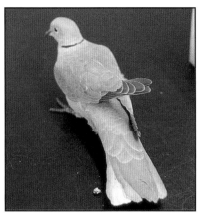

24.5 Adult collared dove with a left shoulder injury. Note the typically 'tilted' wing tip held above the normal right wing tip.

24.5). Kirschner wires and hypodermic needles make good intramedullary pins. Commercially available shuttle pins (Cook, UK) are also useful in pigeons.

Granulating wounds

These are commonly seen as a sequel to trauma or raptor strike (wounds usually on the dorsum). Debridement and primary closure are often impossible. Even with extensive wounds, good results can be achieved with daily cleaning and application of Intra Site gel (Smith & Nephew).

Ruptured crop

This condition, rarely seen in other birds, probably occurs because the crop is often so full and so may be more likely to rupture when traumatized. The birds usually present with a necrotic granulating wound forming a crop fistula. Even if the wound is fresh, it is important not to operate at once as the bruised crop wall margins will necrose, resulting in breakdown. It is recommended that the bird should be stabilized for 2–3 days first; this involves broad-spectrum antibiosis and stomach tubing (via the crop wound into the proventriculus). The crop wall and skin are debrided and repaired in two layers using simple continuous sutures with 3/0 Vicryl (Ethicon).

Infectious diseases

Infectious diseases of pigeons and doves are described in Figure 24.6. External parasites are rarely a problem, with the exception of ticks (Figure 24.7).

Disease	Causal agent	Clinical signs	Diagnosis	Treatment	Comments
Paramyxovirus (Newcastle disease)	Paramyxovirus-1 (PMV-1)	Many, including failure to prehend grain, head tremor, torticollis, polydipsia/polyuria, diarrhoea, deformed eggs	**Notifiable disease**	Recovery can occur in 3–8 weeks with supportive treatment	Birds may be carriers: treatment not recommended as can rapidly spread through rehabilitation unit and affect many avian species
Pigeon pox	Poxvirus	As for gamebirds		Lesions may resolve in few weeks and recovered birds have strong immunity If infection is severe with extensive lesions, birds may need to be euthanased on welfare grounds	Highly contagious so barrier nursing of suspect cases advised
Upper respiratory tract infection (URTI) ('coryza', 'one-eyed cold')	Herpesvirus, poxvirus, PMV-1 (rare), chlamydophilosis, mycoplasmosis, staphylococcosis, streptococcosis, pasteurellosis, trichomoniasis (rare) May also be due to dust irritation or foreign body	Swollen sinuses (uni- or bilateral) Ocular/nasal discharge	Accurate diagnosis essential for accurate treatment Bacteriology, cytology and serology	Presence in differential list of zoonotic agents and some agents highly infectious to other birds, therefore columbids should be admitted and treated with great caution	Environment plays large role in transmission of respiratory disease: bird rooms should be well ventilated; young birds should not be in same airspace as older birds; new birds should be quarantined for at least 10 days before entering unit with other birds

24.6 Infectious diseases of pigeons and doves. (continues) ▶

Disease	Causal agent	Clinical signs	Diagnosis	Treatment	Comments
Joint swelling	*Salmonella* spp. and *E. coli* commonly implicated	Septic polyarthritis Note that single swollen joints may be due to trauma or infection	Culture/sensitivity of septic joint fluid	Antibiosis, ideally on basis of sensitivity results	Treatment should not be attempted if many joints affected or if doubt that affected joint will not return to full function
Trichomoniasis ('canker')	*Trichomonas* spp.	White caseous lesions in mouth, pharynx and crop	Fresh wet preparations of caseous material reveal motile flagellates Important to differentiate from candidiasis and bacterial infections	Metronidazole or carnidazole	If lesions are not too extensive, therapy is usually successful Many birds asymptomatic carriers and organism highly contagious, therefore some recommend treating all cases with single dose of carnidazole on admission Clinical cases should be barrier nursed
Coccidiosis	Various species	Wasting and diarrhoea (latter especially in young birds)	Oocysts in faecal samples	Toltrazuril, clazuril, amprolium or sulfadimethoxine	Many adults carry few organisms with no clinical problems Prevention by good hygiene and by not mixing adults and young birds
Nematodes	*Capillaria* spp. and ascarids common	Weight loss and mucoid diarrhoea (in severe cases) Migration of ascarid larvae through liver may cause sudden death	Ova in faecal samples	Fenbendazole	Advisable to deworm all birds on admission

24.6 (continued) Infectious diseases of pigeons and doves.

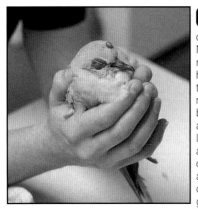

24.7 A tick on the head of a collared dove. Note the intense reaction on the head and around the right eye. Death may result unless broad-spectrum antibiosis (e.g. long-acting amoxicillin or oxytetracycline) and short-acting cortoicosteroids are given promptly.

Therapeutics

The general principles of therapeutics, as detailed in Chapter 2, apply to pigeon and dove casualties. An avian formulary is given in Appendix 1.

Management in captivity

Long-term patients may be kept in a small aviary. Feeding is simple: mixed grain rations are available in small quantities from pet stores and agricultural merchants. These will suffice in the short to medium term for all weaned birds. For long-term patients a poultry pellet may provide a more complete ration. Grit may also be provided.

Rearing of young

Young 'abandoned' birds are often presented. Many of these will be at the squeaker stage (fully developed but with a few tufts of down) and can be reared on chick crumb with a little grain.

Younger birds require a crop milk substitute. There are three options (and as crop milk is semi-solid each recipe should be made up as a paste):

- Chick crumb soaked in water
- Baby cereal (e.g. Milupa), made with boiling water and allowed to cool
- One hard-boiled egg yolk plus three tablespoons each of mixed baby cereal, oatmeal and cornmeal. Mix with milk to a stiff consistency then leave to stand until the mix becomes stiff enough to roll into pellets (Hickman and Guy, 1994).

As it is not uncommon to see rickets in hand-reared squabs, the addition of a calcium/vitamin D_3 supplement (e.g. Nutrobal, Vetark) to these feeds is recommended.

Birds should be fed until the crop is full, then fed again on demand.

Release

Adults

These birds may be released wherever the local area will support them. Often rehabilitators will have a flock of released birds around their premises, which requires understanding neighbours. It is important not to let the situation get out of hand, as control of infectious disease in a large feral flock is impossible.

Young birds

The release of hand-reared orphans may be a problem. They often refuse to leave 'home' and will return even if released far away. This is especially true of the rock dove. Stocker (2000) recommended releasing birds on sea cliffs more than 200 km from the rescue centre. It is important not to imprint young birds during rearing, as this will worsen the problem.

Rehoming racing pigeons

Racing pigeons are often found and presented to veterinary practices or rehabilitators. After the bird has been stabilized, its owner should be contacted as soon as possible. Racing birds are identified by means of a numbered leg band, which should enable the Royal Pigeon Racing Association (see 'Specialist organizations') to provide owner contact details. The information is also sometimes stamped on the primary feathers.

Legal aspects

Rock, stock and turtle doves are protected at all times. Wood pigeons and collared doves may be taken under the terms of a General Licence all year round. All species are regarded as indigenous and so may be held and re-released after treatment (see Chapter 5). Racing pigeons have owners, and both veterinary surgeons and rehabilitators should be cautious about treatment and euthanasia.

Specialist organization

Royal Pigeon Racing Association
The Reddings, Cheltenham, Gloucestershire GL51 6RN
Tel.: 01452 713529

References and further reading

Beynon PH, Forbes NA and Harcourt-Brown NH (eds) (1996) *Manual of Raptors, Pigeons and Waterfowl*. BSAVA, Cheltenham
Hickman M and Guy M (1994) *Care of the Wild, Feathered and Furred*. Robson Books, London
Stocker L (2000) *Practical Wildlife Care*. Blackwell Science, Oxford

25

Small birds

Dick Best

Introduction

Passerines and allied orders (including cuckoos, swifts, kingfishers and woodpeckers) have been grouped together as 'small birds' to form a chapter that will deal, inevitably, with the handling of casualties from a large number of diverse species. Although their natural history in the wild and their husbandry requirements whilst in captivity may differ widely, the approach to their handling and treatment in a veterinary practice or rehabilitation unit is very similar.

Small birds, especially juveniles of the common urban species, form a significant proportion of the total of wildlife casualties presented at rehabilitation units in Britain. In a survey of a limited number of British wildlife rehabilitation units recorded over a 7-year period, 'small birds' represented approximately 25% of all casualties received (BWRC, 1999).

Species found in the British Isles

Figure 25.1 describes the main characteristics of the commoner families of small birds.

Order/Family	Common name	Diet	Feeding strategy	Resident/migrant	Typical habitat
Cuculiformes					
Cuculidae	Cuckoos	Insects	Foraging	Summer migrant	Widespread
Apodiformes					
Apodidae	Swifts	Insects	Aerial feeders	Summer migrants	Widespread but mainly urban breeding
Coraciiformes					
Alcedinidae	Kingfisher	Small fish	Plunge diving	Resident	Inland waters and coastal
Piciformes					
Picidae	Woodpeckers	Insects	Arboreal, also ground feeding	Resident	Mainly woodland, farmland and gardens
Passeriformes					
Alaudidae	Larks	Insects/invertebrates	Ground feeder	Resident/partial migrant	Open grass and farmland
Hirundinidae	Swallows and martins	Insects	Aerial feeders	Summer migrants	Widespread
Motacillidae	Wagtails and pipits	Insects/invertebrates	Ground feeders	Resident and summer migrants	Open land, often close to water
Troglodytidae	Wren	Insects/invertebrates	Foraging	Resident/partial migrant	Widespread
Prunellidae	Dunnock	Insects/invertebrates Seeds	Foraging	Resident	Widespread
Turdidae	Thrushes, blackbird, robin	Insects/invertebrates Berries	Foraging	Resident, partial migrants and winter visitors	Widespread
Sylviidae	Warblers	Insects Seasonal berries	Foraging	Summer migrants	Woodland, scrub, reedbeds
Muscicapidae	Flycatchers	Flying insects	Aerial sorties from perch	Summer migrant	Woodland
Paridae	Tits	Insects, seeds	Foraging	Resident	Widespread
Corvidae	Crows	Carrion, nestlings invertebrates, seeds, fruit	Foraging	Resident	Widespread

25.1 Taxonomy of common British 'small birds', their diets and habitats. (continues) ▶

Order/Family	Common name	Diet	Feeding strategy	Resident/migrant	Typical habitat
Passeriformes continued					
Sturnidae	Starling	Insects/invertebrates Fruit	Foraging	Resident/partial migrant	Widespread
Passeridae	Sparrows	Seeds, insects	Foraging	Resident	Widespread, mostly open country
Fringillidae	Finches	Seeds, insects	Foraging	Resident, winter migrants	Widespread
Emberizidae	Buntings	Seeds, insects	Foraging	Resident, winter migrants	Widespread, mostly open country

25.1 (continued) Taxonomy of common British 'small birds', their diets and habitats.

When faced with a casualty of an unfamiliar species accurate identification would be, in the majority of cases, an advantage and may require reference to a field guide or the help of an experienced ornithologist. If identification of the actual species is not possible, at least identification of the family or genus will give some indication of the bird's natural history. Identification will allow a correct judgement to be made of the natural diet for the species, whether the species is a migrant and, possibly, the age and sex of the individual; all these facts are important in the development of a realistic strategy for the treatment of the casualty (see Chapter 2).

Identifying nestlings and fledglings

Determination of the age of a young bird will indicate whether it has gained the age of independence or needs to be hand-reared. Nestlings will be partially feathered and, when handled, will normally call and gape widely, revealing a bright yellow mouth (Figure 25.2). A recently fledged bird will be fully feathered, with down feathers on the head and back, and usually with a brightly coloured gape-flange in the commissures of the beak.

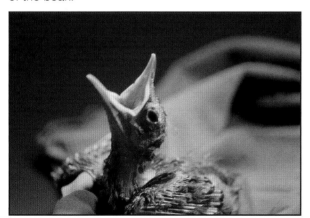

25.2 Nestling blackbird. Nestlings will solicit their parents to feed them by calling and gaping their mouths to expose a brightly coloured mucosa.

Ecology and biology

Figure 25.1 gives details of the natural diet, feeding strategies and natural habitats of the commoner families and genera dealt with in this chapter.

Reproduction

All 'small birds' have altricial and nidicolous young. Their breeding strategy is to produce, in each breeding season, large numbers of offspring of which only a few successful individuals will survive. The majority of losses in these offspring are presumed to be caused by exposure, starvation, disease and predation and many juvenile birds that are brought into captivity, as casualties, are victims of this natural morbidity.

Anatomy and physiology

Anatomy

The structure of birds in this group varies with the lifestyle of each species. For example, the beak shape varies from fine and narrow in a predominantly insectivorous species to thicker and longer in an omnivorous species or heavy and stubby in a predominantly granivorous species (Figure 25.3).

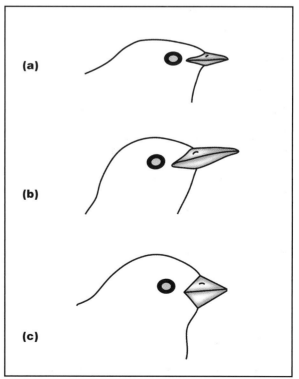

25.3 Typical passerine beak structures: (a) insectivore; (b) omnivore; (c) granivore.

All birds in the orders covered in this chapter have crops, though in some of the Passeriformes (notably the finches) the crops are located laterally, or even dorsally, at the base of the neck.

Aerial-feeding birds have relatively long, thin wings, whereas most other small birds have short rounded wings. Most perching species have a typical configuration of the digits with three forward-facing toes and a single hind toe (anisodactyl); climbing species, notably woodpeckers, have the second and third digits facing forward and the first and fourth digits facing backwards (zygodactyl).

Physiology

A significant feature of all small animals is their low bodyweight in relation to their total body surface and the associated high metabolic rate and thermoneutral range (see Chapter 2).

High energy requirements demand a regular intake of food, especially in small birds with low fat reserves; for example, blue tits (*Parus caeruleus*) may not survive more than 48–72 hours without food (Perrins, 1979). It is important to administer regularly a rich source of energy, such as glucose, to an inappetent passerine. Similarly, to conserve its energy reserves it is important, whilst a bird is in captivity, to maintain the environmental temperature within its thermoneutral range. This for most small birds of less than 50 g will be approximately 25–30°C.

Due to their low circulating blood volume, small birds may develop hypovolaemic shock following even a small haemorrhage.

Healing processes appear to function relatively quickly in these species and, in the absence of complications (such as infection), soft tissue injuries and well aligned fractures resolve rapidly. An aligned fracture to a long bone, for example, may be stable within 10 days.

Feathers

Knowledge of the process by which a damaged or plucked feather is replaced is important in assessing the length of time some casualties have to be retained in captivity. As occurs in all birds, a plucked feather will regrow within 2–3 weeks. Damaged feathers, where the shaft remains in the follicle, will not be replaced until the next natural moult.

Nestlings of small bird species will be naked when hatched and then rapidly grow a plumage of down feathers, which is replaced by the first juvenile plumage before fledging. In the majority of species the body feathers of this first juvenile plumage (but not the main flight feathers of the wing) are replaced during the autumn (juvenile moult) and this plumage will last the bird until its first adult moult (Ginn and Melville, 1983). Hence, damaged flight feathers in juvenile birds may not be replaced until the end of the next breeding season.

It is possible to pluck out a damaged feather to encourage a new one to grow or, in larger species, to replace a damaged feather with an undamaged one by 'imping', a technique commonly used in falconry (see Chapter 22).

Capture, handling and transportation

A general description of the methods of capture, handling and transportation that are suitable for small birds is given in Chapter 2. It is important to emphasize the danger of compromising a small bird's breathing when exerting excessive manual pressure on the body wall. The ideal methods of handling a small bird for examination and treatment are the ringer's hold for birds weighing < 150–200 g (see Figure 2.5a) and the pigeon fancier's hold for larger species (see Figure 2.5b).

Zoonoses

The common risks to handlers are physical injuries (mainly bites and scratches from larger species, especially Corvidae) and the dangers of acquiring zoonotic infections. Diseased wild birds may be clinically affected by potentially zoonotic infections, such as salmonellosis, or may be asymptomatic carriers of pathogens, such as *Campylobacter*, *Salmonella* and *Escherichia coli* (see Chapter 2).

Examination and assessment for rehabilitation

The basic principles of the examination and assessment for rehabilitation of a casualty are described in Chapter 2. The importance of an accurate identification of the species has already been emphasized, as this will give an indication of the following requirements of a casualty in captivity:

- Natural diet (insectivorous, granivorous, omnivorous)
- Habitat and feeding strategy (aerial feeder, arboreal, ground-dwelling)
- Social behaviour (gregarious and non-territorial, solitary and territorial)
- Movements (resident, partial migrant, summer or winter visitor)
- Age (dependent/independent juvenile, or adult).

Early assessment of the casualty's body condition by 'scoring' the pectoral muscle mass and by weighing is important. Figure 25.4 gives the weights of free-living individuals of the commoner species.

Species	Average weight (g)
Common swift (*Apus apus*)	36–50
Green woodpecker (*Picus viridis*)	180–220
House martin (*Delichon urbica*)	15–21
Wren (*Troglodytes troglodytes*)	8–13
Blackbird (*Turdus merula*)	80–110
Blackcap (*Sylvia atricapilla*)	14–20
Great tit (*Parus major*)	16–21
Jackdaw (*Corvus monedula*)	220–270
Carrion crow (*Corvus corone*)	540–600
Starling (*Sturnus vulgaris*)	75–90
House sparrow (*Passer domesticus*)	22–32
Chaffinch (*Fringilla coelebs*)	19–24

25.4 Weight range of free-living individuals of some common species of British 'small birds'.

Euthanasia

A detailed discussion of euthanasia will be found in Chapter 2.

Intravenous injection of an overdose of pentobarbital (see Appendix 1) is possible in most birds weighing over 150 g but for smaller birds the most suitable site is an intrahepatic injection (see Chapter 2). The injection is made with as fine a needle as possible (27 gauge) just under the caudal edge of the sternum, in a cranial direction at approximately 30 degrees to the plane of the sternum and, in a bird of < 50 g, to a depth of at least 1 cm. If the positioning of the injection is accurate, death will ensue rapidly.

Volatile anaesthetic agents can be used in a suitable anaesthetic chamber to euthanase a bird or to induce anaesthesia prior to performing euthanasia by another means.

First aid

A general description of first aid procedures for wildlife casualties is given in Chapter 2. The importance of maintaining a small bird casualty within its thermoneutral range has already been emphasized, as has been the need to administer a source of readily available energy.

Fluid therapy

For very small birds, the most accessible and least stressful route of administration of fluids and glucose for stabilization is orally with a suitable crop tube. Small birds weighing < 30 g can be given no more than 0.5 ml of fluid at a time by gavage, whereas those weighing 100 g may be given up to 2.0 ml.

Casualties weighing > 100 g can be given fluid as an intravenous bolus (approximately 1% of the bird's bodyweight) or, if collapsed, by the intraosseous route. Subcutaneous injections of fluid can be given into the loose skin of the inner thigh of birds of all sizes and repeated as necessary.

First aid therapeutics

Many small bird casualties are the victims of predation and suffer from wounds that are heavily infected. Such casualties are likely to be suffering from hypovolaemic shock and, although intravenous injections might be impractical, treatment with analgesics would be indicated. Early wound treatment and systemic administration of a suitable antibiotic may prevent a fatal septicaemia (see later).

Fracture immobilization

Fractures urgently require immobilization, especially long bone fractures in the wing, to prevent further soft tissue damage. Small birds tolerate their wings being immobilized by taping the flight feathers with adhesive masking or 'autoclave' tape (the adhesive of which does not damage or remain on the plumage).

- Fractures distal to the elbow can be immobilized by taping the primary to the tertiary feathers
- Fractures of the humerus need to be immobilized by holding the wing rigidly against the body with

adhesive tape or conforming/cohesive tape (e.g. Vetwrap, 3M; Co-form and Co-flex, Millpledge) that encircles the body (see Chapter 2)
- Leg fractures that are distal to the stifle can be immobilized successfully using a variety of splints and bandages (see 'Orthopaedic problems' and Chapter 22).

Short-term hospitalization

The requirements for short-term housing of small birds are similar to those needed for long-term housing (see 'Management in captivity').

Anaesthesia and analgesia

A general description of avian anaesthesia and analgesia is given in Chapter 2 and in the avian formulary in Appendix 1. The anaesthetic agent of choice for small birds is inhalation with isoflurane. Masks of a suitable size for small birds can be made from the plastic cases of disposable syringes.

Anaesthesia may be maintained, especially in very small birds (< 50 g), by using the mask but entubation of the trachea is possible with tubes made from soft plastic catheters.

In cases of injury to the head or obstruction of the airways, anaesthesia can be induced and maintained by cannulation of an air sac (see Chapter 2).

Injectable anaesthetics can be used in small birds but are less satisfactory than inhalation methods. Details are given in Chapter 2 and in Appendix 1.

It is especially important to ensure that small birds are kept warm during anaesthesia and recovery. The use of a heat pad during anaesthesia and heated cages for recovery are important, to ensure that the environment of the patient remains within its thermoneutral range (25–30°C for small birds weighing less than 50 g).

Specific conditions

Trauma

Orthopaedic problems

The majority of orthopaedic problems in small birds are likely to be fractures resulting from attacks by predators or in-flight collisions. The basic principles of avian orthopaedics are given in Chapter 2.

Fractures of the carpometacarpus and fractures of either one of the ulna or radius may heal well, if the wing is supported with the flight feathers being taped together in a closed position (see 'First aid' and Chapter 2). Fractures of the humerus and simultaneous fractures of both the radius and ulna usually have a poor prognosis as they are often severely comminuted, open and associated with soft tissue damage. If healing does occur, the resulting callus and scar tissue are likely to compromise the bird's flying ability.

Due to their low bodyweight, small birds are able to support themselves on one leg while a leg fracture is healing. Closed fractures of the femur in small birds will heal with cage rest, especially if the fragments are in reasonable alignment; even poorly aligned fractures may heal but are likely to result in shortening of the limb and development of a large callus. Leg fractures distal to the stifle can be immobilized successfully using a variety of splints and bandages, possibly the most successful design being an Altman splint, which is fashioned from masking tape and, being very light, is well tolerated by most small birds (Figure 25.5).

The opinion is often given that many passerines can survive in the wild with one functioning leg. Although lame individuals are frequently seen in the wild, this may not necessarily mean that that they will survive in the long term or be able to perform all their natural behaviour patterns. Similarly with wing fractures, a bird must not only be able to fly short distances but also be capable of evading predators, migrating and, even for a sedentary species, making long-distance flights in the face of adverse weather. The nature of the healed fracture and the suitability for release should be assessed critically with each individual case.

Cat predation
Displaced and grounded fledglings are highly vulnerable to predation by domestic cats, especially in urban gardens, and such casualties are common with juvenile small birds. A recent survey of a small number of rehabilitation units showed that, during the period April to June, approximately 15% of all bird casualties were recorded as being caused by cat predation (BWRC, unpublished data).

The injuries caused in these attacks vary from a loss of feathers and superficial soft tissue injuries to severe bite wounds that might penetrate deeply into muscle tissue, open the coelomic cavity or cause fractures of ribs, vertebral column and limb bones. Simple superficial skin injuries may resolve quickly, within days, with routine wound management, but feather loss or damage will take much longer to heal. Feathers that have been plucked may regrow within

2–3 weeks but damaged feathers will not regrow until the next moult (see 'Anatomy and physiology').

Minor soft tissue injuries and simple, closed fractures of limb bones may heal well with routine wound management, systemic antibiotic treatment and immobilization of a fracture (see 'Orthopaedic conditions'). However, severe lacerations caused by teeth and claws will inevitably be infected and can cause serious soft tissue and orthopaedic damage. Euthanasia might be considered on humanitarian grounds in very severe cases, especially where the coelomic cavity has been punctured or there is a major orthopaedic problem. If treatment is considered appropriate, supportive therapy should be given together with the simultaneous administration of a systemic antibiotic and analgesic.

The wounds of 'catted' juvenile birds are frequently infected with *Pasteurella multicida*, a common, if not normal, constituent of the oral bacterial flora of the cat, and other bacteria (including *Pseudomonas* spp.) are also involved. Some of these organisms may be resistant to many of the commoner antibiotics used in birds and piperacillin has been found to be very helpful (I. Robinson, personal communication).

Infectious diseases

Viral diseases
Investigations have been made into the possible role of wild birds in the epidemiology of many viral diseases of livestock, both mammalian and avian, such as avian influenza (Capua *et al.*, 2000). In general it appears that, although wild birds can be infected with such pathogens, it is unlikely that they are significant carriers. Wild birds do, however, play a significant role in the epidemiology of arboviruses.

Viral papilloma of finches: Papillomas are occasionally seen on the feet of finches, especially chaffinches (*Fringilla coelebs*) (Blackmore and Keymer, 1969). They vary from small, apparently insignificant nodules

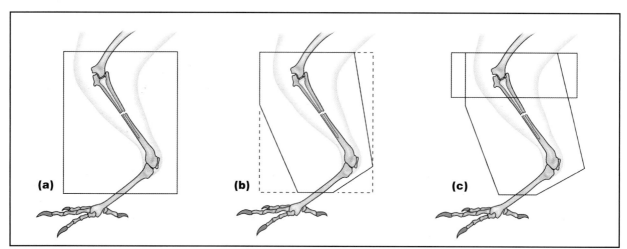

25.5 Altman splint. (a) Two pieces of masking tape are applied either side of the leg and pressed firmly together to form the splint. For effective immobilization, the resulting splint must include as much as possible of the limb above and below the fracture site. (b) Excess tape is cut away from the splint to reduce size and weight. The splint is very well tolerated by most patients. (c) Pieces of tape can be added to the splint around the stifle joint to give added stability. Simple fractures will have formed a callus and immobilized themselves within 2–3 weeks, after which the splint can be removed to allow the bird to regain limb function.

to large growths that distort the feet and cause lameness. Clusters of cases have been recorded. There is no specific treatment and severely affected birds should be euthanased.

Bacterial diseases

Heavy mortalities have been reported amongst flocks of greenfinches and house sparrows feeding at bird tables (Kirkwood *et al.*, 1995; Routh and Sleeman, 1995; Kirkwood, 1998; Pennycott *et al.*, 2002) from which *Salmonella* species, including *S. typhimurium*, were isolated. Birds have been reported as showing loss of body condition, splenomegaly, yellow nodules in the liver, spleen and crop wall, and diffuse crop lesions. These outbreaks are associated with the large numbers of birds congregating in a small area and leading to a heavy contamination of the feeding area. Kirkwood and MacGregor (1997) and Kirkwood (1998) made the following recommendations for the hygiene of garden feeding sites to reduce the risks of infectious disease:

- Place food in small amounts at several sites
- Preferably use suspended feeders, with no sills or flat surfaces
- Bird tables should be cleaned regularly, all surfaces disinfected and any spilled food removed from the ground beneath
- Gloves should be worn when cleaning or handling feeders or bird tables.

Parasites

Ectoparasitic infestations

Many species of ectoparasite have been recorded as infesting 'small birds'. The clinical significance of most infestations, especially in birds that are underweight, is unclear. Biting ectoparasites do play an essential role in the transmission of many potential pathogens and this may be of great significance in migrating birds, which have the ability to carry disease over large distances.

Ticks: Engorged adult female *Ixodes* spp. are frequently found attached to the heads of small birds, especially to the periorbital skin, and their presence may be associated with a severe and often fatal local or systemic reaction. Treatment may be indicated in some cases and ectoparasiticide, anti-inflammatory and antibiotic administration might be helpful, together with the removal of the tick and supportive treatment.

Hippoboscids (flat flies): Mention should also be made of the dipteran louse-fly of the family Hippoboscidae, which is commonly found on small birds, especially hirundines and swifts. It appears to be of little clinical importance, though larger numbers are occasionally found on emaciated birds. As it is a blood-feeding parasite, it is potentially significant in the epidemiology of blood-borne diseases.

Endoparasitic infestations

The majority of endoparasites that have been described in small birds are of doubtful clinical significance. For a discussion on the routine treatment for parasitic infestations in wildlife casualties, see Chapter 2.

Gapeworm: Of the nematode parasites, mention must be made of the gapeworm *Syngamus trachea*, a very common parasite of starlings and members of the Corvidae. It is often associated with respiratory sounds and respiratory distress, especially in young birds that have been presented for other problems, such as trauma. Diagnosis may be made by direct examination of the trachea assisted by pen-torch trans-illumination through the skin and may be confirmed with demonstration of the typical ova (Figure 25.6) either in wet preparations of sputum or in routine faecal examination. Treatment with benzimidazoles or ivermectin in uncomplicated cases is usually successful. The ova are commonly carried in invertebrates, such as earthworms, as transmission hosts, and feeding large numbers of these to hand-reared young birds may present a problem.

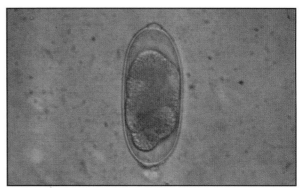

25.6 *Syngamus trachea* egg. This is a common nematode parasite of gamebirds, starlings and members of the crow family. It frequently causes clinical signs of partial tracheal obstruction. The ova are readily demonstrated by direct microscopic examination of pharyngeal mucus and faeces (wet preparations or by flotation techniques).

Other conditions

Grounded swifts

Swifts are a truly aerial species: they feed, roost and even copulate in the air. Once on level ground, even a fit bird will have difficulty in becoming airborne.

During the breeding season fledglings frequently become grounded and, being unable to take off, rapidly become exhausted. In the hand, juvenile birds can be distinguished from adults by white or pale fringes to the wing coverts. Fledglings usually weigh between 34 and 52 g when they first fly at an average age of 42 days. Some may fledge early, especially in periods of poor weather when they might not be fed by the adults, and these may represent a proportion of the 'grounded' young birds (Cramp, 1988). If such birds are in good body condition and weigh within the normal range, they can, if conditions are suitable, be released immediately in an open space (where they can be easily retrieved if not able to fly). If conditions are unsuitable or a bird is in poor condition, it can be retained in captivity for a short time to rest in a dark secluded box and given oral glucose solution before being flight-tested.

Where the casualty is an underweight adult, or is a juvenile and unable to fly, treatment can be considered. However, swifts are highly specialized aerial feeders and although they can be fed for short periods with oral feeding fluids (e.g. Hill's a/d, Hill's Nutrition; Reanimyl, Virbac) or wax moth larvae, long-term captivity rarely results in the release of the casualty. Euthanasia could be considered as an alternative to hospitalization for the majority of cases.

Starvation associated with adverse weather

Birds are able to avoid the worst effects of prolonged adverse weather by migrating. Even species regarded as being non-migratory will move large distances when faced with such problems. Occasionally, in prolonged periods of freezing weather (which usually also involve Continental Europe), large numbers of passerine casualties can be found suffering from starvation due to their inability to find accessible food resources (Figure 25.7).

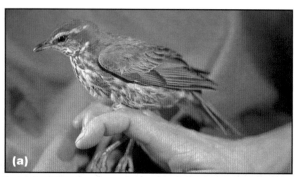
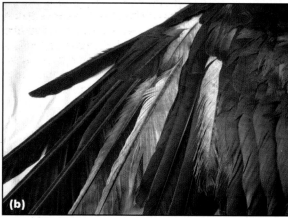
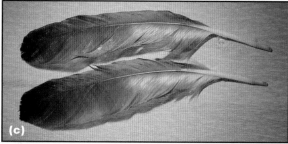

25.7 (a) Redwing. In severe winters large numbers of redwings and fieldfares are forced further west across continental Europe to Britain where, if conditions are no better, they suffer from starvation and may be admitted to rehabilitation units. (b) Juvenile carrion crows are frequently found in an emaciated state and showing lack of pigmentation to the plumage, especially the flight and tail feathers and (c) fretmarks – transverse lines of feather malformation and weakness, assumed to be associated with periods of malnutrition or disease during the development of the feather. ((b) Courtesy of G Cousquer)

Therapeutics

The calculation of an effective dose using allometric scaling and methods of administering medication are discussed in Chapter 2.

For very small birds weighing < 50 g, an intramuscular injection is a painful and stressful procedure and should be avoided whenever possible. Oral dosage by gavage, using medications suitable for that route, may be preferable. Indirect methods of medication, using food or water, are unreliable unless the medicated food can be given in measured amounts.

Management in captivity

Long-term

The basic principles of managing a wildlife casualty in captivity are described in Chapter 2 and the design of accommodation for small bird casualties follows the points outlined in that chapter:

* Security to prevent escape
* Seclusion from disturbance. A standard rectangular breeding cage with a grille front (to which a heat lamp can be fixed), with solid sides, back and roof, and placed as high as possible within the room, will give a small bird a sense of security
* For perching species, a variety of suitably sized perches of natural (and disposable) twigs and branches, or artificial wood or plastic perches that can be thoroughly disinfected
* Floor covered with a substrate that is easily replaced
* The ability to darken the room to assist ease of capture for treatment
* Cage doors small, and well placed to ease capture and prevent escape
* Food and water containers placed so that the casualty can reach them despite its disability.

Feeding

The diet fed to casualties will vary with the species and can be designed along the guidelines given in Figure 25.8. Some birds require specially designed accommodation to encourage their natural feeding behaviour, as follows.

Swifts

Swifts are obligatory aerial insect feeders. They are unlikely to feed on their own and need to be fed by hand with mealworms, wax moth larvae or other insects. Their natural food is small flying insects and an adult returning to feed a nestling is likely to have as many as 1000 insects in a food ball. When roosting, swifts cling to a vertical surface; in captivity, a towel attached to the side of a solid-walled cage provides a suitable perch.

Woodpeckers

Woodpeckers are mainly arboreal, finding most of their food on the trunks and larger branches of trees. In

Dietary groups	Families	Hand-rearing diets	Natural supplements
Insectivores	Cuckoo Swift Woodpeckers Larks Hirundines Wagtails/pipits Wren Flycatchers	Commercial softbill rearing diet Commercial insectivore diet Mealworms, wax worms, maggots, small crickets	Wild insects (adults and larvae), spiders etc Insects caught by sweeping net over long grass
Insectivores/granivores	Dunnock Tits Sparrows Finches Buntings	Commercial softbill rearing diet Commercial insectivore diet Live food as above Small seed mixture	As above Wild seeds (groundsel, seeding grasses)
Fish-eater	Kingfisher	Small fish, available frozen as food for carnivorous fish	
Omnivores	Thrushes Crows Starling	Commercial softbill rearing diet Commercial dogfood/catfood	Wild insects and invertebrates (earthworms)

25.8 Artificial diets and natural supplements for hand-rearing and hospitalization of small birds.

captivity they will use a tree trunk or branch fixed in an upright position. They feed primarily on invertebrates (mainly insects) and suitable insectivore food can be placed in cracks in the trunk.

Rearing of orphans

Juvenile small birds probably form the majority of wildlife casualties presented to rehabilitation units and urban veterinary practices. The point has already been made that, with most species of small birds, their normal breeding strategy is to produce large numbers of offspring each season to offset the high natural mortality, and that many casualties may represent these natural losses.

Juveniles might be presented as nestlings (i.e. young birds not fully feathered and still dependent on their parents) or as fledglings (i.e. fully feathered young that have left the nest, yet are still dependent on their parents for care and protection). Although fledged birds are presented as abandoned or orphaned individuals, in reality it is more likely that they have been displaced and separated from their parents. Many altricial (nest-reared) birds on the point of fledging leave the nest before they can fly and remain for several days in the safety of the tree canopy or surrounding vegetation, where they can be displaced by strong winds or predators. Once on the ground they are flightless and vulnerable; it is in this state that many are found in urban gardens and brought into captivity, often the victims of cat predation.

If a juvenile passerine is uninjured, it might be preferable to return the bird to the location where it was found and place it in the cover of vegetation, possibly within a small, partially closed box to which the adults can gain access. The alternative is to foster it or to keep it in captivity to be reared by hand. Juvenile birds of many species can be fostered into nests holding young of the same age and species and this will often require the cooperation and expertise of local naturalists. Although it might be a concern, it does not appear to be generally true that handling juvenile birds will cause adults to abandon or to reject them.

If returning a young bird to its natal territory is impossible (because the precise site is unknown), or impracticable (the nest site has been destroyed) or no suitable sites for fostering are available, consideration can be given to rearing by hand. Success depends on a sound knowledge of the biology of the species plus endless patience and a realistic approach to the problems involved. These problems include:

- The fact that hand-rearing is very time-consuming
- Finding a substitute for the natural diet
- Encouraging the bird to become independent and to hunt or forage for food successfully
- Preventing the bird from becoming socially imprinted on humans
- Preventing a dependence on an unnatural food.

Throughout the hand-rearing process it is important to ensure that attention is paid to hygiene, by preventing:

- Build-up of food and faecal material on the birds and in their housing
- Cross-contamination between patients
- Zoonotic infections being acquired by handlers.

To prevent social imprinting on human handlers, it is important to minimize the contact with humans and, whenever possible, to rear conspecifics together in groups.

As with all small bird casualties, identification of the species and the approximate age is important (Figure 25.9) so that the correct diet and husbandry can be established. All newly captured juveniles benefit from supportive treatment in the form of heat, fluids and energy. Nestlings require additional heat (brooding)

Approximate age	Distinguishing features	Frequency of feeding
1–4 days	Egg tooth on dorsal tip of upper mandible Naked Eye lids fused for first few days	Every 15 min for at least 12 hours per day
4–7 days	Naked, but early development of 'pin' feathers on wings and tail	Every 30–60 min for at least 12 hours per day Encourage self-feeding
7–14 days	Body feathering complete	
14–21 days	Wing and tail feathering fully grown Fully fledged	Every 2–3 hours for at least 12 hours per day Encourage self-feeding
28–42 days	Able to fly	Should be self-feeding

25.9 Ageing of juvenile small birds and frequency of hand-feeding.

until fully feathered. The optimal environmental temperature for a nestling will vary from approximately 35°C immediately after hatching to 25°C at fledging. Newly admitted patients may be suffering from hypothermia, which may reduce gut motility. Initially, such birds must be given heat to correct the body core temperature, together with fluids and an energy source (see 'First aid') before solid foods are attempted (Ackermann, 2000).

Nestlings need to be kept in a container, such as a plastic box, that will mimic the nest cup. It should be easy to clean and the 'cup' should have a non-slip disposable or washable base to enable the birds to grip. Whilst being fed, most nestlings will instinctively move to the edge of the container to defecate. If the rearing diet is being tolerated by the nestling, it will pass its droppings (faeces and urine) in a mucus-coated faecal sac which, in the wild, would be removed intact by the adults.

Feeding

The growth rate of nestling small birds is phenomenal: a blackbird can grow to a fledgling weighing over 90 g in 14 days. Most small bird nestlings will consume an equivalent of 10–20% of their bodyweight in food each day. Daily monitoring of the bodyweight (taken at the same time each day) gives an indication of the adequacy of the diet and the health of the bird.

Nestlings will normally gape in response to movement over their heads or gentle tapping of the beak or skin around the mouth. If newly acquired nestlings do not gape, they may be stimulated to do so by covering the brooding box with a thick cloth for a while, the removal of which will simulate an adult leaving the nest (Humphries, 1988). The food can be given in a semi-solid consistency, in small amounts on the end of a suitably sized blunt rod or forceps, possibly being dipped into water before being fed (Figure 25.10).

The bird should be fed until its crop is full; however, there is a risk of overfeeding, as some nestlings will still solicit food when their crop is already full. The crop should be allowed to become empty, or nearly empty, before the next feeding. The frequency of feeding will vary with the age of the bird (see Figure 25.9). In the wild, nestlings are fed only during the hours of daylight and are brooded during the night. Larger species, such as the corvids, are fed less frequently and fledge later – for example, 33 days for a carrion crow compared with 14 days for a blackbird.

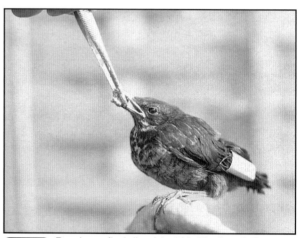

25.10 Rearing a fledgling blackbird by hand. Cats commonly injure fledglings and this bird had an open fracture to a radius, which healed with the help of masking tape support to the wing and antibiotic treatment.

After the age of natural fledging, when wild fledglings would start to forage under the protection of their parents, hand-reared birds should be encouraged to feed on suitable food materials. By the age of independence (averaging 3–4 weeks for most small species) they should be feeding and flying well enough to be released to the wild using a 'soft release' method (see 'Management in captivity and release' and Chapter 3).

The choice of a suitable hand-rearing diet will vary with the species (see Figure 25.9). It must be as varied as practicable to ensure a balanced diet that provides adequate amounts of water, carbohydrate, fat and high quality protein together with vitamins, minerals and trace elements. Many experienced hand-rearers will use a standard rearing food, based on a softbill rearing diet, for the first 7–14 days and then encourage the nestling to start to feed independently, using food items closely matching its natural diet. Diets should include a commercial avian multivitamin and mineral supplement and, for granivorous fledglings, a source of insoluble grit as supplied for use with captive finches.

Release

The general principles of release are dealt with in Chapter 3.

Adults

Short-term casualties can usually be released without any special preparations and, whenever feasible, as close as possible to the site where they were found.

Long-term casualties require preparation for a 'soft release' method. As soon as the casualty is considered fit for release, it should be placed in an aviary situated in a suitable habitat. The casualty is given time to acclimatize itself to the aviary and its new environment. Then, when the conditions are considered suitable, a release-flap is opened and left open so that the bird is able to return to the aviary for supplementary feeding and to roost.

Special problems occur with long-term casualties of migratory species that are hospitalized beyond their normal period of residence. Such casualties must be retained in captivity until the next season, transported to their correct geographical area or, if neither of these alternatives is considered appropriate, euthanased.

Young birds

The release of hand-reared small birds requires the selection of a suitable habitat, known to have a viable wild population of conspecific birds and, therefore, with adequate food resources and free from excessive pressures from predators or human activities. A 'soft release' technique would be preferred, with the bird (or possibly a small group of hand-reared individuals of the same species) being housed in an aviary placed in a suitable site (see 'Management in captivity and release' and Chapter 3).

Legal considerations

Details of the legislation relating to wildlife casualties is given in Chapter 5. Some of the rarer species of small birds breeding in Britain are included in Schedule 4 of the Wildlife and Countryside Act 1981 and need to be registered with DEFRA when kept in captivity. These include kingfisher, redwing and fieldfare.

References and further reading

Ackermann J (2000) Care of orphan birds. *Kirk's Current Veterinary Therapy XIII Small Animal Practice*. WB Saunders, Philadelphia
Blackmore DK and Keymer IF (1969) Cutaneous disease in wild birds in Britain. *British Birds* **62**, 316–331
BWRC (1999) Report on the Wildlife Casualties Recording Scheme 1993–1997. *Rehabilitator* **28**. British Wildlife Rehabilitation Council, c/o RSPCA Wildlife Department, Horsham
Capua I *et al.* (2000) Monitoring for highly pathogenic avian influenza in wild birds in Italy. *Veterinary Record* **147**, 640
Cramp S (1988) *The Birds of the Webstern Palaearctic. Vol.IV.* Oxford University Press, Oxford
Ginn HB and Melville DS (1983) *Moult in Birds*. BTO Guide 19. British Trust for Ornithology, Tring
Humphries PN (1988) Rearing orphan birds. *Companion Animal Practice* **2**(4), 45–49, and (5) 36–38
Jordan WJ and Hughes J (1982) *Care of the Wild*. Macdonald, London
King AS and McLelland J (1984) *Birds – Their Structure and Function*. Baillière Tindall, London
Kirkwood JK (1998) Population density and infectious disease at bird tables. *Veterinary Record* **142**, 468
Kirkwood JK and MacGregor SK (1997) *Infectious Diseases in Garden Birds: Minimising the Risks*. Universities Federation for Animal Welfare, Wheathamstead
Kirkwood JK *et al.* (1995) Garden bird mortalities. *Veterinary Record* **136**, 372
Pennycott TW, Cinderly A, Park A, Mather HA and Foster G (2002) *Salmonella enterica* subspecies *enterica* serotype Typhimurium and *Escherichia coli* O86 in wild birds at two gardens in south-west Scotland. *Veterinary Record* **151**, 563–567
Perrins C (1979) *British Tits*. Collins, London
Perrins C (1987) *Collins New Generation Guide to the Birds of Britain and Europe*. Collins, London
Routh A and Sleeman JM (1995) Greenfinch mortalities. *Veterinary Record* **136**, 500
Stocker L (2000) *Practical Wildlife Care*. Blackwell Science, Oxford
Wildlife Information Network (2002) *UK Wildlife First Aid and Care* (CD-Rom). Royal Veterinary College, London

Acknowledgement

Acknowledgements are due to John Chitty for his helpful comments on this chapter.

26

Reptiles, amphibians and fish

John E. Cooper

Introduction

Only a small number of species of reptiles and amphibians are now found in the UK.

Reptiles

The three species of snake found in the UK are the grass snake (*Natrix natrix*), adder or viper (*Vipera berus*) and smooth snake (*Coronella austriaca*). The lizard species are the common or viviparous lizard (*Lacerta vivipara*), sand lizard (*Lacerta agilis*) and slow worm (*Anguis fragilis*).

The largest of the snakes is the grass snake (Figure 26.1a), which can reach a length of a metre or more and which can usually be recognized by the yellow ring around its neck, though this varies considerably in colour and conspicuousness. The adder, Britain's only poisonous snake, is usually characterized by a dark diamond zig-zag down its back. The smooth snake is rare and most unlikely to be presented as a casualty, except in the area around Bournemouth and Southampton (the New Forest).

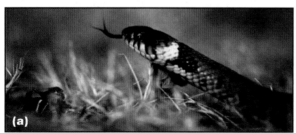

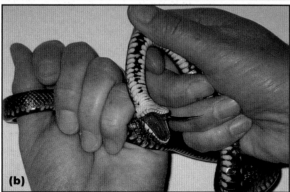

26.1 (a) The grass snake (*Natrix natrix*) is easily identified by the yellow band around the neck. (Courtesy of C Seddon.) (b) Grass snakes may sham death and appear as injured or dying to the inexperienced. (Courtesy of ME Cooper.)

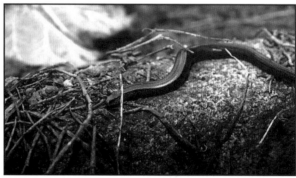

26.2 Slow worm (*Anguis fragilis*), a legless lizard. (Courtesy of C Seddon.)

The slow worm, although a lizard, is legless (Figure 26.2) and is occasionally mistaken for a snake; it is small (35 cm or less in length) and shiny and it has eyelids so that, unlike snakes, it can blink.

If in doubt over identification, the advice of an experienced herpetologist or local naturalist should be sought. There are also many useful field guides and keys (e.g. Arnold and Burton, 1978).

Amphibians

The indigenous frog species in the UK is the common frog (*Rana temporaria*; Figure 26.3). The edible frog (*R. esculenta*) and the marsh or laughing frog (*R. ridibunda*) are thought to be introduced species.

Toads and newts found in the UK are the common toad (*Bufo bufo*; Figure 26.4a), the rare and localized natterjack toad (*B. calamita*; Figure 26.4b), the common or smooth newt (*Triturus vulgaris*), palmate newt (*T. helvetica*) and great-crested newt (*T. cristata*).

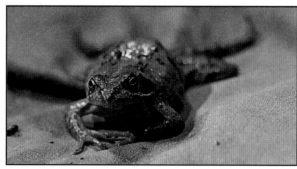

26.3 Common frog (*Rana temporaria*). Frogs are distinguished from toads by their smooth skin. This casualty had been attacked by a domesticated cat, a common cause of injury.

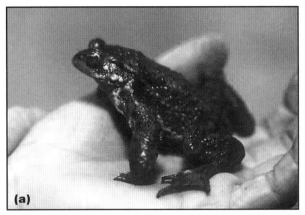

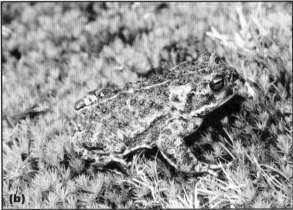

26.4 Some British toads. (a) Common toad (*Bufo bufo*). Courtesy of C. Seddon.) (b) Natterjack toad (*Bufo calamita*). (Courtesy of P Dawson.)

Fish

There are dozens of species of fish in Britain, some of them indigenous and others introduced, and hybrids abound. A useful key for north European species is Wheeler (1978). Those to be covered in this chapter are the teleosts (bony fish), and the groups of particular importance to rehabilitators are generally members of the Carassidae (carp family), Anguillidae (eels) and Gasterophilidae (sticklebacks). Occasionally a rehabilitation centre may receive a sick or injured marine specimen that may be a cartilaginous (rather than bony) fish, such as a small shark.

Ecology and biology

Reptiles, amphibians and fish, although often lumped together as 'cold-blooded' or 'ectothermic' animals, are very different taxonomically and biologically. All three groups are vertebrates and therefore show some similarities in anatomy and physiology, but their lifestyles are very diverse and this is reflected in their biology and ecology. For clarity, the biology of the three groups will be discussed in reverse order, starting with fish.

Fish

Most species of fish are entirely aquatic and all British species depend upon gills for respiration. Their health and welfare are, therefore, very much influenced by the quality of the water in which they live. The majority of British species lay eggs and none has a larval stage; a few produce live young. The skin of fish is made up of the normal layers of epidermis and dermis, but scales are a characteristic feature; fish scales (in contrast to those of reptiles) are mesodermal in origin.

Amphibians

Amphibians are essentially terrestrial animals that must return to the water to breed. As a result, their life cycle consists of eggs that hatch into larvae (tadpoles), which ultimately metamorphose into young adults.

Dependence on water or a damp environment is a feature of all British amphibians. The common toad, which has a relatively thick epidermis, is less susceptible to desiccation than are the three species of newt, which have a thin epidermis. Small species are more vulnerable than are large. The skin of all amphibians is mucous and very sensitive to physical or chemical damage. The immature amphibian depends very much upon the quality of the water in which it lives in order to remain in good health. The reliance of the tadpole on water quality tends to become less as it matures and starts to breathe with lungs rather than external or internal gills.

Reptiles

British reptiles are entirely terrestrial animals, though all species can swim if necessary and the grass snake is frequently found in or near water because of its penchant for amphibians and fish.

The skin of reptiles is heavily keratinized and serves as a defence against trauma and desiccation.

Reptiles have no larval stage. Some, such as the grass snake, lay eggs, while others, such as the adder and viviparous lizard, produce live young.

Environment

The ectothermic nature of reptiles, amphibians and fish means that they are almost entirely dependent on behavioural strategies in order to maintain their body temperatures within a preferred optimum temperature zone (POTZ). The POTZ of most British reptiles lies within the range of 22–30°C (Cooper and Jackson, 1981). The range is lower for amphibians (15–30°C) and fish (10–20°C).

All three groups thermoregulate by moving to a warmer or colder location as necessary. This trait is best illustrated by reptiles; thus, a lizard will sun itself in order to raise its body temperature and then retreat to a shady spot or hole in the ground when there is a danger of its temperature exceeding the top of the POTZ. The indigenous British reptiles all tend to inhabit relatively warm localities where they are able to thermoregulate and reproduce. Amphibians do not usually bask – indeed, the structure of their skin would make this a hazardous practice – but they too move from place to place, seeking the temperature and other environmental cues that they require. Fish also move from one area of water to another; they will favour shade or sunlit areas according to their requirements.

Feeding

All British reptiles are carnivorous but their diet ranges from small rodents (adder) through lizards (smooth snake) to insects and molluscs (lizards).

Adult amphibians are also carnivorous, primarily taking invertebrates, but the immature stages of amphibians (tadpoles) are herbivorous for the first part of their life when they are aquatic and bear gills.

Some species of fish are obligate carnivores; others may be omnivores or plant-eaters.

Physiology

Ectothermy

Both the veterinary surgeon and the rehabilitator must be aware of the importance of the POTZ and make adequate provision for it. Most body functions are carried out optimally if the animal is within its POTZ; thus, for instance, digestive and liver enzymes are most likely to function efficiently and antibody production is maximized. Where the POTZ is not known, the provision in captivity of a temperature gradient (see later) is wise (Beynon *et al.*, 1992).

The absorption, metabolism and excretion of therapeutic agents is temperature-dependent and the frequency of dosing (medicating) reptiles, amphibians and fish is influenced by this.

Capture, handling and transportation

The handling, transportation and care of reptiles, amphibians and fish must always take the following into account:

- The inability of all these animals to control their body temperature by internal means
- The particular vulnerability of amphibians and fish to desiccation and skin damage
- The sensitivity of fish and larval amphibians to hypoxia and other deleterious effects if water quality is poor.

Of the three groups, the reptiles are the least vulnerable to damage because they bear a thick protective layer of epidermis; however, this is more readily traumatized when the animal is sloughing (shedding) its skin. Amphibians have a sensitive integument that can very easily be damaged by rough handling or other factors and so also do fish, which may at the very least lose mucus and the protection that this offers or, worse, have scales damaged, permitting infection to enter and osmotic disturbances to arise.

- All handling, particularly forcible restraint, should be kept to a minimum
- Amphibians and fish should be kept moist and, preferably, handled only with a soft net or, in an emergency, a damp towel or teacloth (Porter, 1989).

Human safety

The only species of venomous reptile in Britain, the adder, is not highly venomous but its bite can very occasionally cause death in a young, old or debilitated individual. Handling equipment such as snake sticks and tongs may be needed, but sick or injured adders can often be scooped or swept into a bucket or other suitable container. Those who handle adders regularly should have access to appropriate antivenom, either by carrying it themselves or by ensuring that it is kept at a local hospital or medical practice. It should only be administered in an emergency.

British toads can present a hazard on account of bufotoxin, which is a product of the parotid glands and can prove irritating and damaging to broken skin, conjunctiva or mucous membranes. A damaged or stressed toad will often produce copious quantities of such parotid material and therefore the wearing of gloves, appropriately moistened, when dealing with such animals is strongly advised.

None of the British fish is significantly toxic to humans but some species, such as sticklebacks, bear sharp spines, and certain fish (e.g. eels) will readily bite.

Zoonoses are covered below.

Handling

In an emergency, most of the British reptiles and amphibians can be held in the hand and thus transported, at least for a short distance. There are some important considerations:

- The adder is a venomous species, which makes this method unsuitable (but see below)
- Amphibians do not tolerate comfortably warm, dry surfaces; therefore, prolonged handling can be deleterious
- Some amphibians, notably toads, can produce both skin and (more importantly) parotid secretions
- All three species of British lizard can lose their tails (autotomy); a new tail will grow but every attempt should be made to avoid such tail loss.

There are also legal considerations when handling wild protected species (see below). As a general rule, a casualty reptile, amphibian or fish is likely to be either so severely injured or sick that it is easily captured, or virtually impossible to locate and to catch. Most injuries will either kill such a small animal or have only relatively minor effects.

Transportation

Transportation presents relatively few difficulties but the legal considerations (see Chapter 5) must be borne in mind.

Reptiles

Reptiles are best carried in a cloth or canvas bag, which can be protected from insults by being placed within a solid box container for long journeys. The bag should be cleaned after each use. If an adder is being transported, particular care needs to be taken since it is possible for the animal to bite through the cloth.

Amphibians

Amphibians can be transported in a similar way to reptiles but it is preferable to place damp vegetation, such as moss, within the bag or to dowse the bag in water at intervals. Tadpoles need to be transported in water but great care has to be taken not to overcrowd or to damage them. Tadpoles at the final stage of their metamorphosis are particularly susceptible to rough handling or desiccation and can easily drown.

Fish

Fish and the tadpoles of amphibians are often best carried, initially at any rate, in the water from which they came, care being taken to ensure that it is also of the same temperature (see later).

Attention may need to be paid to the provision of adequate oxygen, especially for those species (e.g. salmonids) that have a high requirement. An oxygen source (such as a cylinder with a reducing valve) can be used if available, or crude oxygenation can be achieved by pouring in water from a height to produce a 'flowing' effect. Alternatively, the fish can be anaesthetized with a low dose of either benzocaine or tricaine methane sulphonate, both of which will reduce its oxygen demand. The oxygen-carrying capacity of water is increased if its temperature is lowered (in an emergency this can be achieved by adding ice cubes) but a sudden drop in temperature can, in itself, be a stressor.

Zoonoses

Zoonoses of reptile and amphibian origin are well recognized. Some that may be acquired from reptiles have been publicized in the context of keeping these animals as pets.

Casualty reptiles, amphibians and fish can harbour and spread a whole range of bacteria, particularly Gram-negative organisms. Some of these are opportunists (e.g. *Pseudomonas* spp.) that may take advantage of an immunocompromised host or may enter an existing wound.

The key to prevention of spread of zoonoses is good hygiene. It is wise in any rehabilitation centre or veterinary practice that deals with casualties to have and to use in-house codes of practice and protocols that will minimize the risk of spread of zoonoses and provide some protection if there is such an occurrence (see Chapter 5).

Examination and assessment for rehabilitation

Assessment of ectothermic vertebrates for rehabilitation has not been addressed in detail but Latas (2000), working in the USA, provided an excellent 'general plan' for evaluating such species, including triage protocols for given situations.

Reptiles, amphibians and fish need to be handled for a detailed examination. Since many species are small, use of a hand lens or magnifying loupe is recommended, particularly to search for small skin lesions.

Light anaesthesia may prove a great asset – especially for the adder, which is venomous, and with lizards, which may shed their tail (see above) during the handling process.

A substantial proportion of those that are submitted as casualties are in a poor state of health and die soon after. This is largely related to their small size and to their susceptibility to dehydration and other factors following injuries, burns and the like.

Euthanasia

Euthanasia is an important option and should be considered at an early stage. Methods of euthanasia for these three groups have been investigated in some detail since the seminal report on the subject by UFAW/WSPA (1989). It is now clear that ectothermic animals need special consideration because reception – and probably awareness – of painful stimuli in such species may continue long after the animal is assumed to be dead.

Physical methods of killing are to be preferred (see Chapter 2) but this should involve destruction of brain. Decapitation while the animal is still conscious must not be carried out except in dire emergencies and should be followed by destruction of the brain. Other techniques may also be used, including an overdose of an appropriate agent such as pentobarbital (by the intravenous or intraperitoneal route) or isoflurane or halothane (by inhalation).

Amphibians can be particularly difficult to kill (Stocker, 2000). When large numbers are involved – for instance, if a pond is polluted or there is an epizootic amongst frogs – it may be necessary to use a chamber and to kill the animals *en masse* with benzocaine. Similar methods are used for fish.

Great care must always be taken to ensure that the animal is truly dead before disposal of the body and this is not always easy to assess. The development of rigor mortis is perhaps the most reliable sign.

First aid procedures

The indications for first aid in these animals are often similar to those in other species but the key in both amphibians and fish is hydration – total immersion in clean, well oxygenated water (fish), or partial immersion in such water, possibly coupled with regular spraying (amphibians). Fluids can also be given to reptiles and amphibians by mouth – oesophageal or gastric lavage.

Physical injuries are common in these casualties. Control of haemorrhage is vital and the prompt administration of fluids is usually necessary. The intravenous, intraperitoneal or intraosseous routes are particularly useful and permit rapid absorption, but they depend upon some skill and on knowledge of the anatomy of the species. Alternatively, a subcutaneous injection can be given. Few reliable data exist on the quantities of fluid needed but a useful basic guide is to give up to 5% of the animal's bodyweight over 12 hours.

Burns and other skin lesions can rapidly prove fatal in small reptiles, and covering such wounds with an adhesive drape (e.g. Opsite, Smith & Nephew) is recommended. Liquid Skin (Boots) has been used to treat wounds in toads (H. Berman, personal communication).

Other first aid measures for all ectothermic species consist of providing the animal with an environment that is within its POTZ, together with an appropriate relative humidity.

Like other wild animals, free-living reptiles, amphibians and fish that come into captivity are highly susceptible to stressors and these should be minimized by providing a suitable environment, including substrate, and hiding places such as tubes or half flower pots. Colour changes, such as marked pallor, are often a sign of stress, especially in amphibians and fish.

Anaesthesia and analgesia

Anaesthesia

Anaesthesia of reptiles and amphibians has developed remarkably since the early 1980s and methods available are detailed in a number of modern texts (Frye, 1991; Beynon *et al.*, 1992; Mader, 1996).

Isoflurane, induced with a facemask or an anaesthetic chamber, is the anaesthetic agent of choice for terrestrial species. Isoflurane may not always be available and in such cases other volatile liquids, such as halothane, are appropriate. In the field injectable anaesthetic agents, such as ketamine, are often used.

Fish and aquatic amphibians are best anaesthetized using benzocaine (which has first to be dissolved in acetone) or tricaine methane sulphonate (MS222, which should be buffered). Both agents are absorbed from the water by the gills or skin and their use is discussed in more detail in Meredith and Redrobe (2002) and Wildgoose (2001). Recovery is accelerated by bubbling oxygen through the water (fish), by spraying it on the gills (fish and immature amphibians), or by applying it to the skin (immature and adult amphibians).

Analgesia

Analgesics have not been properly evaluated for these groups (Bennett, 1998). A certain amount of pain relief can be achieved by supportive measures, such as irrigating the skin of amphibians that have dermal lesions and by provision of a hiding place for a fish with a damaged tail fin or operculum. In reptiles, analgesics can be tried, using agents that are efficacious in birds (e.g. carprofen), but there has to be a careful balance between administering an agent of doubtful efficacy and the stress that may be caused to the animal in carrying out the administration.

Specific conditions

Many diseases are recognized in captive reptiles, amphibians and fish. Far less is known about conditions that occur in the wild, though there are scattered papers and reports, mainly based on individual cases (see References and further reading).

The main conditions of relevance are:

- Physical injuries, including those caused by trauma, burns, hyperthermia, hypothermia or exposure to irritant or corrosive chemicals (Figure 26.5)
- Infectious diseases due to bacteria, fungi, viruses and various parasites.

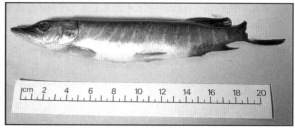

26.5 This pike (*Esox lucius*) had traumatic damage to its tail fin due to attack by an unknown predator. Following veterinary treatment, the fish was returned to the wild. (Courtesy of ME Cooper.)

Trauma

Many reptiles and amphibians are killed on the roads and substantial numbers are injured in gardens as a result of strimming or mowing, or by entanglement with nylon netting (Anon., 2002), or where piles of grass cuttings or rubbish in which reptiles and amphibians have taken refuge are set on fire and the animals suffer from burns or perish.

Infectious diseases

These can affect all three groups of animals (but there is a particularly rich volume of literature on the infectious diseases of fish). Casualties are usually presented as individual cases but from time to time there may be an epizootic of infectious disease (e.g. bacterial diseases of frogs or fish) or mortality due to extensive chemical pollution. In such instances it is important to approach the problem on a 'group' basis and to pay attention to the animals' environment (see Chapter 4).

Gram-negative bacteria, such as *Aeromonas*, *Pseudomonas* and *Citrobacter* species, are an important cause of disease. For example, 'redleg' (probably the best known disease of frogs and other amphibians) is usually attributable to *Aeromonas hydrophila*. However, the infectious agent is likely to be secondary to stressors, which can range from social aggression to poor water quality. Skin lesions will permit the ingress of such pathogens.

Surgical procedures

Reptiles

Surgical techniques in reptiles are based on those used for reptiles in captivity. The British reptile fauna comprises relatively small species and therefore some surgical techniques that are feasible in larger animals are either not practicable or are difficult to perform. One important consideration is that the heavily keratinized skin can make incisions difficult and healing is often protracted, especially during hibernation. Strong sutures with a long half-life are usually required.

Amphibians

In the case of amphibians, some surgical procedures are similar to those used in reptiles, birds and mammals. Caution must be exercised because of the susceptibility of frogs, newts and their allies to desiccation and the fact that the surgical approach to other parts of the body is usually through the skin. Damaged epithelium – for example, because of the use of alcohol-based disinfectants – can easily serve as a portal of entry for infection or precipitate loss of fluids and electrolytes.

Fish

Surgery on fish is well documented. More details may be found in different editions of the *BSAVA Manual of Exotic Pets* (e.g. Beynon and Cooper, 1991; Meredith and Redrobe, 2002) and in the *BSAVA Manual of Ornamental Fish, 2nd edition* (Wildgoose, 2001).

Therapeutics

- Reptiles can be dosed orally, per cloacam or by a number of parenteral routes – subcutaneous, intramuscular, intravenous, intraperitoneal and intraosseous
- In amphibians, an additional route that proves useful for both immature and older adult animals is absorption through the skin or gills
- Fish are usually treated by administering the agent in the water, in food, topically, or by injection (intraperitoneal, intramuscular or occasionally intravenous).

Various therapeutic agents have been employed successfully in reptiles and amphibians over the years but in very few countries are these licensed for use in such species. Larval amphibians in many respects resemble fish, and proprietary medicines available to aquarists, such as malachite green, can sometimes be used to treat them.

Medication of fish presents fewer problems because some agents are licensed for these species and there is a body of knowledge about the use of both prescription-only and proprietary medicines.

Information on some of the therapeutic agents that can be used in reptiles, amphibians and fish are given in various texts (e.g. Beynon and Cooper, 1991; Wildgoose, 2001; Meredith and Redrobe, 2002).

Some agents that are used are fairly basic. Fluids are a key part of stabilizing an animal that has an injury or an infectious disease. Many other simple treatments are regularly used by herpetologists and ichthyologists; some of these may need to be used in circumstances where facilities and funding are limited. However, care must always be taken. For example, iodine preparations have an important part to play on skin wounds of reptiles, but similar wounds in amphibians are more safely treated using a slightly hypertonic salt solution or an appropriately diluted disinfectant.

Management in captivity

Information on feeding, housing and behavioural problems can be found in standard textbooks (Frye, 1991; Butcher, 1992; Beynon *et al.*, 1992; Mader, 1996).

Reptiles and amphibians are usually housed in a glass or plastic-sided vivarium (which can be fashioned from an aquarium), provided with a temperature and humidity gradient, and appropriate substrates (Porter, 1989). Fish need an aquarium, bath or other watertight container and their water may require oxygenation.

Rearing of orphans

This is not applicable to reptiles and fish because their young are independent and usually present no particular problems as such.

'Orphaned' amphibians are different. Immature amphibians, certainly those found in Britain, are tadpoles and these exhibit a number of differences from the adults. For much of their life they have gills rather than lungs and they are susceptible to such factors as drying-out of ponds or pollution. The rearing of tadpoles is not particularly difficult but requires an understanding of the biology and natural history of the species. Young tadpoles are essentially herbivorous, feeding on vegetable matter (chopped lettuce can be useful in captivity), but as they metamorphose they become carnivorous, requiring meat or earthworms. Cannibalism can take place.

Release

Pre-release health monitoring is essential and some information is to be found in Cooper (1990), Corbett (1990) and Latas (2000). Health monitoring protocols prior to release of reptiles, amphibians and fish are discussed in Woodford (2001).

Publications on release of ectothermic vertebrates are sparse (Cooper, 1990), and most available information is derived from studies on movement of animals for 'conservation' reasons. The factors involved in the translocation of great-crested newts were evaluated by Oldham and Humphries (2000), while Cooke (2001) described how translocation of the great-crested newt had evolved as part of a conservation strategy for the species. Reptiles and amphibians face many hazards when released, not all of which may be apparent beforehand; for example, unusual mortality in sand lizards in Dorset was found to be due to predation by woodpeckers (Phelps, 2001).

Post-release monitoring

Description and marking for subsequent recognition or identification is a well established procedure in field biology. Often the simplest method of recognition is to record, with a photograph or drawing, the animal's body coloration and pattern.

The marking of fish presents problems for various reasons, including concerns about the effect of such techniques on survival and welfare. Methods include the attachment of tags and marking of scales.

Telemetry is a valuable aid to the identification and tracking of fish and reptiles. It can involve either external or internal application of a transmitter: the former is generally to be preferred but even this may adversely affect normal behaviour and prejudice survival in the wild.

Techniques for marking amphibians tend to be less sophisticated and some (e.g. toe clipping) should definitely not be carried out on casualties, as there is strong evidence that this is deleterious – as well as raising ethical questions about welfare.

Legal aspects

In addition to general legal aspects (see Chapter 5), some of which are applicable to reptiles, amphibians and fish, there is specific legislation that relates to these animals. The smooth snake, sand lizard, natterjack toad and great-crested newt are given special protection under the Wildlife and Countryside Act. Most other species cannot be offered for sale without a licence and several species may not be intentionally killed or injured. The adder is included in the Schedule to the Dangerous Wild Animals Act, which means that rehabilitators who are not veterinary surgeons (who, if giving treatment, are exempt from the provisions of the Dangerous Wild Animals Act) must hold a licence from the local authority if they hold an adder in captivity.

Fish are also covered by legislation relating to health (e.g. notifiable diseases) and to fishing (see Chapter 5).

Specialist organizations

Association for the Study of Reptiles and Amphibians (ASRA)
Cotswold Wildlife Park, Burford, Oxon OX8 4JW

British Chelonia Group (BCG)
1577 Bristol Road South, Longbridge, Birmingham B45 9UA

British Herpetological Society
c/o Zoological Society of London, Regent's Park, London NW1 4RY

CEFAS Weymouth Laboratory
Barrack Road, The Nothe, Weymouth, Dorset DT4 8UB

Institute of Aquaculture
University of Stirling, Stirling FK9 4LA

References and further reading

Anon. (2002) *Frogs and Toads – the Facts*. RSPCA, Horsham
Arnold EN and Burton JA (1978) *A Field Guide to the Reptiles and Amphibians of Britain and Europe*. Collins, London
Bennett RA (1998) Pain and analgesia in reptiles and amphibians. *Proceedings of the AAZV/AAWV Joint Conference*, p. 461
Beynon PH and Cooper JE (eds) (1991) *Manual of Exotic Pets*. BSAVA, Cheltenham
Beynon PH, Lawton MPC and Cooper JE (eds) (1992) *Manual of Reptiles*. BSAVA, Cheltenham
Butcher RL (ed.) (1992) *Manual of Ornamental Fish*. BSAVA, Cheltenham
Cooke AS (2001) A case study in the evolution of crested newt conservation. *Herpetological Bulletin* **78**, 16–20
Cooper JE (1990) Reptiles and amphibians. In: *Proceedings of the Third Symposium of the British Wildlife Rehabilitation Council*, ed. T Thomas, pp. 76–77. RSPCA, Horsham
Cooper JE and Jackson OF (eds) (1981) *Diseases of the Reptilia*. Academic Press, London
Corbett KF (1990) Rescue and relocation of British reptiles. In: *Proceedings of the Third Symposium of the British Wildlife Rehabilitation Council*, ed. T Thomas, pp. 58–60. RSPCA, Horsham
Frye FL (1991) *Biomedical and Surgical Aspects of Captive Reptile Husbandry*. Krieger, Melbourne, Florida
Latas PJ (2000) Evaluation of reptiles and amphibians for release, rehabilitation or adoption. *Journal of Wildlife Rehabilitation* **23**(3), 13–21
Mader DR (ed.) (1996) *Reptile Medicine and Surgery*. WB Saunders, Philadelphia
Meredith A and Redrobe S (eds) (2002) *BSAVA Manual of Exotic Pets, 4th edn*. BSAVA, Gloucester
Oldham RS and Humphries (2000) Evaluating the success of great crested newt (*Triturus cristatus*) translocation. *Herpetological Journal* **10**, 183–190
Phelps T (2001) *Lacerta agilis* (sand lizard): unusual mortality at site in South East Dorset. *Herpetological Bulletin* **78**, 31–32
Porter V (1989) *Animal Rescue*. Ashford, Southampton
Stocker L (2000) *Practical Wildlife Care*. Blackwell Science, Oxford
UFAW/WSPA (1989) *Euthanasia of Amphibians and Reptiles*. Report of a Joint Working Party. Universities Federation for Animal Welfare, Potters Bar
Wheeler A (1978) *Key to the Fishes of Northern Europe*. Frederick Warne, London
Wildgoose WH (ed.) (2001) *BSAVA Manual of Ornamental Fish, 2nd edn*. BSAVA, Gloucester
Woodford MH (ed.) (2001) *Quarantine and Health Screening Protocols for Wildlife Prior to Translocation and Release in to the Wild*. Office International des Epizooties (OIE), Veterinary Specialist Group/International Union for the Conservation of Nature (VSG/IUCN), Care for the Wild International and European Association of Zoo and Wildlife Veterinarians (EAZWV), Paris

Acknowledgements

I am grateful to Mr Henry Berman and Mr Peter Dawson, who read and commented on early drafts of this chapter. The latter also very kindly provided the photograph of the natterjack toad.

Appendix 1

Avian formulary

The following dosages are given only as guidelines, with the information being collated from a variety of sources. No responsibility can be taken by the authors for the accuracy of this information.

None of the following therapeutic agents has a product licence for use in wildlife (see Chapter 5). LA = long-acting.

More accurate dosage can be calculated by allometric scaling (see Chapter 2) using the following formula:

$$E = (W/1000)^{0.75} \times D$$

where E = dose of medicine in mg, W = bodyweight of bird in (g) and D = dose for small mammals in (mg/kg).

Drug and formulation	Dosage	Comments
Antibacterial agents		
Amoxicillin 150 mg/ml short- and long-acting injectable suspensions	150 mg/kg i.m. q8–12h (q24h for long-acting preparation)	
Amoxicillin/clavulanate 175 mg/ml injectable suspension 50, 250, 500 mg tablets and 50 mg/ml oral suspension	35 mg/kg i.m. q24h 150 mg/kg orally q8–12h	
Carbenicillin 100 mg/ml injectable solution	100–200 mg/kg i.v., i.m. q12h	
Cefalexin 180 mg/ml injectable suspension 50, 250, 600 mg tablets and 100 mg/ml oral suspension	35–100 mg/kg i.m., orally q6–8h	
Doxycycline 20, 100 mg capsules 260 mg/sachet soluble powder	15–50 mg/kg orally q12–24h 130 mg/l drinking water	Drug of choice for chlamydophilosis
Enrofloxacin 25 mg/ml injectable solution	10–15 mg/kg i.m., orally q24h	Irritant, causing tissue damage when injected i.m. and s.c. Oral dosing may cause regurgitation
Marbofloxacin 20 mg/ml injectable solution 5, 20, 80 mg tablets	10 mg/kg i.m., orally q24h	Less irritant than enrofloxacin
Oxytetracycline 200 (LA) mg/ml injectable solution Tablets and oral powders	50–100 mg/kg i.m. q12–24h 50 mg/kg orally q8h	
Piperacillin sterile powder for reconstitution	100–200 mg/kg i.m. q8–12h	Reconstituted drug can be deep frozen and stored as small aliquots in 1 ml syringes. (I. Robinson, pers. comm.)
Trimethoprim/sulphonamide 240 mg active ingredients/ml solution 120 and 480 mg tablets	8 mg/kg i.m. q12h 20–50 mg/kg orally q12h	Do not use in dehydrated birds
Tylosin 50 mg/ml injectable solution	20–40 mg/kg i.m., s.c. q8–12h	▶

Avian formulary

Drug and formulation	Dosage	Comments
Antifungal agents		
Amphotericin B 50 mg vials 100 mg/ml oral suspension	1.0 mg/kg i.v. q8h for 7 days also intratracheally for 12 days then alternate days for 5 weeks 1.0 mg/kg orally q12h	Aspergillosis Oral and enteric candidiasis
F10 (combination of quaternary ammonium compound and biguanide complex disinfectants)	Used for nebulization at concentrations between 1:200 and 1:500	Claimed to be of value for prophylaxis and therapy of aspergillosis
Itraconazole 100 mg capsules 10 mg/ml oral syrup	5–10 mg/kg orally q24h for 7–10 days for prophylaxis and q12h for 4–6 weeks for therapy	Aspergillosis
Nystatin 100,000 IU/ml oral suspension	300,00 IU/kg orally q12h for 5–7 days	Candidiasis
Anti-inflammatory and analgesic agents		
Buprenorphine 0.3 mg/ml injectable solution	0.1 mg/kg i.v., i.m. q12h	Also has a sedative effect
Butorphanol 0.5 mg/ml injectable solution	2–4 mg/kg i.v., i.m., orally q24h	Also has a sedative effect
Carprofen 50 mg/ml injectable solution	5–10 mg/kg i.v., i.m. q24h	
Dexamethasone sodium phosphate 2 mg/kg injectable solution	1–2 mg/kg i.v. or 2–4 mg/kg i.m. q24h	Corticosteroid (including topical) preparations should be used with care as they have been linked with several disease syndromes (Hess, 2001). Use for a short course (48 hours) Dexamethasone phenylproprionate should be avoided due to its long half-life Products containing triamcinolone should be avoided due to its extremely high potency
Hydrocortisone sodium succinate 100 mg powder for reconstitution	10 mg/kg i.v	For the treatment of shock
Ketoprofen 10 mg/ml injectable solution	2–4 mg/kg i.m. q24h	
Meloxicam 5 mg/ml injectable solution 1.5 mg/ml oral suspension	0.2 mg/kg i.m. q24h 0.2 mg/kg (2 drops/kg) orally q24h	Reported to be well tolerated for long periods of administration
Prednisolone sodium succinate 10 mg/ml injectable solution	11–25 mg/kg i.v.	For the treatment of shock
Anthelmintics		
Fenbendazole 2.5% and 10% suspensions	20–50 mg/kg orally; may repeat in 10 days	For capillariasis (and cestodes) dose for 3–5 consecutive days It has been reported that pigeons and doves may be susceptible to doses as low as 20 mg/kg given on 3 consecutive days
Ivermectin 10 mg/ml injectable solution	0.2 mg/kg i.m., s.c., orally	Also active against ectoparasites Dilute 1:50 in propylene glycol, 1.0 ml/kg oral or percutaneous administration
Levamisole 75 mg/ml solution	20–50 mg/kg orally	May administer in drinking water for 3 consecutive days
Praziquantel 56.8 mg/ml injectable solution 50 mg tablets	7.5 mg/kg i.m. 5–10 mg/kg orally q2–4 wks	Active against cestodes Also active against trematodes at 10 mg/kg s.c or orally q24h for 14 days

▶

Drug and formulation	Dosage	Comments
Antiprotozoal agents		
Amprolium 3.4% oral solution	25 mg/kg orally q24h for 7 days (28 ml/4.5 litres drinking water)	Coccidiosis
Carnidazole 10 mg tablets	20 mg/kg orally	Flagellate infections
Chloroquine 200 mg tablets	15 mg/kg orally q24h for 7 days	Haematozoan infections Initial dose 25 mg/kg orally (may include 0.75 mg/kg primaquine on day 1)
Clazuril 2.5 mg tablets	5–10 mg/kg orally every 3rd day for 3 treatments	Coccidiosis
Dimetridazole 40% w/w powder	3 g/4.5 litres drinking water for 7 days	Flagellate infections (From 2002 licence withdrawn for administration to gamebirds) May cause toxicity (nervous signs – tremors, ataxia) in small birds
Mefloquine 275 mg tablets	50 mg/kg orally q24h for 7 days	Haematozoan infections May give together with chloroquine at 15 mg/kg orally q24h
Metronidazole 5 mg/ml injectable solution 20 mg and 500 mg tablets	10 mg/kg i.m. q12h 20–50 mg/kg orally q12h	Flagellate infections May cause toxicity (nervous signs – tremors, ataxia) in small birds
Pyrimethamine 25 mg tablets	0.5 mg/kg orally q12h for 30 days	Haematozoan infections – *Leucocytozoon*
Sulfadimethoxine 100 mg per 4 g sachet	Dissolve one sachet in 2 litres of drinking water for 5 days	Coccidiosis
Toltrazuril 25 mg/ml oral solution	10 mg/kg orally alternate days for 3 treatments Gamebirds: Dose in drinking water for 2 consecutive days	Coccidiosis
Trimethoprim/sulphonamide 240 mg active ingredients/ml solution 120, 480 mg tablets	12–60 mg/kg i.m. q12h 20–50 mg/kg orally q12h	Coccidial and haematozoan infections
Ectoparasiticides		
Fipronil 0.25% w/v spray	Spray beneath plumage to skin. Repeat after 2–4 weeks	Alcohol base might damage feather structure
Ivermectin 10 mg/ml injectable solution	0.2 mg/kg i.m., orally	Also dilute 1:50 in propylene glycol, 1.0 ml/kg orally or percutaneous administration
Permethrin various dusting powders and sprays	Apply beneath plumage	
Poison antidotes		
Atropine 0.6 mg/ml injectable solution	0.2–0.4 mg/kg i.m. q3–4h	For organophosphate poisoning (see Chapter 22)
Pralidoxime 200 mg/ml injectable solution	10–20 (or 100) mg/kg i.m. q8–12h as needed	For organophosphate poisoning (see Chapter 22)
Sodium calcium edetate (EDTA) 250 mg/ml injectable solution	62.6 mg/kg q8–24h (depending on level of toxicity)	For lead poisoning (see Chapter 20) Administered diluted to 5% solution in an isotonic glucose/saline preparation and given i.v. or undiluted i.m. or s.c. ▶

Drug and formulation	Dosage	Comments
Poison antidotes continued		
Penicillamine 50, 125, 250 mg tablets	15–30 mg/kg tid orally	For lead poisoning (see Chapter 20) Given as an adjunct to injectable drugs. Higher doses may lead to gastrointestinal side effects. To be given on an empty proventriculus
Succimer (DMSA)	25–35 mg/kg bid orally for 5 days in each week for 3–5 weeks	For lead poisoning (see Chapter 20) Fewer side effects than penicillamine
Sedative and anaesthetic agents		
Diazepam 5 mg/ml injectable solution	0.5–1.0 mg/kg i.v., i.m. q6–8h as needed	As a sedative for convulsing bird
Ketamine 100 mg/ml injectable solution	20–50 mg/kg i.m., i.v.	Effective alone for sedation but in combination with other agents will produce good analgesia and muscle relaxation
Ketamine plus xylazine 20 mg/ml injectable solution	5 mg/kg ketamine + 1–4 mg/kg xylazine i.m.	Reversal with yohimbine 0.1 mg/km i.m.
Ketamine plus medetomidine 1 mg/ml injectable solution	3–5 mg/kg ketamine + 150–300 µg/kg medetomidine i.v. (preferably) or i.m.	Gives 30 minutes surgical anaesthesia. Birds are standing 10 minutes following reversal with 750–1500 µg /kg (i.e. the same volume) of atipamezole
Alphaxolone/alphadolone (Saffan) 12 mg total steroids/ml	5–10 mg/kg i.v.(preferably) or i.m.	Especially useful for inducing anaesthesia in larger waterfowl
Miscellaneous agents		
Doxapram 20 mg/ml injectable solution	10 mg/kg i.v., i.m.	Respiratory stimulant
Furosemide 50 mg/ml injectable solution	2 mg/kg i.v., i.m.	Diuretic

References

Hess L (2001) Possible complications associated with topical corticosteroid use in birds. In: *Proceedings of the 22nd Annual Conference and Expo of the Association of Avian Veterinarians, Orlando, 22-24 August*, pp. 29—32

Appendix 2

Useful addresses

This list contains organizations and associations concerned with the care of animals, their welfare or conservation plus government departments and official bodies for licensing, permits and advice. Species-specific groups are listed at the end of the relevant chapter.

Agricultural Department (Welsh Office)
Crown Buildings, Cathays Park, Cardiff CF1 3NQ

Animal Welfare Foundation
c/o British Veterinary Association, 7 Mansfield Street, London W1M 0AT

Association of British Wild Animal Keepers
2A Northcote Road, Clifton, Bristol BS8 3HB

British Bird Council
1577 Bristol Road South, Longbridge, Birmingham B45 9UA

British Veterinary Zoological Society (BVZS)
c/o British Veterinary Association, 7 Mansfield Street, London WIG 9NQ

British Wildlife Rehabilitation Council
c/o Wildlife Department, RSPCA, Wilberforce Way, Horsham, West Sussex

CITES (Convention on International Trade in Endangered Species) Secretariat
International Environment House, Chemin des Anémones, CH-1219 Châtelaine, Geneva, Switzerland
www.cites.org

Countryside Council for Wales
Plas Penrhos, Ffordd Penrhos, Bangor, Gwynnedd LL57 2LQ

Department for the Environment, Food and Rural Affairs (DEFRA)
Nobel House, 17 Smith Square, London SW1P 3JR
www.defra.gov.uk

Department of Agriculture and Fisheries for Scotland (DAFS)
Pentland House, 47 Robbss Loan, Edinburgh ED14 1TW

English Nature
Northminster House, Peterborough PE1 1UA

The Environment Agency
Rio House, Waterside Drive, Aztec West, Almondsbury, Bristol BS32 4HD

Institute of Zoology
Zoological Society of London, Regents Park, London NW1 4RY

The Mammal Society
15 Cloisters House, 8 Battersea Park Road, London SW5 4BG
www.mammal.org.uk

The People's Trust for Endangered Species
15 Cloisters House, 8 Battersea Park Road, London SW5 4BG
www.ptes.org.uk

Royal Society for the Prevention of Cruelty to Animals (RSPCA)
Wildlife Department, Wilberforce Way, Horsham, West Sussex

RSPCA Wildlife Hospitals:
- Stapeley Grange, London Road, Stapeley, Nantwich, Cheshire CW5 7JW
- Station Road, East Winch, King's Lynn, Norfolk PE32 1NR
- West Hatch, Taunton, Somerset TA3 5RT

Scottish Natural Heritage
2–5 Anderson Place, Edinburgh EH6 5NP

Scottish Society for the Prevention of Cruelty to Animals (SSPCA)
Braehead Mains, 603 Queensferry Road, Edinburgh EH4 6EA

Ulster Society for the Prevention of Cruelty to Animals
Knockdean, 11 Drumview Road, Lisburn, Co Antrim, BT27 6YF

Universities Federation for Animal Welfare (UFAW)
The Old School, Brewhouse Hill, Wheathampstead, Herts AL4 8AN

Wildlife Hospitals Trust (St Tiggywinkle's)
1 Pemberton Close, Aviesbury, Bucks HP21 7NY

Wildlife Incident Unit
Central Science Laboratories, Sand Hutton, York YO4 1LZ
Tel: 0800 321 600
(for advice regarding pesticides used against wild birds and mammals)

Wildlife Information Network
Royal Veterinary College, Royal College Street, London NW1 0UT

Appendix 3

Common and scientific names

Mammals

Common name	Scientific name
American mink	*Mustela vison*
American river otter	*Lutra canadensis*
Arctic fox	*Alopex lagopus*
Asian small-clawed otter	*Aonyx cinerea*
Atlantic white-sided dolphin	*Lagenorhynchus acutus*
Badger	*Meles meles*
Bank vole	*Clethrionomys glareolus*
Barbastelle bat	*Barbastella barbastellus*
Bechstein's bat	*Myotis bechsteinii*
Big brown bat	*Eptesicus fuscus*
Black rat	*Rattus rattus*
Blue hare	*Lepus timidus*
Bottlenose dolphin	*Tursiops truncatus*
Brandt's bat	*Myotis brandtii*
Brown hare	*Lepus europaeus*
Brown long-eared bat	*Plecotus auritus*
Brown rat	*Rattus norvegicus*
Carsac fox	*Vulpes corsac*
Chinese water deer	*Hydropotes inermis*
Common dolphin	*Delphinus delphis*
Common dormouse	*Muscardinus avellanarius*
Common rat	*Rattus norvegicus*
Common seal	*Phoca vitulina vitulina*
Common shrew	*Sorex araneus*
Common vole	*Microtus arvalis*
Cottontail	*Sylvilagus floridanus*
Daubenton's bat	*Myotis daubentonii*
Edible dormouse	*Myoxus (Glis) glis*
Eurasian badger	*Meles meles*
Eurasian otter	*Lutra lutra*
European beaver	*Castor fiber*
European hedgehog	*Erinaceus europaeus*
European mole	*Talpa europaea*
European rabbit	*Oryctolagus cuniculus*
Fallow deer	*Dama dama*
Fat dormouse	*Myoxus (Glis) glis*
Field vole	*Microtus agrestis*
Fox	*Vulpes vulpes*
Greater horseshoe bat	*Rhinolophus ferrumequinum*
Greater white-toothed shrew	*Crocidura russula*
Grey long-eared bat	*Plecotus austriacus*
Grey seal	*Halichoerus grypus*
Grey squirrel	*Sciurus carolinensis*
Harbour porpoise	*Phocoena phocoena*
Harbour seal	*Phoca vitulina vitulina*
Harp seal	*Phoca groenlandica*

Common name	Scientific name
Harvest mouse	*Micromys minutus*
Hazel dormouse	*Muscardinus avellanarius*
Hooded seal	*Cystophara cristata*
House mouse	*Mus musculus*
Irish hare	*Lepus timidus*
Killer whale	*Orcinus orca*
Leisler's bat	*Nyctalus leisleri*
Lesser horseshoe bat	*Rhinolophus hipposideros*
Lesser white-toothed shrew	*Crocidura suaveolens*
Little brown bat	*Myotis lucifugus*
Long-finned pilot whale	*Globicephala melas*
Mexican free-tailed bat	*Tadarida brasiliensis*
Minke whale	*Balaenoptera acutorostrata*
Mountain hare	*Lepus timidus*
Mouse-eared bat	*Myotis myotis*
Nathusius' pipistrelle	*Pipistrellus nathusii*
Natterer's bat	*Myotis nattereri*
Noctule bat	*Nyctalus noctula*
Orca	*Orcinus orca*
Pine marten	*Martes martes*
Pipistrelle bat	*Pipistrellus pipistrellus* and *P. pygmaeus*
Polecat	*Mustela putorius*
Pygmy shrew	*Sorex minutus*
Red deer	*Cervus elaphus*
Red fox	*Vulpes vulpes*
Red squirrel	*Sciurus vulgaris*
Reeves muntjac	*Muntiacus reevesi*
Ringed seal	*Phoca hispida*
Risso's dolphin	*Grampus griseus*
River otter	*Lutra canadensis*
Roe deer	*Capreolus capreolus*
Serotine bat	*Eptesicus serotinus*
Short-tailed vole	*Microtus agrestis*
Sika deer	*Cervus nippon*
Stoat	*Mustela erminea*
Striped dolphin	*Stenella coeruleoalba*
Varying hare	*Lepus timidus*
Water shrew	*Neomys fodiens*
Water vole	*Arvicola terrestris*
Weasel	*Mustela nivalis*
Whiskered bat	*Myotis mystacinus*
White-beaked dolphin	*Lagenorhynchus albirostris*
Wildcat	*Felis silvestris*
Wood mouse	*Apodemus sylvaticus*
Yellow-necked mouse	*Apodemus flavicollis*

Birds

Common name	Scientific name
Arctic tern	*Sterna paradisaea*
Barn owl	*Tyto alba*
Barnacle goose	*Branta leucopsis*
Bewick's swan	*Cygnus columbianus*
Black grouse	*Lyrurus tetrix*
Black-necked grebe	*Podiceps nigricollis*
Black-throated diver	*Gavia arctica*
Blackbird	*Turdus merula*
Blackcap	*Sylvia atricapilla*
Black-headed gull	*Larus ridibundas*
Blue tit	*Parus caeruleus*
Brent goose	*Branta bernicla*
British storm petrel	*Hydrobates pelagicus*
Canada goose	*Branta canadensis*
Capercaillie	*Tetrao urogallus*
Carrion crow	*Corvus corone*
Chaffinch	*Fringilla coelebs*
Chukar partridge	*Alectoris chukar*
Collared dove	*Streptopelia decaocto*
Common buzzard	*Buteo buteo*
Common gull	*Larus canus*
Common kestrel	*Falco tinnunculus*
Common pheasant	*Phasianus colchicus*
Common quail	*Coturnix coturnix*
Common scoter	*Mellanita nigra*
Common snipe	*Gallinago gallinago*
Common swift	*Apus apus*
Common tern	*Sterna hirundo*
Coot	*Fulica atra*
Cormorant	*Phalacrocorax carbo*
Corncrake	*Crex crex*
Eider	*Somateria mollissima*
English partridge	*Perdix perdix*
Eurasian sparrow hawk	*Accipiter nisus*
Feral pigeon	*Columba livia*
Fieldfare	*Turdus pilaris*
Fulmar	*Fulmarus glacialis*
Golden eagle	*Aquila chrysaetos*
Goldeneye	*Buchephala clangula*
Goosander	*Mergus merganser*
Great black-backed gull	*Larus marinus*
Great crested grebe	*Podiceps cristatus*
Great northern diver	*Gavia immer*
Great tit	*Parus major*
Green woodpecker	*Picus viridis*
Grey partridge	*Perdix perdix*
Grey heron	*Ardea cinerea*
Greylag goose	*Anser anser*
Guillemot	*Uria aalga*
Herring gull	*Larus argentatus*
House martin	*Delichon urbica*
House sparrow	*Passer domesticus*

Common name	Scientific name
Jackdaw	*Corvus monedula*
Kingfisher	*Alcedo atthis*
Kittiwake	*Rissa tridactyla*
Lesser black-backed gull	*Larus fuscus*
Little egret	*Egretta garzetta*
Little grebe	*Tachybaptus ruficollis*
Little owl	*Athena noctua*
Little tern	*Sterna albifrons*
Mallard	*Anas platyrhynchos*
Manx shearwater	*Puffinus puffinus*
Moorhen	*Gallinula chlorpus*
Mute swan	*Cygnus olor*
Northern gannet	*Sula bassana*
Peregrine	*Falco peregrinus*
Pink-footed goose	*Anser brachyrhynchus*
Pintail	*Anas acuta*
Pochard	*Aythya ferina*
Ptarmigan	*Lagopus mutus*
Puffin	*Fratercula artica*
Racing pigeon	*Columba livia*
Razorbill	*Alca torda*
Red grouse	*Lagopus lagopus*
Red kite	*Milvus milvus*
Red-breasted merganser	*Mergus serrator*
Red-legged partridge	*Alectoris rufa*
Red-throated diver	*Gavia stellata*
Redwing	*Turdus iliacus*
Robin	*Erithacus rubercula*
Rock dove	*Columba livia*
Sandwich tern	*Sterna sandvicensis*
Scaup	*Aythya marila*
Shag	*Phalacrocorax aristotelis*
Shelduck	*Tadoma tadoma*
Shoveler	*Anas clypeata*
Skylark	*Alauda arvensis*
Slavonian grebe	*Podiceps auritus*
Smew	*Mergus albellus*
Starling	*Sturnus vulgaris*
Stock dove	*Columba oenas*
Swallow	*Hirundo rustica*
Tawny owl	*Strix aluco*
Teal	*Anas crecca*
Thrush	*Turdus philomelos*
Tufted duck	*Aythya fuligula*
Turtle dove	*Streptopelia turtur*
Water rail	*Rallus aquaticus*
White-fronted goose	*Anser albifrons*
Whooper swan	*Cygnus cygnus*
Wigeon	*Anas penelope*
Wood pigeon	*Columba palumbus*
Woodcock	*Scolopax rusticola*
Wren	*Troglodytes troglodytes*

Common and scientific names

Other

Common name	Scientific name	Common name	Scientific name
Adder	*Vipera berus*	Marsh frog	*Rana ridibunda*
American red-eared terrapin	*Pseudemys scripta elegans*	Natterjack toad	*Bufo calamita*
Common frog	*Rana temporaria*	Palmate newt	*Triturus helvetica*
Common newt	*Triturus vulgaris*	Pike	*Esox lucius*
Common lizard	*Lacerta vivipara*	Sand lizard	*Lacerta agilis*
Common toad	*Bufo bufo*	Slow worm	*Anguis fragilis*
Edible frog	*Rana esculenta*	Smooth newt	*Triturus vulgaris*
European pond tortoise	*Emys orbicularis*	Smooth snake	*Coronella austriaca*
Grass snake	*Natrix natrix*	Viper	*Vipera berus*
Great-crested newt	*Triturus cristata*	Viviparous lizard	*Lacerta vivipara*
Laughing frog	*Rana ridibunda*	Waxworm	*Galleria mellonella*

A glossary of terms as used in this book

Allometric scaling
A method of examining, amongst similar organisms, the effects of size on various natural processes, including clinical pharmacology

Altricial
Used to describe birds or mammals that are helpless when young and dependent on their parents for food

Anisodactyl
Commonest arrangement of toes on a bird's foot: three toes pointing forward and one toe (digit I) pointing backwards

Caecotroph
Soft mucus-covered caecal pellets passed (usually at night) and immediately ingested from the anus as a normal part of cellulose digestion in lagomorphs (known as caecotrophy, coprophagy)

Calamus
The hollow shaft of a contour feather, embedded in the follicle

Congenerics
Individuals of the same genus

Conspecifics
Individuals of the same species

Coprodaeum
Cranial compartment of the avian cloaca that receives the rectum

Creance (falconry term)
A long line attached to the bird during training that allows the bird to fly short distances to the trainer

Crepuscular
Active at dusk and dawn, when the light level is low

Diastema
The gap in rodents/herbivores between the incisors and molar teeth

Dysrexia
A reduction in normal appetite

Ectothermic
'Cold-blooded'. Maintains body temperature by absorbing heat from the environment or by insulating itself so that body temperature is maintained

Endothermic
'Warm-blooded'. Having a stable body temperature that is generally independent of the temperature of the surrounding environment

Euthanasia
Painless killing to relieve unnecessary suffering

Gentles
Larvae of blowflies (maggots) produced commercially for angling bait

Gut-loading
Feeding prey animals, such as mealworms, with nutritional supplements to increase their nutritional value

Hack (falconry term)
To return or "hack" a raptor back to the wild. Young trained raptors may be allowed to fly freely for a period before being trained for the hunting season

Hack flight or aviary (falconry term)
An aviary from which a raptor is released after a period of acclimatization and familiarization and to which it may return for supplementary feeding and security whilst it gains confidence and fitness

Hard release
Release to the wild without any special preparation or familiarization with the release site

Heterothermic
see **Ectothermic**

Homeothermic
see **Endothermic**

Imping
The process of replacing a damaged primary, secondary or tail feather by gluing a suitably trimmed replacement feather on to a peg fixed within the shaft of the remnant of the damaged feather

Imprinting
Rapid learning very early in an animal's social development that results in strong behavioural patterns of attraction

Induced ovulation
Ovulation that occurs following a stimulus, usually copulation

_K_-selection
Breeding strategy whereby few offspring are produced but are given intense parental attention, with low juvenile mortality

Mantling
Behaviour of raptors: stretching of wings to cover food whilst plucking/feeding to protect from rivals

Mealworm
Larva of _Tenebrio_ spp. beetles, used as food for insectivorous animals in captivity

Melon
A rounded waxy mass found in the head of some dolphins and toothed whales that is thought to play a part in the focusing of sound signals

Milk oil
An antimicrobial fatty acid produced by an enzymatic reaction on the doe's milk in the suckling rabbit's stomach, which controls the gastrointestinal microbial contents of suckling rabbits and protects them from enteric infection

Mist-netting
Lengths of fine-meshed nylon nets strung between poles to catch flying birds, as used by bird-ringers

Glossary

Necropsy
A post-mortem examination, usually of a whole animal; also used to describe the post-mortem examination of tissues or organs

Nidicolous
Used to describe young birds that remain within the nest, usually until fully fledged

Nidifugous
Used to describe young birds that leave the nest, usually as soon as they are mobile

Pelagic
Found in the open sea

Pinkies
Young rodents before they have grown hair or opened their eyes

Poikilothermic
see **Ectothermic**

Precocial
Used to describe some animals that display independent activity at birth, especially young birds that are hatched covered with down and with open eyes

Rhamphotheca
The hard keratinized sheath that covers the bone of the beak in most birds

Riparian
Living along or near the bank of a river

Soft release
Process of releasing an animal to the wild whereby it is confined in accommodation at the release site, allowed freedom after a period of acclimatization and then encouraged to return for supplementary food and security. The accommodation is removed once the animal has reached a state of independence

Sweep net
Hand net used by entomologists to collect insects from grass sward

Thermoneutral range
The range of environmental temperatures within which a homeothermic animal needs to expend no energy to maintain a stable body temperature

Velvet
A covering of fragile, highly vascular skin covering the bone of a newly growing antler, which is shed once antler growth is complete.

Ventriculus
Gizzard

Vibrissae
Whiskers

Zygodactyl
Arrangement of the toes: two facing forward (digits II and III) and two backwards (digits I and IV)

Index

287

Index

Index

Index

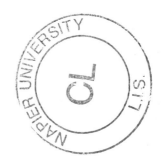

BSAVA Manual of
Exotic Pets
Fourth edition

Edited by
Anna Meredith MA VetMB
CertLAS CertZooMed MRCVS
and
Sharon Redrobe BSc BVetMed
CertLAS CertZooMed MRCVS

Completely revised and expanded
NEW edition

Detailed overview of biology and husbandry

Handling and restraint described
and illustrated

Clinical examination and diagnostics

Problem-oriented approach to diseases

Common surgical procedures

Additional chapters address anatomy,
physiology and imaging

Drug formularies

30 international contributors

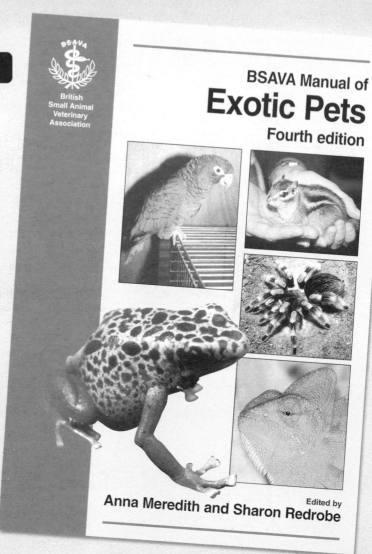

BSAVA Manual of
Exotic Pets
Fourth edition

Anna Meredith and Sharon Redrobe

Edited by

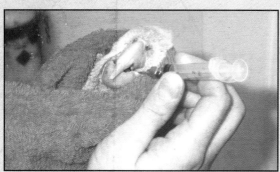

312 pages. Extensively illustrated in colour
ISBN: 0 905214 47 1

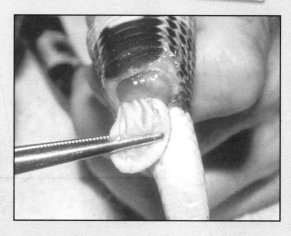

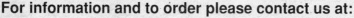

For information and to order please contact us at:

British Small Animal Veterinary Association • Woodrow House
1 Telford Way • Waterwells Business Park • Quedgeley • Gloucester • GL2 2AB
Tel: 01452 726709 • e-mail: publications@bsava.com • www.bsava.com